611.018022 G2443c 2014
Gartner, Leslie P., 1943-
Color atlas and text of
histology

Sixth Edition

Color Atlas and Text of

Histology

D1194520

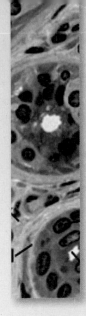

Sixth Edition

Color Atlas and Text of
Histology

LESLIE P. GARTNER, PH.D.
Professor of Anatomy (Retired)
Department of Biomedical Sciences
Baltimore College of Dental Surgery
Dental School
University of Maryland
Baltimore, Maryland

JAMES L. HIATT, PH.D.
Professor Emeritus
Department of Biomedical Sciences
Baltimore College of Dental Surgery
Dental School
University of Maryland
Baltimore, Maryland

. Wolters Kluwer | Lippincott Williams & Wilkins
Health

Philadelphia · Baltimore · New York · London
Buenos Aires · Hong Kong · Sydney · Tokyo

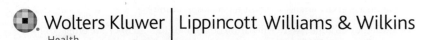
CUYAHOGA COMMUNITY COLLEGE
METROPOLITAN CAMPUS LIBRARY

Acquisitions Editor: Crystal Taylor
Product Manager: Catherine Noonan
Vendor Manager: Bridgett Dougherty
Art Director: Jennifer Clements
Marketing Manager: Joy Fisher-Williams
Designer: Joan Wendt
Compositor: SPi Global

Sixth Edition

Copyright © 2014, 2009, 2006, 2000, 1994, 1990 Lippincott Williams & Wilkins, a Wolters Kluwer business.

351 West Camden Street   Two Commerce Square
Baltimore, MD 21201   2001 Market Street
                                  Philadelphia, PA 19103

Printed in China

Translations:
Chinese (Taiwan): Ho-Chi Book Publishing Company
Chinese (Mainland China): Liaoning Education Press/CITIC
Chinese (Simplified Chinese): CITIC/Chemical Industry Press
French: Wolters Kluwer France
Greek: Parissianos
Indonesian: Binarupa Publisher
Italian: Masson Italia; EdiSES
Japanese: Igaku-Shoin; Medical Sciences International (MEDSI)
Korean: E*Public, Co., Ltd
Portuguese: Editora Guanabara Koogan
Russian: Logosphera
Spanish: Editorial Medica Panamericana; Gestora de Derechos Autorales; Libermed Verlag
Turkish: Gunes Bookshops

All rights reserved. This book is protected by copyright. No part of this book may be reproduced or transmitted in any form or by any means, including as photocopies or scanned-in or other electronic copies, or utilized by any information storage and retrieval system without written permission from the copyright owner, except for brief quotations embodied in critical articles and reviews. Materials appearing in this book prepared by individuals as part of their official duties as U.S. government employees are not covered by the above-mentioned copyright. To request permission, please contact Lippincott Williams & Wilkins at Two Commerce Square, 2001 Market Street, Philadelphia, PA 19103, via email at permissions@lww.com, or via website at lww.com (products and services).

Library of Congress Cataloging-in-Publication Data
Gartner, Leslie P., 1943-
   Color atlas and text of histology / Leslie P. Gartner, James Hiatt. — 6th ed.
     p. ; cm.
   Includes index.
   Rev. ed. of: Color atlas of histology / Leslie P. Gartner, James L. Hiatt. 5th ed. c2009.
   ISBN 978-1-4511-1343-3
   I. Hiatt, James L., 1934- II. Gartner, Leslie P., 1943-. Color atlas and text of histology. III. Title.
   [DNLM: 1. Histology—Atlases. QS 517]
   611'.0180222—dc23

                                                                 2012031983

DISCLAIMER
Care has been taken to confirm the accuracy of the information present and to describe generally accepted practices. However, the authors, editors, and publisher are not responsible for errors or omissions or for any consequences from application of the information in this book and make no warranty, expressed or implied, with respect to the currency, completeness, or accuracy of the contents of the publication. Application of this information in a particular situation remains the professional responsibility of the practitioner; the clinical treatments described and recommended may not be considered absolute and universal recommendations.

The authors, editors, and publisher have exerted every effort to ensure that drug selection and dosage set forth in this text are in accordance with the current recommendations and practice at the time of publication. However, in view of ongoing research, changes in government regulations, and the constant flow of information relating to drug therapy and drug reactions, the reader is urged to check the package insert for each drug for any change in indications and dosage and for added warnings and precautions. This is particularly important when the recommended agent is a new or infrequently employed drug.

Some drugs and medical devices presented in this publication have Food and Drug Administration (FDA) clearance for limited use in restricted research settings. It is the responsibility of the health care provider to ascertain the FDA status of each drug or device planned for use in their clinical practice.

The publishers have made every effort to trace the copyright holders for borrowed material. If they have inadvertently overlooked any, they will be pleased to make the necessary arrangements at the first opportunity.

To purchase additional copies of this book, call our customer service department at (800) 638-3030 or fax orders to (301) 223-2320. International customers should call (301) 223-2300.

Visit Lippincott Williams & Wilkins on the Internet: http://www.lww.com. Lippincott Williams & Wilkins customer service representatives are available from 8:30 am to 6:00 pm, EST.

RRS1211

To my wife Roseann, my daughter Jen,
and my mother Mary
LPG

To my wife Nancy and my children
Drew, Beth, and Kurt
JLH

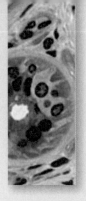

Preface

We are very pleased to be able to present the sixth edition of our *Color Atlas and Text of Histology*, an atlas that has been in continuous use since its first publication as a black and white atlas in 1987. The success of that atlas prompted us to revise it considerably, retake all of the images in full color, change its name, and publish it in 1990 under the title *Color Atlas of Histology*. In the past 22 years, the Atlas has undergone many changes. We added color paintings, published a corresponding set of Kodachrome slides, and added histophysiology to the text. The advent of high-resolution digital photography allowed us to reshoot all of the photomicrographs for the fourth edition, and we created a CD-ROM that accompanied and was packaged with our Atlas. For the fifth edition, we updated the *Interactive Color Atlas of Histology* and made it available to the student on the Lippincott Williams & Wilkins Website, http://thePoint.lww.com, that could be accessed from anywhere in the world via an Internet connection. The online Atlas contained every photomicrograph and electron micrograph and accompanying legends present in the Atlas. The student had the capability to study selected chapters or to look up a particular item via a keyword search. Images could be viewed with or without labels and/or legends, enlarged using the "zoom" feature, and compared side-by-side to other images. Also, the updated software allowed students to self-test on all labels using the "hotspot" mode, facilitating learning and preparation for practical examinations. For examination purposes, the online Atlas contained over 300 additional photomicrographs with more than 700 interactive fill-in and true/false questions organized in a fashion to facilitate the student's learning and preparation for practical exams. Additionally, we have included approximately 100 USMLE Step I format multiple choice questions, based on photomicrographs created specifically for the questions, which can be accessed in test or study mode.

We are grateful to the many faculty members throughout the world who have assigned our Atlas to their students whether in its original English or in its translated form, which now counts 11 languages. We have received many compliments and constructive suggestions not only from faculty members but also from students, and we tried to incorporate those ideas into each new edition. One suggestion that we have resisted, however, was to change the order of the chapters. There were several faculty members who suggested a number of varied sequences; they all made sense to us, and it would have been very easy for us to adopt any one of the suggested chapter orders. However, we feel partial to and very comfortable with the classical sequence that we adopted so many years ago; it is just as valid and logical an arrangement as all the others that were suggested and, in the final analysis, we felt that instructors can simply tell their classes to use the chapters of the Atlas in a different sequence without harming the coherence of the material.

Major changes have been introduced in this, the sixth edition. The most exciting change is that we have completely rewritten and enhanced the textual material to such an extent that it can be used not only as an Atlas but also as an abbreviated textbook, which necessitated the title change to indicate that major alteration; therefore, the new title of the sixth edition is *Color Atlas and Text of Histology*. Additionally, we have enlarged the trim size of the book to its current size of 8½ × 11 inches, which permitted us to enlarge the photomicrographs so that the student can see details of the images to advantage. We have created new tables for each chapter. We have also included a new feature in the form of an Appendix that describes and illustrates many of the common stains used in the preparation of histological specimens. Probably the second most exciting change that we have introduced into this edition is the expansion of the Clinical Considerations components, many of which are now illustrated with histopathological images that we were graciously permitted to borrow from: Rubin, R., Strayer, D, et al., eds: *Rubin's Pathology. Clinicopathologic Foundations of Medicine*, 5th ed. Baltimore, Lippincott, Williams & Wilkins, 2008; Mills, S.E. editor, Carter, D. Greenson, J.K. Reuter, V.E. Stoler, M.H. eds. *Sternberger's Diagnostic Surgical Pathology*, 5th ed., Philadelphia, Lippincott, Williams & Wilkins, 2010; and Mills, S.E., ed: *Histology for Pathologists*, 3rd ed. Philadelphia, Lippincott, Williams & Wilkins, 2007.

As in the previous editions, most of the photomicrographs of this book are of tissues stained with hematoxylin and eosin. All indicated magnifications in light and electron micrographs are original magnifications. Many of the sections were prepared from plastic-embedded specimens, as noted. Most of the exquisite electron micrographs included in this book were kindly provided by our colleagues throughout the world as identified in the legends.

As with all of our textbooks, the Color Atlas and Text of Histology has been written with the student in mind; thus the material is complete but not esoteric. We wish to help the student learn and enjoy histology, not be overwhelmed by it. Furthermore, this book is designed not only for use in the laboratory but also as preparation for both didactic and practical examinations. Although we have attempted to be accurate and complete, we know that errors and omissions may have escaped our attention. Therefore, we welcome criticisms, suggestions, and comments that could help improve this book. Please address them to LPG21136@yahoo.com.

Leslie P. Gartner
James L. Hiatt

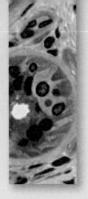

Acknowledgments

We would like to thank Todd Smith for the rendering of the outstanding full-color plates and thumbnail figures, Jerry Gadd for his paintings of blood cells, and our many colleagues who provided us with electron micrographs. We are especially thankful to Dr. Stephen W. Carmichael of the Mayo Medical School for his suggestions concerning the suprarenal medulla and Dr. Cheng Hwee Ming of the University of Malaya Medical School for his comments on the distal tubule of the kidney. Additionally, we are grateful to our good friends at Lippincott Williams & Wilkins, including our always cheerful, and exceptionally helpful, Product Manager, Catherine Noonan; Senior Acquisitions Editor, Crystal Taylor; Art Director, Jennifer Clements; and Editorial Assistant, Amanda Ingold. Finally, we wish to thank our families again for encouraging us during the preparation of this work. Their support always makes the labor an achievement.

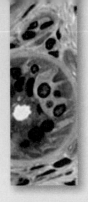

Reviewers

Ritwik Baidya, MBBS, MS
Professor
Anatomy & Embryology
Saba University School of Medicine
Saba, Dutch Caribbeans

Roger J. Bick, MMedEd, MBS
Course Director for Histology
Associate Professor of Pathology
University of Texas Medical School at Houston
Houston, Texas

Marc J. Braunstein, MD, PhD
Internal Medicine Resident
Hofstra North Shore LIJ School of Medicine
Hempstead, New York

Paul Johnson
Neurology Resident
University of Washington
Seattle, Washington

Sonia Lazreg
Medical Student
Mount Sinai School of Medicine
New York, New York

David J. Orlicky, PhD
Associate Professor
University of Colorado at Denver and Health
    Sciences Center
Denver, Colorado

Guy Sovak, PEng, BSc, MSc, PhD
Assistant Professor
Coordinator Special Projects
Department of Anatomy
Canadian Memorial Chiropractic College
Toronto, Canada

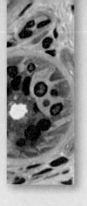

Contents

CHAPTER 19 **Special Senses**   **454**

Sixth Edition

Color Atlas and Text of
Histology

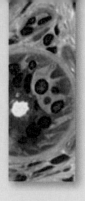

1 THE CELL

CHAPTER OUTLINE

Cells not only constitute the basic units of the human body but also function in executing all of the activities that the body requires for its survival. Although there are more than 200 different cell types, most cells possess common features, which permit them to perform their varied responsibilities. The living component of the cell is the **protoplasm,** which is subdivided into the **cytoplasm** and the **nucleoplasm** (see Graphics 1-1 and 1-2). The protoplasm also contains nonliving material such as crystals and pigments.

CYTOPLASM

Plasmalemma

Cells possess a membrane, the **plasmalemma,** that provides a selective, structural barrier between the cell and the outside world. This phospholipid bilayer with **integral** and **peripheral proteins** and **cholesterol** embedded in it functions

- in cell-cell recognition,
- in exocytosis and endocytosis,
- as a receptor site for signaling molecules, such as **G proteins** (Table 1-1), and
- as an initiator and controller of the secondary messenger system.

Materials may enter the cell by several means, such as

- **pinocytosis** (nonspecific uptake of molecules in an aqueous solution),
- **receptor-mediated endocytosis** (specific uptake of substances, such as low density lipoproteins), or
- **phagocytosis** (uptake of particulate matter).

Secretory products may leave the cell by two means, **constitutive** or **regulated secretion.**

- **Constitutive secretion,** using non–clathrin-coated vesicles, is the default pathway that does not require an extracellular signal for release, and thus, the secretory product (e.g., procollagen) leaves the cell in a continuous fashion.
- **Regulated secretion** requires the presence of clathrin-coated storage vesicles whose contents (e.g., pancreatic enzymes) are released only after the initiation of an extracellular signaling process.

The fluidity of the plasmalemma is an important factor in the processes of membrane synthesis, endocytosis, exocytosis, as well as in **membrane trafficking** (see Graphic 1-3)—conserving the membrane as it is transferred through the various cellular compartments. The degree of fluidity is influenced

- directly by temperature and the degree of unsaturation of the fatty acyl tails of the membrane phospholipids and
- indirectly by the amount of cholesterol present in the membrane.

Ions and other hydrophilic molecules are incapable of passing across the lipid bilayer; however, small nonpolar molecules, such as oxygen and carbon dioxide, as well as uncharged polar molecules, such as water and glycerol, all diffuse rapidly across the lipid bilayer. Specialized multipass integral proteins, known, collectively, as **membrane transport proteins**, function in the transfer of substances such as ions and hydrophilic molecules across the plasmalemma. There are two types of such proteins: ion channels and carrier proteins. Transport across the cell membrane may be

- **passive** down an ionic or concentration gradient (**simple diffusion**) or
- **facilitated diffusion** via ion channel or carrier proteins (no energy required) or
- **active** only via carrier proteins (energy required, usually against a gradient).

Ion channel proteins possess an aqueous pore and may be **ungated** or **gated.** The former are always open, whereas gated ion channels require the presence of a stimulus (alteration in voltage, mechanical stimulus, presence of a ligand, G protein, neurotransmitter substance, etc.) that opens the gate. These **ligands** and **neurotransmitter substances** are types of signaling molecules. **Signaling molecules** are either hydrophobic (lipid soluble) or hydrophilic and are used for cell-to-cell communication.

- Lipid-soluble molecules diffuse through the cell membrane to activate **intracellular messenger systems** by binding to receptor molecules located in either the cytoplasm or the nucleus.
- Hydrophilic signaling molecules initiate a specific sequence of responses by binding to **receptors** (integral proteins) embedded in the cell membrane.

Carrier proteins, unlike ion channels, can permit the passage of molecules with or without the expenditure of energy. If the material is to be transported against a concentration gradient, then carrier proteins can utilize ATP-driven methods or sodium ion concentration differentials to achieve the desired movement. Unlike ion channels, the materials to be transported bind to the internal aspect of the carrier protein. The material may be transported

- individually (**uniport**) or
- in concert with another molecule (coupled transport) and the two substances may travel
  - in the same direction (**symport**) or
  - in opposite directions (**antiport**).

TABLE 1-1 • Functions and Examples of Heterotrimeric G Proteins*

Type	Function	Examples
G_s	Activates adenylate cyclase, leading to formation of cAMP thus activating protein kinases	Binding of epinephrine to β-adrenergic receptors increases cAMP levels in cytosol.
G_i	Inhibits adenylate cyclase, preventing formation of cAMP, thereby protein kinases are not activated	Binding of epinephrine to α_2-adrenergic receptors decreases cAMP levels in cytosol.
G_q	Activates phospholipase C, leading to formation of inositol triphosphate and diacylglycerol, permitting the entry of calcium into the cell which activates protein kinase C	Binding of antigen to membrane-bound IgE causes the release of histamine by mast cells.
G_o	Opens K^+ channels, allowing potassium to enter the cell and closes Ca^{2+} channels thereby calcium movement in or out of the cell is inhibited	Inducing contraction of smooth muscle
G_{olf}	Activates adenylate cyclase in olfactory neurons which open cAMP-gated sodium channels	Binding of odorant to G protein–linked receptors initiates generation of nerve impulse.
G_t	Activates cGMP phosphodiesterase in rod cell membranes, leading to hydrolysis of cGMP resulting in the hyperpolarization of the rod cell plasmalemma	Photon activation of rhodopsin causes rod cells to fire.
$G_{12/13}$	Activates Rho family of GTPases which control the formation of actin and the regulation of the cytoskeleton	Facilitating cellular migration

*cAMP, cyclic adenosine monophosphate; cGMP, cyclic guanosine monophosphate; IgE, immunoglobulin E

Cells possess a number of distinct organelles, many of which are formed from membranes that are similar to but not identical with the biochemical composition of the plasmalemma.

Mitochondria

Mitochondria (see Graphic 1-2) are composed of an outer and an inner membrane with an intervening compartment between them known as the **intermembrane space**. The inner membrane is folded to form flat, shelf-like structures (or tubular in steroid-manufacturing cells) known as **cristae** and encloses a viscous fluid-filled space known as the **matrix space.** Mitochondria

- function in the **generation of ATP,** utilizing a chemiosmotic coupling mechanism that employs a specific sequence of enzyme complexes and proton translocator systems (**electron transport chain** and the ATP-synthase containing **elementary particles**) embedded in their cristae
- generate heat in **brown fat** instead of producing ATP
- also assist in the **synthesis** of certain **lipids** and **proteins;** they possess the enzymes of the **TCA cycle (Krebs' cycle), circular DNA** molecules, and matrix granules in their matrix space
- increase in number by undergoing **binary fission.**

Ribosomes

Ribosomes are small, bipartite, nonmembranous organelles that exist as individual particles that do not coalesce with each other until protein synthesis begins. The two subunits are of unequal size and constitution. The large subunit is 60S and the small subunit is 40S in size (see Table 1-2). Each subunit is composed of proteins and r-RNA, and together they function as an interactive "workbench" that not only provides a surface upon which protein synthesis occurs but also as a catalyst that facilitates the synthesis of proteins.

Endoplasmic Reticulum

The **endoplasmic reticulum** is composed of tubules, sacs, and flat sheets of membranes that occupy much of the

TABLE 1-2 • Ribosome Composition

Subunit	Size	Number of Proteins	Types of rRNA
Large	60S	49	5S 5.8S 28S
Small	40S	33	18S

rRNA, ribosomal ribonucleic acid; S, Svedberg units

intracellular space (see Graphic 1-2). There are two types of endoplasmic reticula, smooth and rough.

- **Smooth endoplasmic reticulum** functions in the synthesis of **cholesterols** and **lipids** as well as in the **detoxification** of certain drugs and toxins (such as barbiturates and alcohol). Additionally, in skeletal muscle cells, this organelle is specialized to sequester and release calcium ions and thus regulate muscle contraction and relaxation.
- The **rough endoplasmic reticulum** (RER), whose cytoplasmic surface possesses receptor molecules for ribosomes and signal recognition particles (SRPs) (known as **ribophorins** and **docking protein**, respectively), is continuous with the **outer nuclear membrane**. The RER functions in the **synthesis** and **modification of proteins** that are to be **packaged,** as well as in the synthesis of membrane lipids and proteins.

Protein synthesis requires the code-bearing mRNA, amino acid–carrying tRNAs, and ribosomes (see Graphic 1-4). Proteins that will not be packaged are synthesized on **ribosomes** in the cytosol, whereas **noncytosolic proteins** (secretory, lysosomal, and membrane proteins) are synthesized on ribosomes on the **rough endoplasmic reticulum.** The complex of mRNA and ribosomes is referred to as a **polysome.**

- The **signal hypothesis** states that mRNAs that code for noncytosolic proteins possess a constant initial segment, the **signal codon,** which codes for a **signal protein.**
- As the mRNA enters the cytoplasm, it becomes associated with the small subunit of a ribosome. The small subunit has a binding site for mRNA as well as three binding sites (A, P, and E) for tRNAs.
  1. Once the initiation process is completed, the **start codon** (AUG for the amino acid methionine) is recognized, and the **initiator tRNA** (bearing methionine) is attached to the **P site** (peptidyl-tRNA-binding site), the large subunit of the ribosome, which has corresponding A, P, and E sites, becomes attached, and protein synthesis may begin.
  2. The next codon is recognized by the proper acylated tRNA, which then binds to the **A site** (aminoacyl-tRNA binding site). Methionine is uncoupled from the initiator tRNA (at the P site), and a **peptide bond** is formed between the two amino acids (forming a **dipeptide**) so that the tRNA at the P site loses its amino acid and the tRNA at the A site now has two amino acids attached to it. The formation of this peptide bond is catalyzed by the enzyme **peptidyl transferase**, a part of the large ribosomal subunit.

  3. As the peptide bond is formed, the large subunit shifts in relation to the small subunit and the attached tRNA's wobble just enough to cause them to move just a little bit, so that the initiator tRNA (that lost its amino acid at the P site) moves to the **E site** (exit site) and the tRNA that has two amino acids attached to it moves from the A site to the P site freeing the A site.
  4. As this shifting occurs, the small ribosomal subunit moves the space of a single codon along the mRNA, so that the two ribosomal subunits are once again aligned with each other and the A site is located above the next codon on the mRNA strand.
  5. As a new tRNA with its associated amino acid occupies the A site (assuming that its anticodon matches the newly exposed codon of the mRNA), the initiator RNA drops off the E site, leaving the ribosome. The dipeptide is uncoupled from the tRNA at the P site, and a peptide bond is formed between the dipeptide and the new amino acid, forming a tripeptide.
  6. The empty tRNA again moves to the E site to fall off the ribosome, as the tRNA bearing the tripeptide moves from the A site to the P site. In this fashion, the peptide chain is elongated to form the signal protein.

The cytosol contains proteins known as **signal recognition particles (SRPs).**

- SRP binds to the signal protein, inhibits the continuation of protein synthesis, and the entire polysome proceeds to the RER.
- A **signal recognition particle receptor**, a transmembrane protein located in the membrane of the RER, recognizes and properly positions the polysome.
- The docking of the polysome results in the movement of the SRP-ribosome complex to a protein translocator, a pore in the RER membrane.
- The large subunit of the ribosome binds to and forms a tight seal with the protein translocator, aligning the pore in the ribosome with the pore in the protein translocator.
- The signal recognition particle and SRP receptor leave the polysome, permitting protein synthesis to resume, and the forming protein chain can enter the RER cisterna through the aqueous channel that penetrates the protein translocator.
- During this process, the enzyme **signal peptidase**, located in the RER cisterna, cleaves signal protein from the growing polypeptide chain.
- Once protein synthesis is complete, the two ribosomal subunits fall off the RER and return to the cytosol.

The newly synthesized protein is modified in the RER by glycosylation, as well as by the formation of disulfide bonds, which transforms the linear protein into a globular form.

Golgi Apparatus, *cis*-Golgi Network, and the *trans*-Golgi Network

The **Golgi apparatus (complex)** is composed of a specifically oriented cluster of vesicles, tubules, and flattened membrane-bounded cisternae. Each Golgi complex has

- a convex entry face, known as the *cis* **face** closer to the nucleus, and
- a concave exit face, known as the *trans* **face** oriented toward the cell membrane.
- Between the *cis* face and the *trans* face are several intermediate cisternae, known as the **medial face** (see Graphic 1-2).

The Golgi complex not only **packages** but also **modifies** macromolecules synthesized on the surface of the RER. Newly synthesized proteins pass from the region of the RER, known as the **transitional endoplasmic reticulum**, to

- the **vesicular-tubular cluster (VTC,** formerly referred to as the ERGIC), by **transfer vesicles** whose membrane is covered by protein coatomer II (COPII) and are, therefore, also known as coatomer II–coated vesicles. From the VTC, the proteins are delivered to
- the *cis*-Golgi network, probably via COPI-coated (coatomer I) vesicles.
- The proteins continue to travel to the *cis*, medial, and *trans* faces of the Golgi apparatus (probably) by COPI-coated vesicles (or, according to some authors, via cisternal maturation).
- Lysosomal oligosaccharides are phosphorylated in the VTC and/or in the *cis* face;
- mannose groups are removed and galactose and sialic acid (**terminal glycosylation**) are added in the medial face, whereas
- selected amino acid residues are phosphorylated and sulfated in the *trans* face.

Sorting and the final **packaging** of the macromolecules are the responsibility of the *trans*-**Golgi network (TGN).**

- Mannose 6-phosphate receptors in the TGN recognize and package enzymes destined for lysosomes.
  - These **lysosomal enzymes** leave the TGN in clathrin-coated vesicles.
- **Regulated secretory proteins** are separated and are also packaged in clathrin-coated vesicles.
- **Membrane proteins** and proteins destined for constitutive (unregulated) transport are packaged in non–clathrin-coated vesicles.

It should be noted that material can travel through the Golgi complex in an **anterograde fashion,** as just described, as well as in a **retrograde fashion,** which occurs in situations such as when escaped proteins that are residents of the RER or of a particular Golgi face have to be returned to their compartments of origin in COPI-coated vesicles.

Endosomes

Endosomes are intermediate compartments within the cell, utilized in the destruction of endocytosed, phagocytosed, or autophagocytosed materials as well as in the formation of lysosomes. Endosomes

- possess **proton pumps** in their membranes, which pump H^+ into the endosome, thus acidifying the interior of this compartment.
- are intermediate stages in the formation of lysosomes.

Receptors permit the endocytosis of a much greater concentration of ligands than would be possible without receptors. This process is referred to as **receptor-mediated endocytosis** and involves the formation of a **clathrin-coated endocytic vesicle,** which, once within the cell, sheds its clathrin coat and fuses with an **early endosome.**

- **Early endosomes** are located at the periphery of the cell and contain receptor-ligand complexes, and their acidic contents (pH 6) are responsible for the uncoupling of receptors from ligands.
- The receptors are usually carried into a system of tubular vesicles, the **recycling endosomes,** from which the receptors are returned to the plasmalemma, whereas the ligands are translocated to late endosomes located deeper in the cytoplasm.
- Within **late endosomes,** the pH is even more acidic (pH 5.5). Many investigators have suggested that early endosomes mature into late endosomes by the fusion of vesicles with one another as well as with late endosomes that have been formed earlier.

Lysosomes

Lysosomes are formed by the utilization of **late endosomes** as an intermediary compartment.

- Both lysosomal membranes and lysosomal enzymes are packaged in the TGN and
- are delivered in separate **clathrin-coated vesicles** to late endosomes, forming **endolysosomes,** which then mature to become **lysosomes.**

These membrane-bounded vesicles whose proton pumps are responsible for their very acidic interior (pH 5.0) contain various **hydrolytic enzymes** that function in **intracellular digestion.** They

- degrade certain macromolecules as well as phagocytosed particulate matter (**phagolysosomes**) and autophagocytosed material (**autophagolysosomes**).

- Frequently, the indigestible remnants of lysosomal degradation remain in the cell, enclosed in vesicles referred to as **residual bodies.**
- The lysosomal membrane maintains its integrity possibly because the luminal aspects of the membrane proteins are glycosylated to a much greater extent than those of other membranes thus preventing the degradation of the membrane.

Peroxisomes

Peroxisomes are membrane-bounded organelles housing **oxidative enzymes** such as **urate oxidase, D-amino acid oxidase,** and **catalase.** These organelles function

- in the formation of free radicals (e.g., superoxides), which destroy various substances, and
- in the protection of the cell by degrading hydrogen peroxide by catalase.
- They also function in **detoxification** of certain toxins and in elongation of some fatty acids during **lipid synthesis.**

Most of the proteins intended for inclusions into peroxisomes are synthesized in the cytosol rather than on the RER. All peroxisomes are formed by **fission** from preexisting peroxisomes.

Proteasomes

Proteasomes are small, barrel-shaped organelles that function in the degradation of cytosolic proteins. There are two types of proteasomes, the **larger 26S** and the **smaller 20S.** The practice of cytosolic proteolysis is highly regulated, and the candidate protein must be tagged by several **ubiquitin** molecules before it is permitted to be destroyed by the 26S proteasome system. The 20S proteasome degrades proteins that are **oxidized** by reactive oxygen species to form protein carbonyls.

Cytoskeleton

The **cytoskeleton** is composed of a filamentous array of proteins that act not only as the structural framework of the cell but also to **transport** material within it from one region of the cell to another and provide it with the capability of **motion** and cell division. Components of the cytoskeleton include

- **microtubules** (consisting of α- and β-tubulins arranged in 13 protofilaments),
- **thin** (actin) **filaments** (also known as **microfilaments**). Thin filaments function in the movement of cells from one place to another as well as in the movement of regions of the cell with respect to itself.
- **Intermediate filaments** are thicker than thin and thinner than thick filaments. They function in providing a structural framework to the cell and resisting mechanical stresses placed on cells (Table 1-3).
- **Thick filaments,** included here although not traditionally considered to be part of the cytoskeleton, are composed of myosin, and they interact with thin filaments to facilitate cell movement either along a surface or movement of cellular regions with respect to the cell.

TABLE 1-3 • Major Intermediate Filaments

Type	Location	Function
Keratin	Epithelial cells Cells of hair and nails	Support; tension bearing; withstands stretching; associated with desmosomes, hemidesmosomes, and tonofilaments; immunological marker for epithelial tumors
Vimentin	Mesenchymal cells, chondroblasts, fibroblasts, endothelial cells	Structural support, forms cage-like structure around nucleus; immunological marker for mesenchymal cell tumors
Desmin and vimentin	Muscle: skeletal, smooth, cardiac	Links myofibrils to myofilaments; desmin is an immunological marker for tumors arising in muscle.
GFAP* and vimentin	Astrocytes, oligodendrocytes, Schwann cells, and neurons	Support; GFAP is an immunological marker for glial tumors.
Neurofilaments	Neurons	Support of axons and dendrites, immunological marker for neurological tumors
Lamins A, B, and C	Lines nuclear envelopes of all cells	Organizes and assembles nuclear envelope, maintains organization of nuclear chromatin

GFAP, glial fibrillar acidic protein

Microtubules are also associated with proteins, known as **microtubule-associated proteins (MAPs)**, which permit organelles, vesicles, and other components of the cytoskeleton to bind to microtubules.

- Most microtubules originate from **the microtubule-organizing center** of the cell, located in the vicinity of the Golgi apparatus.
- These elements of the cytoskeleton are pathways for intracellular translocation of organelles and vesicles, and during cell division, chromosomes are moved into their proper locations.
- Two important MAPs, **kinesin** and **dynein**, are motor proteins that facilitate anterograde and retrograde intracellular vesicular and organelle movement, respectively.
- The **axoneme** of cilia and flagella, as well as a framework of centrioles, are formed mostly of microtubules.

Inclusions

Cytoplasmic **inclusions,** such as **lipids, glycogen, secretory granules,** and **pigments,** are also consistent constituents of the cytoplasm. Many of these inclusions are transitory in nature, although some pigments, for example, **lipofuscin,** are permanent residents of certain cells.

NUCLEUS

The **nucleus** is enclosed by the **nuclear envelope,** composed of an **inner** and an **outer nuclear membrane** with an intervening **perinuclear cistern** (see Graphic 1-2). The outer nuclear membrane is studded with **ribosomes** and is continuous, in places, with the **rough endoplasmic reticulum.** In areas the inner and outer membranes fuse with each other, forming circular profiles, known as

- **nuclear pores** that permit communication between the nucleoplasm and the cytoplasm.

- These perforations of the nuclear envelope are guarded by protein assemblies which, together with the perforations, are known as **nuclear pore complexes,** providing regulated passageways for the transport of materials in and out of the nucleus.

The nucleus houses **chromosomes** and is the location of **RNA synthesis.**

- **mRNA** and **tRNA,** as well as **microRNA,** are transcribed in the nucleus,
- whereas **rRNA** is transcribed in the region of the nucleus known as the **nucleolus.**

The nucleolus is also the site of assembly of ribosomal proteins and rRNA into the small and large subunits of **ribosomes.** These ribosomal subunits enter the cytosol separately.

CELL CYCLE

The **cell cycle** is governed by the cell cycle control system that not only ensures the occurrence of the correct sequence of events in a timely fashion but also monitors and controls them. The cell cycle is subdivided into four phases, G_1, S, G_2, and M.

- During the presynthetic phase, G_1, the cell increases its size and organelle content.
- During the **S phase,** DNA (plus histone and other chromosome-associated protein) synthesis and centriole replication occur.
- During G_2, ATP is accumulated, centriole replication is completed, and tubulin is accumulated for spindle formation. G_1, S, and G_2 are also referred to as **interphase.**
- **M** represents **mitosis,** which is subdivided into prophase, prometaphase, metaphase, anaphase, and telophase (see Table 1-4). The result is the division of the cell and its genetic material into two identical daughter cells.

The sequence of events in the cell cycle is controlled by a number of trigger proteins, known as **cyclin-dependent kinases** and **cyclins.**

TABLE 1-4 • Stages of Mitosis

Stage	DNA Content	Identifying Characteristics
Prophase	DNA content doubles in the S phase of interphase (4n); also, centrioles replicate.	Nuclear envelope begins to disappear and the nucleolus disappears. Chromosomes have been replicated and each chromosome is composed of two sister chromatids attached to each other at centromere. Centrioles migrate to opposite poles where they act as microtubule-organizing centers and give rise to spindle fibers and astral rays.
Prometaphase	DNA complement is 4n.	Nuclear envelope disappears. Kinetochores, additional microtubule-organizing centers, develop at centromeres and kinetochore microtubules form.
Metaphase	DNA complement is 4n.	Chromosomes align at the equatorial plate of the mitotic spindle.
Anaphase	DNA complement is 4n.	Sister chromatids separate at centromere and each chromatid migrates to an opposite pole of the cell along the microtubule, a process known as karyokinesis. In late anaphase, a cleavage furrow begins to form.
Telophase	Each new daughter cell contains a single complement of DNA (2n).	Deepening of the cleavage furrow restricts the continuity between the two developing daughter cells forming the midbody. The two daughter cells separate from each other, a process known as cytokinesis. Nuclear envelope reforms, nucleoli reappear, and chromosomes disperse, forming new interphase nucleus in each daughter cell.

CLINICAL CONSIDERATIONS

Lysosomal Storage Diseases

Certain individuals suffer from **lysosomal storage diseases**, which involve a hereditary deficiency in the ability of their lysosomes to degrade the contents of their endolysosomes. One of the best-characterized examples of these diseases is **Tay-Sachs disease** that occurs mostly in children whose parents are descendants of Northeast European Jews. Since the lysosomes of these children are unable to catabolize GM2 gangliosides, due to hexoaminidase deficiency, their neurons accumulate massive amounts of this ganglioside in endolysosomes of ever increasing diameters. As the endolysosomes increase in size, they obstruct neuronal function and the child dies by the third year of life.

Zellweger's Disease

Zellweger's disease is an inherited autosomal recessive disorder that interferes with normal peroxisomal biogenesis whose characteristics include renal cysts, hepatomegaly, jaundice, hypotonia of the muscular system, and cerebral demyelination resulting in psychomotor retardation.

Cancer

Recent studies have suggested that most **cancers** arise not from mutations in individual genes but from the formation of aneuploidy. In fact, within the same tumor, the chromosomal configurations of individual cells vary greatly, and the DNA content of the cells may be 50% to 200% of the normal somatic cell. It is interesting to note that in the apparently chaotic reshuffling and recombination of chromosomes in cancer cells, there appears to be an order, as in Burkitt's lymphoma, where chromosomes 3, 13, and 17 usually displayed translocations and chromosomes 7 and 20 were usually missing segments.

Hereditary Hemochromatosis

Excessive iron storage in **hereditary hemochromatosis**, untreated, can be a lethal disorder. The individual absorbs too much iron, which accumulates in the parenchymal cells of vital organs such as the liver, pancreas, and heart. Because it may affect organs in different sequence, the symptoms vary and diagnosis may be difficult. Testing the blood levels for high concentration of ferritin and transferrin can provide definitive diagnosis, which can be confirmed by genetic testing. Since this is a hereditary disorder, the close relatives of the positive individual should also undergo genetic testing.

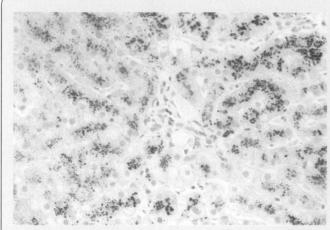

In the case of the liver, displayed in this photomicrograph of a Prussian blue-stained specimen, the lysosomes of hepatocytes are congested by large accumulations of iron (appearing as small, granular deposits). (Reprinted with permission from Rubin R, Strayer D, et al., eds. Rubin's Pathology. Clinicopathologic Foundations of Medicine, 5th ed., Baltimore: Lippincott, Williams & Wilkins, 2008. p. 19.)

Hydropic Swelling

When cells become injured by coming into contact with toxins, are placed in areas of low or high temperature or low oxygen concentration, as well as being exposed to various inimical conditions, their cytoplasm swells and

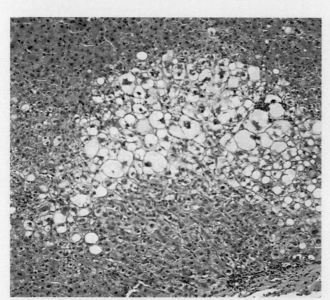

This light photomicrograph of a liver of a patient with toxic hepatic injury displays hydropic swelling. Note that the affected cells are enlarged with accumulations of fluid, but the nuclei of most cells appear to be at their normal location. The cells at the periphery seem to be healthy. (Reprinted with permission from Rubin R, Strayer D, et al., eds. Rubin's Pathology. Clinicopathologic Foundations of Medicine, 5th ed., Baltimore: Lippincott, Williams & Wilkins, 2008. p. 9.)

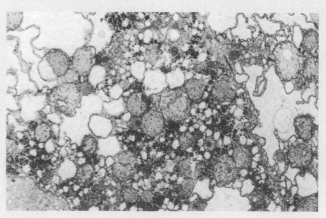

An electron micrograph of a liver with hydropic swelling displays enlarged cisternae of the endoplasmic reticulum that cause the liver cells to be swollen. (Reprinted with permission from Rubin R, Strayer D, et al., eds. Rubin's Pathology. Clinicopathologic Foundations of Medicine, 5th ed., Baltimore: Lippincott, Williams & Wilkins, 2008. p. 9.)

takes on a pale appearance. This characteristic is usually reversible and is called **hydropic swelling**. Usually, the nuclei occupy their normal position, their organelle content remains unaltered, but the organelles are located farther away from each other, and viewed with the electron microscope, it is noted that the cisternae of their endoplasmic reticulum are dilated.

Genital Herpes Infection

One of the most common sexually transmitted diseases, **herpes simplex virus** (**HSV-2, genital herpes**) infection of the cervix (although **HSV-1**, usually associated with cold sores on the lips and, occasionally, the eyes, can also

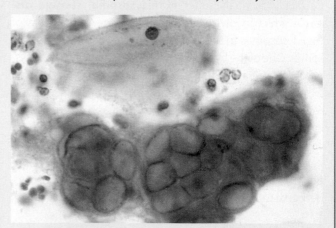

Note the healthy epithelial cell with its pink cytoplasm with its healthy-appearing nucleus. The infected epithelial cells possess multiple nuclei with "ground glass" appearance and with peripherally located chromatin. (Reprinted with permission from Rubin R, Strayer, D, et al., eds. Rubin's Pathology. Clinicopathologic Foundations of Medicine, 5th ed., Baltimore: Lippincott, Williams & Wilkins, 2008. p. 1268.)

be a causative factor). Usually, infection by herpes simplex virus displays the presence of painful blisters that discharge a clear fluid, form a scab within a week or so, and disappear. During this episode, the genital area in females is painful and urination may be accompanied by a burning feeling. However, if the affected region is the cervix or the vagina, the pain may be much less severe. When the blisters break, the fluid within them is filled with HSV and the individual is infectious. Subsequent to the outbreak of the blistering, the virus retreats, along nerve fibers, into the ganglion and remains there until the next episode. HSV infections cannot be cured, but the severity of the pain and the duration of the episode can be lessened by antiviral agents.

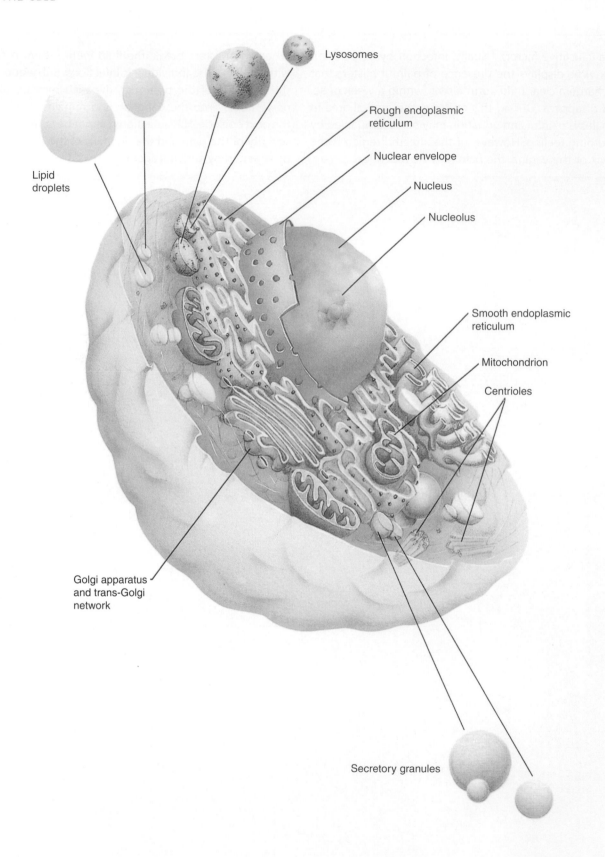

Lysosomes

Rough endoplasmic
reticulum

Nuclear envelope

Nucleus

Nucleolus

Lipid
droplets

Smooth endoplasmic
reticulum

Mitochondrion

Centrioles

Golgi apparatus
and trans-Golgi
network

Secretory granules

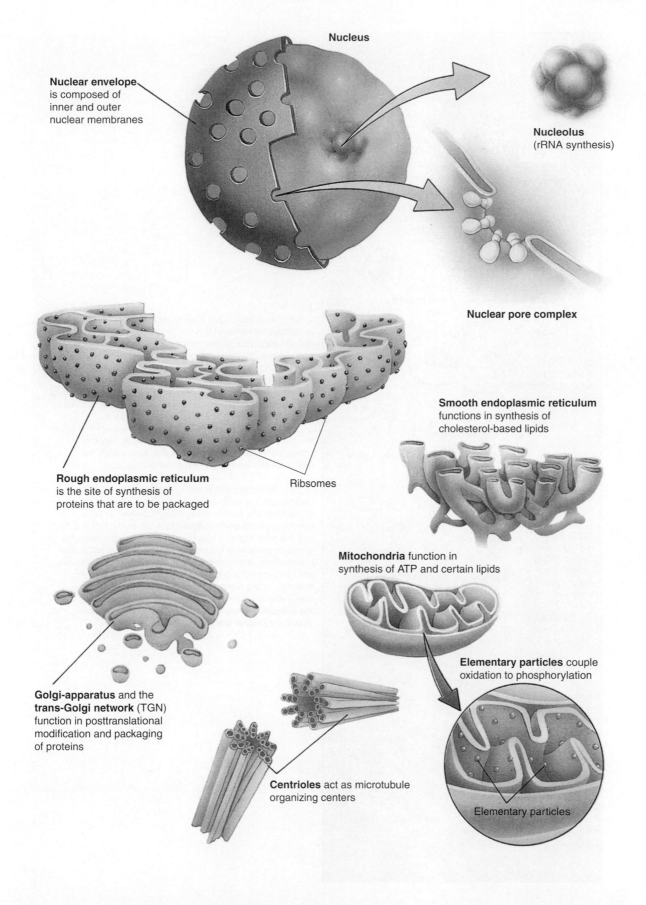

Nucleus

Nuclear envelope is composed of inner and outer nuclear membranes

Nucleolus (rRNA synthesis)

Nuclear pore complex

Rough endoplasmic reticulum is the site of synthesis of proteins that are to be packaged

Ribsomes

Smooth endoplasmic reticulum functions in synthesis of cholesterol-based lipids

Golgi-apparatus and the **trans-Golgi network** (TGN) function in posttranslational modification and packaging of proteins

Centrioles act as microtubule organizing centers

Mitochondria function in synthesis of ATP and certain lipids

Elementary particles couple oxidation to phosphorylation

Elementary particles

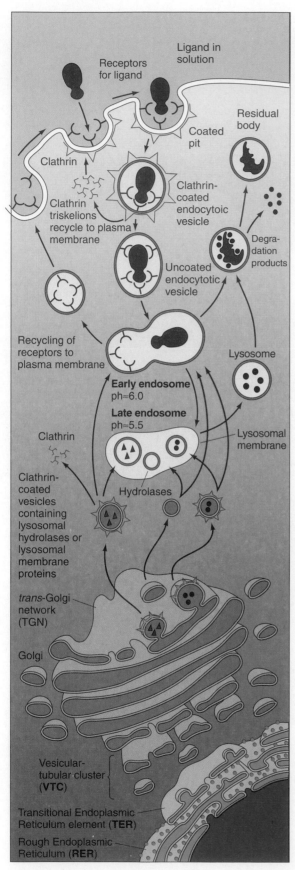

Signaling molecules bind to **receptors** (integral proteins) embedded in the cell membrane and initiate a specific sequence of responses. Receptors permit the endocytosis of a much greater concentration of ligands than would be otherwise possible. This process, **receptor-mediated endocytosis**, involves the formation of **clathrin-coated endocytic vesicles**. Once within the cell, the vesicle sheds its clathrin coat and fuses with an early endosome (pH $\cong$ 6) where the receptor is uncoupled from the ligand. The receptors are carried from the early endosome into a system of tubular vesicles, known as the **recycling endosome**, from which the receptors are returned to the cell membrane.

The ligand is transferred by the use of multivesicular bodies from the early endosome to another system of vesicles, late endosomes, located deeper in the cytoplasm. **Late endosomes** are more acidic (pH $\cong$ 5.5) and it is here that the ligand begins to be degraded. Late endosomes receive lysosomal hydrolases and lysosomal membranes, and in that fashion late endosomes probably are transformed into lysosomes (pH $\cong$ 5.0). Hydrolytic enzymes of the lyosomes degrade the ligand, releasing the usable substances for utilization by the cell, whereas the indigestible remnants of the ligand may remain in vesicles, **residual bodies**, within the cytoplasm.

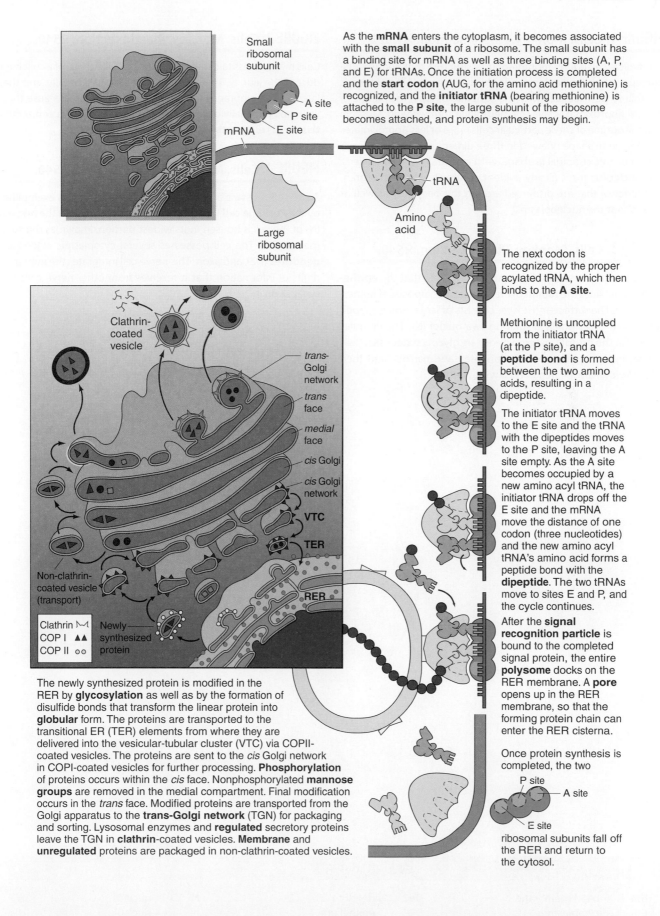

Small ribosomal subunit

A site
P site
E site

mRNA

Large ribosomal subunit

As the **mRNA** enters the cytoplasm, it becomes associated with the **small subunit** of a ribosome. The small subunit has a binding site for mRNA as well as three binding sites (A, P, and E) for tRNAs. Once the initiation process is completed and the **start codon** (AUG, for the amino acid methionine) is recognized, and the **initiator tRNA** (bearing methionine) is attached to the **P site**, the large subunit of the ribosome becomes attached, and protein synthesis may begin.

tRNA

Amino acid

The next codon is recognized by the proper acylated tRNA, which then binds to the **A site**.

Methionine is uncoupled from the initiator tRNA (at the P site), and a **peptide bond** is formed between the two amino acids, resulting in a dipeptide.

The initiator tRNA moves to the E site and the tRNA with the dipeptides moves to the P site, leaving the A site empty. As the A site becomes occupied by a new amino acyl tRNA, the initiator tRNA drops off the E site and the mRNA move the distance of one codon (three nucleotides) and the new amino acyl tRNA's amino acid forms a peptide bond with the **dipeptide**. The two tRNAs move to sites E and P, and the cycle continues.

After the **signal recognition particle** is bound to the completed signal protein, the entire **polysome** docks on the RER membrane. A **pore** opens up in the RER membrane, so that the forming protein chain can enter the RER cisterna.

Once protein synthesis is completed, the two

P site
A site
E site

ribosomal subunits fall off the RER and return to the cytosol.

Clathrin-coated vesicle

trans-Golgi network
trans face
medial face
cis Golgi
cis Golgi network
VTC
TER
RER

Non-clathrin-coated vesicle (transport)

Clathrin ⋈
COP I ▲▲
COP II ∘∘

Newly synthesized protein

The newly synthesized protein is modified in the RER by **glycosylation** as well as by the formation of disulfide bonds that transform the linear protein into **globular** form. The proteins are transported to the transitional ER (TER) elements from where they are delivered into the vesicular-tubular cluster (VTC) via COPII-coated vesicles. The proteins are sent to the *cis* Golgi network in COPI-coated vesicles for further processing. **Phosphorylation** of proteins occurs within the *cis* face. Nonphosphorylated **mannose groups** are removed in the medial compartment. Final modification occurs in the *trans* face. Modified proteins are transported from the Golgi apparatus to the **trans-Golgi network** (TGN) for packaging and sorting. Lysosomal enzymes and **regulated** secretory proteins leave the TGN in **clathrin**-coated vesicles. **Membrane** and **unregulated** proteins are packaged in non-clathrin-coated vesicles.

PLATE 1-1 · Typical Cell

FIGURE 1. Cells. Monkey. Plastic section. ×1,323.

The typical cell is a membrane-bound structure that consists of a **nucleus** (N) and **cytoplasm** (C). Although the cell membrane is too thin to be visualized with the light microscope, the outline of the cell approximates the cell membrane (*arrowheads*). Observe that the outline of these particular cells more or less approximates a rectangle in shape. Viewed in three dimensions, these cells are said to be tall, cuboidal in shape, with a centrally placed nucleus. The **nucleolus** (n) is clearly evident, as are the chromatin granules (*arrows*) that are dispersed around the periphery as well as throughout the nucleoplasm.

FIGURE 3. Cells. Monkey. Plastic section. ×540.

Cells come in a variety of sizes and shapes. Note that the **epithelium** (E) that lines the **lumen** of the bladder is composed of numerous layers. The surface-most layer consists of large, dome-shaped cells, some occasionally displaying two **nuclei** (N). The granules evident in the cytoplasm (*arrowhead*) are glycogen deposits. Cells deeper in the epithelium are elongated and narrow, and their nuclei (*arrow*) are located in their widest region

FIGURE 2. Cells. Monkey. Plastic section. ×540.

Cells may possess tall, thin morphologies, like those of a collecting duct of the kidney. Their **nuclei** (N) are located basally, and their lateral cell membranes (*arrowheads*) are outlined. Because these cells are epithelially derived, they are separated from **connective tissue** (CT) **elements** by a **basal membrane** (BM).

FIGURE 4. Cells. Monkey. Plastic section. ×540.

Some cells possess a rather unusual morphology, as exemplified by the **Purkinje cell** (PC) of the cerebellum. Note that the **nucleus** (N) of the cell is housed in its widest portion, known as the soma (perikaryon). The cell possesses several cytoplasmic extensions, **dendrites** (De), and axon. This nerve cell integrates the numerous digits of information that it receives from other nerve cells that synapse on it.

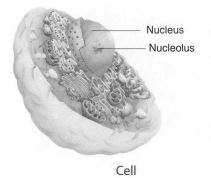

— Nucleus
— Nucleolus

Cell

KEY

BM	basal membrane	**De**	dendrite	**N**	nucleus
C	cytoplasm	**E**	epithelium	**n**	nucleolus
CT	connective tissue	**L**	lumen	**PC**	Purkinje cell

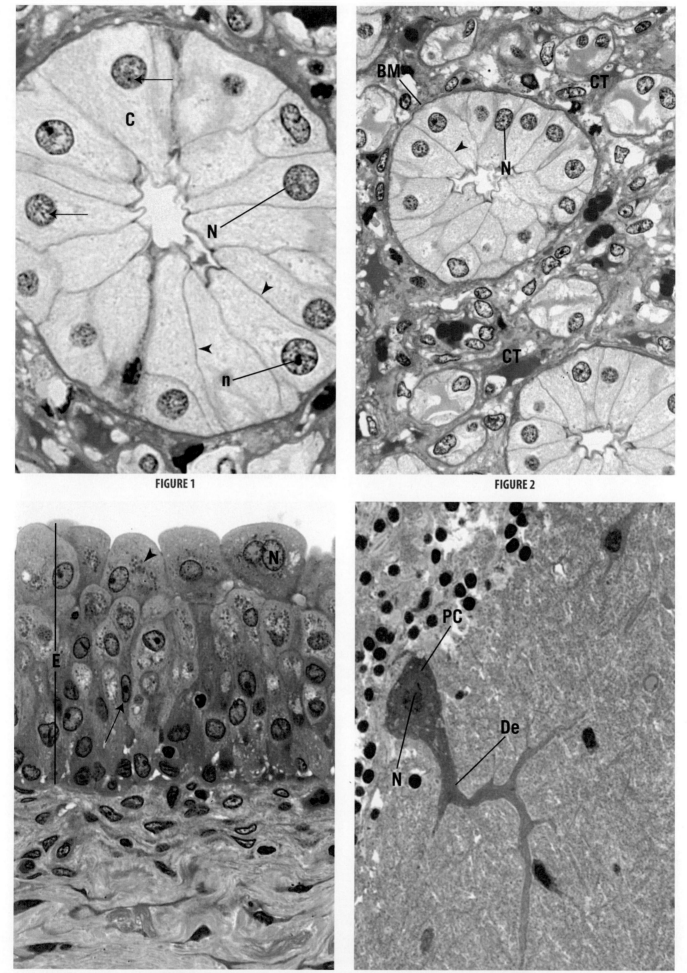

FIGURE 1

FIGURE 2

FIGURE 3

FIGURE 4

PLATE 1-1 • Typical Cell

PLATE 1-2 • Cell Organelles and Inclusions

FIGURE 1. Nucleus and Nissl bodies. Spinal cord. Human. Paraffin section. ×540.

The motor neurons of the spinal cord are multipolar neurons because they possess numerous processes arising from an enlarged **soma** (S), which houses the **nucleus** (N) and various organelles. Observe that the nucleus displays a large, densely staining **nucleolus** (n). The cytoplasm also presents a series of densely staining structures known as **Nissl bodies** (NB), which have been demonstrated by electron microscopy to be RER. The staining intensity is due to the presence of ribonucleic acid of the ribosomes studding the surface of the RER.

FIGURE 3. Zymogen granules. Pancreas. Monkey. Plastic section. ×540.

The exocrine portion of the pancreas produces enzymes necessary for proper digestion of ingested food materials. These enzymes are stored by the pancreatic cells as **zymogen granules** (ZG) until their release is effected by hormonal activity. Note that the parenchymal cells are arranged in clusters known as **acini** (Ac), with a central lumen into which the secretory product is released. Observe that the zymogen granules are stored in the apical region of the cell, away from the basally located **nucleus** (N). *Arrows* indicate the lateral cell membranes of adjacent cells of an acinus.

FIGURE 2. Secretory products. Mast cell. Monkey. Plastic section. ×540.

The **connective tissue** (CT) subjacent to the epithelial lining of the small intestines is richly endowed with **mast cells** (MC). The granules (*arrows*) of mast cells are distributed throughout their cytoplasm and are released along the entire periphery of the cell. These small granules contain histamine and heparin, as well as additional substances. Note that the **epithelial cells** (EC) are tall and columnar in morphology and that **leukocytes** (Le) are migrating, via intercellular spaces, into the **lumen** (L) of the intestines. *Arrowheads* point to terminal bars, junctions between epithelial cells. The **brush border** (BB) has been demonstrated by electron microscopy to be microvilli.

FIGURE 4. Mucous secretory products. Goblet cells. Large intestines. Monkey. Plastic section. ×540.

The glands of the large intestine house **goblet cells** (GC), which manufacture a large amount of mucous material that acts as a lubricant for the movement of the compacted residue of digestion. Each goblet cell possesses an expanded apical portion, the **theca** (T), which contains the secretory product of the cell. The base of the cell is compressed and houses the **nucleus** (N) as well as the organelles necessary for the synthesis of the mucus—namely, the RER and the Golgi apparatus. *Arrows* indicate the lateral cell membranes of contiguous goblet cells.

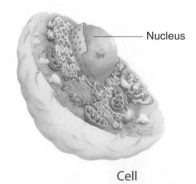

Nucleus

Cell

KEY

AC	acinus	L	lumen	NB	Nissl body
BB	brush border	Le	leukocyte	S	soma
CT	connective tissue	MC	mast cell	T	theca
EC	epithelial cell	N	nucleus	ZG	zymogen granule
GC	goblet cell	n	nucleolus		

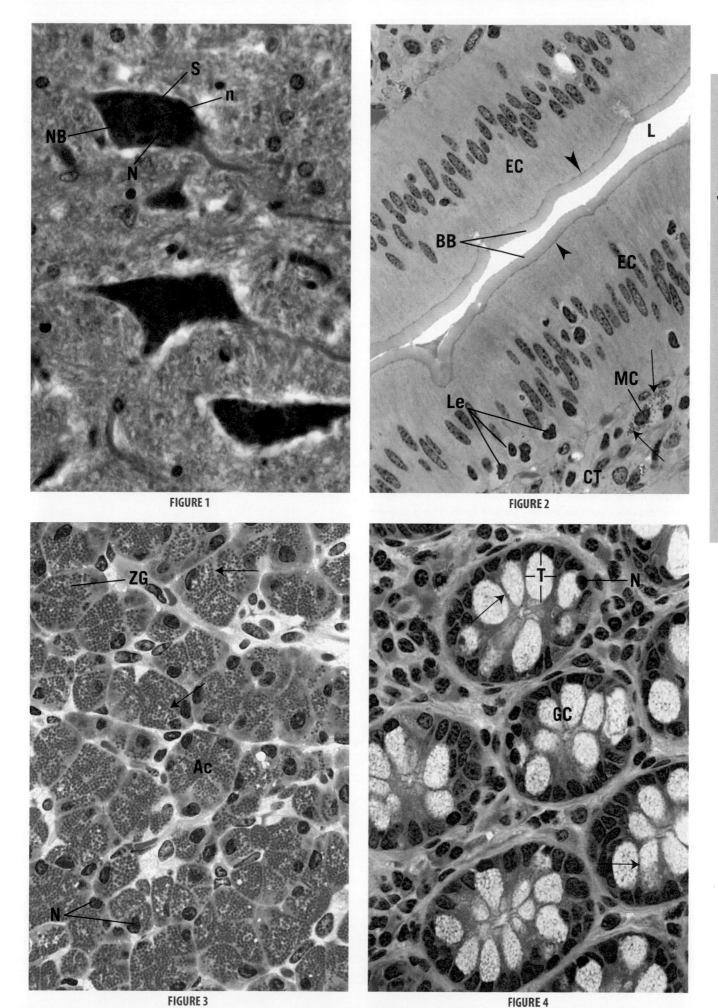

PLATE 1-2 · Cell Organelles and Inclusions

FIGURE 1

FIGURE 2

FIGURE 3

FIGURE 4

PLATE 1-3 · Cell Surface Modifications

FIGURE 1. Brush border. Small intestines. Monkey. Plastic section. ×540.

The cells lining the **lumen** (L) of the small intestine are columnar cells, among which are numerous mucus-producing **goblet cells** (GC). The columnar cells' function is absorbing digested food material along their free, apical surface. To increase their free surface area, the cells possess a **brush border** (BB), which has been demonstrated by electron microscopy to be microvilli—short, narrow, finger-like extensions of plasmalemma-covered cytoplasm. Each microvillus bears a glycocalyx cell coat, which also contains digestive enzymes. The core of the microvillus contains longitudinally arranged actin filaments as well as additional associated proteins.

FIGURE 3. Stereocilia. Epididymis. Monkey. Plastic section. ×540.

The lining of the epididymis is composed of tall, columnar **principal cells** (Pi) and short **basal cells** (BC). The principal cells bear long stereocilia (*arrows*) that protrude into the lumen. It was believed that stereocilia were long, nonmotile, cilia-like structures. However, studies with the electron microscope have shown that stereocilia are actually long microvilli that branch as well as clump with each other. The function, if any, of stereocilia within the epididymis is not known. The lumen is occupied by numerous spermatozoa, whose dark heads (*asterisks*) and pale flagella (*arrowhead*) are clearly discernible. Flagella are very long, cilia-like structures used by the cell for propulsion.

FIGURE 2. Cilia. Oviduct. Monkey. Plastic section. ×540.

The lining of the oviduct is composed of two types of epithelial cells: bleb-bearing **peg cells** (pc), which probably produce nutritional factors necessary for the survival of the gametes, and pale **ciliated cells** (CC). Cilia (*arrows*) are long, motile, finger-like extensions of the apical cell membrane and cytoplasm that transport material along the cell surface. The core of the cilium, as shown by electron microscopy, contains the axoneme, composed of microtubules arranged in a specific configuration of nine doublets surrounding a central pair of individual microtubules.

FIGURE 4. Intercellular bridges. Skin. Monkey. Plastic section. ×540.

The epidermis of thick skin is composed of several cell layers, one of which is the stratum spinosum shown in this photomicrograph. The cells of this layer possess short, stubby, finger-like extensions that interdigitate with those of contiguous cells. Before the advent of electron microscopy, these intercellular bridges (*arrows*) were believed to represent cytoplasmic continuities between neighboring cells; however, it is now known that these processes merely serve as regions of desmosome formation so that the cells may adhere to each other.

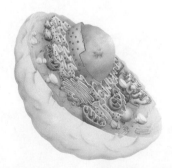

Cell

KEY					
BB	brush border	GC	goblet cell	Pi	principal cell
BC	basal cell	L	lumen		
CC	ciliated cell	pc	peg cell		

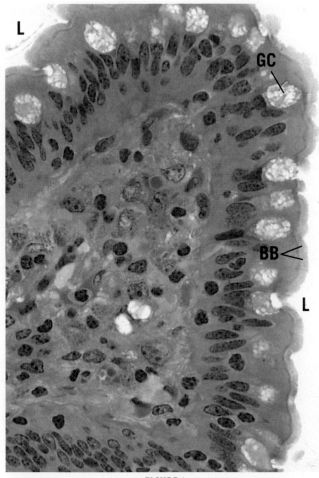

FIGURE 1

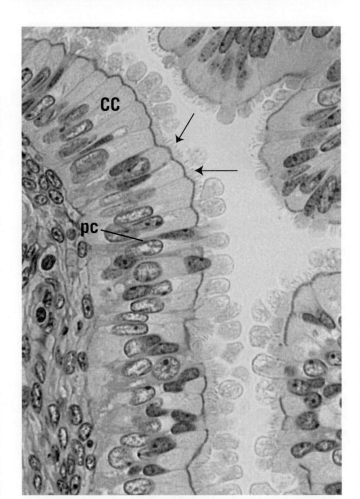

FIGURE 2

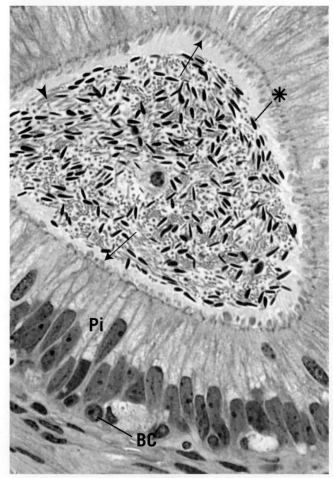

FIGURE 3

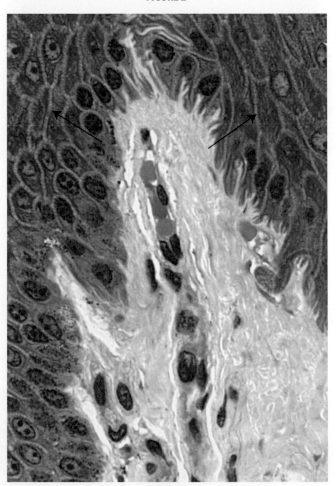

FIGURE 4

PLATE 1-3 • Cell Surface Modifications

PLATE 1-4 • Mitosis, Light and Electron Microscopy

FIGURE 1. Mitosis. Whitefish blastula. Paraffin section. ×270.

This photomicrograph of whitefish blastula shows different stages of mitosis. The first mitotic stage, **prophase** (P), displays the short, thread-like chromosomes (*arrow*) in the center of the cell. The nuclear membrane is no longer present. During **metaphase** (M), the chromosomes line up at the equatorial plane of the cell. The chromosomes begin to migrate toward the opposite poles of the cell in early **anaphase** (A) and proceed farther and farther apart as anaphase progresses (*arrowheads*). Note the dense regions, **centrioles** (c), toward which the chromosomes migrate.

FIGURE 3. Mitosis. Mouse. Electron microscopy. ×9423.

Neonatal tissue is characterized by mitotic activity, in which numerous cells are in the process of proliferation. Observe that the interphase **nucleus** (N) possesses a typical **nuclear envelope** (NE), perinuclear chromatin (*asterisk*), nucleolus, and nuclear pores. A cell that is undergoing the mitotic phase of the cell cycle loses its nuclear membrane and nucleolus, whereas its **chromosomes** (Ch) are quite visible. These chromosomes are no longer lined up at the equatorial plate but are migrating to opposite poles, indicating that this cell is in the early to mid-anaphase stage of mitosis. Observe the presence of cytoplasmic organelles, such as mitochondria, RER, and Golgi apparatus.

FIGURE 2. Mitosis. Whitefish blastula. Paraffin section. ×540.

During the early telophase stage of mitotic division, the **chromosomes** (Ch) have reached the opposite poles of the cell. The cell membrane constricts to separate the cell into the two new daughter cells, forming a cleavage furrow (*arrowheads*). The spindle apparatus is visible as parallel, horizontal lines (*arrow*) that eventually form the midbody. As telophase progresses, the two new daughter cells will uncoil their chromosomes, and the nuclear membrane and nucleoli will become reestablished.

KEY

A	anaphase	M	metaphase	P	prophase
C	centriole	N	nucleus		
Ch	chromosome	NE	nuclear envelope		

PLATE 1-4 • Mitosis, Light and Electron Microscopy

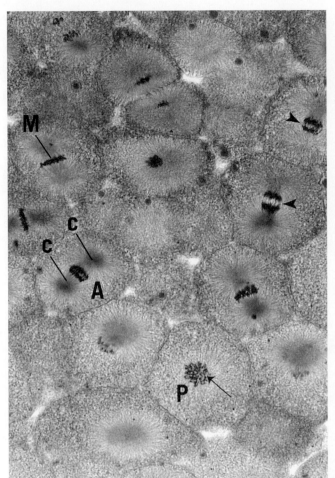

FIGURE 1

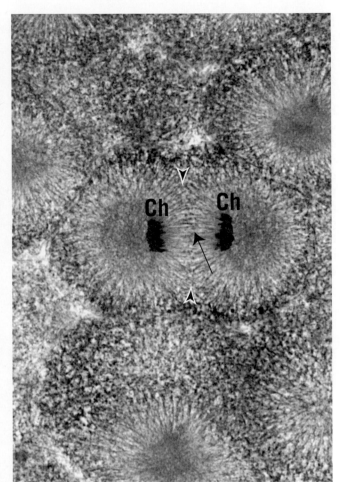

FIGURE 2

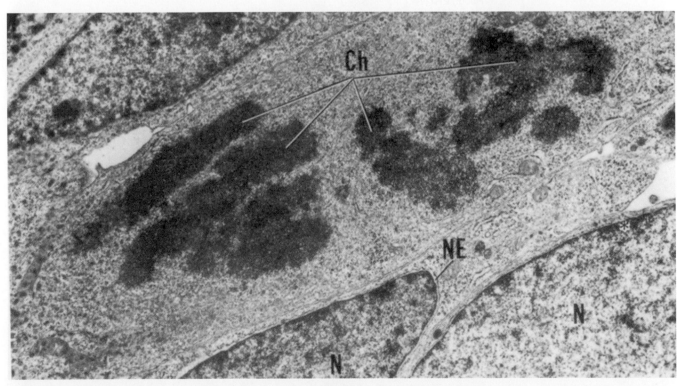

FIGURE 3

PLATE 1-5 · Typical Cell, Electron Microscopy

FIGURE 1. Typical cell. Pituitary. Rat. Electron microscopy. ×8936.

The gonadotrophs of the pituitary gland provide an excellent example of a typical cell because they house many of the cytoplasmic organelles possessed by most cells. The cytoplasm is limited by a cell membrane (*arrowheads*) that is clearly evident, especially where it approximates the plasmalemma of the adjacent electron-dense cells. **Mitochondria** (m) are not numerous but are easily recognizable, especially in longitudinal sections, because their cristae (*arrows*) are arranged in a characteristic fashion. Because this cell actively manufactures a secretory product that must be packaged and delivered outside of the cell, it possesses a well-developed **Golgi apparatus** (GA), positioned near the **nucleus** (N). Observe that the Golgi is formed by several stacks of flattened membranes. Additionally, this cell is well-endowed with **rough endoplasmic reticulum**, indicating active protein synthesis. The cytoplasm also displays secretory products (*asterisks*), which are transitory inclusions.

The nucleus is bounded by the typical **nuclear envelope** (NE), consisting of a ribosome-studded outer nuclear membrane and an inner nuclear membrane. The peripheral chromatin and chromatin islands are clearly evident, as is the **nucleolus-associated chromatin** (NC). The clear area within the nucleus is the nucleoplasm representing the fluid component of the nucleus. The **nucleolus** (n) presents a sponge-like appearance composed of electron-lucent and electron-dense materials, suspended free in the nucleoplasm. The electron-dense region is composed of the pars granulosa and the pars fibrosa, whereas the electron-lucent region is probably the nucleoplasm in which the nucleolus is suspended. (From Stokreef JC, Reifel CW, Shin SH. A possible phagocytic role for folliculo-stellate cells of anterior pituitary following estrogen withdrawal from primed male rats. *Cell Tissue Res* 1986;243:255–261.)

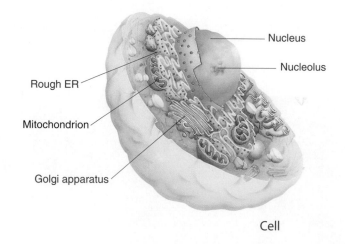

Rough ER

Mitochondrion

Golgi apparatus

Nucleus

Nucleolus

Cell

KEY

GA	Golgi apparatus	**n**	nucleolus	**NE**	nuclear envelope
m	mitochondrion	**NC**	nucleolus-associated	**rER**	rough endoplasmic
N	nucleus		chromatin		reticulum

PLATE1-5 • Typical Cell, Electron Microscopy

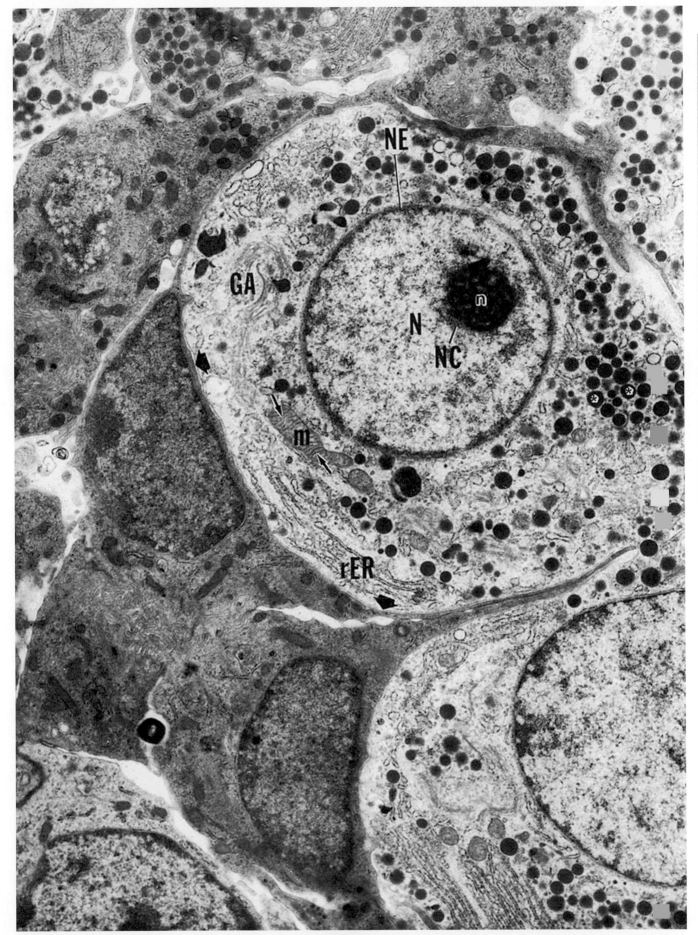

FIGURE 1

PLATE 1-6 • Nucleus and Cytoplasm, Electron Microscopy

FIGURE 1. Nucleus and cytoplasm. Liver. Mouse. Electron microscopy. ×44,265.

The **nucleus** (N) displays its nucleoplasm and **chromatin** (c) to advantage in this electron micrograph. Note that the inner (*arrowheads*) and outer (*double arrows*) membranes of the nuclear envelope fuse to form **nuclear pores** (NP). The RER is richly endowed by **ribosomes** (r). Note the presence of numerous **mitochondria** (m), whose double membrane and **cristae** (Cr) are quite evident.

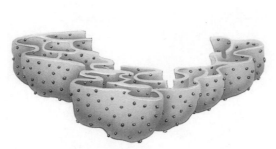

Rough endoplasmic reticulum

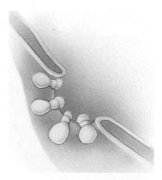

Nuclear pore complex

PLATE 1-6 · Nucleus and Cytoplasm, Electron Microscopy

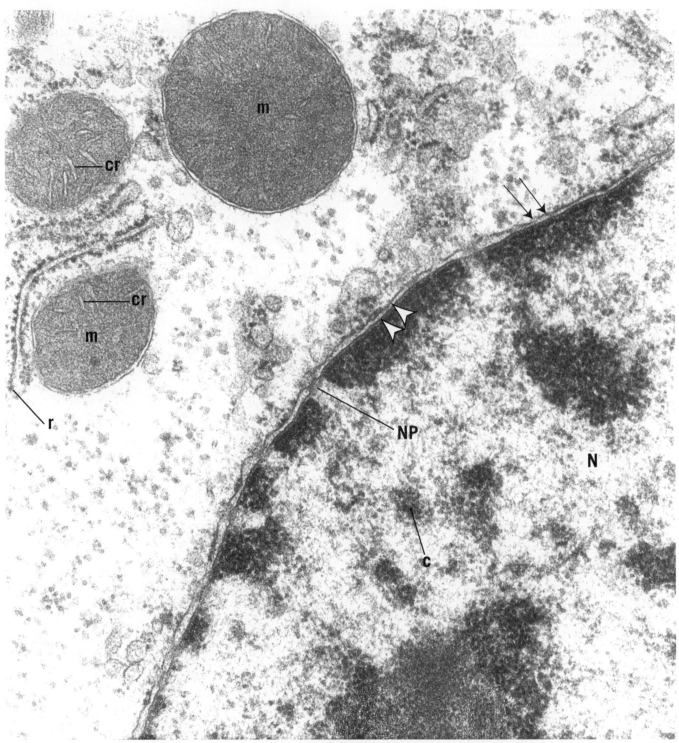

FIGURE 1

PLATE 1-7 • Nucleus and Cytoplasm, Electron Microscopy

FIGURE 1. Nucleus and cytoplasm. Liver. Mouse. Electron microscopy. ×20,318.

This electron micrograph of a liver cell displays the **nucleus** (N), with its condensed **chromatin** (c), as well as many cytoplasmic organelles. Note that the **mitochondria** (m) possess electron-dense matrix granules (*arrows*) scattered in the matrix of the intercristal spaces. The perinuclear area presents the **Golgi apparatus** (GA), which is actively packaging material in **condensing vesicles** (CV). The **rough endoplasmic reticulum** is obvious due to its **ribosomes** (R), whereas the **smooth endoplasmic reticulum** is less obvious.

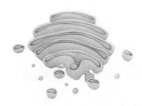

Golgi apparatus

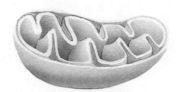

Mitochondrion

PLATE 1-7 · Nucleus and Cytoplasm, Electron Microscopy

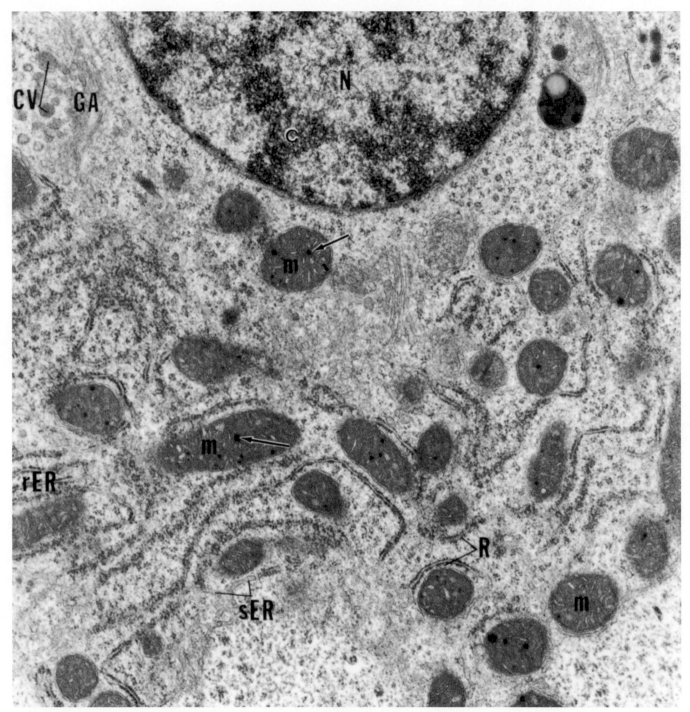

FIGURE 1

PLATE 1-8 · Golgi Apparatus, Electron Microscopy

FIGURE 1. Golgi apparatus. Mouse. Electron microscopy. ×28,588.

The extensive Golgi apparatus of this secretory cell presents several flattened membrane-bound **cisternae** (Ci), stacked one on top of the other. The convex face (*cis* face) (ff) receives **transfer** **vesicles** (TV) derived from the RER. The concave, ***trans*-Golgi network** (mf), releases **condensing vesicles** (CV), which house the secretory product. (From Gartner LP, Seibel W, Hiatt JL, et al. A fine-structural analysis of mouse molar odontoblast maturation. *Acta Anat (Basel)* 1979;103:16–33.)

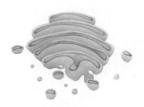

Golgi apparatus

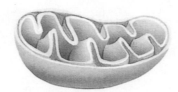

Mitochondrion

PLATE 1-8 · Golgi Apparatus, Electron Microscopy

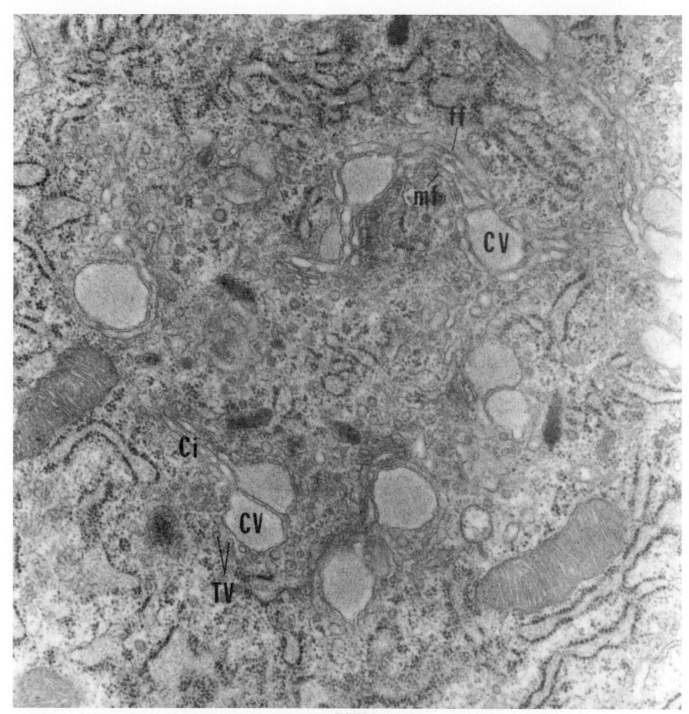

FIGURE 1

PLATE 1-9 · Mitochondria, Electron Microscopy

FIGURE 1. Mitochondria. Electron microscopy. ×69,500.

The basal aspect of this cell presents several mitochondria. The outer membrane of each mitochondrion is smooth, whereas its inner membrane is folded to form **cristae** (Cr) as is evident in the longitudinally sectioned mitochondrion.

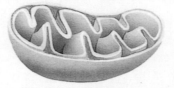

Mitochondrion

PLATE 1-9 · Mitochondria, Electron Microscopy

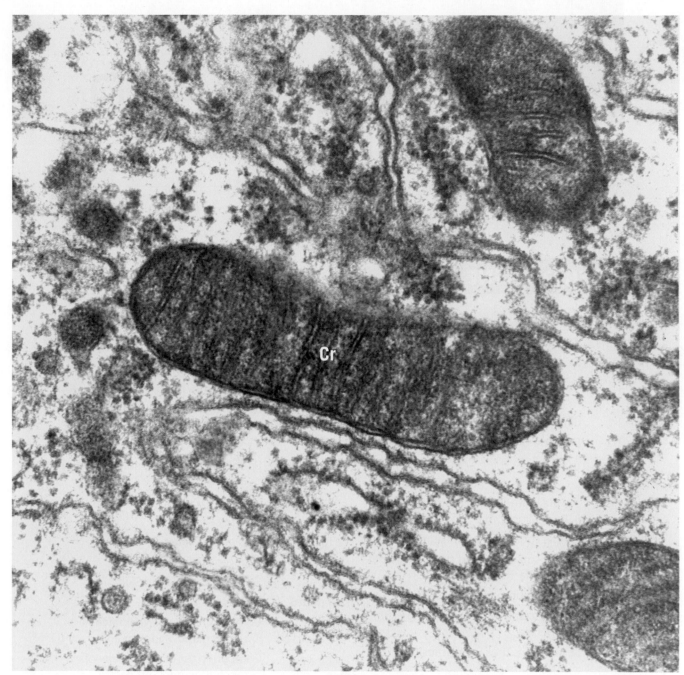

FIGURE 1

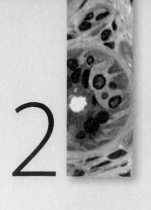

2 EPITHELIUM AND GLANDS

Epithelium is one of the four basic tissues of the body and is derived from all three germ layers. It is composed of very closely packed, contiguous cells, with very little or no extracellular material in the extracellular spaces. Epithelia either form membranes that are represented as sheets covering the body surface and lining its internal surface or occur as secretory elements known as glands. Almost always, epithelia and their derivatives are separated from underlying or surrounding connective tissues by a thin, noncellular layer, the **basement membrane**. This is usually composed of two regions, the epithelially derived **basal lamina** and the connective tissue–derived **lamina reticularis**.

> Viewed with the light microscope, the narrow acellular structure interposed between an epithelium and the underlying connective tissue is known as the basement membrane. The same structure, when viewed with the electron microscope, has been resolved to have three components, lamina lucida, lamina densa (both manufactured by epithelial cells), and lamina reticularis (manufactured by cells of connective tissue). The two epithelially derived components are collectively known as the basal lamina. Recently, many investigators have stopped using the term basement membrane and substituted the term basal lamina for both light and electron microscopic descriptions. In this atlas, we continue to use basement membrane for light microscopic and basal lamina for electron microscopic descriptions. Additionally, certain cells, such as muscle cells and Schwann cells, invest themselves with an acellular material that resembles a basal lamina, and that will be referred to as an external lamina.

EPITHELIUM

Epithelial Membranes

Epithelial membranes are avascular, deriving their nutrients by diffusion from blood vessels in the adjacent connective tissues. These membranes can

- cover a surface,
- line a cavity, or
- line a tube.

Surfaces covered may be dry, as the outer body surface, or wet, as the covering of the ovary. However, all lining epithelia have a wet surface (e.g., those lining the body cavities, blood vessels, gastrointestinal tract).

Membranes that line serous body cavities are referred to as **mesothelia**, whereas those lining blood and lymph vessels and the chambers of the heart are known as **endothelia**.

Epithelial membranes are classified according to the shape of the most superficial cell layer, which may be **squamous** (flat), **cuboidal**, or **columnar**, as observed when sectioned perpendicular to the exposed surface of the membrane. Moreover, the number of cell layers composing the epithelium also determines its classification (Table 2-1), in that

- a single layer of cells constitutes a **simple epithelium**,
- whereas two or more layers of cells are referred to as a **stratified epithelium**.

In a simple epithelium, all of the cells contact the basal lamina and reach the free surface. In **pseudostratified epithelia** (which may or may not possess cilia or stereocilia), however, all of the cells contact the basal lamina, although some cells are much shorter than others and do not reach the free surface. Therefore, this is a simple epithelium that appears to be stratified.

Stratified squamous epithelium (SE) may be

- **keratinized**,
- **nonkeratinized**, or
- **parakeratinized**.

Since stratified squamous epithelium is the thickest of the epithelia, as a barrier, it affords the greatest protection of the body from the external milieu. In order to enhance this protection, stratified squamous epithelium may possess an outer surface composed of dying or dead epithelial cells and then the epithelium is known as parakeratinized or keratinized, respectively. The stratified epithelium lining much of the urinary tract is known as **transitional epithelium**; its free surface is characterized by large, dome-shaped cells (Table 2-1).

Epithelial membranes possess numerous functions, which include

- protection from mechanical abrasion, chemical penetration, and bacterial invasion;
- reduction of friction;
- absorption of nutrients as a result of its polarized cells that are capable of performing vectorial functions;
- secretion;
- excretion of waste products;
- synthesis of various proteins, enzymes, mucins, hormones, and a myriad of other substances;
- receiving sensory signals from the external (or internal) milieu; and
- **forming glands** whose function is **secreting** enzymes, hormones, lubricants, or other products;

TABLE 2-1 • Classification of Epithelia

Type	Surface Cell Shape	Examples (Some)
Simple		
Simple squamous	Flattened	Lining blood and lymphatic vessel walls (endothelium), pleural and abdominal cavities (mesothelium)
Simple cuboidal	Cuboidal	Lining ducts of most glands
Simple columnar	Columnar	Lining much of digestive tract, gall bladder
Pseudostratified	All cell rest on basal lamina with only some reaching the surface. Cells that reach the surface are columnar.	Lining of nasal cavity, trachea, bronchi, epididymis
Stratified		
Stratified squamous (nonkeratinized)	Flattened (with nuclei)	Lining mouth, esophagus, vagina
Stratified squamous (keratinized)	Flattened (without nuclei)	Epidermis of the skin
Stratified cuboidal	Cuboidal	Lining ducts of sweat glands
Stratified columnar	Columnar	Conjunctiva of eye, lining some large excretory ducts
Transitional	Large dome-shaped cells when bladder is empty, flattened when bladder is distended	Lining renal calyces, renal pelvis, ureter, urinary bladder, proximal portion of urethra

- and movement of material along the epithelial sheet (such as mucus along the respiratory tract) by the assistance of specialized structures, known as cilia.

Epithelial cells usually undergo regular turnover because of their function and location. For example, cells of the epidermis that are sloughed from the surface originated approximately 28 days earlier by mitosis from cells of the basal layers. Other cells, such as those lining the small intestine, are replaced every few days. Still others continue to proliferate until adulthood is reached, at which time the mechanism is shut down. However, when large numbers of cells are lost, for example, because of injury, certain mechanisms trigger the proliferation of new cells to restore the cell population.

Epithelial cells may present specializations along their various surfaces (see Graphic 2-1). These surfaces are **apical** (microvilli, stereocilia, cilia, and flagella), **lateral or basolateral** (junctional complexes, zonula occludens, zonula adherens, macula adherens, gap junctions), and **basal** (hemidesmosomes and basal lamina).

Apical Surface Modifications

Microvilli are closely spaced, finger-like extensions of the cell membrane that increase the surface area of cells that function in absorption and secretion. Dense clusters of microvilli are evident in light micrographs, as a striated or brush border.

- The core of each microvillus possesses a cluster of 15 or so microfilaments (actin filaments) that are embedded in **villin** at the tip of the microvillus and are anchored in the terminal web of the cell.
- The actin filaments are linked to each other by **fimbrin** and **fascin** and to the membrane of the microvillus by **myosin** I. Where the actin filaments are anchored in the terminal web myosin II, molecules abound, and these assist in the spreading of the microvilli apart to increase the intervillous spaces and facilitate absorption or secretion.

Stereocilia are located in the epididymis as well as in a few limited regions of the body. They were named cilia because of their length; however, electron micrography proved them to be elongated microvilli whose functions are, as yet, unknown.

- The core of these stereocilia is composed of actin filaments that are bound to one another by **fimbrin** and to the membrane of the stereocilia by **erzin**.

Cilia are elongated, motile, plasmalemma-covered extensions of the cytoplasm that move material along the cell surface.

- Each cilium arises from a centriole (**basal body**) and possesses an **axoneme** core composed of nine pairs of peripheral (doublets) and two single, centrally placed microtubules (singlets).
- Microtubules of the doublets possess **dynein** arms with ATPase activity, which functions in energizing ciliary motion.
  - Each doublet is composed of a complete microtubule, **microtubule A**, consisting of 13 protofilaments, and a
  - **microtubule B**, composed of only 10 protofilaments.
  - Microtubule A shares three of its protofilaments with microtubule B.
- The two singlets are surrounded by a **central sheet**, composed of an elastic material
- each doublet is attached to the central sheet by a **radial spoke**, also composed of an elastic material
  - **nexin bridges** bind adjacent doublets to each other.

Basolateral Surface Modifications (see Graphic 2-1)

Junctional complexes, which occupy only a minute region of the basolateral cell surfaces, are visible with light microscopy as **terminal bars**, structures that encircle the entire cell. Terminal bars are composed of three components:

- **zonula occludens** (tight or occluding junction),
- **zonula adherens** (adhering junction), and
- **macula adherens** (desmosomes, also adhering junction).

The first two encircle the cell, whereas desmosomes do not. Additionally, another type of junction, the **gap junction**, permits two cells to communicate with each other.

- **Zonulae occludentes** are formed in such a fashion that the plasma membranes of the two adjoining cells are very close to each other and the transmembrane proteins of the two cells contact each other in the extracellular space.

- There are a number of transmembrane proteins that participate in the formation of the zonula occludens, **claudins, occludins, junctional adhesion molecules, ZO-1, ZO-2**, and **ZO-3** proteins, among others.
- Although all of these proteins are necessary to exclude material from traversing the paracellular route, it is the **claudins** that form a physical barrier that cannot be penetrated.
  - Some claudins possess aqueous channels that are designed to permit the movement of ions, water, and some very small molecules.
  - These proteins are preferentially adherent to the P-face (protoplasmic face) of the membrane and form characteristic ridges evident in freeze fracture preparation, whereas the E-face (extracellular face) presents corresponding grooves.

The zonulae occludentes are also responsible from preventing integral proteins of the cell from migrating from the apical surface to the basolateral surface and vice versa.

- In **zonulae adherentes,** the plasma membranes of adjacent epithelial cells are farther apart than in the region of the zonula adherens.
  - **Cell adhesion molecules (CAMs)** are the most significant components of adhering junctions of epithelial cells and in the zonulae adherentes the calcium-dependent proteins are known as **E-cadherins**.
  - The cytoplasmic moiety of the E-cadherins has binding sites for **catenins**, which, in turn, bind to **vinculin** and **α-actinin** that are capable of forming bonds with the thin filaments of the cytoskeleton.
  - In the presence of calcium in the extracellular space, the two epithelial cells adhere to each other and the adherence is reinforced by the cytoskeleton of the two cells.

The zonulae adherentes reinforce and stabilize the zonulae occludentes as well as distribute stresses across the epithelial sheet.

- **Maculae adherentes (desmosomes)** resemble spot welding that holds the two cells together; thus, they are not continuous structures like the two zonulae discussed above, but discrete entities.
  - Desmosomes are composed of an intracellular **attachment plaque**, consisting of **plakophilins, plakoglobins,** and **desmoplakins**, that adheres to the cytoplasmic aspect of the two adjacent cell membranes as mirror images.

○ Intermediate filaments enter and leave the plaques, resembling hairpins.

○ Embedded into the plaques are transmembrane, calcium-dependent cadherins, **desmogleins** and **desmocollins**.

▪ The extracellular moieties of desmogleins and desmocollins contact those of the adjacent cell and in the presence of calcium attach the two cells to each other.

• At **gap junctions** (communicating junctions, **nexus**), the two cell membranes are very close to each other, about 2 nm apart.

○ Interposed within the cell membrane of each cell and meeting each other are **connexons** composed of six subunits, known as a **connexins**; these multipass proteins form a cylindrical structure with a central pore.

○ A connexon of one cell matches the connexon of the other cell and thus forms an aqueous channel, about 2 nm in diameter, between the two cells that permits water, ions, and molecules smaller than 1 kDa in size to traverse the channel and go from one cell into the next.

○ Each cell has the ability to open or close the channel, and this regulation is calcium as well as pH dependent. In this fashion, a healthy cell can shut off communication with a cell that may be damaged.

Basal Surface Modifications (see Graphic 2-1)

The basal cell membrane of the cell is affixed to the basal lamina by adhering junctions known as the hemidesmosomes.

• A **hemidesmosome** resembles half of a desmosome, but its biochemical composition and clinical significance demonstrate enough dissimilarity that hemidesmosomes are no longer viewed as being merely a half of a desmosome.

○ A hemidesmosome has an intracellular plaque, composed mostly of **plectin, BP230,** and **erbin**.

○ Intermediate filaments terminate in the plaque, by interacting with BP230 and plectin.

○ Hemidesmosomes also possess transmembrane protein components, known as **integrin molecules** whose cytoplasmic moiety is embedded in the plaque and is attached to it by interacting with BP230 and erbin.

○ The extracellular region of the integrin molecules contacts laminin and type IV collagen of the basal lamina and binds to them if extracellular calcium is present.

○ In this manner, hemidesmosomes assist in the anchoring of epithelial sheets to the adjacent basal lamina.

• The three components of the basement membrane, when viewed with the electron microscope, are the lamina lucida, lamina densa (collectively known as the basal lamina), and the lamina reticularis.

○ The **lamina lucida** is that region of the basal lamina that houses the extracellular moieties of the transmembrane **laminin receptors, integrin** and **dystroglycans** molecules and the glycoproteins **laminin, entactin,** and **perlacans**.

○ The **lamina densa** is composed of **type IV collagen**, coated by laminin, entactin, and perlacan on its epithelial surface, and **fibronectin** on the lamina reticularis surface. Additionally, two other **collagen types, XV and XVIII**, are also present in the lamina densa. The lamina densa adheres to the **lamina reticularis**.

○ The **lamina reticularis** composed mostly of **type III collagen**, proteoglycans, glycoproteins, and slender elastic fibers, by **anchoring fibers (type VII collagen)** and **microfibrils (fibrillin)**.

Basal laminae function as structural supports for the epithelium, as molecular filters (e.g., in the renal glomerulus), in regulating the migration of certain cells across epithelial sheaths (e.g., preventing entry to fibroblasts but permitting access to lymphoid cells), in epithelial regeneration (e.g., in wound healing where it forms a surface along which regenerating epithelial cells migrate), and in cell-to-cell interactions (e.g., formation of myoneural junctions).

GLANDS

Most glands are formed by epithelial downgrowths into the surrounding connective tissue.

• Glands that deliver their secretions onto the epithelial surface do so via ducts and are known as **exocrine glands.**

• Glands that do not maintain a connection to the outside (ductless) and whose secretions enter the vascular system for delivery are known as **endocrine glands**.

The secretory cells of a gland are referred to as its **parenchyma** and are separated from surrounding connective tissue and vascular elements by a basement membrane.

• Exocrine glands are classified according to various parameters, for example, morphology of their

TABLE 2-2 • Exocrine Gland Characteristics

Cellular Composition	Example
Unicellular (single cell)	Goblet cell
Multicellular (more than one cell)	Submandibular gland

Duct Form	Example
Simple (unbranched)	Sweat gland
Compound (branched)	Mammary gland

Type of Secretion	Example
Serous (watery)	Parotid gland
Mucus (viscous)	Palatal glands
Mixed (serous and mucus)	Sublingual gland

Mode of Secretion	Example
Merocrine (only secretory product released)	Parotid gland
Apocrine (secretory product along with a portion of cell cytoplasm)	Lactating mammary gland (according to some authors)
Holocrine (cell dies and becomes the secretion)	Sebaceous gland

functional units, branching of their ducts, types of secretory products they manufacture, and the method whereby their component cells release secretory products (Table 2-2).

- The classification of endocrine glands is much more complex, but morphologically, their secretory units either are composed of **follicles** or are arranged in **cords** and clumps of cells (see Graphic 2-2).

CLINICAL CONSIDERATIONS

Bullous Pemphigoid

Bullous pemphigoid, a rare autoimmune disease, is caused by autoantibodies binding to some of the protein components of hemidesmosomes. Individuals afflicted with this disease exhibit skin blistering of the groin and axilla about the flexure areas and often in the oral cavity. Fortunately, it can be controlled by steroids and immunosuppressive drugs.

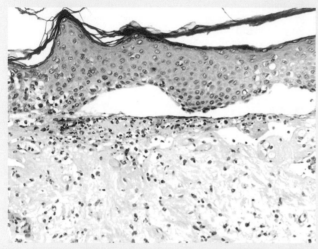

Bullous pemphigoid. Note that the epidermis is lifted from the dermis, a characteristic of bullous pemphigoid because the hemidesmosomes are attacked by the immune system thus separating the epidermis from the underlying dermis, which displays the presence of an inflammatory infiltrate of neutrophils, lymphocytes, and eosinophils. (Reprinted with permission from Mills SE, Carter D, Greenson JK, Reuter VE, Stoler MH, eds. Sternberger's Diagnostic Surgical Pathology, 5th ed. Philadelphia: Lippincott Williams & Wilkins. 2010. p. 17.)

Pemphigus Vulgaris

Pemphigus vulgaris is an autoimmune disease, caused by autoantibodies binding to some of the components of desmosomes. This disease causes blistering and is usually found occurring in middle-aged individuals. It is a relatively dangerous disease since the blistering can easily lead to infections. Frequently, this disease also responds to steroid therapy.

Tumor Formation

Under certain pathologic conditions, mechanisms that regulate cell proliferation do not function properly; thus, epithelial proliferation gives rise to tumors that may be benign if they are localized, or malignant if they wander from their original site and metastasize (seed) to another area of the body and continue to proliferate. Malignant tumors that arise from surface epithelium are termed carcinomas, whereas those developing from glandular epithelium are called adenocarcinomas.

Metaplasia

Epithelial cells are derived from certain germ cell layers, possess a definite morphology and location, and perform specific functions; however, under certain pathological conditions, they may undergo metaplasia, transforming into another epithelial cell type. An example of such metaplasia occurs in the lining epithelium of the oral cavity of individuals who smoke or use chewing tobacco as well as in Barrett's esophagus, where the long-term gastric reflux causes the epithelium of the lower portion of the esophagus to resemble the cardiac stomach but with the presence of goblet cells rather than surface lining cells.

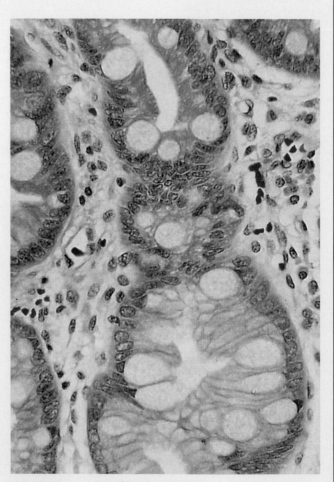

Metaplasia in a case of Barrett's esophagus. Note that the normal esophageal epithelium, stratified squamous nonkeratinized, has been replaced by a simple columnar epithelium resembling that of the cardiac stomach but rich in goblet cells. (Reprinted with permission from Mills SE. Histology for Pathologists, 3rd ed. Philadelphia. Lippincott Williams & Wilkins, 2007. p. 580.)

Cholera

Cholera toxins cause the release of tremendous volumes of fluid from the individual afflicted by that disease. The toxin attacks the zonulae occludentes by disturbing the proteins ZO-1 and ZO-2, thereby disrupting the zonulae occludentes and permitting the paracellular movement of water and electrolytes. The patient has uncontrolled diarrhea and subsequent fluid and electrolyte loss. If the fluids and salts are not replaced in a timely manner, the patient dies.

Psoriasis Vulgaris

Psoriasis affects approximately 2% of the population and may have a familial trait. It usually begins its course between 10 and 40 years of age, and it first appears as patches of dry skin that is raised and is reddish in color on the knees, scalp, elbows, back, or the buttocks. It is believed to be an immune disorder that causes a higher than normal mitotic activity of the cells of the stratified squamous keratinized epithelium, the epidermis, of the skin. In most individuals, this condition has no symptoms other than the unsightly appearance of the skin. In some individuals, however, the condition is accompanied by pain and/or itching, or both.

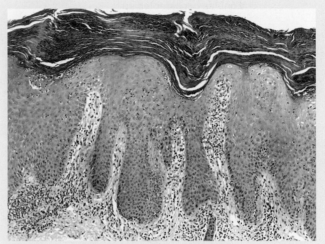

The normal keratinized stratified squamous epithelium of skin of this patient is greatly modified. Note that the stratum spinosum layer is greatly thickened and the cells of the stratum corneum appear to possess nuclei. Higher magnification of that area, however (not shown), demonstrates that the nuclei belong to neutrophils that invaded the epithelium. Also, note the absence of the strata granulosum and lucidum, which confirms that this specimen is not taken from regions of thick skin, namely, the palm of the hand or the sole of the foot. The large number of nuclei present in the papillary layer of the dermis belong to lymphocytic infiltrate. (Reprinted with permission from Mills SE, Carter D, et al., eds. Sternberg's Diagnostic Surgical Pathology, 5th ed. Philadelphia: Lippincott, Williams & Wilkins, 2010. p. 6.)

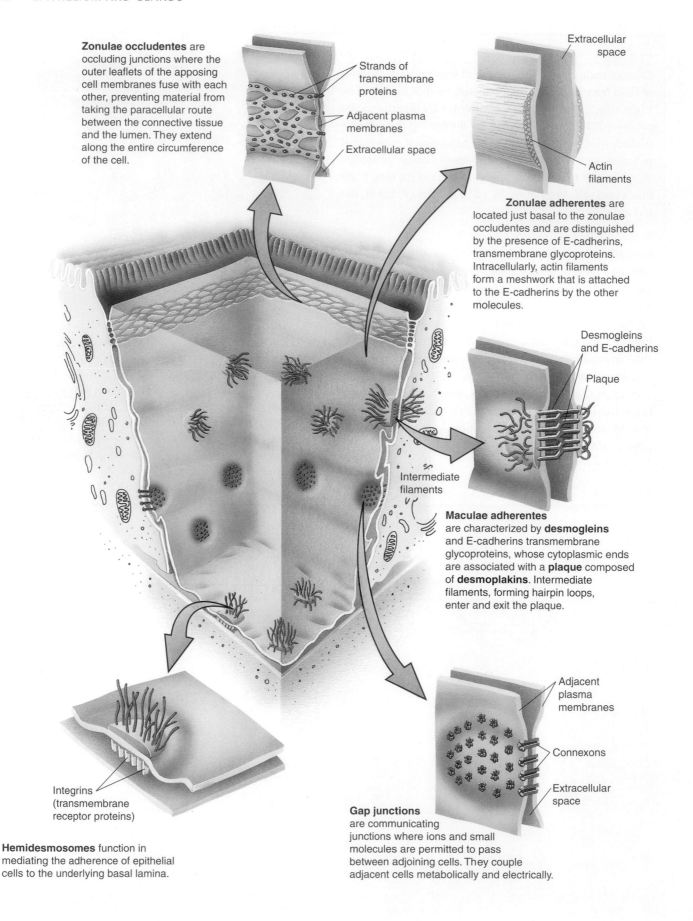

Zonulae occludentes are occluding junctions where the outer leaflets of the apposing cell membranes fuse with each other, preventing material from taking the paracellular route between the connective tissue and the lumen. They extend along the entire circumference of the cell.

Strands of transmembrane proteins

Adjacent plasma membranes

Extracellular space

Extracellular space

Actin filaments

Zonulae adherentes are located just basal to the zonulae occludentes and are distinguished by the presence of E-cadherins, transmembrane glycoproteins. Intracellularly, actin filaments form a meshwork that is attached to the E-cadherins by the other molecules.

Desmogleins and E-cadherins

Plaque

Intermediate filaments

Maculae adherentes are characterized by **desmogleins** and E-cadherins transmembrane glycoproteins, whose cytoplasmic ends are associated with a **plaque** composed of **desmoplakins**. Intermediate filaments, forming hairpin loops, enter and exit the plaque.

Integrins (transmembrane receptor proteins)

Hemidesmosomes function in mediating the adherence of epithelial cells to the underlying basal lamina.

Adjacent plasma membranes

Connexons

Extracellular space

Gap junctions are communicating junctions where ions and small molecules are permitted to pass between adjoining cells. They couple adjacent cells metabolically and electrically.

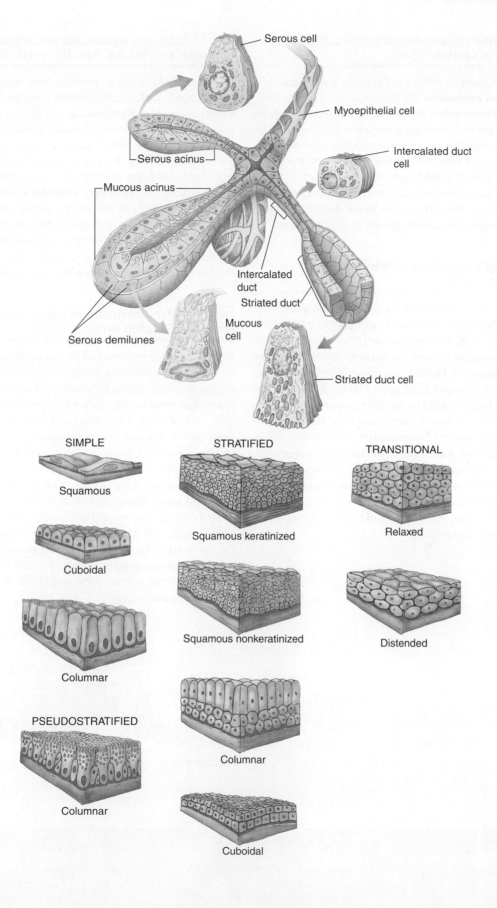

Serous cell

Myoepithelial cell

Serous acinus

Intercalated duct cell

Mucous acinus

Intercalated duct

Striated duct

Mucous cell

Serous demilunes

Striated duct cell

SIMPLE

Squamous

Cuboidal

Columnar

PSEUDOSTRATIFIED

Columnar

STRATIFIED

Squamous keratinized

Squamous nonkeratinized

Columnar

Cuboidal

TRANSITIONAL

Relaxed

Distended

PLATE 2-1 • Simple Epithelia and Pseudostratified Epithelium

FIGURE 1. Simple squamous epithelium. Kidney. Monkey. Plastic section. ×540.

The lining of the **lumen** (L) of this small arteriole is composed of a **simple squamous epithelium** (SE) (known as the endothelium). The cytoplasm of these cells is highly attenuated and can only be approximated in this photomicrograph as a thin line (between the *arrowheads*). The boundaries of two contiguous epithelial cells cannot be determined with the light microscope. The **nuclei** (N) of the squamous epithelial cells bulge into the lumen, characteristic of this type of epithelium. Note that some of the nuclei appear more flattened than others. This is due to the degree of agonal contraction of the **smooth muscle** (M) cells of the vessel wall.

FIGURE 3. Simple columnar epithelium. Monkey. Plastic section. ×540.

The simple columnar epithelium of the duodenum in this photomicrograph displays a very extensive **brush border** (MV) on the apical aspect of the cells. The **terminal web** (TW), where microvilli are anchored, appears as a dense line between the brush border and the apical cytoplasm. Distinct dots (*arrowheads*) are evident, which, although they appear to be part of the terminal web, are actually terminal bars, resolved by the electron microscope to be junctional complexes between contiguous cells. Note that the cells are tall and slender, and their **nuclei** (N), more or less oval in shape, are arranged rather uniformly at the same level in each cell. The basal aspects of these cells lie on a basal membrane (*arrows*), separating the epithelium from the **connective tissue** (CT). The round **nuclei** (rN) noted within the epithelium actually belong to leukocytes migrating into the **lumen** (L) of the duodenum. A few **goblet cells** (GC) are also evident.

FIGURE 2. Simple squamous and simple cuboidal epithelia. x.s. Kidney. Paraffin section. ×270.

The medulla of the kidney provides ideal representation of simple squamous and simple cuboidal epithelia. Simple squamous epithelium, as in the previous figure, is easily recognizable due to flattened but somewhat bulging **nuclei** (N). Note that the cytoplasm of these cells appears as thin, dark lines (between *arrowheads*); however, it must be stressed that the dark lines are composed of not only attenuated cells but also the surrounding basal membranes. The **simple cuboidal epithelium** (CE) is very obvious. The lateral cell membranes (*arrow*) are clearly evident in some areas; even when they cannot be seen, the relationships of the round nuclei permit an imaginary approximation of the extent of each cell. Note that simple cuboidal cells, in *section*, appear more or less like small squares with centrally positioned nuclei.

FIGURE 4. Pseudostratified columnar epithelium with cilia. Paraffin section. ×270.

The first impression conveyed by this epithelium from the nasal cavity is that it is stratified, being composed of at least four layers of cells; however, careful observation of the *inset* (×540) demonstrates that these are closely packed cells of varying heights and girth, each of which is in contact with the basal membrane. Here, unlike in the previous photomicrograph, the **nuclei** (N) are not uniformly arranged, and they occupy about three-fourths of the epithelial layer. The location and morphology of the nuclei provide an indication of the cell type. The short **basal cells** (BCs) display small, round to oval nuclei near the basal membrane. The tall, ciliated cells (*arrows*) possess large, oval nuclei. The **terminal web** (TW) supports tall, slender **cilia** (C), which propel mucus along the epithelial surface. The connective tissue is highly vascularized and presents good examples of simple squamous epithelia (*arrowheads*) that compose the endothelial lining of **blood** (BV) and **lymph vessels** (LV).

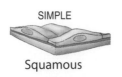
SIMPLE
Squamous

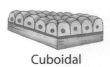
Cuboidal

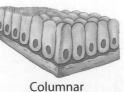
Columnar

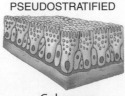
PSEUDOSTRATIFIED
Columnar

KEY

BC	basal cell	**GC**	goblet cell	**N**	nucleus
BV	blood vessel	**L**	lumen	**rN**	round nucleus
C	cilia	**LV**	lymph vessel	**SE**	simple squamous epithelium
CE	simple cuboidal epithelium	**M**	smooth muscle	**TW**	terminal web
CT	connective tissue	**MV**	brush border		

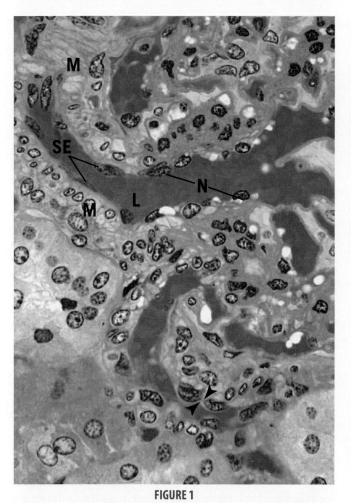

FIGURE 1

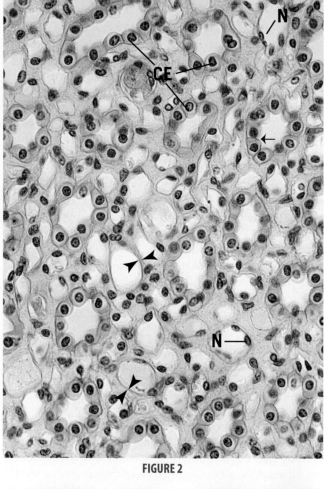

FIGURE 2

PLATE 2-1 • Simple Epithelia and Pseudostratified Epithelium

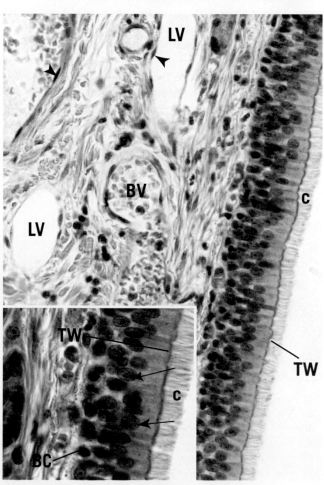

FIGURE 3

FIGURE 4

PLATE 2-2 • Stratified Epithelia and Transitional Epithelium

FIGURE 1. Stratified cuboidal epithelium. Monkey. Plastic section. ×540.

Stratified cuboidal epithelium is characterized by two or more layers of cuboid-shaped cells, as illustrated in this photomicrograph of a sweat gland duct. The **lumen** (L) of the duct is surrounded by cells whose cell boundaries are not readily evident, but the layering of the **nuclei** (N) demonstrates that this epithelium is truly stratified. The epithelium of the duct is surrounded by a **basal membrane** (BM). The other thick tubular profiles are tangential sections of the **secretory** (s) portions of the sweat gland, composed of simple cuboidal epithelium. Note the presence of a **capillary** (Cp), containing a single red blood cell, and the bulging nucleus (*arrow*) of the epithelial cell constituting the endothelial lining. The large empty space in the lower right-hand corner of this photomicrograph represents the lumen of a **lymph vessel** (LV) whose endothelial lining presents a flattened nucleus bulging into the lumen. Note that more cytoplasm is evident near the pole of the nucleus (*arrowhead*) than elsewhere.

FIGURE 3. Stratified squamous keratinized epithelium. Skin. Paraffin section. ×132.

The palm of the hand is covered by a thick stratified squamous keratinized epithelium. The definite difference between this and the preceding photomicrograph is the thick layer of nonliving cells containing **keratin** (K), which functions in protecting the deeper living cells and tissues from abrasion, desiccation, and invasion by bacterial flora. Although the various layers of this epithelium are examined in greater detail in Chapter 11, certain features need to be examined here. Note that the interdigitation between the connective tissue **dermal ridges** (P) and the **epithelial ridges** (R) provides a larger surface area for adhesion and providing nutrients than would be offered by a merely flat interface. The **basal membrane** (BM) is a definite interval between the epithelium and the connective tissue. The basal layer of this epithelium, composed of cuboidal cells, is known as the stratum germinativum, which possesses a high mitotic activity. Cells originating here press toward the surface and, while on their way, change their morphology, manufacture proteins, and acquire different names. Note the **duct** (D) of a sweat gland piercing the base of an epidermal ridge as it continues toward the outside (*arrows*).

FIGURE 2. Stratified squamous nonkeratinized epithelium. Plastic section. ×270.

The lining of the esophagus provides a good example of stratified squamous nonkeratinized epithelium. The lack of vascularity of the epithelium, which is approximately 30 to 35 cell layers thick, is clearly evident. Nourishment must reach the more superficial cells via diffusion from blood vessels of the **connective tissue** (CT). Note that the deepest cells, which lie on the basal membrane and are known as the **basal layer** (BL), are actually cuboidal in shape. Due to their mitotic activity, they give rise to the cells of the epithelium, which, as they migrate toward the surface, become increasingly flattened. By the time they reach the surface, to be sloughed off into the **esophageal lumen** (EL), they are squamous in morphology. The endothelial lining of a vessel is shown as scattered **nuclei** (N) bulging into the **lumen** (L), providing an obvious contrast between stratified and simple squamous epithelia.

FIGURE 4. Transitional epithelium. Bladder. Monkey. Plastic section. ×132.

The urinary bladder, as most of the excretory portion of the urinary tract, is lined by a specialized type of stratified epithelium—the transitional epithelium. This particular specimen was taken from an empty, relaxed bladder, as indicated by the large, **round**, dome-**shaped** (rC) **cells**, some of which are occasionally binucleated (*arrow*), abutting the **lumen** (L). The epithelial cells lying on the **basal membrane** (BM) are quite small but increase in size as they migrate superficially and begin to acquire a pear shape. When the bladder is distended, the thickness of the epithelium decreases and the cells become flattened, more squamous-like. The connective tissue-epithelium interface is flat, with very little interdigitation between them. The **connective tissue** (CT) is very vascular immediately deep to the epithelium, as is evident from the sections of the **arterioles** (A) and **venules** (V) in this field. Observe the simple squamous endothelial linings of these vessels, characterized by their bulging nuclei (*arrowheads*).

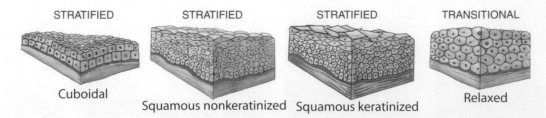

STRATIFIED — Cuboidal

STRATIFIED — Squamous nonkeratinized

STRATIFIED — Squamous keratinized

TRANSITIONAL — Relaxed

KEY

A	arteriole	**EL**	esophageal lumen	**R**	epithelial ridge
BL	basal layer	**K**	keratin	**rC**	round-shaped cell
BM	basal membrane	**L**	lumen	**S**	secretory portion
CP	capillary	**LV**	lymph vessel	**V**	venule
CT	connective tissue	**N**	nucleus		
D	duct	**P**	dermal ridge		

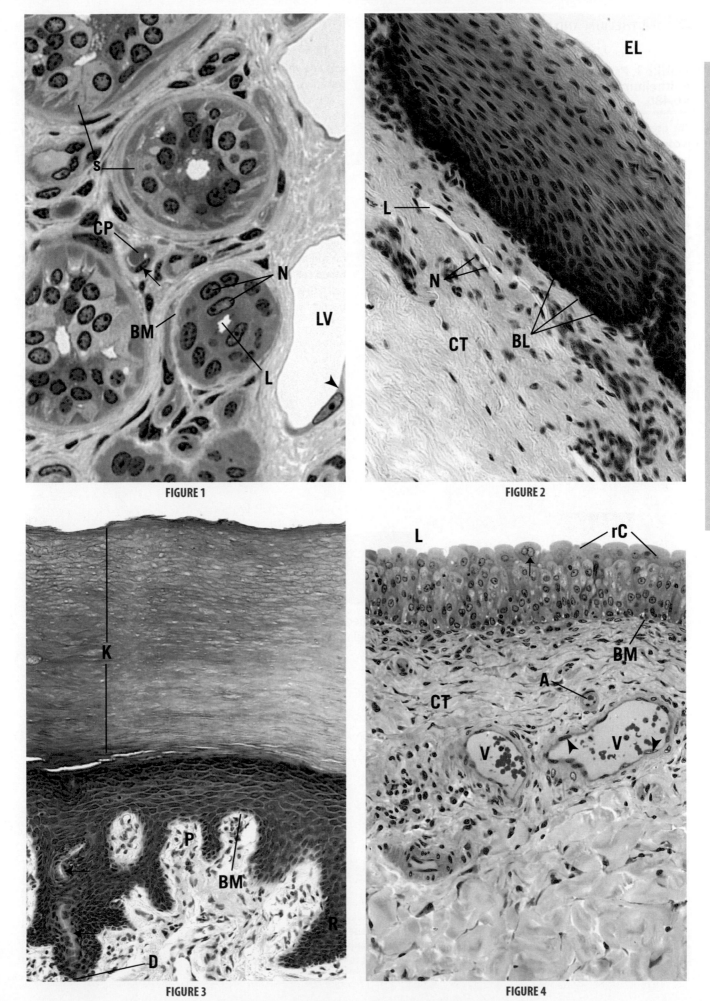

PLATE 2-2 • Stratified Epithelia and Transitional Epithelium

FIGURE 1

FIGURE 2

FIGURE 3

FIGURE 4

PLATE 2-3 · Pseudostratified Ciliated Columnar Epithelium, Electron Microscopy

FIGURE 1. Pseudostratified ciliated columnar epithelium. Hamster trachea. Electron microscopy. ×6,480.

The pseudostratified ciliated columnar epithelium of the trachea is composed of several types of cells, some of which are presented here. Since this is an oblique section through the epithelium, it is not readily evident here that all of these cells touch the **basal lamina** (BL). Note that the pale-staining **ciliated cells** (CC) display **rough endoplasmic reticulum** (rER), **mitochondria** (M), **Golgi apparatus** (G), and numerous **cilia (C)** interspersed with **microvilli** (MV). Each cilium, some of which are seen in cross section, displays its plasma membrane and its **axoneme** (A). The cilia are anchored in the terminal web via their **basal bodies** (BB). The mitochondria appear to be concentrated in this area of the cell. The second cell types to be noted are the **mucous cells** (MC),

also known as goblet cells. These cells produce a thick, viscous secretion, which appears as **secretory granules** (SG) within the apical cytoplasm. The protein moiety of the secretion is synthesized on the **rough endoplasmic reticulum** (rER), whereas most of the carbohydrate groups are added to the protein in the **Golgi apparatus** (G). The mucous cells are nonciliated but do present short, stubby **microvilli** (MV) on their apical surface. When these cells release their secretory product, they change their morphology. They no longer contain secretory granules, and their microvilli become elongated and are known as brush cells. They may be recognized by the filamentous structures within the supranuclear cytoplasm. The lower right-hand corner of this electron micrograph presents a portion of a **capillary** (Ca) containing a **red blood cell** (RBC). Observe that the highly attenuated **endothelial cell** (EC) is outside of but very close to the **basal lamina** (BL) of the tracheal epithelium. (Courtesy of Dr. E. McDowell.)

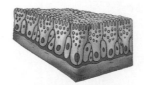

Pseudostratified columnar epithelium

KEY

A	axoneme	**CC**	ciliated cell	**MV**	microvillus
BB	basal body	**EC**	endothelial cell	**RBC**	red blood cell
BL	basal lamina	**G**	Golgi apparatus	**rER**	rough endoplasmic
C	cilium	**M**	mitochondrion		reticulum
Ca	capillary	**MC**	mucous cell	**SG**	secretory granule

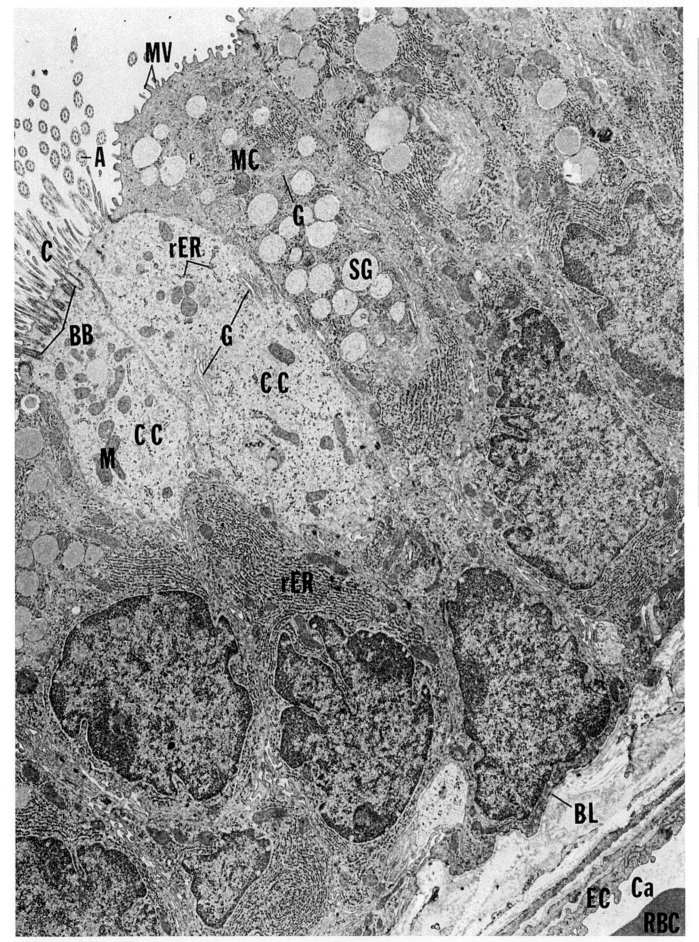

FIGURE 1

PLATE 2-4 • Epithelial Junctions, Electron Microscopy

FIGURE 1. Epithelial junction. Human. Electron microscopy. ×27,815.

This electron micrograph represents a thin section of an intercellular canaliculus between clear cells of a human eccrine sweat gland stained with ferrocyanide-reduced osmium tetroxide. A tight junction (*arrows*) separates the lumen of the **intercellular canaliculus** (IC) from the basolateral intercellular space. Observe the **nucleus** (N). (From Briggman JV, Bank HL, Bigelow JB, Graves JS, Spicer SS. Structure of the tight junctions of the human eccrine sweat gland. *Am J Anat* 1981;162:357–368.)

FIGURE 2. Epithelial junction. Zonula occludens. Human. Electron microscopy. ×83,700.

This is a freeze fracture replica of an elaborate tight junction along an intercellular canaliculus between two clear cells. Note the smooth transition from a region of wavy, nonintersecting, densely packed junctional elements to an area of complex anastomoses. At the step fracture (*arrows*), it can be seen that the pattern of ridges on the E-face corresponds to that of the grooves on the P-face of the plasma membrane of the adjacent clear cell. In certain areas (*arrowheads*), several of the laterally disposed, densely packed junctional elements are separated from the luminal band. The direction of platinum shadowing is indicated by the *circled arrow*. (From Briggman JV, Bank HL, Bigelow JB, Graves JS, Spicer SS. Structure of the tight junctions of the human eccrine sweat gland. *Am J Anat* 1981;162:357–368.)

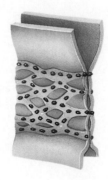

Zonulae occludentes

PLATE 2-4 • Epithelial Junctions, Electron Microscopy

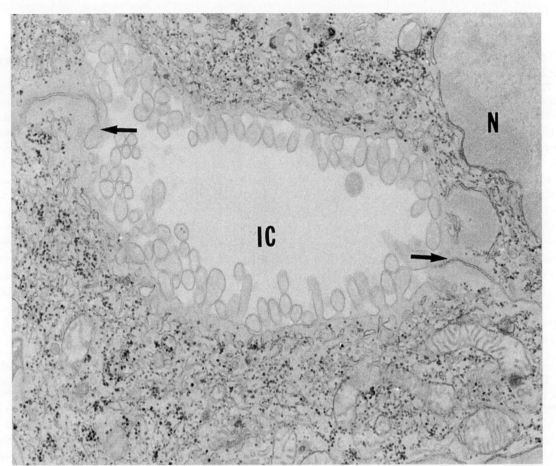

FIGURE 1

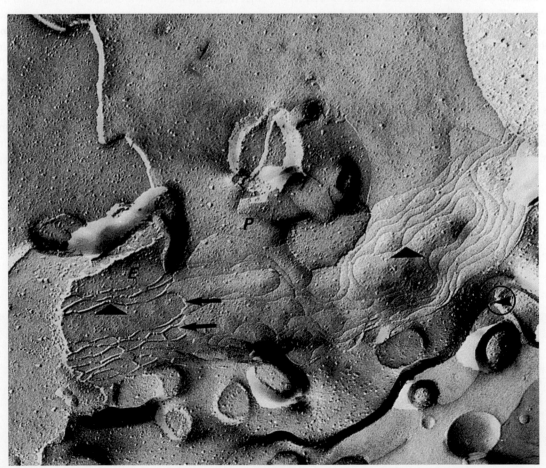

FIGURE 2

PLATE 2-5 · Glands

FIGURE 1. Goblet cells. Ileum. Monkey. Plastic section. ×270.

Goblet cells are unicellular exocrine glands that are found interspersed among simple columnar and pseudostratified columnar epithelia. This photomicrograph of an ileal villus displays numerous **goblet cells** (GC) located among the **simple columnar epithelial cells** (EC). The brush border (*arrowhead*) of the columnar cells is only scantly present on the goblet cells. The expanded apical region of the goblet cell is known as the **theca** (T) and is filled with **mucin** (m), which, when released into the lumen of the gut, coats and protects the intestinal lining. The lower right-hand corner of the simple columnar epithelium was sectioned somewhat obliquely through the nuclei of the epithelial cells, producing the appearance of a stratified epithelium (*asterisk*). Looking at the epithelium above the *double arrows*, however, it is clearly simple columnar. The occasional **round nuclei** (rN) are those of lymphocytes migrating through the epithelium into the **lumen** (L). Figure 2 is a higher magnification of the *boxed area*.

FIGURE 3. Sebaceous gland. Scalp. Paraffin section. ×132.

Sebaceous glands are usually associated with hair follicles. They discharge their sebum into the follicle, although in certain areas of the body they are present independent of hair follicles. These glands, surrounded by slender connective tissue **capsules** (Ca), are pear-shaped saccules with short ducts. Each saccule is filled with large, amorphous cells with nuclei in various states of degeneration (*arrows*). The periphery of the saccule is composed of small, cuboidal **basal cells** (BC), which act in a regenerative capacity. As the cells move away from the periphery of the saccule, they enlarge and increase their cytoplasmic **fat** (f) content. Near the duct, the entire cell degenerates and becomes the **secretion** (se). Therefore, sebaceous glands are classified as simple, branched, acinar glands with a holocrine mode of secretion. **Smooth muscles** (M), arrector pili, are associated with sebaceous glands. Observe the **secretory** (s) and **duct** (D) portions of a sweat gland above the sebaceous gland.

FIGURE 2. Goblet cells. Ileum. Monkey. Plastic section. ×540.

This photomicrograph is a higher magnification of the *boxed area* of the previous figure, demonstrating the light microscopic morphology of the goblet cell. The **mucin** (m) in the expanded **theca** (T) of the goblet cell has been partly precipitated and dissolved during the dehydration procedure. The **nucleus** (N) of the goblet cell is relatively dense due to the condensed chromatin. Between the nucleus and the theca is the **Golgi zone** (GZ), where the protein product of the cell is modified and packaged into secretory granules for delivery. The **base** (b) of the goblet cell is slender, almost as if it were "squeezed in" between neighboring columnar epithelial cells, but it touches the **basal membrane** (BM). The terminal web and brush border of the goblet cell are greatly reduced but not completely absent (*arrowheads*). The **round nuclei** (rN) belong to leukocytes migrating through the epithelium into the **lumen** (L) of the ileum.

FIGURE 4. Eccrine sweat glands. Skin. Paraffin section. ×270.

Eccrine sweat glands are the most numerous glands in the body, and they are extensively distributed. The glands are simple, unbranched, and coiled tubular, producing a watery solution. The **secretory portion** (s) of the gland is composed of a simple cuboidal type of epithelium with two cell types, a lightly staining cell that makes up most of the secretory portion and a darker staining cell that usually cannot be distinguished with the light microscope. Surrounding the secretory portion are **myoepithelial cells** (MC), which, with their numerous branching processes, encircle the secretory tubule and assist in expressing the fluid into the ducts. The **ducts** (D) of sweat glands are composed of a stratified cuboidal type of epithelium, whose cells are smaller than those of the secretory unit. In histologic sections, therefore, the ducts are always darker than the secretory units. The large, empty-looking spaces are **adipose** (fat) **cells** (AC). Note the numerous small blood vessels (*arrows*) in the vicinity of the sweat gland.

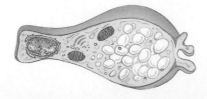

Goblet cell

KEY					
AC	adipose cell	F	fat	rN	round nucleus
b	base	GC	goblet cell	S	secretory
BC	basal cell	GZ	Golgi zone	Se	secretion
BM	basal membrane	L	lumen	T	theca
Ca	capsule	M	smooth muscle		
D	duct	m	mucin		
EC	simple columnar epithelial cell	MC	myoepithelial cell		
		N	nucleus		

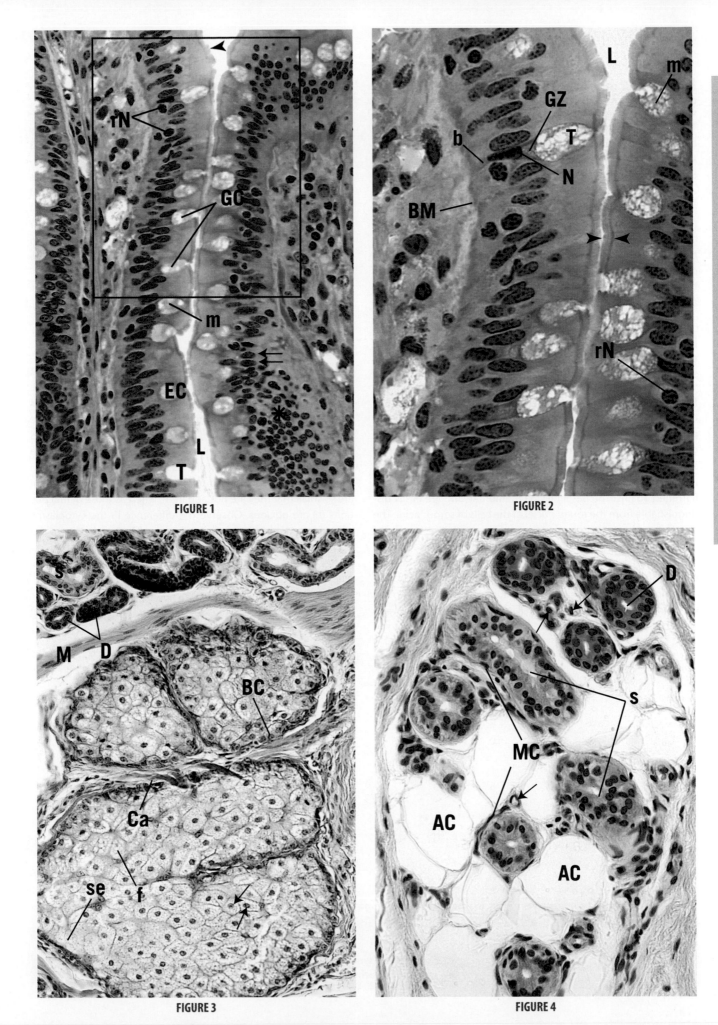

PLATE 2-5 · Glands

FIGURE 1

FIGURE 2

FIGURE 3

FIGURE 4

PLATE 2-6 · Glands

FIGURE 1. Compound tubuloacinar (alveolar) serous gland. Pancreas. Monkey. Plastic section. ×540.

This is a photomicrograph of the exocrine portion of the pancreas, a compound tubuloacinar (alveolar) serous gland. The duct system of this gland is studied in Chapter 15 on the Digestive System. Only its secretory cells are considered at this point. Each acinus, when sectioned well, presents a round appearance with a small central **lumen** (L), with the secretory cells arranged like a pie cut into pieces. The **connective tissue** (CT) investing each acinus is flimsy in the pancreas. The secretory cells are more or less trapezoid-shaped, with a round, basally situated **nucleus** (N). The cytoplasm contains numerous **zymogen granules** (ZG), which are the membrane-bound digestive enzymes packaged by the Golgi apparatus.

FIGURE 3. Compound tubuloacinar (alveolar) mixed gland. Sublingual gland. Monkey. Plastic section. ×540.

The sublingual gland is a mostly mucous, compound tubuloacinar gland that contains many mucous tubules and acini. These profiles of mucous acini are well represented in this photomicrograph. Note the open **lumen** (L) bordered by several trapezoid-shaped cells whose lateral plasma membranes are clearly evident (*double arrows*). The **nuclei** (N) of these mucous cells appear to be flattened against the basal plasma membrane and are easily distinguishable from the round nuclei of the cells of serous acini. The cytoplasm appears to possess numerous vacuole-like structures that impart a frothy appearance to the cell. The serous secretions of this gland are derived from the few serous cells that appear to cap the mucous units, known as **serous demilunes** (SD). The secretory products of the serous demilunes gain entrance to the lumen of the secretory unit via small intercellular spaces between neighboring mucous cells.

FIGURE 2. Compound tubuloacinar (alveolar) mucous glands. Soft palate. Paraffin section. ×132.

The compound tubuloacinar glands of the palate are purely mucous and secrete a thick, viscous fluid. The secretory acini of this gland are circular in section and are surrounded by fine **connective tissue** (CT) elements. The **lumina** (L) of the mucous acini are clearly distinguishable, as are the trapezoid-shaped **parenchymal cells** (PC), which manufacture the viscous fluid. The **nuclei** (N) of the trapezoid-shaped cells are dark, dense structures that appear to be flattened against the basal cell membrane. The cytoplasm has an empty, frothy appearance, which stains a light grayish-blue with hematoxylin and eosin.

FIGURE 4. Compound tubuloacinar (alveolar) mixed gland. Submandibular gland. Monkey. Plastic section. ×540.

The submandibular gland is a compound tubuloacinar gland that produces a mixed secretion, as does the sublingual gland of the previous figure. However, this gland contains many purely **serous acini** (SA) and very few purely mucous ones, namely, because the mucous acini are capped by **serous demilunes** (SD). Also, this gland possesses an extensive system of **ducts** (D). Note that the cytoplasm of the serous cells appears to be blue when stained with hematoxylin and eosin. Also notice that the lumina of the acini are so small that they are not apparent, whereas those of mucous units (L) are obvious. Observe the difference in the cytoplasms of serous and mucus-secreting cells as well as the density of the nuclei of individual cells. Finally, note that the lateral cell membranes (*arrows*) of mucus-producing cells are clearly delineated, whereas those of the serous cells are very difficult to observe.

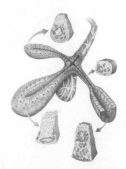

Salivary gland

KEY					
CT	connective tissue	N	nucleus	SD	serous demilunes
D	duct	PC	parenchymal cell	ZG	zymogen granules
L	lumen	SA	serous acini		

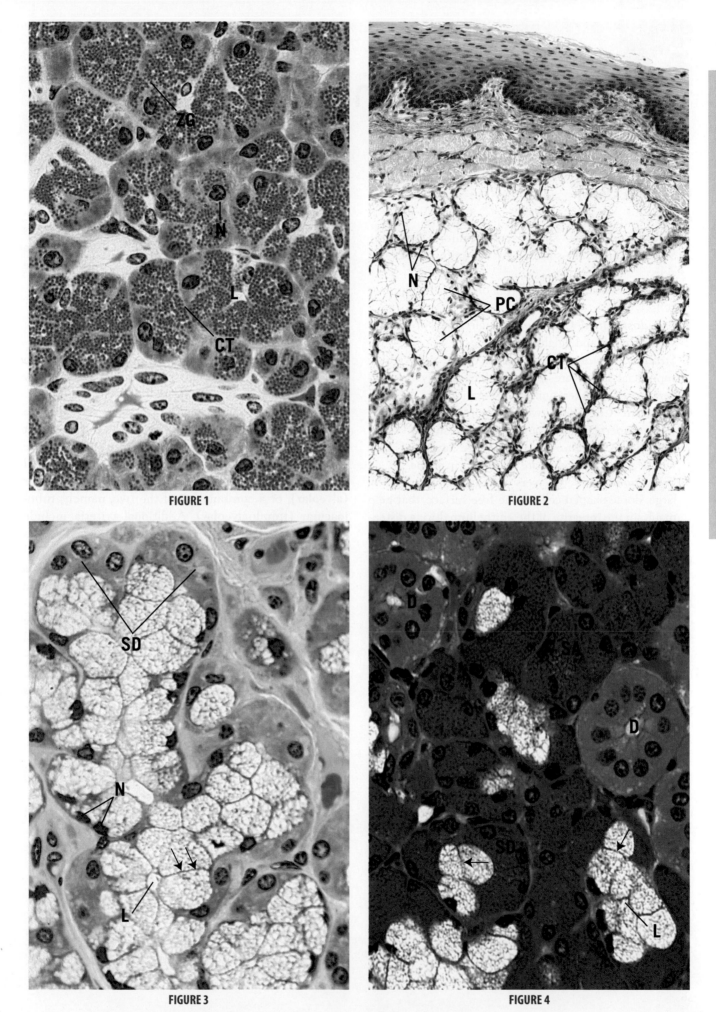

PLATE 2-6 · Glands

FIGURE 1

FIGURE 2

FIGURE 3

FIGURE 4

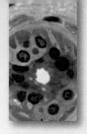

Chapter Summary

I. EPITHELIUM

A. Types

1. *Simple Squamous*—single layer of uniform flat cells.
2. *Simple Cuboidal*—single layer of uniform cuboidal cells.
3. *Simple Columnar*—single layer of uniform columnar cells.
4. *Pseudostratified Columnar*—single layer of cells of varied shapes and heights.
5. *Stratified Squamous*—several layers of cells whose superficial layers are flattened. These may be non-keratinized, parakeratinized, or keratinized.
6. *Stratified Cuboidal*—two or more layers of cells whose superficial layers are cuboidal in shape.
7. *Stratified Columnar*—two or more layers of cells whose superficial layers are columnar in shape.
8. *Transitional*—several layers of cells, characterized by large, dome-shaped cells at the free surface, that help maintain the integrity of the epithelium during distention of the various components of the urinary tract.

B. General Characteristics

1. Free Surface Modifications

Cells may possess **microvilli** (brush border, striated border), short finger-like projections that increase the surface area of the cell; **stereocilia** (long anastomosing microvilli), which are only found in a few places in the body such as in the epididymis; and **cilia**, which are long, motile projections of the cell with a 9 + 2 microtubular substructure (**axoneme**).

2. Lateral Surface Modifications

For the purposes of adhesion, the cell membranes form junctional complexes involving the lateral plasmalemma of contiguous cells. These junctions are known as **desmosomes** (maculae adherentes), **zonulae occludentes**, and **zonulae adherentes**. For the purpose of intercellular communication, the lateral cell membranes form **gap junctions** (nexus, septate junctions).

3. Basal Surface Modifications

The basal cell membrane that lies on the basal membrane forms **hemidesmosomes** to assist the cell to adhere to the underlying connective tissue.

4. Basal Membrane

The **basement membrane** of light microscopy is composed of an epithelially derived **basal lamina** (which has two parts, **lamina densa** and **lamina lucida**) and a **lamina reticularis** derived from connective tissue, which may be absent.

II. GLANDS

A. Exocrine Glands

Exocrine glands, which deliver secretions into a system of ducts to be conveyed onto an epithelial surface, may be **unicellular** (goblet cells) or **multicellular**.

Multicellular glands may be classified according to the branching of their **duct system**. If the ducts are not branched, the gland is **simple**; if they are branched, the gland is **compound**. Moreover, the three-dimensional shape of the secretory units may be **tubular, acinar (alveolar)**, or a combination of the two, namely, **tubuloacinar (tubuloalveolar)**. Additional criteria include (1) the **type** of secretory product produced: **serous** (parotid, pancreas), **mucous** (palatal glands), and **mixed** (sublingual, submandibular), possessing serous and mucous acini and **serous demilunes**, and (2) the **mode of secretion**: **merocrine** (only the secretory product is released, as in the parotid gland), **apocrine** (the secretory product is accompanied by some of the apical cytoplasm, as perhaps in mammary glands), and **holocrine** (the entire cell becomes the secretory product, as in the sebaceous gland, testes, and ovary). Glands are subdivided by connective tissue septa into lobes and lobules, and the ducts that serve them are interlobar, intralobar, interlobular, and intralobular (striated, intercalated).

Myoepithelial (basket) cells are ectodermally derived myoid cells that share the basal lamina of the glandular parenchyma. These cells possess long processes that surround secretory acini and, by occasional contraction, assist in the delivery of the secretory product into the system of ducts.

B. Endocrine Glands

Endocrine glands are ductless glands that release their secretion into the bloodstream. These glands are described in Chapter 10.

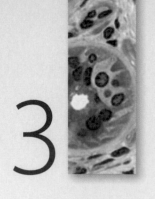

3 | CONNECTIVE TISSUE

Connective tissues encompass the major structural constituents of the body. Although seemingly diverse, structurally and functionally they possess many shared qualities; therefore, they are considered in a single category. Most connective tissues are derived from mesoderm, which form the multipotential mesenchyme from which bone, cartilage, tendons, ligaments, capsules, blood and hematopoietic cells, and lymphoid cells develop. Functionally, connective tissues serve in support, defense, transport, storage, and repair, among others. Connective tissues, unlike epithelia, are composed mainly of

- **extracellular elements** and
- a limited number of **cells**.

They are classified mostly on the basis of their nonliving components rather than on their cellular constituents. Although the precise ordering of the various subtypes differs from author to author, the following categories are generally accepted:

- Embryonic connective tissues
  - Mesenchymal
  - Mucous
- Adult connective tissues
  - Connective tissue proper
    - Loose (areolar)
    - Reticular
    - Adipose
    - Dense irregular
    - Dense regular
      - Collagenous
      - Elastic
- Specialized connective tissues
  - Supporting tissues
    - Cartilage
    - Bone
  - Blood

EXTRACELLULAR MATRIX

The extracellular matrix of connective tissue proper may be subdivided into **fibers, amorphous ground substance,** and **extracellular fluid.**

Fibers

Three types of fibers are recognized histologically: collagen, reticular, and elastic.

- **Collagen,** the most abundant of the fibers, is inelastic and is composed of a staggered array of the protein **tropocollagen,** composed of three α chains. Interestingly, every third amino acid is **glycine,** and a significant amount of **proline, hydroxyproline, lysine,** and **hydroxylysine** constitutes much of the tropocollagen subunit.

- Since **glycine** is a very small amino acid, the three α chains can form a tight helix as they wrap around each other.
- The hydrogen bonds of **hydroxyproline** residues of individual α chains hold the three chains together to maintain the stability of the tropocollagen molecule.
- **Hydroxylysine** residues hold the tropocollagen molecules to each other to form collagen fibrils.

Currently, there are at least 25 different types of collagens that are known, depending on the amino acid composition of their α chains. The most common collagens are

- type I (dermis, bone, capsules of organs, fibrocartilage, dentin, cementum),
- type II (hyaline and elastic cartilages),
- type III (reticular fibers),
- type IV (lamina densa of the basal lamina),
- type V (placenta), and
- type VII (anchoring fibrils of the basal lamina).

With the exception of type IV, all collagen fibers display a **67-nm periodicity** as the result of the specific arrangement of the tropocollagen molecules.

Synthesis of collagen occurs on the rough endoplasmic reticulum (RER), where polysomes possess different mRNAs coding for the three α **chains (preprocollagens).**

Within the RER cisternae, specific proline and lysine residues are **hydroxylated,** and hydroxylysine residues are **glycosylated.**

Each α chain possesses **propeptides (telopeptides)** located at both amino and carboxyl ends. These propeptides are responsible for the precise **alignment** of the α chains, resulting in the formation of the **triple helical procollagen** molecule.

Coatomer-coated transfer vesicles convey the procollagen molecules to the **Golgi apparatus** for modification, mostly the addition of carbohydrate side chains. Subsequent to transfer to the **trans-Golgi network,** the **procollagen** molecule is exocytosed (via non–clathrin-coated vesicles), and the propeptides are cleaved by the enzyme **procollagen peptidase,** resulting in the formation of tropocollagen.

Tropocollagen molecules self-assemble, forming fibrils with 67-nm characteristic banding (see Graphic 3-1). Type IV collagen is composed of procollagen rather than tropocollagen subunits, hence the absence of periodicity and fibril formation in this type of collagen.

- **Reticular fibers** (once believed to have different composition) are thin, branching, carbohydrate-coated fibers composed of type III collagen that form delicate networks around smooth muscle cells, certain epithelial cells, adipocytes, nerve fibers, and blood vessels.

○ They also constitute the structural framework of certain organs, such as the liver and the spleen.

○ As a result of the carbohydrate coat, when stained with silver stain, the silver preferentially deposits on these fibers giving them a brown to black appearance in the light microscope.

- **Elastic fibers,** as their name implies, are highly elastic and may be stretched to about 150% of their resting length without breaking.

  ○ They are composed of an amorphous protein, **elastin,** surrounded by a **microfibrillar** component, consisting of **fibrillin.**

  ○ The elasticity of elastin is due to its lysine content in that four lysine molecules, each belonging to a different elastin chain, form covalent **desmosine crosslinks** with one another.

  ○ These links are highly deformable and can stretch as tensile forces are applied to them. Once the tensile force ceases, the elastic fibers return to their resting length.

  ○ Elastic fibers do not display a periodicity and are found in regions of the body that require considerable flexibility and elasticity.

Amorphous Ground Substance

The **amorphous ground substance** constitutes the gel-like matrix in which the fibers and cells are embedded and through which extracellular fluid diffuses. Ground substance is composed of glycosaminoglycans (GAGs), proteoglycans, and glycoproteins.

- **Glycosaminoglycans (GAGs)** are linear polymers of repeating disaccharides, one of which is always a **hexosamine** and the other is a **hexuronic acid.** All of the GAGs, with the exception of **hyaluronic acid,** are sulfated and, thus, possess a predominantly **negative charge.** The major GAGs constituents are **hyaluronic acid, chondroitin 4-sulfate, chondroitin 6-sulfate, dermatan sulfate,** and **heparan sulfate** (see Table 3-1).

- **Proteoglycans** are composed of a protein core to which GAGs are covalently bound. Many of these proteoglycan molecules are also linked to hyaluronic acid, forming massive molecules, such as **aggregans aggregate,** of enormous electrochemical **domains** that attract osmotically active cations (e.g., Na^+), forming hydrated molecules that provide a gel-like consistency to connective tissue proper and function in resisting

TABLE 3-1 • Types of Glycosaminoglycans (GAGs)

GAGs	Sulfated	Repeating Disaccharides	Linked to Core Protein	Location
Hyaluronic acid	No	D-Glucuronic acid-beta-1,3-N-acetyl-D-glucosamine	No	Most connective tissue, synovial fluid, cartilage, dermis, vitreous humor, umbilical cord
Keratan sulfate I and II	Yes	Galactose-beta-1,4-N-acetyl-D-glucosamine-6-SO$_4$	Yes	Cornea (keratan sulfate I), Cartilage (keratan sulfate II)
Heparan sulfate	Yes	D-Glucuronic acid-beta-1,3-N-acetyl galactosamine L-Iduronic acid-2 or -SO$_4$-beta-1,3-N-acetyl-D-galactosamine	Yes	Blood vessels, lung, basal lamina
Heparin (90%) Heparin (10%)	Yes	L-Iduronic acid-beta-1,4-sulfo-D-glucosamine-6-SO$_4$ D-Glucuronic acid-beta-1,4-N-acetylglucosamine-6-SO$_4$	No	Mast cell granule, liver, lung, skin
Chondroitin 4-sulfate	Yes	D-Glucuronic acid-beta-1,3-N-acetylgalactosamine-6-SO$_4$	Yes	Cartilage, bone, cornea, blood vessels
Chondroitin 6-sulfate	Yes	D-Glucuronic acid-beta-1,3-N-acetylgalactosamine-6-SO$_4$	Yes	Cartilage, Wharton's jelly, blood vessels
Dermatan sulfate	Yes	L-Iduronic acid-alpha-1,3-N-acetylglucosamine-4-SO$_4$	Yes	Heart valves, skin, blood vessels

compression and slowing down the flow of extracellular fluid, thus permitting more time for the exchange of materials by the cells and retarding the spread of invading microorganisms.

- **Glycoproteins** have also been localized in connective tissue proper. The best characterized are laminin, fibronectin, chondronectin, osteonectin, entactin, and tenascin.
  - ○ Laminin and entactin are derived from epithelial cells, and tenascin is made by glial cells of the embryo, whereas the remainder are manufactured by cells of connective tissue.
  - ○ Many cells possess **integrins,** transmembrane proteins, with receptor sites for one or more of these glycoproteins. Moreover, glycoproteins also bind to collagen, thus facilitating cell adherence to the extracellular matrix.

The basement membrane, interposed between epithelia and connective tissues, is described in Chapter 2, Epithelium and Glands.

Extracellular Fluid

Extracellular fluid (tissue fluid) is the fluid component of blood, similar to plasma, that percolates throughout the ground substance, carrying nutrients, oxygen, signaling molecules, and other blood-borne materials to and carbon dioxide and waste products from cells. Extracellular fluid leaves the vascular supply at the arterial end of the capillaries and returns into the circulatory system at the venous end of capillaries, the venules, and the excess fluid enters lymphatic capillaries.

CELLS

The following are cells of connective tissue proper—or more accurately, loose (areolar) connective tissue (see Graphic 3-2).

- **Fibroblasts,** the predominant cell type, are responsible for the **synthesis** of collagen, elastic and reticular fibers, and much, if not all, of the ground substance.
  - ○ The morphology of these cells appears to be a function of their synthetic activities, and therefore, resting (or inactive fibroblasts) cells were often referred to as fibrocytes, a term that is rapidly disappearing from the literature.
- **Macrophages (histiocytes)** are derived from monocytes in bone marrow. They migrate to the connective tissue and function in ingesting **(phagocytosing)** foreign particulate matter. These cells also participate in enhancing the immunologic activities of lymphocytes.

- **Plasma cells** are the major cell type present during **chronic inflammation.** These cells are derived from a subpopulation of lymphocytes and are responsible for the synthesis and release of humoral antibodies.
- **Mast cells** are usually observed in the vicinity of small blood vessels, although the relationship between them is not understood.
  - ○ These cells house numerous metachromatic granules containing **histamine**, which is a smooth muscle contractant, and **heparin**, which is an anticoagulant.
  - ○ Mast cells also release **eosinophilic** and **neutrophilic chemotactic factors** and **leukotriene** among their agents (see Table 3-2).
  - ○ Because of the presence of immunoglobulins on the external surface of the mast cell plasmalemma, these cells, in sensitized individuals, may become degranulated (i.e., release their granules) and release membrane-derived factors, resulting in **anaphylactic reactions** or even in life-threatening anaphylactic shock.
- **Pericytes** are also associated with minute blood vessels, but much more closely than are mast cells, since they share the basal laminae of the endothelial cells.
  - ○ Pericytes are believed to be **contractile cells** that assist in the regulation of blood flow through the capillaries.
  - ○ Additionally, they may also be **pluripotential cells,** which assume the responsibilities of mesenchymal cells in adult connective tissue.
- **Fat cells (adipocytes)** may form small clusters or aggregates in loose connective tissue. They **store lipids** and form adipose tissue, which protects, insulates, and cushions organs of the body (see Adipose Tissue below).
- **Leukocytes** (white blood cells) leave the bloodstream and enter the connective tissue spaces. Here they assume various functions, which are discussed in Chapter 5.

CONNECTIVE TISSUE TYPES

- **Mesenchymal** and **mucous connective tissues** are limited to the embryo.
  - ○ Mesenchymal connective tissue consists of mesenchymal cells and fine reticular fibers interspersed in a semifluid matrix of ground substance.
  - ○ Mucous connective tissue is more viscous in consistency, contains collagen bundles and numerous fibroblasts, and is found deep to the fetal skin and in the umbilical cord (where it is known as Wharton's jelly), surrounding the umbilical vessels.

TABLE 3-2 • Mast Cells Factors and Functions

Substance	Intracellular Source	Action
Primary mediators		
Histamine	Granules	Vasodilator; increases vascular permeability; causes contraction of bronchial smooth muscle; increases mucus production
Heparin	Granules	Anticoagulant; inactivates histamine
ECF	Granules	Attractant for eosinophils to site of inflammation
NCF	Granules	Attractant for neutrophils to site of inflammation
Aryl sulfate	Granules	Inactivates leukotriene C_4, limiting inflammatory response
Chondroitin sulfate	Granules	Binds and inactivates histamine
Neutral proteases	Granules	Protein cleavage to activate complement; increases inflammatory response
Secondary mediators		
Prostaglandin D_2	Membrane lipid	Causes contraction of bronchial smooth muscle; increases mucus secretion; vasoconstriction
Leukotrienes C_4, D_4, E_4	Membrane lipid	Vasodilators; increases vascular permeability; contraction of bronchial smooth muscle
Bradykinins	Membrane lipid	Causes vascular permeability; responsible for pain sensation
Thromboxane A_2	Membrane lipid	Causes platelet aggregation; vasoconstriction
Platelet-activating factor	Activated by phospholipase A_2	Attracts neutrophils and eosinophils; causes vascular permeability; contraction of bronchial smooth muscle

ECF, eosinophil chemotactic factor; NCF, neutrophil chemotactic factor.

- **Loose (areolar) connective tissue** is distributed widely, since it constitutes much of the superficial fascia and invests neurovascular bundles. The cells and intercellular elements described above help form this more or less amorphous, watery tissue.
- **Reticular connective tissue** forms a network of thin reticular fibers that constitute the structural framework of bone marrow and many lymphoid structures, as well as a framework enveloping certain cells.
- **Adipose tissue** is composed of fat cells, reticular fibers, and a rich vascular supply. There are two types of adipose tissue, white (unilocular) and brown (multilocular).
  - ○ **Unilocular adipose tissue** is composed of fat cells, reticular fibers, and a rich vascular supply.
    - ▪ Cells of **unilocular adipose tissue** store triglycerides in a single, large fat droplet that occupies most of the cell. These cells make the enzyme **lipoprotein lipase,** which is transported to the luminal surface of the capillary endothelial cell membrane, where it hydrolyzes chylomicrons and very low density lipoproteins.
    - ▪ The fatty acids and monoglycerides are transported to the adipocytes, diffuse into their cytoplasm, and are reesterified into triglycerides.
    - ▪ **Hormone-sensitive lipase,** activated by **cAMP,** hydrolyzes the stored lipids into fatty acids and glycerol, which are released from the cell as the need arises, to enter the capillaries for distribution to the remainder of the body.
    - ▪ Unilocular adipose tissue acts as a depot for fat, a thermal insulator, and a shock absorber.
  - ○ **Multilocular adipose tissue** is rare in the adult human. It is present in the neonate, as well as in animals that hibernate.
    - ▪ Cells of multilocular adipose tissue possess numerous droplets of lipid in their cytoplasm and a rich supply of mitochondria.
    - ▪ These mitochondria are capable of uncoupling oxidation from phosphorylation, and instead of producing adenosine triphosphate (ATP), they release heat, thus arousing the animal from hibernation.
- **Dense irregular connective tissue** consists of coarse, almost haphazardly arranged bundles of collagen fibers interlaced with few elastic and reticular fibers. The chief cellular constituents are fibroblasts, macrophages, and occasional mast cells. The dermis of the skin and capsules of some organs are composed of dense irregular connective tissue.
- **Dense regular connective tissue** may be composed either of thick, parallel arrays of collagenous fibers, as in tendons and ligaments, or of parallel bundles of elastic fibers, as in the ligamentum nuchae, the ligamentum flava, and the suspensory ligament of the penis. The cellular constituents of both dense regular collagenous and dense regular elastic connective tissues are almost strictly limited to fibroblasts.

CLINICAL CONSIDERATIONS

Keloid Formation

The body responds to wounds, including those caused by surgical intervention, by forming scars that repair the damage first with weak type III collagen that is later replaced by type I collagen, which is much stronger. Some individuals, especially African Americans, form an overabundance of collagen in the healing process, thus developing elevated scars called keloids. The collagen fibers in keloids are much larger, more eosinophilic—said to have a "glassy" appearance—than the normal, fibrillar, collagen. Moreover, keloids are hypocellular, although they frequently display clusters of fibroblasts distributed among the large, glassy collagen fiber bundles.

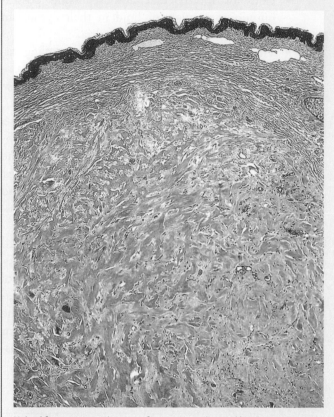

Keloid formation at the site of injury is evidenced by the excessively thick layer of the dermis whose large, eosinophilic, type I collagen fibers are clearly apparent. (Reprinted with permission from Mills SE, Carter D, Greenson JK, Reuter VE, Stoler MH, eds. Sternberger's Diagnostic Surgical Pathology, 5th ed., 2010. Figure 1.54. p. 29.)

Scurvy

Scurvy, a condition characterized by bleeding gums and loose teeth among other symptoms, results from a vitamin C deficiency. Vitamin C is necessary for hydroxylation of proline for proper tropocollagen formation giving rise to fibrils necessary for maintaining teeth in their bony sockets.

Marfan's Syndrome

Patients with Marfan's syndrome, a genetic defect in chromosome 15 that codes for fibrillin, possess undeveloped elastic fibers in their body and are predisposed to rupture of the aorta. Histologically, the aortas of a large portion of individuals with Marfan's syndrome display *cystic medial degeneration*, a condition where the fenestrated membranes as well as the smooth muscles of the tunica media are reduced in quantity or are partially absent. In individuals with a less severe condition of *cystic medial degeneration*, the fenestrated membranes are less well organized, the smooth muscle cells are fewer in number, and the connective tissue is richer in ground substance than in normal aortas.

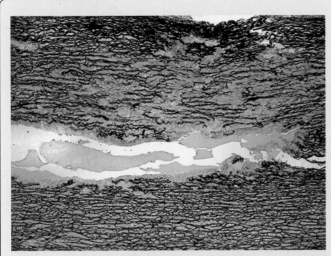 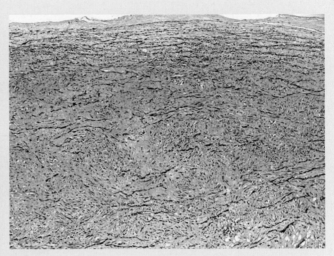

A: Cystic medial degeneration, evident in the media of this aorta from a patient exhibiting Marfan's syndrome, displays that the fenestrated membrane and smooth muscle cells have been replaced by amorphous ground substance. **B**: A less severe case of cystic medial degeneration is displayed in this patient. The tunica media evidences disorganized fenestrated membranes and smooth muscle fibers as well as an increase in the amorphous ground substance. (Reprinted with permission from Mills SE, Carter D, Greenson JK, Reuter VE, Stoler MH, eds. Sternberger's Diagnostic Surgical Pathology, 5th ed. Philadelphia: Lippincott Williams & Wilkins, 2010. Figures 30.1A and B. P. 1228)

Edema

The release of histamine and leukotrienes from mast cells during an inflammatory response elicits increased capillary permeability, resulting in an excess accumulation of extracellular fluid and, thus, gross swelling (edema).

Obesity

There are two types of obesity—hypertrophic obesity, which occurs when adipose cells increase in size from storing fat (adult onset), and hyperplastic obesity, which is characterized by an increase in the number of adipose cells resulting from overfeeding a new-born for a few weeks after birth. This type of obesity is usually lifelong.

Systemic Lupus Erythematosus

Systemic lupus erythematosus is an autoimmune connective tissue disease that results in the inflammation in the connective tissue elements of certain organs as well as of tendons and joints. The symptoms depend on the type and number of antibodies present and can be anywhere from mild to severe and, due to the variety of symptoms, lupus may resemble other conditions such as growing pains, arthritis, epilepsy, and even psychologic diseases. The characteristic symptoms include facial and skin rash, sores in the oral cavity, joint pains and inflammation, kidney malfunction, neurologic conditions, anemia, thrombocytopenia, and fluid on the lungs.

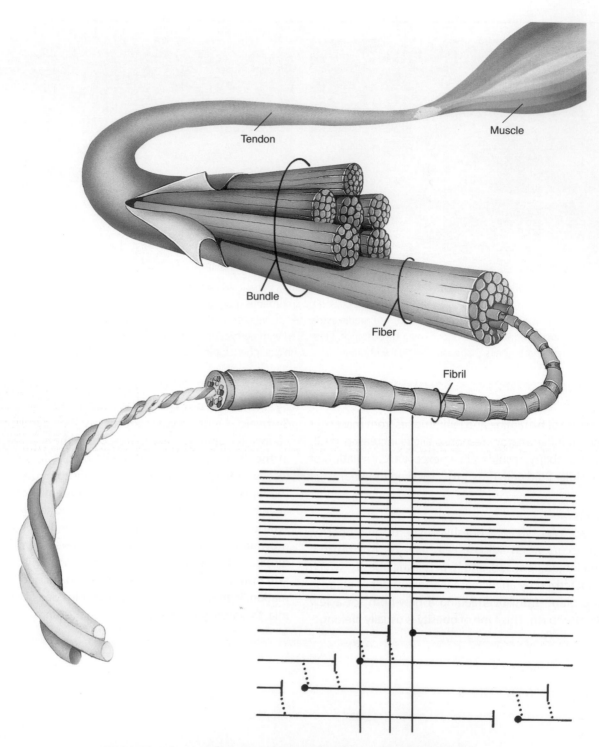

Tendon

Muscle

Bundle

Fiber

Fibril

Each collagen fiber bundle is composed of smaller fibrils, which in turn consist of aggregates of **tropocollagen molecules**. Tropocollagen molecules self-assemble in the extracellular environment in such a fashion that there is a gap between the tail of the one and the head of the succeeding molecule of a single row. As fibrils are formed, tails of tropocollagen molecules overlap the heads of tropocollagen molecules in adjacent rows. Additionally, the **gaps** and **overlaps** are arranged so that they are in register with those of neighboring (but not adjacent) rows of tropocollagen molecules. When stained with a heavy metal, such as osmium, the stain preferentially precipitates in the gap regions, resulting in the repeating **light** and **dark** banding of collagen.

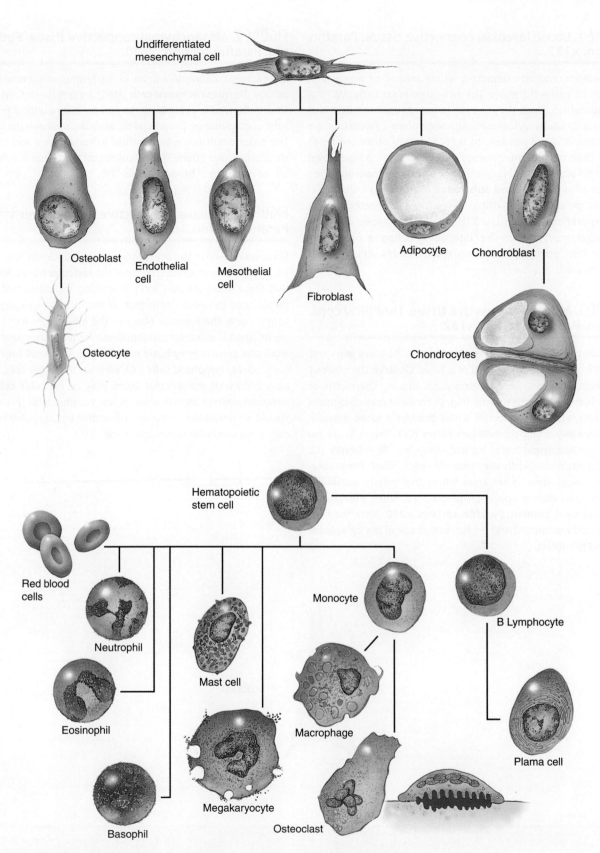

Undifferentiated mesenchymal cell

Osteoblast

Endothelial cell

Mesothelial cell

Fibroblast

Adipocyte

Chondroblast

Osteocyte

Chondrocytes

Hematopoietic stem cell

Red blood cells

Neutrophil

Eosinophil

Basophil

Mast cell

Megakaryocyte

Monocyte

Macrophage

Osteoclast

B Lymphocyte

Plama cell

* The cells on this page are not represented in proportion to their actual diameters.

PLATE 3-1 • Embryonic and Connective Tissue Proper I

FIGURE 1. Loose (areolar) connective tissue. Paraffin section. ×132.

This photomicrograph depicts a whole mount of mesentery, through its entire thickness. The two large **mast cells** (MC) are easily identified, since they are the largest cells in the field and possess a granular cytoplasm. Although their cytoplasms are not visible, it is still possible to recognize two other cell types due to their nuclear morphology. **Fibroblasts** (F) possess oval nuclei that are paler and larger than the nuclei of **macrophages** (M). The semifluid **ground substance** (GS) through which tissue fluid percolates is invisible, since it was extracted during the preparation of the tissues. However, two types of fibers, the thicker, wavy, ribbon-like, interlacing **collagen fibers** (CF) and the thin, straight, branching **elastic fibers** (EF), are well demonstrated.

FIGURE 3. Mucous connective tissue. Umbilical cord. Human. Paraffin section. ×132.

This example of mucous connective tissue (Wharton's jelly) was derived from the umbilical cord of a fetus. Observe the obvious differences between the two embryonic tissues. The matrix of mesenchymal connective tissue (Fig. 2) contains no collagenous fibers, whereas this connective tissue displays a loose network of haphazardly arranged **collagen fibers** (CF). The cells are no longer mesenchymal cells; instead, they are **fibroblasts** (F), although morphologically they resemble each other. The empty-looking spaces (*arrows*) are areas where the ground substance was extracted during specimen preparation. *Inset.* **Fibroblast. Umbilical cord. Human. Paraffin section. ×270**. Note the centrally placed **nucleus** (N) and the fusiform shape of the **cytoplasm** (c) of this fibroblast.

FIGURE 2. Mesenchymal connective tissue. Fetal pig. Paraffin section. ×540.

Mesenchymal connective tissue of the fetus is very immature and cellular. The **mesenchymal cells** (MeC) are stellate-shaped to fusiform cells, whose **cytoplasm** (c) can be distinguished from the surrounding matrix. The **nuclei** (N) are pale and centrally located. The ground substance is semifluid in consistency and contains slender reticular fibers. The vascularity of this tissue is evidenced by the presence of **blood vessels** (BV).

FIGURE 4. Reticular connective tissue. Silver stain. Paraffin section. ×270.

Silver stain, used in the preparation of this specimen, was deposited on the carbohydrate coating of the **reticular fibers** (RF). Note that these fibers are thin, long, branching structures that ramify throughout the field. Note that in this photomicrograph of a lymph node, the reticular fibers in the lower right-hand corner are oriented in a circular fashion. These form the structural framework of a cortical **lymphatic nodule** (LN). The small round cells are probably **lymphoid cells** (LC), whereas the larger cells, closely associated with the reticular fibers, may be **reticular cells** (RC), although definite identification is not possible with this stain. It should be noted that reticular connective tissue is characteristically associated with lymphatic tissue.

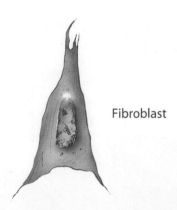

Fibroblast

KEY							
BV	blood vessel	**GS**	ground substance	**MeC**	mesenchymal cell
C	cytoplasm	**LC**	lymphoid cell	**N**	nucleus
CF	collagen fiber	**LN**	lymphatic nodule	**RC**	reticular cell
EF	elastic fiber	**M**	macrophage	**RF**	reticular fiber
F	fibroblast	**MC**	mast cell		

PLATE 3-1 • Embryonic and Connective Tissue Proper I

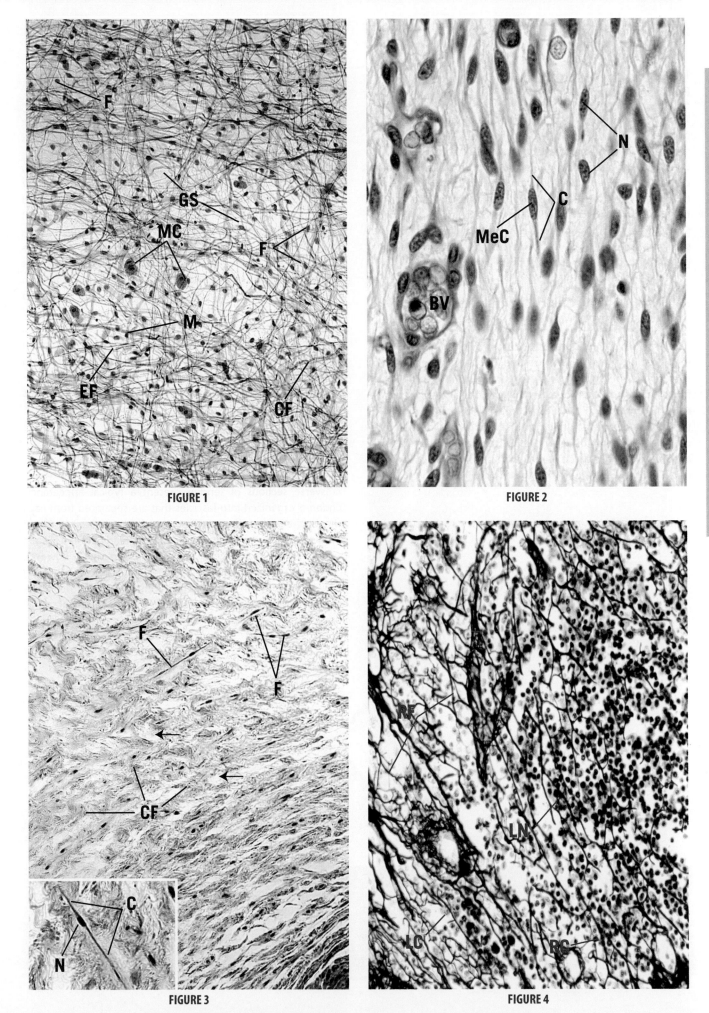

FIGURE 1

FIGURE 2

FIGURE 3

FIGURE 4

PLATE 3-2 • Connective Tissue Proper II

FIGURE 1. Adipose tissue. Hypodermis. Monkey. Plastic section. ×132.

This photomicrograph of adipose tissue is from monkey hypo-dermis. The **adipocytes** (A), or fat cells, appear empty due to tis-sue processing that dissolves fatty material. The **cytoplasm** (c) of these cells appears as a peripheral rim, and the **nucleus** (N) is also pressed to the side by the single, large **fat droplet** (FD) within the cytoplasm. Fat is subdivided into lobules by **septa** (S) of connec-tive tissue conducting **vascular elements** (BV) to the adipocytes. Fibroblast nuclei (*arrows*) are clearly evident in the connective tis-sue septa. Note the presence of the secretory portions of a **sweat gland** (SG) in the upper aspect of this photomicrograph.

FIGURE 3. Dense regular collagenous connective tissue. l.s. Tendon. Monkey. Plastic section. ×270.

Tendons and ligaments present the most vivid examples of dense regular collagenous connective tissue. This connective tissue type is composed of regularly oriented parallel **bundles of collagen fibers** (CF), where individual bundles are demarcated by parallel rows of **fibroblasts** (F). Nuclei of these cells are clearly evident as thin, dark lines, whereas their **cytoplasm** (c) is only somewhat dis-cernible. With hematoxylin and eosin, the collagen bundles stain a more or less light shade of pink with parallel rows of dark blue nuclei of fibroblasts interspersed among them.

FIGURE 2. Dense irregular collagenous connective tissue. Palmar skin. Monkey. Plastic section. ×132.

The dermis of the skin provides a good representation of dense irregular collagenous connective tissue. The thick, coarse, inter-twined bundles of **collagen fibers** (CF) are arranged in a haphaz-ard fashion. Although this tissue has numerous **blood vessels** (BV) and **nerve fibers** (NF) branching through it, it is not a very vascular tissue. Dense irregular connective tissue is only sparsely supplied with cells, mostly fibroblasts and macrophages, whose **nuclei** (N) appear as dark dots scattered throughout the field. At this magni-fication, it is not possible to identify the cell types with any degree of accuracy. The large epithelial structure in the upper center of the field is the **duct** (d) of a sweat gland. At higher magnification (*Inset*, ×540), the coarse bundles of collagen fibers are composed of a conglomeration of **collagen fibrils** (Cf) intertwined around each other. The three cells, whose **nuclei** (N) are clearly evident, cannot be identified with any degree of certainty, even though the **cytoplasm** (c) of the two on the left-hand side is visible. It is possible that they are macrophages, but without employing spe-cial staining techniques, the possibility of their being fibroblasts cannot be ruled out.

FIGURE 4. Dense regular collagenous connective tissue. x.s. Tendon. Paraffin section. ×270.

Transverse sections of tendon present a typical appearance. Tendon is organized into fascicles that are separated from each other by the **peritendineum** (P) surrounding each fascicle. **Blood vessels** (BV) may be observed in the peritendineum. Collagen bundles within the fascicles are regularly arranged; however, shrinkage due to preparation causes an artifactual layering (*arrows*), although in some preparations swelling of the tissue results in a homogenous appearance. The nuclei of **fibroblasts** (F) appear to be strewn about in a haphazard manner.

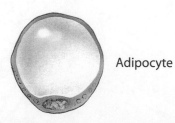

Adipocyte

KEY

A	adipocyte	D	duct	P	peritendineum
BV	blood vessel	F	fibroblast	S	septum
C	cytoplasm	FD	fat droplet	SG	sweat gland
CF	collagen fibril	N	nucleus		
CF	bundle of collagen fibers	NF	nerve fiber		

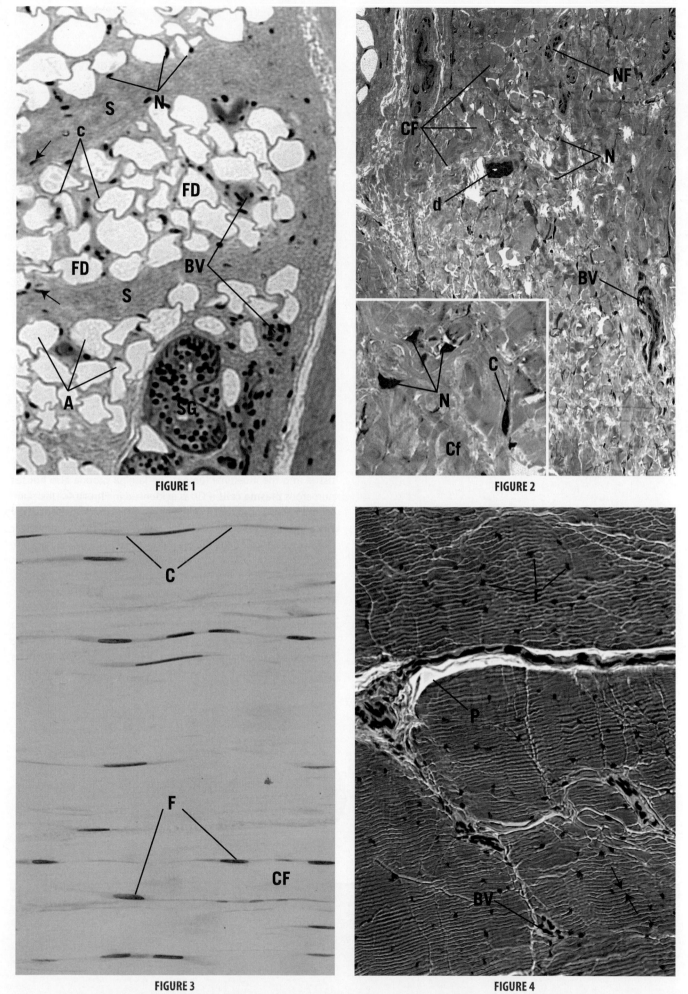

PLATE 3-2 • Connective Tissue Proper II

FIGURE 1

FIGURE 2

FIGURE 3

FIGURE 4

PLATE 3-3 · Connective Tissue Proper III

FIGURE 1. Dense regular elastic connective tissue. l.s. Paraffin section. ×132.

This longitudinal section of dense regular elastic tissue demonstrates that the **elastic fibers** (EF) are arranged in parallel arrays. However, the fibers are short and are curled at their ends (*arrows*). The white spaces among the fibers represent the loose connective tissue elements that remain unstained. The cellular elements are composed of parallel rows of flattened fibroblasts. These cells are also unstained and cannot be distinguished in this preparation.

FIGURE 3. Elastic laminae (membranes). Aorta. Paraffin section. ×132.

The wall of the aorta is composed of thick, concentrically arranged **elastic membranes** (EM). Since these sheet-like membranes wrap around within the wall of the aorta, in transverse sections they present discontinuous, concentric circles, which in this photomicrograph are represented by more or less parallel, wavy, dark lines (*arrows*). The connective tissue material between membranes is composed of ground substance, **collagen fibers** (CF), and reticular fibers. Also present are fibroblasts and smooth muscle cells, whose nuclei may be discerned.

FIGURE 2. Dense regular elastic connective tissue. x.s. Paraffin section. ×132.

A transverse section of dense regular elastic connective tissue displays a characteristic appearance. In some areas the fibers present precise cross-sectional profiles as dark dots of various diameters (*arrows*). Other areas present oblique sections of these fibers, represented by short linear profiles (*arrowhead*). As in the previous figure, the white spaces represent the unstained loose connective tissue elements. The large clear area (*middle left*) is also composed of loose connective tissue surrounding **blood vessels** (BV).

FIGURE 4. Mast cells, plasma cells, macrophages.

Mast cells (MC) are conspicuous components of connective tissue proper, **Figure 4a** (Tendon. Monkey. Plastic section. ×540), although they are only infrequently encountered. Note the round to oval nucleus and numerous small granules in the cytoplasm. Observe also, among the bundles of **collagen fibers** (CF), the nuclei of several fibroblasts. **Mast cells** are very common components of the subepithelial connective tissue (lamina propria) of the digestive tract, **Figure 4b** (Jejunum. Monkey. Plastic section. ×540). Note the **basal membrane** (BM) separating the connective tissue from the **simple columnar epithelium** (E), whose nuclei are oval in shape. The denser, more amorphous nuclei (*arrows*) belong to lymphoid cells, migrating from the connective tissue into the intestinal lumen. The lamina propria also houses numerous **plasma cells** (PC), as evidenced in **Figure 4c** (Jejunum. Monkey. Plastic section. ×540). Plasma cells are characterized by clock face ("cartwheel") nuclei, as well as by a clear paranuclear Golgi zone (*arrowhead*). **Figure 4d** (Macrophage. Liver, injected. Paraffin section. ×270) is a photomicrograph of liver that was injected with india ink. This material is preferentially phagocytosed by macrophages of the liver, known as **Kupffer cells** (KC). These cells appear as dense, black structures in the liver sinusoids; vascular channels are represented by clear areas (*arrow*). An individual Kupffer cell (*Inset*. Paraffin section. ×540) displays the **nucleus** (N) as well as the granules of india ink (*arrowhead*) in its cytoplasm.

Mast cell

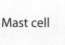

Plasma cell

KEY

BM	basal membrane	EF	elastic fiber	KC	Kupffer cell
BV	blood vessel	EM	elastic membrane	N	nucleus
CF	collagen fiber	MC	mast cell	PC	plasma cell

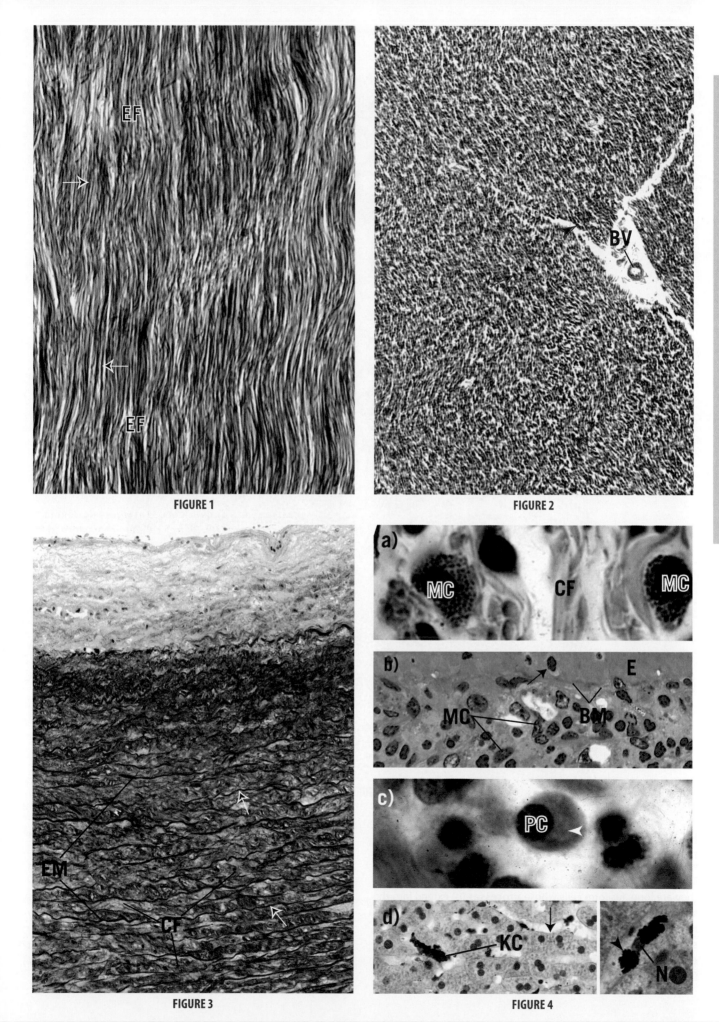

PLATE 3-3 · Connective Tissue Proper III

FIGURE 1

FIGURE 2

FIGURE 3

FIGURE 4

PLATE 3-4 · Fibroblasts and Collagen, Electron Microscopy

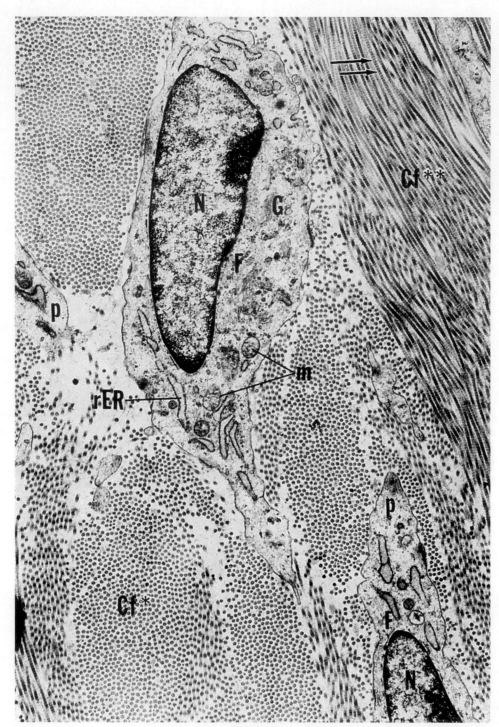

FIGURE 1

FIGURE 1. Fibroblast. Baboon. Electron microscopy. ×11,070.

This electron micrograph of **fibroblasts** (F) demonstrates that they are long, fusiform cells whose **processes** (p) extend into the surrounding area, between bundles of collagen fibrils. These cells manufacture collagen, reticular and elastic fibers, and the ground substance of connective tissue. Therefore, they are rich in organelles, such as **Golgi apparatus** (G), **rough endoplasmic reticulum** (rER), and **mitochondria** (m); however, in the quiescent stage, as in tendons, where they no longer actively synthesize the intercellular elements of connective tissue, the organelle population of fibroblasts is reduced in number, and the plump, euchromatic **nucleus** (N) becomes flattened and heterochromatic. Note that the bundles of **collagen fibrils** (Cf) are sectioned both transversely (*asterisk*) and longitudinally (*double asterisks*). Individual fibrils display alternating transverse dark and light banding (*arrows*) along their length. The specific banding results from the ordered arrangement of the tropocollagen molecules constituting the collagen fibrils. (From Simpson D, Avery B. J Periodontol 1974;45:500–510.)

PLATE 3-5 • Mast Cell, Electron Microscopy

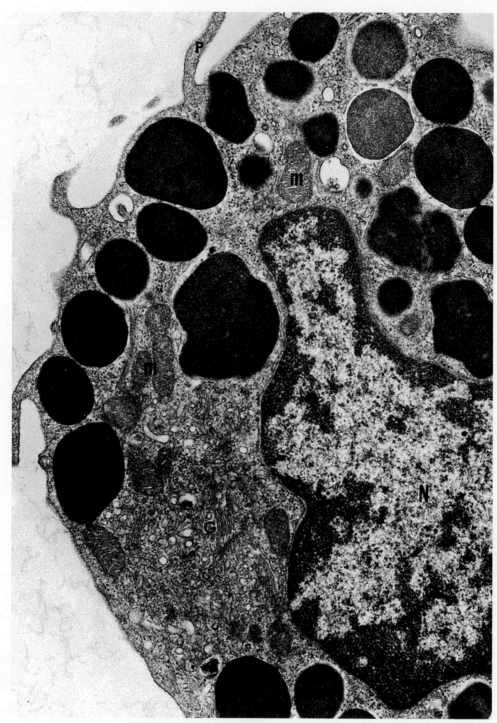

FIGURE 1

FIGURE 1.   Mast cell. Rat. Electron microscopy. ×14,400.

This electron micrograph of a rat peritoneal mast cell displays characteristics of this cell. Note that the **nucleus** (N) is not lobulated, and the cell contains organelles, such as **mitochondria** (m) and **Golgi apparatus** (G). Numerous **processes** (p) extend from the cell. Observe that the most characteristic component of this cell is that it is filled with numerous membrane-bound **granules** (Gr) of more or less uniform density. These granules contain heparin, histamine, and serotonin (although human mast cells do not contain serotonin). Additionally, mast cells release a number of unstored substances that act in allergic reactions. (From Lagunoff D. Contributions of electron microscopy to the study of mast cells. J Invest Dermatol 1972;58:296–311.)

PLATE 3-6 · Mast Cell Degranulation, Electron Microscopy

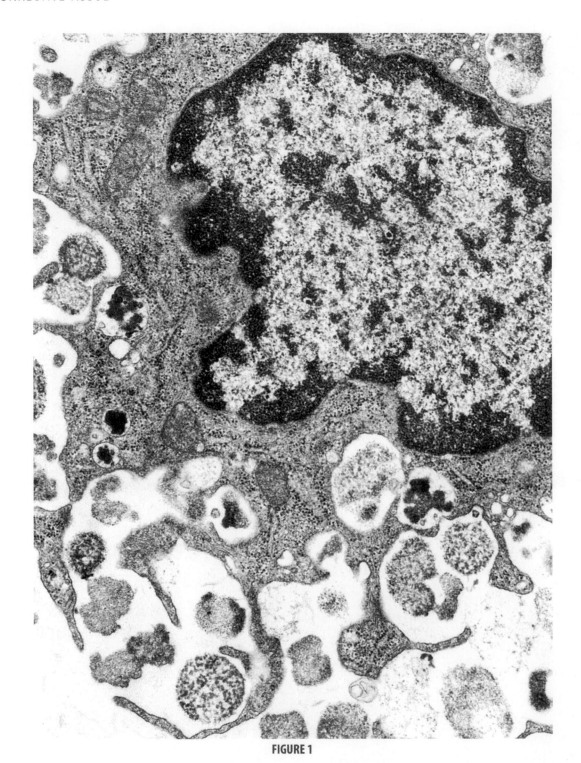

FIGURE 1

FIGURE 1.   Mast cell degranulation. Rat. Electron microscopy. ×20,250.

Mast cells possess receptor molecules on their plasma membrane, which are specific for the constant region of IgE antibody molecules. These molecules attach to the mast cell surface and, as the cell comes in contact with those specific antigens to which it was sensitized, the antigen binds with the active regions of the IgE antibody. Such antibody-antigen binding on the mast cell surface causes degranulation, that is, the release of granules, as well as the release of the unstored substances that act in allergic reactions. Degranulation occurs very quickly but requires both ATP and calcium. Granules at the periphery of the cell are released by fusion with the cell membrane, whereas granules deeper in the cytoplasm fuse with each other, forming convoluted intracellular canaliculi that connect to the extracellular space. Such a canaliculus may be noted in the bottom left-hand corner of this electron micrograph. (From Lagunoff D. Contributions of electron microscopy to the study of mast cells. J Invest Dermatol 1972;58:296–311.)

PLATE 3-7 • Developing Fat Cell, Electron Microscopy

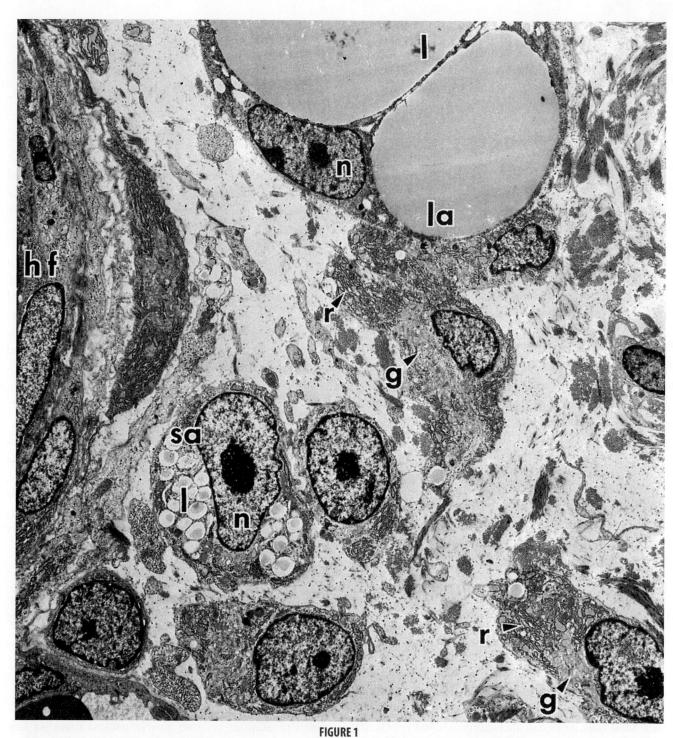

FIGURE 1

FIGURE 1. Developing fat cell. Rat. Electron microscopy. ×3,060.

This electron micrograph from the developing rat hypodermis displays a region of the developing **hair follicle** (hf). The peripheral aspect of the hair follicle presents a **small adipocyte** (sa) whose **nucleus** (n) and nucleolus are clearly visible. Although white adipose cells are unilocular, in that the cytoplasm of the cell contains a single, large droplet of lipid, during development lipid begins to accumulate as small **droplets** (l) in the cytoplasm of the small adipocyte. As the fat cell matures to become a **large adipocyte** (la), its **nucleus** (n) is displaced peripherally, and the lipid **droplets** (l)

fuse to form several large droplets, which will eventually coalesce to form a single, central fat deposit. The nucleus displays some alterations during the transformation from small to large adipocytes, in that the nucleolus becomes smaller and less prominent. Immature adipocytes are distinguishable, since they possess a well-developed **Golgi apparatus** (g) that is actively functioning in the biosynthesis of lipids. Moreover, the **rough endoplasmic reticulum** (r) presents dilated cisternae, indicative of protein synthetic activity. Note the capillary, whose lumen displays a red blood cell in the lower left-hand corner of this photomicrograph. (From Hausman G, Campion D, Richardson R, Martin R. Adipocyte development in the rat hypodermis. Am J Anat 1981;161:85–100.)

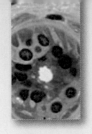

Chapter Summary

I. EMBRYONIC CONNECTIVE TISSUE

A. Mesenchymal Connective Tissue

1. Cells

Stellate to spindle-shaped **mesenchymal cells** have processes that touch one another. Pale scanty cytoplasm with large clear nuclei. Indistinct cell membrane.

2. Extracellular Materials

Delicate, empty-looking matrix, containing fine **reticular fibers.** Small blood vessels are evident.

B. Mucous Connective Tissue

1. Cells

Fibroblasts, with their numerous flattened processes and oval nuclei, constitute the major cellular component. In section, these cells frequently appear spindle-shaped, and resemble or are identical with mesenchymal cells when viewed with a light microscope.

2. Extracellular Materials

When compared with mesenchymal connective tissue, the extracellular space is filled with coarse **collagen bundles,** irregularly arranged, in a matrix of precipitated jelly-like material.

II. CONNECTIVE TISSUE PROPER

A. Loose (Areolar) Connective Tissue

1. Cells

The most common cell types are **fibroblasts,** whose spindle-shaped morphology closely resembles the next most numerous cells, the **macrophages.** The oval nuclei of macrophages are smaller, darker, and denser than those of fibroblasts. **Mast cells,** located in the vicinity of blood vessels, may be recognized by their size, the numerous small granules in their cytoplasm, and their large, round, centrally located nuclei. Occasional **fat cells** resembling round, empty spaces bordered by a thin rim of cytoplasm may also be present. When sectioned through its peripherally squeezed, flattened nucleus, a fat cell has a ring-like appearance.

Additionally, in certain regions such as the subepithelial connective tissue (lamina propria) of the intestines, plasma cells and leukocytes are commonly found. **Plasma cells** are small, round cells with round, acentric nuclei, whose chromatin network presents a clock face (cartwheel) appearance. These cells also display a clear, paranuclear Golgi zone. **Lymphocytes, neutrophils,** and occasional **eosinophils** also contribute to the cellularity of loose connective tissue.

2. Extracellular Materials

Slender bundles of long, ribbon-like bands of **collagen fibers** are intertwined by numerous thin, straight, long, branching **elastic fibers** embedded in a watery matrix of **ground substance,** most of which is extracted by dehydration procedures during preparation. **Reticular fibers,** also present, are usually not visible in sections stained with hematoxylin and eosin.

B. Reticular Connective Tissue

1. Cells

Reticular cells are found only in reticular connective tissue. They are stellate in shape and envelop the reticular fibers, which they also manufacture. They possess large, oval, pale nuclei, and their cytoplasm is not easily visible with the light microscope. The other cells in the interstitial spaces are **lymphocytes, macrophages,** and other **lymphoid cells.**

2. Extracellular Materials

Reticular fibers constitute the major portion of the intercellular matrix. With the use of a silver stain, they are evident as dark, thin, branching fibers.

C. Adipose Tissue

1. Cells

Unlike other connective tissues, adipose tissue is composed of adipose cells so closely packed together that the normal spherical morphology of these cells becomes distorted. Groups of fat cells are subdivided into lobules by thin sheaths of loose connective tissue septa housing **mast cells, endothelial cells** of blood vessels, and other components of **neurovascular elements.**

2. Extracellular Materials

Each fat cell is invested by **reticular fibers,** which, in turn, are anchored to the **collagen fibers** of the connective tissue septa.

D. Dense Irregular Connective Tissue

1. Cells

Fibroblasts, macrophages, and cells associated with **neurovascular bundles** constitute the chief cellular elements.

2. Extracellular Materials

Haphazardly oriented thick, wavy bundles of **collagen fibers,** as well as occasional **elastic** and **reticular fibers** are found in dense irregular connective tissue.

E. Dense Regular Collagenous Connective Tissue

1. Cells

Parallel rows of flattened **fibroblasts** are essentially the only cells found here. Even these are few in number.

2. Extracellular Materials

Parallel fibers of densely packed **collagen** are regularly arranged in dense regular collagenous connective tissue.

F. Dense Regular Elastic Connective Tissue

1. Cells

Parallel rows of flattened fibroblasts are usually difficult to distinguish in preparations that use stains specific for elastic fibers.

2. Extracellular Materials

Parallel bundles of thick **elastic fibers,** surrounded by slender elements of loose connective tissue, comprise the intercellular components of dense regular elastic connective tissue.

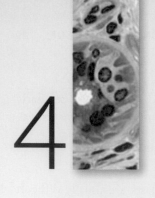

4 CARTILAGE AND BONE

Cartilage and bone form the supporting tissues of the body. In these specialized connective tissues, as in other connective tissues, the extracellular elements dominate their microscopic appearance.

CARTILAGE

Cartilage forms the supporting framework of certain organs, the articulating surfaces of bones, and the greater part of the fetal skeleton, although most of that will be replaced by bone (see Graphic 4-2).

- There are three types of cartilage in the body, namely, hyaline cartilage, elastic cartilage, and fibrocartilage (see Table 4-1).

Cartilage is a nonvascular, strong, and somewhat pliable structure composed of a firm matrix of **proteoglycans** whose main **glycosaminoglycans** are chondroitin-4-sulfate and chondroitin-6-sulfate. The fibrous and cellular components of cartilage are embedded in this matrix. The fibers are either solely collagenous or a combination of elastic and collagenous, depending on the cartilage type.

The cellular components are the

- **chondrocytes,** which are housed individually in small spaces known as **lacunae.**
- **chondroblasts** and **chondrogenic cells,** both of which are located in the **perichondrium.**

Most cartilage is surrounded by a dense irregular collagenous connective tissue membrane, the **perichondrium,** which has an outer fibrous layer and an inner chondrogenic layer.

- The outer **fibrous layer**, although poor in cells, is composed mostly of fibroblasts and collagen fibers.
- The inner cellular or **chondrogenic layer** is composed of chondroblasts and chondrogenic cells. The latter give rise to chondroblasts, cells that are responsible for secreting the **cartilage matrix.** It is from this layer that the cartilage may grow **appositionally.**
- As the chondroblasts secrete matrix and fibers around themselves, they become incarcerated in their own secretions and are then termed chondrocytes.
  - These **chondrocytes,** at least in young cartilage, possess the capacity to undergo cell division, thus contributing to the growth of the cartilage from within **(interstitial growth).**
  - When this occurs, each lacuna may house several chondrocytes and is referred to as a cell nest **(isogenous group).**
  - In order for these cells to manufacture type II collagen and the other components of the cartilage matrix, these cells need **Sox9,** a transcription factor.

- **Hyaline cartilage** is surrounded by a well-defined **perichondrium.** The type II collagen fibers of the matrix of this cartilage are mostly very fine and are, therefore, fairly well masked by the surrounding **glycosaminoglycans,** giving the matrix a smooth, glassy appearance. The acidic nature of the proteoglycans, combined with the enormous size of the proteoglycan-hyaluronic acid complex, results in these molecules possessing huge **domains** and tremendous capacity for binding cations and water. Additionally, the matrix contains **glycoproteins** that help the cells maintain contact with the intercellular matrix. Hyaline cartilage is present at the articulating surfaces of most bones, the C rings of the trachea, and the laryngeal, costal, and nasal cartilages, among others.
- **Elastic cartilage** also possesses a perichondrium. The matrix, in addition to the type II collagen fibers, contains a wealth of coarse elastic fibers that impart to it a characteristic appearance. This cartilage is located in areas like the epiglottis, external ear and ear canal, and some of the smaller laryngeal cartilages.
- **Fibrocartilage** differs from elastic and hyaline cartilage in that it has no perichondrium. Additionally, the chondrocytes are smaller and are usually oriented in parallel longitudinal rows. The matrix of this cartilage contains a large number of thick type I collagen fiber bundles between the rows of chondrocytes. Fibrocartilage is present in only a few places, namely, in some symphyses, the eustachian tube, intervertebral (and some articular) discs, and certain areas where tendons insert into bone (Table 4-1).

BONE

Bone has many functions, including support, protection, mineral storage, and hemopoiesis. At the specialized cartilage-covered ends, it permits articulation or movement. Bone is a vascular connective tissue consisting of cells and calcified extracellular materials, known as the matrix. The calcified matrix is composed of

- Sixty five percent minerals (mostly **calcium hydroxyapatite crystals)**
- Thirty five percent organic matter **(type I collagen, sulfated glycoproteins,** and **proteoglycans)** including bound water.

The presence of these crystals makes bone the body's storehouse of calcium, phosphate, and other inorganic ions. Thus, bone is in a dynamic state of flux, continuously gaining and losing inorganic ions to maintain the body's calcium and phosphate homeostasis.

Bone may be sponge-like (cancellous) or dense (compact).

TABLE 4-1 • Cartilage Types, Characteristics, and Locations

Type	Characteristics	Perichondrium	Locations (Major Samples)
Hyaline	Chondrocytes arranged in groups within a basophilic matrix containing type II collagen	Usually present except at articular surfaces	Articular ends of long bones, ventral rib cartilage, templates for endochondral bone formation
Elastic	Chondrocytes compacted in matrix containing type II collagen and elastic fibers	Present	Pinna of ear, auditory canal, laryngeal cartilages
Fibrocartilage	Chondrocytes arranged in rows in an acidophilic matrix containing type I collagen bundles in rows	Absent	Intervertebral discs, pubic symphysis

- **Cancellous bone**, like that present inside the epiphyses (heads) of long bones, is always surrounded by compact bone.
  - Cancellous bone has large, open spaces surrounded by thin, anastomosing plates of bone.
    - The large spaces are **marrow spaces,** and the plates of bones are **trabeculae** composed of several layers or **lamellae**.
- **Compact bone** is much denser than cancellous bone. Its spaces are much reduced in size, and its lamellar organization is much more precise and thicker.
  - **Compact** bone is always covered and lined by soft connective tissues.
  - The marrow cavity is lined by an **endosteum** composed of **osteoprogenitor cells** (previously known as osteogenic cells), **osteoblasts,** and occasional **osteoclasts.**
  - The periosteum covering the outer surface of compact bone is composed of an
    - outer fibrous layer consisting mainly of collagen fibers and populated by fibroblasts.
    - The inner osteogenic layer consists of some collagen fibers and mostly osteoprogenitor cells and their progeny, the osteoblasts.
    - The periosteum is affixed to bone via **Sharpey's fibers,** collagenous bundles trapped in the calcified bone matrix during ossification.

Cells of Bone

Bone possesses four types of cells: osteoprogenitor cells, osteoblasts, osteocytes, and osteoclasts.

- **Osteoprogenitor cells** give rise to osteoblasts under the influence of transforming growth factor-β and bone morphogenic protein. However, under hypoxic conditions, osteoprogenitor cells become chondrogenic cells; therefore, these two cells are really the

same cell that expresses different factors under differing oxygen tension.
- **Osteoblasts** elaborate bone matrix, become surrounded by the matrix they synthesized, and calcify the matrix via **matrix vesicles** that they release.
  - When osteoblasts are quiescent, they lose much of their protein synthetic machinery and resemble osteoprogenitor cells.
  - Osteoblasts function not only in the control of bone matrix mineralization but also in the formation, recruitment, and maintenance of osteoclasts as well as for the initiation of bone resorption.
  - Osteoblasts express alkaline phosphatase on their cell membranes.
  - Osteoblasts possess **parathyroid receptors** on their cell membrane, and in the presence of **parathormone**, they release **macrophage colony–stimulating factor** that induces the formation of osteoclast precursors.
  - Additionally, osteoblasts have expressed on their cell surface **RANKL (receptor for activation of nuclear factor kappa B ligand)**, a molecule that when contacted by the preosteoclast's surface-bound **RANK** induces preosteoclasts to differentiate into osteoclasts.
  - Osteoblasts release **osteoclast-stimulating factor** which activates osteoclasts to begin resorbing bone.
  - In order for the osteoclast to attach to bone in a secure fashion, they form a sealing zone on the bone surface, and the formation of this tight adherence is facilitated by another osteoblast-derived factor, **osteopontin**.
  - But before the osteoclast can adhere to the bone surface, the osteoblasts must resorb the noncalcified bone matrix that covers the bone surface, and then the osteoblast must leave to provide an available bone surface for the osteoclasts.

- **Osteocytes** are osteoblasts trapped in the matrix that they have synthesized. Two transcription factors have been implicated in the transformation of osteoblasts to osteocytes, namely, **Cbfa1/Runx2** and **osterix**. Both of these factors are essential for the normal development of mammalian skeleton. As the differentiation occurs, the membrane-bound alkaline phosphatase is no longer expressed.
  - They occupy **lacunae**, lenticular-shaped spaces, and possess long osteocytic processes that are housed in tiny canals or tunnels known as **canaliculi.**
  - Osteocytes are responsible for the maintenance of bone.
  - Their cytoplasmic processes contact and form **gap junctions** with processes of other osteocytes within canaliculi; thus, these cells sustain a communication network.
  - Large population of osteocytes are able to respond to blood calcium levels as well as to **calcitonin** and **parathormone,** released by the thyroid and parathyroid glands, respectively.
  - Thus, osteocytes are responsible for the short-term calcium and phosphate homeostasis of the body.
- **Osteoclasts,** large, multinucleated cells derived from monocyte precursors are responsible for the resorption of bone. As they remove bone, they appear to occupy a shallow cavity, **Howship's lacuna (subosteoclastic compartment).** Osteoclasts have four regions:
  - the **basal zone**, housing nuclei and organelles of the cell;
  - the **ruffled border**, composed of finger-like processes that are suspended in the subosteoclastic compartment where the resorption of bone is actively proceeding;
    - The ruffled border possesses many **proton pumps** that deliver hydrogen ions from the osteoclast into the subosteoclastic compartment.
    - Additionally, **aquapores** and **chloride channels** permit the delivery of water and chloride ions, respectively, forming a concentrated solution of HCl in the subosteoclastic compartment, thus decalcifying bone.
    - Enzymes are delivered via vesicles into the subosteoclastic compartment to degrade the organic components of bone.
    - The by-products of degradation are endocytosed by endocytic vesicles and are used by the osteoclast or are exocytosed into the extracellular space where they enter the vascular system for distribution to the rest of the body.
  - the **vesicular zone**, housing numerous vesicles that ferry material out of the cell and into the cell from the subosteoclastic compartment; and

- the **clear zone**, where the osteoclast forms a seal with the bone, isolating the subosteoclastic compartment from the external milieu.

The osteoclast **cell membrane** also possesses **calcitonin receptors;**
  - when calcitonin is bound to the receptors, these cells become inhibited; they stop bone resorption, leave the bone surface, and dissociate into individual cells or disintegrate and are eliminated by macrophages.
  - Cooperation between osteoclasts and osteoblasts is responsible not only for the formation, remodeling, and repair of bone but also for the long-term maintenance of calcium and phosphate homeostasis of the body.

Since bone, unlike cartilage, is a vascular hard tissue whose blood vessels penetrate and perforate it, canaliculi eventually open into channels known as **haversian canals,** housing the blood vessels, in order to exchange cellular waste material for nutrients and oxygen and to convey nutrients, hormones, and other necessary substances to and from the osteocytes.

- Each haversian canal with its surrounding lamellae of bone containing canaliculi radiating to it from the osteocytes trapped in the lacunae is known as an **osteon** or **haversian canal system.**
- Haversian canals, which more or less parallel the longitudinal axis of long bones, are connected to each other by **Volkmann's canals.**

The bony lamellae of compact bone are organized into four lamellar systems: **external** and **internal circumferential lamellae, interstitial lamellae,** and the **osteons** (see Graphic 4-1).

Osteogenesis

Histogenesis of bone occurs via either intramembranous or endochondral ossification.

- **Intramembranous ossification** arises in a richly vascularized mesenchymal membrane where **mesenchymal cells** differentiate into osteoblasts (possibly via osteoprogenitor cells), which begin to elaborate bone matrix, thus forming trabeculae of bone.
  - As more and more trabeculae form in the same vicinity, they will become interconnected.
  - As they fuse with each other, they form **cancellous bone,** the peripheral regions of which will be remodeled to form **compact bone.**
  - The surfaces of these trabeculae are populated with osteoblasts.
  - Frequently, an additional cell type, the **osteoclast,** may be present.

- These large, multinucleated cells derived from **monocyte precursors** are found in shallow depressions on the trabecular surface **(Howship's lacunae)** and function to resorb bone.
  - It is through the integrated interactions of these cells and osteoblasts that bone is remodeled.
- The region of the mesenchymal membrane that does not participate in the ossification process will remain the soft tissue component of bone (i.e., periosteum, endosteum).

Newly formed bone is called **primary** or **woven bone,** since the arrangement of collagen fibers lacks the precise orientation present in older bone. The integrated interaction between osteoblasts and osteoclasts will act to replace the woven bone with **secondary** or **mature bone.**

- **Endochondral ossification,** responsible for the formation of long and short bones, relies on the presence of a hyaline cartilage model that is used as a template on and within which bone is made (see Graphic 4-2).
  - Cartilage does not become bone; instead, a **bony subperiosteal collar** is formed (via intramembranous ossification) around the midriff of the cartilaginous template. This collar increases in width and length.
  - The **chondrocytes** in the center of the template hypertrophy and resorb some of their matrix, thus enlarging their lacunae so much that some lacunae become confluent.
  - The **hypertrophied chondrocytes,** subsequent to assisting in calcification of the cartilage, degenerate and die.
  - The newly formed spaces are invaded by the **periosteal bud** (composed of blood vessels, mesenchymal cells, and osteoprogenitor cells).
  - **Osteoprogenitor cells** differentiate into **osteoblasts,** and these cells elaborate a bony matrix on the surface of the calcified cartilage.
  - As the subperiosteal bone collar increases in thickness and length, osteoclasts resorb the calcified

cartilage-calcified bone complex, leaving an enlarged space, the future marrow cavity (which will be populated by marrow cells).
  - The entire process of ossification will spread away from this primary ossification center, and eventually most of the cartilage template will be replaced by bone, forming the **diaphysis** of a long bone.
  - The formation of the **bony epiphyses** (secondary ossification centers) occurs in a modified fashion so that a cartilaginous covering may be maintained at the articular surface.

The growth in length of a long bone is due to the presence of epiphyseal plates of cartilage located between the epiphysis and the diaphysis.

Bone Remodeling

Adult bone is a continuously being remodeled to compensate for changes in the forces being placed on it. As the remodeling of compact bone occurs, haversian canal systems have to be modified by osteoclastic resorption followed by osteoblastic bone formation. Since this progression takes place completely within the substance of compact bone, it is frequently called **internal remodeling.** The haversian canal system is being remodeled by what is known as a **bone remodeling unit,** which has two components: **resorption cavity (cutting cone)** and **lamellar formation (closing zone).**

- A **resorption cavity** is formed as osteoclasts enter the haversian canal and begin resorbing bone. Osteoclastic activity is followed by an invasion by capillaries, osteoprogenitor cells, and osteoblasts.
- Once the osteoclastic activity ceases, the osteoprogenitor cells divide, forming osteoblasts, which manufacture **lamellae of bone** until a new haversian canal system is completed.
- The process of integrated bone resorption and bone replacement is known as **coupling.**

CLINICAL CONSIDERATIONS

Cartilage Degeneration

Hyaline cartilage begins to degenerate when the chondrocytes hypertrophy and die, a natural process but one that accelerates with aging. This results in decreasing mobility and joint pain.

Vitamin Deficiency

- **Deficiency in Vitamin A** inhibits proper bone formation and growth, while an excess accelerates ossification of the epiphyseal plates producing small stature.
- **Deficiency in Vitamin D**, which is essential for absorption of calcium from the intestine, results in poorly calcified (soft) bone—rickets in children and osteomalacia in adults. When in excess, bone is resorbed.
- **Deficiency in Vitamin C**, which is necessary for collagen formation, produces scurvy—resulting in poor bone growth and repair.

Hormonal Influences on Bone

Calcitonin inhibits bone matrix resorption by altering osteoclast function, thus preventing calcium release. Parathyroid hormone activates osteoblasts to secrete osteoclast-stimulating factor, thus activating osteoclasts to increase bone resorption resulting in increased blood calcium levels. If in excess, bones become brittle and are susceptible to fracture.

Paget's Disease of Bone

Paget's disease of bone is a generalized skeletal disease that usually affects older people. Often, the disease has a familial component, and its results are thickened, but softer, bones of the skull and extremities. It is usually asymptomatic and is frequently discovered after radiographic examination prescribed for other reasons or as a result of blood chemistry showing elevated alkaline phosphatase levels.

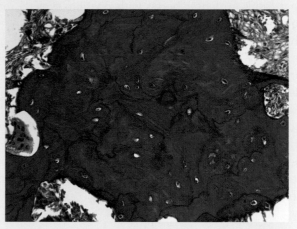

Note that the cement lines that surround haversian canal systems are well defined but irregular in morphology. The osteocytes in their lacunae as well as the peripheral osteoblasts, along with the large osteoclasts in their Howship's lacunae are clearly evident. (Reprinted with permission from Rubin R, Strayer D, et al., eds. Rubin's Pathology. Clinicopathologic Foundations of Medicine, 5th ed. Baltimore: Lippincott Williams & Wilkins, 2008. p. 1120.)

Osteoporosis

Osteoporosis is a decrease in bone mass arising from lack of bone formation or from increased bone resorption. It occurs commonly in old age because of decreased growth hormone and in postmenopausal women because of decreased estrogen secretion. In the latter, estrogen binding to receptors on osteoblasts stimulate the secretion of bone matrix. Without sufficient estrogen, osteoclastic activity reduces bone mass without the concomitant formation of bone, therefore making the bones more liable to fracture.

Osteopetrosis

Osteopetrosis is a constellation of heritable disorders that result in denser bones with possible skeletal malformations. The disease may be the early onset type or the delayed onset type. The early onset type may begin in infancy and can result in early death due to anemia, uncontrollable bleeding, and rampant infection. The delayed onset type of osteopetrosis may be quite mild exhibiting no clinical symptoms, but thickening of the bones and slight facial deformities may be evident. As the bones become thicker the diameters of the foramina become smaller and nerves passing through those constricted openings may become compressed and cause considerable pain.

Osteomalacia

Osteomalacia is a condition in the adult that resembles rickets that occurs in children who have depressed vitamin D levels and, consequently, cannot absorb enough calcium in their gastrointestinal tract. This condition is difficult to diagnose because initially the patient presents with nonspecific symptoms that range from aches and pains to muscle weakness. Once advanced stages of osteomalacia are reached, the symptoms include deep bone pain, difficulty in walking, and bone fractures. Histologic pictures of cancellous bone present overly thin trabeculae of bone with prominent Howship's lacunae occupied by osteoclasts and the presence of exceptionally thick osteoid over the thin calcified bony trabeculae and spicules.

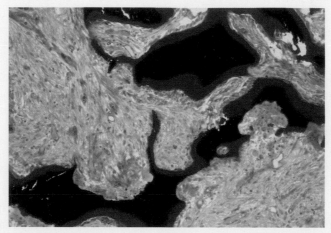

Observe the large marrow spaces and the thin calcified bone (black) in the histologic image of osteomalacia. Note the very thick osteoid (magenta-colored homogeneous material) covering the calcified bony trabeculae. Osteoclastic activity is apparent in the scalloped indentation on the middle right of the image. (Reprinted with permission from Rubin R, Strayer D, et al., eds., Rubin's Pathology. Clinicopathologic Foundations of Medicine, 5th ed. Baltimore: Lippincott Williams & Wilkins, 2008, p. 1117.)

Chondrosarcoma

Chondrosarcoma, a malignant tumor that develops in existing cartilage or bone, is more frequently present in males and is one of the most common cancers of bone. There are three types of chondrosarcoma, depending on their location. The most common type is known as **central chondrosarcoma** because it develops in the marrow cavity, and patients are usually in their 40s or 50s when the tumor makes its appearance; the next most common is **peripheral chondrosarcoma,** because it makes it initial appearance outside and then invades the bone, and patients are usually in their early 20s; the least common form is known as the **juxtacortical chondrosarcoma**, it begins its development in the region of the metaphysis and invades the bone, and patients suffering from this type of chondrosarcoma are in their mid 40s. The clinical symptom is pain localized to the site of the lesion, and histologic examinations display the presence of malignant chondrocytes in a matrix that resembles that of hyaline cartilage.

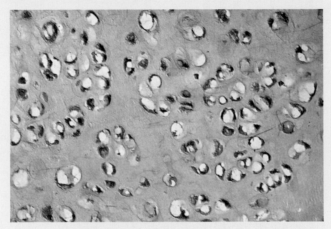

Observe the dense population of atypical chondrocytes dispersed within the hyaline cartilage–like matrix in this section from a patient suffering from chondrosarcoma. (Reprinted with permission from Rubin R, Strayer D, et al., eds., Rubin's Pathology. Clinicopathologic Foundations of Medicine, 5th ed. Baltimore: Lippincott Williams & Wilkins, 2008. p. 1128.)

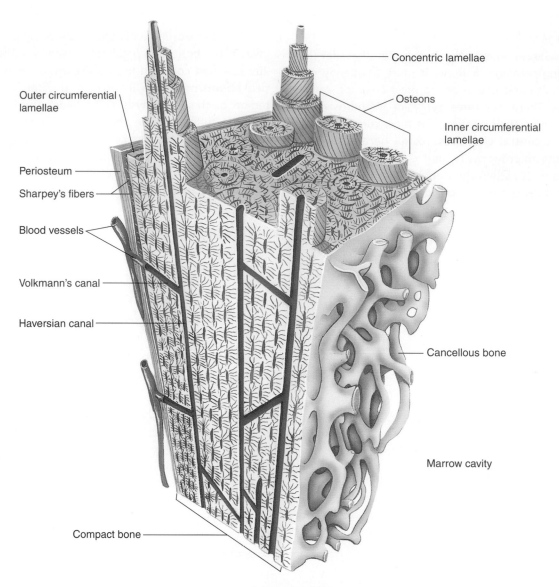

Concentric lamellae

Osteons

Inner circumferential lamellae

Outer circumferential lamellae

Periosteum

Sharpey's fibers

Blood vessels

Volkmann's canal

Haversian canal

Cancellous bone

Marrow cavity

Compact bone

Compact Bone

Compact bone is surrounded by dense irregular collagenous connective tissue, the **periosteum**, which is attached to the **outer circumferential lamellae** by **Sharpey's fibers**. Blood vessels of the periosteum enter the bone via larger nutrient canals or small **Volkmann's canals**, which not only convey blood vessels to the **Haversian canals** of **osteons** but also interconnect adjacent Haversian canals. Each osteon is composed of concentric lamellae of bone whose collagen fibers are arranged so that they are perpendicular to those of contiguous lamellae. The **inner circumferential lamellae** are lined by endosteal lined cancellous bone that protrudes into the marrow cavity.

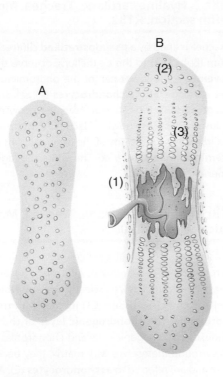

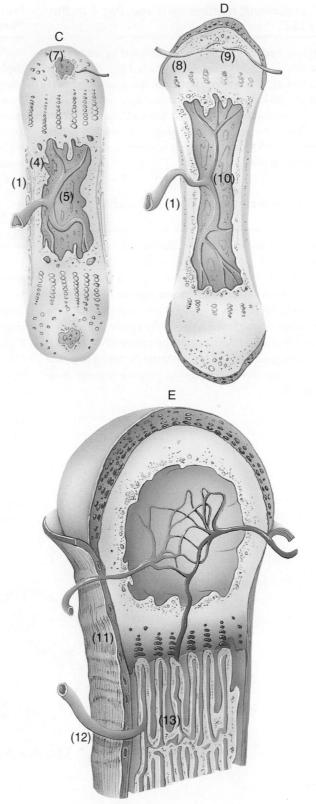

Endochondral Bone Formation

A. Endochondral bone formation requires the presence of a hyaline cartilage model.

B. Vascularization of the diaphysis perichondrium (2) results in the transformation of chondrogenic cells to osteogenic cells, resulting in the formation of a **subperiosteal bone collar** (1) (via intramembranous bone formation), which quickly becomes perforated by osteoclastic activity. Chondrocytes in the center of the cartilage hypertrophy (3), and their lacunae become confluent.

C. The subperiosteal bone collar (1) increased in length and width, the confluent lacunae are invaded by the **periosteal bud** (4), and osteoclastic activity forms a primitive marrow cavity (5) whose walls are composed of calcified cartilage-calcified bone complex. The epiphyses display the beginning of **secondary ossification centers** (7).

D and E. The subperiosteal bond collar (1) has become sufficiently large to support the developing long bone, so that much of the cartilage has been resorbed, with the exception of the **epiphyseal plate** (8) and the covering of the epiphyses (9). Ossification in the epiphyses occurs from the center (10), thus the vascular periosteum (11) does not cover the cartilaginous surface. Blood vessels (12) enter the **epiphyses**, without vascularizing the cartilage, to constitute the vascular network (13) around which spongy bone will be formed.

PLATE 4-1 • Embryonic and Hyaline Cartilages

FIGURE 1. Embryonic hyaline cartilage. Pig. Paraffin section. ×132.

The developing hyaline cartilage is surrounded by **embryonic connective tissue** (ECT). Mesenchymal cells have participated in the formation of this cartilage. Note that the developing **perichondrium** (P), investing the cartilage, merges both with the embryonic connective tissue and with the cartilage. The chondrocytes in their lacunae are round, small cells packed closely together (*arrow*), with little intervening homogeneously staining matrix (*arrowheads*).

FIGURE 3. Hyaline cartilage. Rabbit. Paraffin section. ×270.

The perichondrium is composed of **fibrous** (F) and **chondrogenic** (CG) layers. The former is composed of mostly collagenous fibers with a few fibroblasts, whereas the latter is more cellular, consisting of **chondroblasts** and **chondrogenic cells** (*arrows*). As chondroblasts secrete matrix, they become surrounded by the intercellular substance and are consequently known as **chondrocytes** (C). Note that chondrocytes at the periphery of the cartilage are small and elongated, whereas those at the center are large and ovoid to round (*arrowhead*). Frequently, they are found in **isogenous groups** (IG).

FIGURE 2. Hyaline cartilage. Trachea. Monkey. Paraffin section. ×132.

The trachea is lined by **a pseudostratified ciliated columnar epithelium** (Ep). Deep to the epithelium, observe the large, blood-filled **vein** (V). The lower half of the photomicrograph presents hyaline cartilage whose **chondrocytes** (C) are disposed in **isogenous groups** (IG) indicative of interstitial growth. Chondrocytes are housed in spaces known as lacunae. Note that the territorial matrix (*arrow*) in the vicinity of the lacunae stains darker than the interterritorial matrix (*asterisk*). The entire cartilage is surrounded by **a perichondrium** (P).

FIGURE 4. Hyaline cartilage. Trachea. Monkey. Plastic section. ×270.

The pseudostratified ciliated columnar epithelium displays numerous goblet cells (*arrows*). The cilia, appearing at the free border of the epithelium, are clearly evident. Note how the subepithelial **connective tissue** (CT) merges with the **fibrous perichondrium** (F). The **chondrogenic layer** of the perichondrium (Cg) houses chondrogenic cells and chondroblasts. As chondroblasts surround themselves with matrix, they become trapped in lacunae and are referred to as **chondrocytes** (C). At the periphery of the cartilage, the chondrocytes are flattened, whereas toward the interior they are round to oval. Due to the various histologic procedures, some of the chondrocytes fall out of their lacunae, which then appear as empty spaces. Although the **matrix** (M) contains many collagen fibrils, they are masked by the glycosaminoglycans; hence, the matrix appears homogeneous and smooth. The proteoglycan-rich lining of the lacunae is responsible for the more intense staining of the territorial matrix, which is particularly evident in Figures 2 and 3.

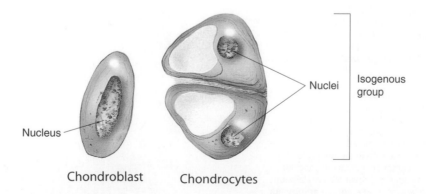

Nucleus

Chondroblast

Nuclei

Isogenous group

Chondrocytes

KEY					
C	chondrocyte	ECT	embryonic connective tissue	IG	isogenous group
Cg	chondrogenic perichondrium	Ep	pseudostratified ciliated columnar epithelium	M	matrix
CT	connective tissue	F	fibrous perichondrium	P	perichondrium
				V	vein

PLATE 4-1 · Embryonic and Hyaline Cartilages

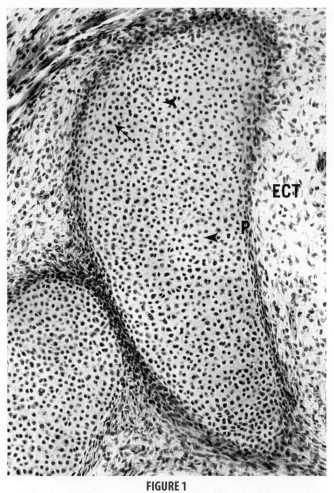

FIGURE 1

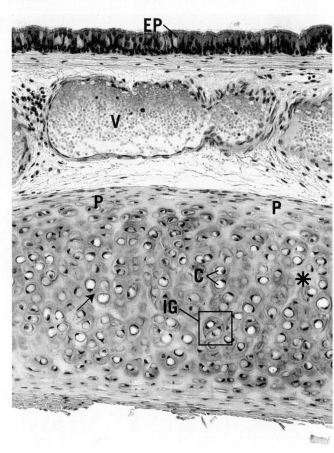

FIGURE 2

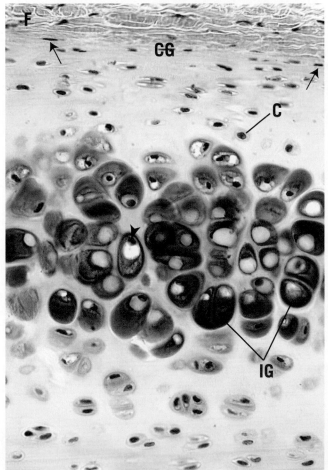

FIGURE 3

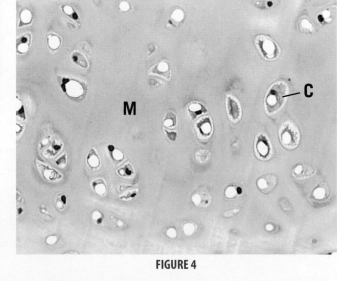

FIGURE 4

PLATE 4-2 · Elastic and Fibrocartilages

FIGURE 1. Elastic cartilage. Epiglottis. Human. Paraffin section. ×132.

Elastic cartilage, like hyaline cartilage, is enveloped by a **peri-chondrium** (P). **Chondrocytes** (C), which are housed in lacunae (*arrow*), have shrunk away from the walls, giving the appearance of empty spaces. Occasional lacunae display two chondrocytes (*asterisk*), indicative of interstitial growth. The matrix has a rich **elastic fiber** (E) component that gives elastic cartilage its characteristic appearance as well as contributing to its elasticity. The *boxed area* appears at a higher magnification in Figure 3.

FIGURE 3. Elastic cartilage. Epiglottis. Human. Paraffin section. ×540.

This is a high magnification of the *boxed area* in Figure 1. The **chondrocytes** (C) are large, oval to round cells with acentric **nuclei** (N). The cells accumulate lipids in their cytoplasm, often in the form of lipid droplets, thus imparting to the cell a "vacuolated" appearance. Note that the **elastic fibers** (E) mask the matrix in some areas and that the fibers are of various thicknesses, especially evident in cross-sections (*arrows*).

FIGURE 2. Elastic cartilage. Epiglottis. Human. Paraffin section. ×270.

This higher magnification of the perichondrial region of Figure 1 displays the outer **fibrous** (F) and inner **chondrogenic** (CG) regions of the perichondrium. Note that the chondrocytes (*arrow*) immediately deep to the chondrogenic layer are more or less flattened and smaller than those deeper in the cartilage. Additionally, the amount and coarseness of the elastic fibers increase adjacent to the large cells.

FIGURE 4. Fibrocartilage. Intervertebral disc. Human. Paraffin section. ×132.

The **chondrocytes** (C) of fibrocartilage are aligned in parallel rows, lying singly in individual lacunae. The nuclei of these chondrocytes are easily observed, whereas their cytoplasm is not as evident (*arrow*). The matrix contains thick bundles of **collagen fibers** (CF), which are arranged in a more or less regular fashion between the rows of cartilage cells. Unlike elastic and hyaline cartilages, fibrocartilage is not enveloped by a perichondrium.

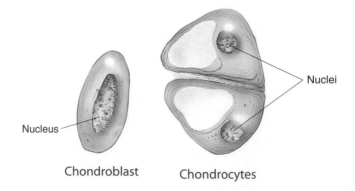

Nucleus

Chondroblast

Nuclei

Chondrocytes

KEY						
C	chondrocyte	**E**	elastic fiber	**N**	nucleus
CF	collagen fiber	**F**	fibrous perichondrium	**P**	perichondrium
Cg	chondrogenic perichondrium				

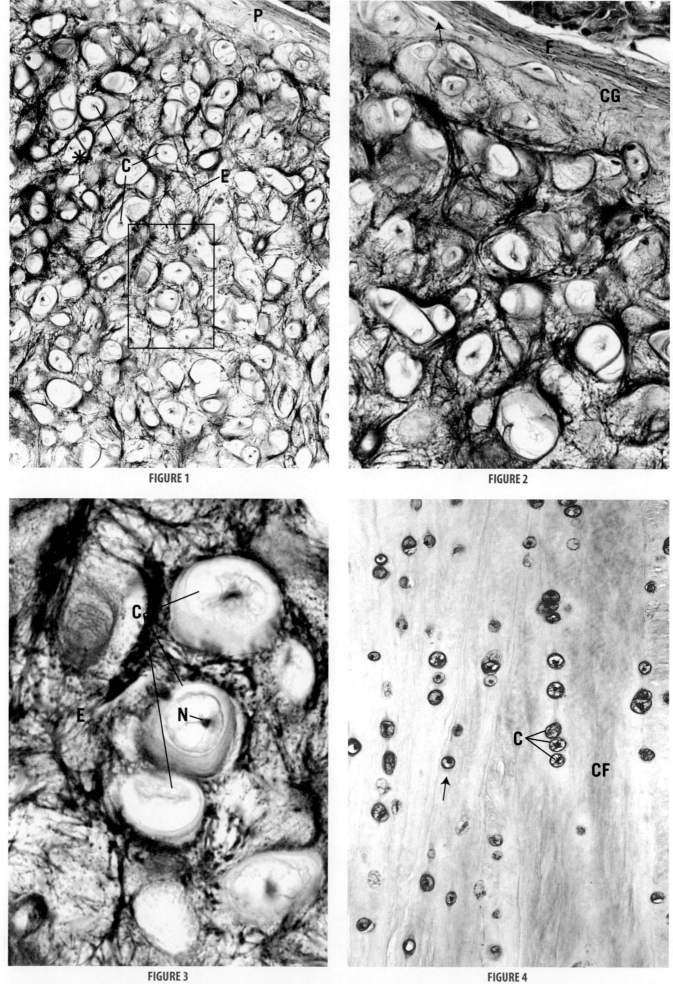

PLATE 4-2 · Elastic and Fibrocartilages

FIGURE 1

FIGURE 2

FIGURE 3

FIGURE 4

PLATE 4-3 · Compact Bone

FIGURE 1. Decalcified compact bone. Human. Paraffin section. ×132.

Cross section of decalcified bone, displaying **skeletal muscle** (SM) fibers that will insert a short distance from this site. The outer **fibrous periosteum** (FP) and the inner **osteogenic periosteum** (OP) are distinguishable due to the fibrous component of the former and the cellularity of the latter. Note the presence of the **inner circumferential** (IC) **lamellae, osteons** (Os), and interstitial lamellae (*asterisk*). Also observe the **marrow** (M) occupying the marrow cavity, as well as the endosteal lining (*arrow*).

FIGURE 3. Decalcified compact bone. Human. Paraffin section. ×540.

A small osteon is delineated by its surrounding cementing line (*arrowheads*). The lenticular-shaped **osteocytes** (Oc) occupy flattened spaces, known as lacunae. The lacunae are lined by uncalcified osteoid matrix. *Inset.* **Decalcified compact bone. Human. Paraffin section. ×540.** A haversian canal of an osteon is shown to contain a small **blood vessel** (BV) supported by slender connective tissue elements. The canal is lined by flattened **osteoblasts** (Ob) and, perhaps, **osteogenic cells** (Op).

FIGURE 2. Decalcified compact bone. Human. Paraffin section. ×132.

This is a cross section of decalcified compact bone, displaying **osteons** or **haversian canal systems** (Os) as well as **interstitial lamellae** (IL). Each osteon possesses a central **haversian canal** (HC), surrounded by several **lamellae** (L) of bone. The boundary of each osteon is visible and is referred to as a cementing line (*arrowheads*). Neighboring haversian canals are connected to each other by **Volkmann's canals** (VC), through which blood vessels of osteons are interconnected to each other.

FIGURE 4. Undecalcified ground compact bone. x.s. Human. Paraffin section. ×132.

This specimen was treated with India ink to accentuate some of the salient features of compact bone. The **haversian canals** (HC) as well as the lacunae (*arrows*) appear black in the figure. Note the connection between two osteons at top center, known as **Volkmann's canal** (VC). The canaliculi appear as fine, narrow lines leading to the haversian canal as they anastomose with each other and with lacunae of other osteocytes of the same osteon.

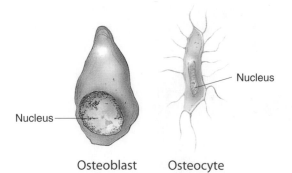

Nucleus

Nucleus

Osteoblast   Osteocyte

KEY

BV	blood vessel	L	lamella	OP	osteogenic periosteum
FP	fibrous periosteum	M	marrow	Os	osteon
HC	haversian canal	Ob	osteoblast	SM	skeletal muscle fiber
IC	inner circumferential lamella	Oc	osteocyte	VC	Volkmann's canal
IL	interstitial lamella	Op	osteogenic cell		

PLATE 4-3 • Compact Bone

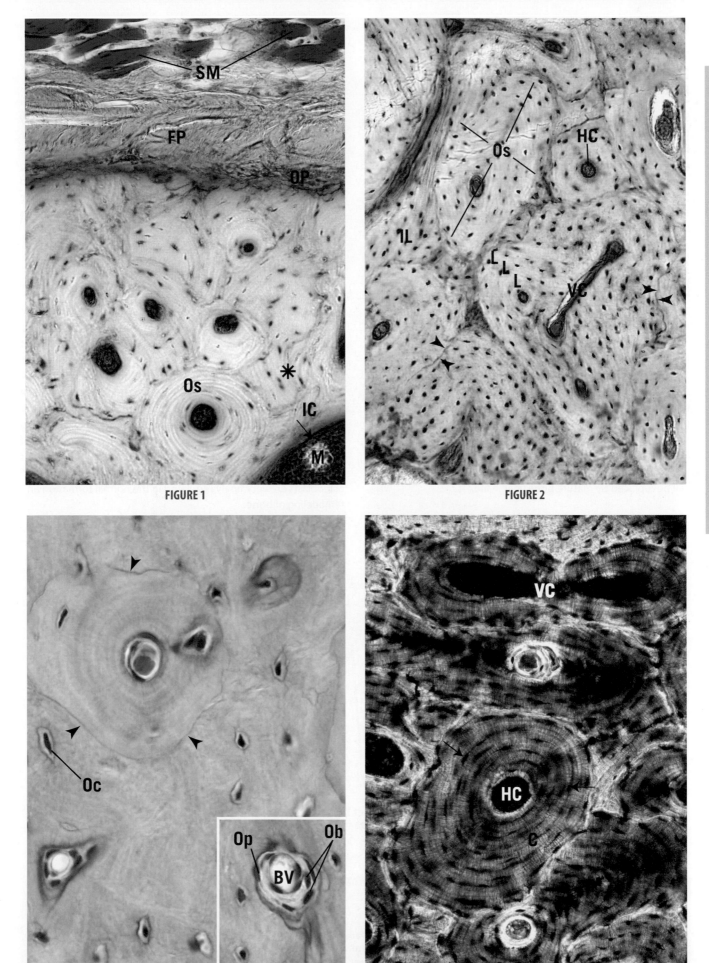

FIGURE 1

FIGURE 2

FIGURE 3

FIGURE 4

PLATE 4-4 · Compact Bone and Intramembranous Ossification

FIGURE 1. Undecalcified ground bone. x.s. Human. Paraffin section. ×270.

This transverse section of an osteon clearly displays the **lamellae** (L) of bone surrounding the **haversian canal** (HC). The cementing line acts to delineate the periphery of the osteon. Note that the **canaliculi** (C) arising from the peripheral-most lacunae usually do not extend toward other osteons. Instead, they lead toward the haversian canal. Canaliculi, which appear to anastomose with each other and with lacunae, house long osteocytic processes in the living bone.

FIGURE 3. Intramembranous ossification. Pig skull. Paraffin section. ×270.

This photomicrograph of intramembranous ossification is taken from the periphery of the bone-forming region. Note the developing **periosteum** (P) in the upper right-hand corner. Just deep to this primitive periosteum, **osteoblasts** (Ob) are differentiating and are elaborating **osteoid** (Ot), as yet uncalcified bone matrix. As the osteoblasts surround themselves with bone matrix, they become trapped in their lacunae and are known as **osteocytes** (Oc). These osteocytes are more numerous, larger, and more ovoid than those of mature bone, and the organization of the collagen fibers of the bony matrix is less precise than that of mature bone. Hence, this bone is referred to as immature (primary) bone, and it will be replaced by mature bone later in life.

FIGURE 2. Intramembranous ossification. Pig skull. Paraffin section. ×132.

The anastomosing **trabeculae** (T) of forming bone appear darkly stained in a background of **embryonic connective tissue** (ECT). Observe that this connective tissue is highly vascular and that the bony trabeculae are forming primitive **osteons** (Os) surrounding large, primitive **haversian canals** (HC), whose center is occupied by **blood vessels** (BV). Observe that the **osteocytes** (Oc) are arranged somewhat haphazardly. Every trabecula is covered by **osteoblasts** (Ob).

FIGURE 4. Intramembranous ossification. Pig skull. Paraffin section. ×540.

This photomicrograph is taken from an area similar to those of Figures 2 and 3. This trabecula demonstrates several points, namely, that **osteoblasts** (Ob) cover the entire surface and that **osteoid** (Ot) is interposed between calcified bone and the cells of bone and appears lighter in color. Additionally, note that the osteoblast marked with the *asterisk* is apparently trapping itself in the matrix it is elaborating. Finally, note the large, multinuclear cells, **osteoclasts** (Ocl), which are in the process of resorbing bone. The activity of these large cells results in the formation of Howship's lacunae (*arrowheads*), which are shallow depressions on the bone surface. The interactions between osteoclasts and osteoblasts are very finely regulated in the normal formation and remodeling of bone.

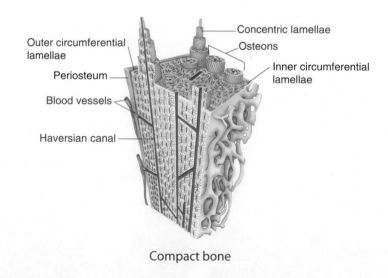

Compact bone

KEY						
BV	blood vessel	**L**	lamella	**Os**	osteon
C	canaliculus	**Ob**	osteoblast	**Ot**	osteoid
ECT	embryonic connective tissue	**Oc**	osteocyte	**P**	periosteum
HC	haversian canal	**Ocl**	osteoclast	**T**	trabecula

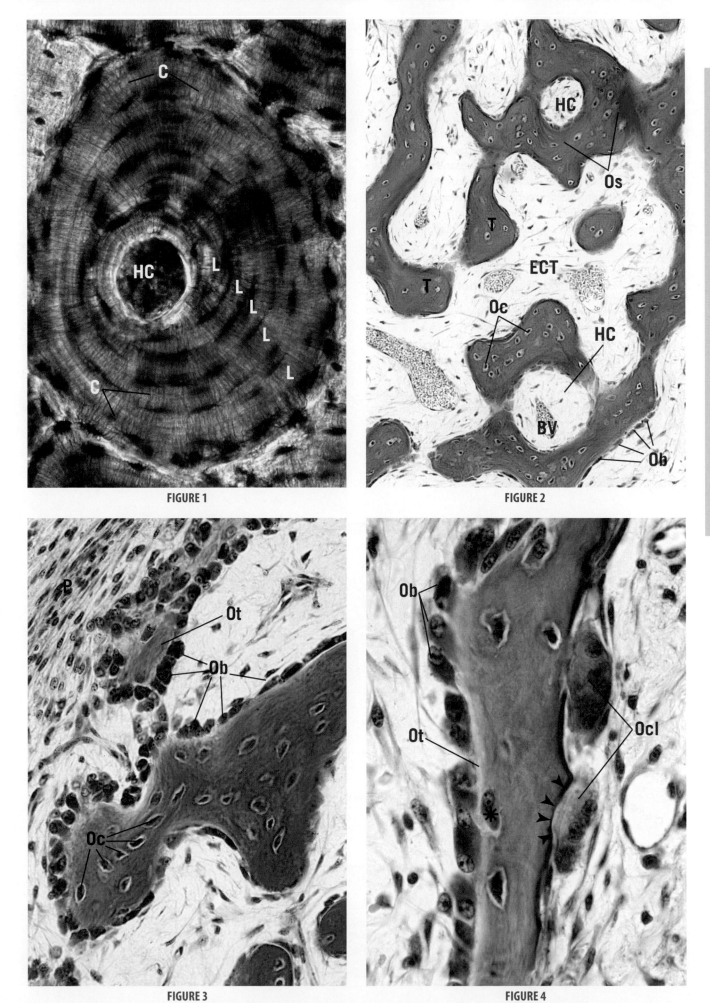

PLATE 4-4 • Compact Bone and Intramembranous Ossification

FIGURE 1

FIGURE 2

FIGURE 3

FIGURE 4

PLATE 4-5 · Endochondral Ossification

FIGURE 1.   Epiphyseal ossification center. Monkey. Paraffin section. ×14.

Most long bones are formed by the endochondral method of ossification, which involves the replacement of a cartilage model by bone. In this low-power photomicrograph, the **diaphysis** (D) of the lower phalanx has been replaced by bone, and the medullary cavity is filled with **marrow** (M). The **epiphysis** (E) of the same phalanx is undergoing ossification and is the **secondary center of ossification** (2°), thereby establishing the **epiphyseal plate** (ED). The **trabeculae** (T) are clearly evident on the diaphyseal side of the epiphyseal plate.

FIGURE 2.   Endochondral ossification. l.s. Monkey. Paraffin section. ×14.

Much of the cartilage has been replaced in the diaphysis of this forming bone. Note the numerous **trabeculae** (T) and the developing **bone marrow** (M) of the medullary cavity. Ossification is advancing toward the **epiphysis** (E), in which the secondary center of ossification has not yet appeared. Observe the **periosteum** (P), which appears as a definite line between the subperiosteal bone collar and the surrounding connective tissue. The *boxed area* is represented in Figure 3.

FIGURE 3.   Endochondral ossification. Monkey. Paraffin section. ×132.

This montage is a higher magnification of the *boxed area* of Figure 2. The region where the periosteum and perichondrium meet is evident (*arrowheads*). Deep to the periosteum is the **subperiosteal bone collar** (BC), which was formed via intramembranous ossification. Endochondral ossification is evident within the cartilage template. Starting at the top of the montage, note how the chondrocytes are lined up in long columns (*arrows*), indicative of their intense mitotic activity at the future epiphyseal plate region. In the epiphyseal plate, this will be the **zone of cell proliferation** (ZP). The chondrocytes increase in size in the **zone of cell maturation and hypertrophy** (ZH) and resorb some of their lacunar walls, enlarging them to such an extent that some of the lacunae become confluent. The chondrocytes die in the **zone of calcifying cartilage** (ZC). The presumptive medullary cavity is being populated by bone marrow, osteoclastic and osteogenic cells, and blood vessels. The osteogenic cells are actively differentiating into osteoblasts, which are elaborating bone on the calcified walls of the confluent lacunae. At the bottom of the photomicrograph, observe the bone-covered trabeculae of calcified cartilage (*asterisks*).

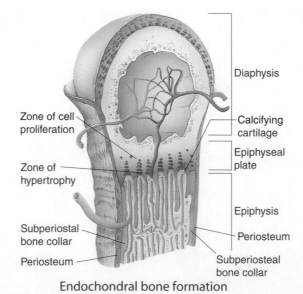

Endochondral bone formation

KEY					
BC	subperiosteal bone collar	P	periosteum	ZC	zone of calcifying cartilage
D	diaphysis	2°	secondary center of	ZH	zone of cell maturation and
E	epiphysis		ossification		hypertrophy
ED	epiphyseal plate	T	trabecula	ZP	zone of proliferation
M	marrow				

PLATE 4-5 · Endochondral Ossification

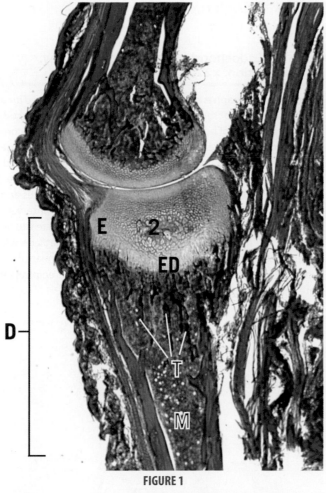

FIGURE 1

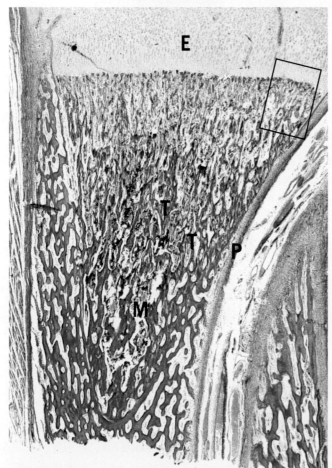

FIGURE 2

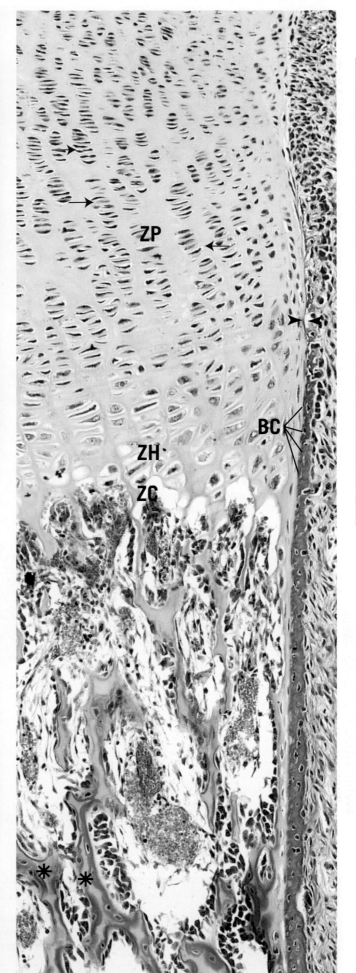

FIGURE 3

PLATE 4-6 • Endochondral Ossification

FIGURE 1. Endochondral ossification. Monkey. Paraffin section. ×132.

This photomicrograph is a higher magnification of a region of Plate 4-5, Figure 3. Observe the multinucleated osteoclast (*arrowheads*) resorbing the bone-covered trabeculae of calcified cartilage. The **subperiosteal bone collar** (BC) and the **periosteum** (P) are clearly evident, as is the junction between the bone collar and the cartilage (*arrows*). The medullary cavity is being established and is populated by **blood vessels** (BV), osteogenic cells, osteoblasts, and hematopoietic cells.

FIGURE 3. Endochondral ossification. x.s. Monkey. Paraffin section. ×196.

A cross section of the region of endochondral ossification presents many round spaces in calcified cartilage that are lined with bone (*asterisks*). These spaces represent confluent lacunae in the cartilage template, where the chondrocytes have hypertrophied and died. Subsequently, the cartilage-calcified and the invading osteogenic cells have differentiated into osteoblasts (*arrowheads*) and lined the calcified cartilage with bone. Since neighboring spaces were separated from each other by calcified cartilage walls, bone was elaborated on the sides of the walls. Therefore, these trabeculae, which in longitudinal section appear to be stalactite-like structures of bone with a calcified cartilaginous core, are, in fact, spaces in the cartilage template that are lined with bone. The walls between the spaces are the remnants of cartilage between lacunae that became calcified and form the substructure upon which bone was elaborated. Observe the forming **medullary cavity** (MC), housing **blood vessels** (BV), **hematopoietic tissue** (HT), osteogenic cells, and osteoblasts (*arrowheads*). The **subperiosteal bone collar** (BC) is evident and is covered by a **periosteum,** whose two layers, **fibrous** (FP) and **osteogenic** (Og), are clearly discernible.

PROPERTY OF LIBRARY
SOUTH UNIVERSITY CLEVELAND CAMPUS
WARRENSVILLE HEIGHTS, OH 44128

FIGURE 2. Endochondral ossification. Monkey. Paraffin section. ×270.

This photomicrograph is a higher magnification of the *boxed area* in Figure 1. Note that the trabeculae of calcified cartilage are covered by a thin layer of bone. The darker staining bone (*arrow*) contains osteocytes, whereas the lighter staining **calcified cartilage** (CC) is acellular, since the chondrocytes of this region have died, leaving behind empty lacunae that are confluent with each other. Observe that **osteoblasts** (Ob) line the trabecular complexes and that they are separated from the calcified bone by thin intervening **osteoid** (Ot). As the subperiosteal bone collar increases in thickness, the trabeculae of bone-covered calcified cartilage will be resorbed so that the cartilage template will be replaced by bone. The only cartilage that will remain will be the epiphyseal plate and the articular covering of the epiphysis.

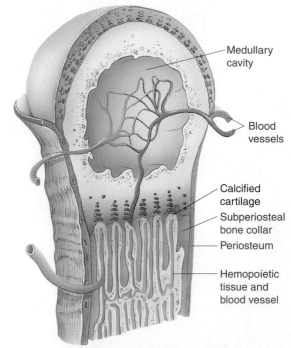

Endochondral bone formation

KEY					
BC	subperiosteal bone collar	**HT**	hematopoietic tissue	**Og**	osteogenic periosteum
BV	blood vessel	**MC**	medullary cavity	**Ot**	osteoid
CC	calcified cartilage	**Ob**	osteoblast	**P**	periosteum
FP	fibrous periosteum				

PLATE 4-6 · Endochondral Ossification

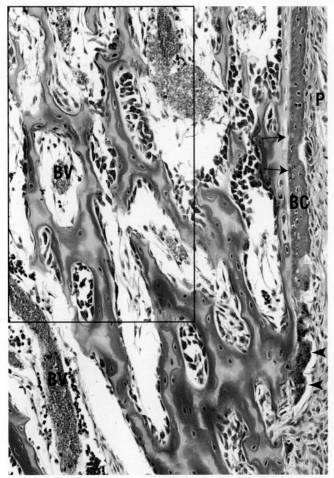

FIGURE 1

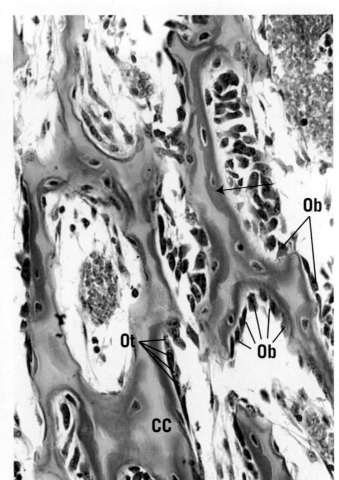

FIGURE 2

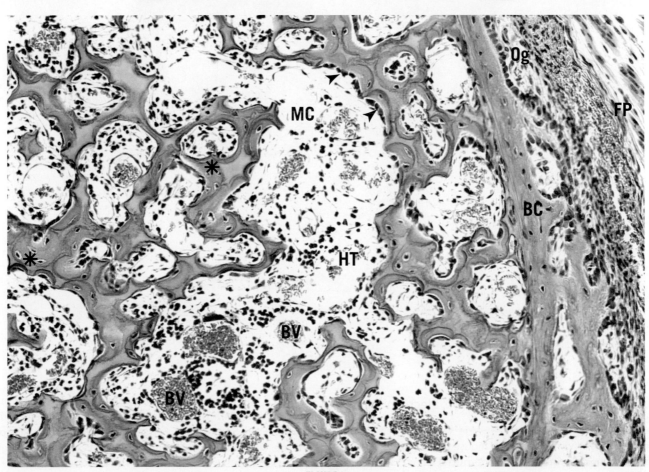

FIGURE 3

PLATE 4-7 • Hyaline Cartilage, Electron Microscopy

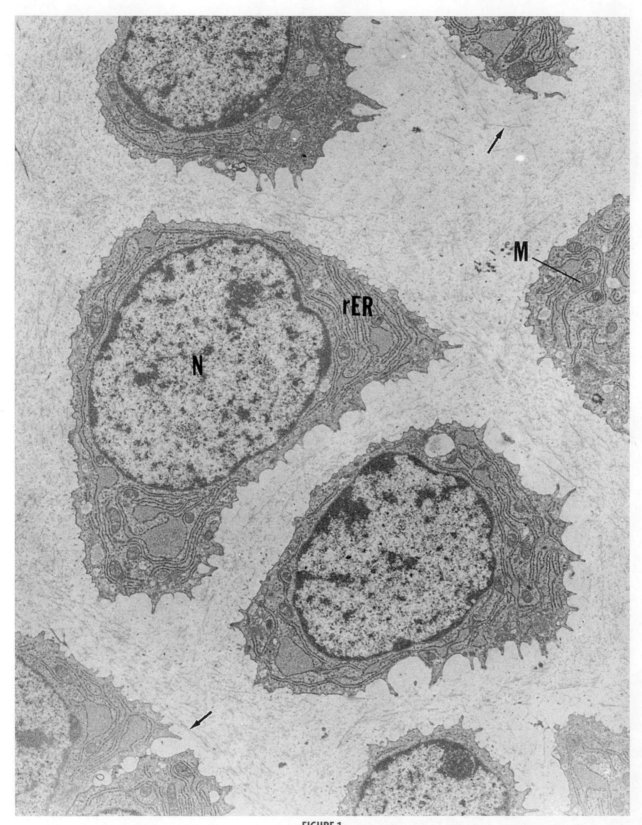

FIGURE 1

FIGURE 1. Hyaline cartilage. Mouse. Electron microscopy. ×6,120.

The hyaline cartilage of a neonatal mouse trachea presents chondrocytes, whose centrally positioned **nuclei** (N) are surrounded with a rich **rough endoplasmic reticulum** (rER) and numerous **mitochondria** (M). The matrix displays fine collagen fibrils (*arrows*). (From Seegmiller R, Ferguson C, Sheldon H. Studies on cartilage, VI: a genetically determined defect in tracheal cartilage. J Ultrastruct Res 1972;38:288–301.)

PLATE 4-8 • Osteoblasts, Electron Microscopy

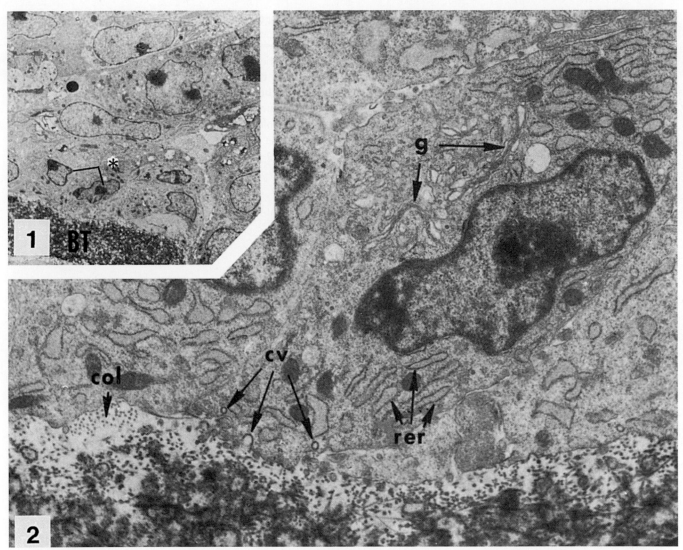

FIGURE 1 and 2

FIGURE 1. Osteoblasts from long bone. Rat. Electron microscopy. ×1,350.

This low-magnification electron micrograph displays numerous fibroblasts and osteoblasts in the vicinity of a **bony trabecula** (BT). The osteoblasts (*asterisk*) are presented at a higher magnification in Figure 2. (From Ryder M, Jenkins S, Horton J. The adherence to bone by cytoplasmic elements of osteoclast. J Dent Res 1981;60:1349–1355.)

FIGURE 2. Osteoblasts. Rat. Electron microscopy. ×9,450.

Osteoblasts, at higher magnification, present well-developed **Golgi apparatus** (g), extensive **rough endoplasmic reticulum** (rer), and several **coated vacuoles** (cv) at the basal cell membrane. Observe the cross sections of **collagen fibers** (col) in the bone matrix. (From Ryder M, Jenkins S, Horton J. The adherence to bone by cytoplasmic elements of osteoclast. J Dent Res 1981;60:1349–1355.)

PLATE 4-9 • Osteoclast, Electron Microscopy

FIGURE 1a. Osteoclast from long bone. Rat. Electron microscopy. ×1,800.

Two nuclei of an osteoclast are evident in this section. Observe that the cell is surrounding a bony surface (*asterisk*). The region of the nucleus marked by an *arrowhead* is presented at a higher magnification in Figure 1B.

FIGURE 2. Osteoclasts. Human. Paraffin section. ×600.

The nuclei (N) of these multinuclear cells are located in their **basal region** (BR), away from **Howship's lacunae** (HL). Note that the **ruffled border** (*arrowheads*) is in intimate contact with Howship's lacunae. (Courtesy of Dr. J. Hollinger.)

FIGURE 1b. Osteoclast. Rat. Electron microscopy. ×10,800.

This is a higher magnification of a region of Figure 1A. Note the presence of the **nucleus** (N) and its **nucleolus** (n), as well as the **ruffled border** (RB) and **clear zone** (CZ) of the osteoclast. Numerous **vacuoles** (v) of various sizes may be observed throughout the cytoplasm. (From Ryder M, Jenkins S, Horton J. The adherence to bone by cytoplasmic elements of osteoclast. J Dent Res 1981;60:1349–1355.)

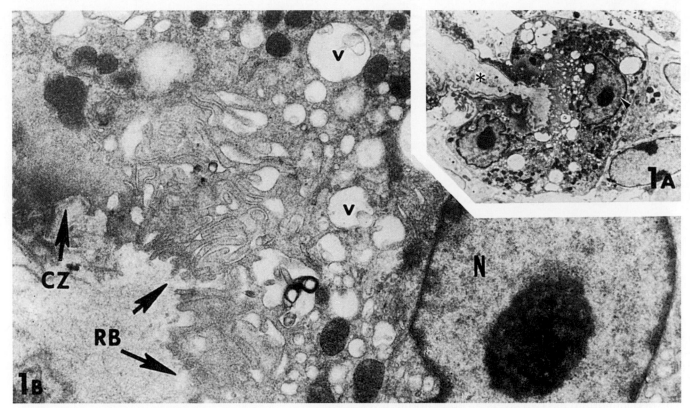

FIGURE 1

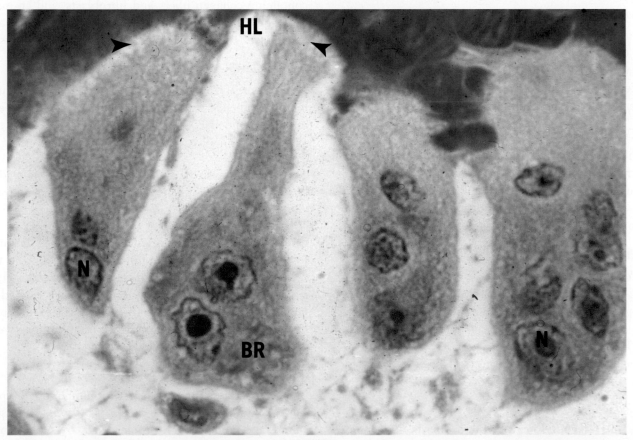

FIGURE 2

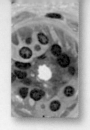

Chapter Summary

I. CARTILAGE

A. Embryonic Cartilage

1. Perichondrium

The **perichondrium** is very thin and cellular.

2. Matrix

The **matrix** is scanty and smooth in appearance.

3. Cells

Numerous, small, round **chondrocytes** are housed in small spaces in the matrix. These spaces are known as **lacunae.**

B. Hyaline Cartilage

1. Perichondrium

The perichondrium has two layers, an outer **fibrous layer**, which contains collagen and fibroblasts, and an inner **chondrogenic layer,** which contains **chondrogenic cells** and **chondroblasts.**

2. Matrix

The **matrix** is smooth and basophilic in appearance. It has two regions, the **territorial (capsular) matrix,** which is darker and surrounds **lacunae**, and the **interterritorial (intercapsular) matrix**, which is lighter in color. The collagen fibrils are masked by the ground substance.

3. Cells

Either **chondrocytes** are found individually in **lacunae** or there may be two or more chondrocytes (**isogenous group**) in a lacuna. The latter case signifies **interstitial growth. Appositional growth** occurs just deep to the perichondrium and is attributed to **chondroblasts.**

C. Elastic Cartilage

1. Perichondrium

The perichondrium is the same in elastic cartilage as in hyaline cartilage, but also has elastic fibers.

2. Matrix

The **matrix** contains numerous dark **elastic fibers** in addition to the **collagen fibrils.**

3. Cells

The cells are **chondrocytes, chondroblasts,** and **chondrogenic cells,** as in hyaline cartilage.

D. Fibrocartilage

1. Perichondrium

The perichondrium is usually absent.

2. Matrix

The **ground substance** of matrix is very scanty. Many thick collagen bundles are located between parallel rows of chondrocytes.

3. Cells

The **chondrocytes** in fibrocartilage are smaller than those in hyaline or elastic cartilage, and they are arranged in parallel longitudinal rows between bundles of thick collagen fibers.

II. BONE

A. Decalcified Compact Bone

1. Periosteum

The **periosteum** has two layers, an outer **fibrous layer**, containing **collagen fibers** and **fibroblasts**, and an inner **osteogenic layer**, containing **osteoprogenitor cells** and **osteoblasts.** It is anchored to bone by **Sharpey's fibers.**

2. Lamellar Systems

Lamellar organization consists of **outer** and **inner circumferential lamellae, osteons (haversian canal systems),** and **interstitial lamellae.**

3. Endosteum

The **endosteum** is a thin membrane that lines the **medullary cavity,** which contains **yellow** or **white bone marrow.**

4. Cells

Osteocytes are housed in small spaces called **lacunae. Osteoblasts** and **osteoprogenitor cells** are found in the osteogenic layer of the periosteum, in the endosteum, and lining haversian canals. **Osteoclasts** are located in **Howship's lacunae** along resorptive surfaces of bone. **Osteoid,** noncalcified bone matrix, is interposed between the cells of bone and the calcified tissue.

5. Vascular Supply

Blood vessels are found in the periosteum, in the marrow cavity, and in the haversian canals of osteons. Haversian canals are connected to each other by Volkmann's canals.

B. Undecalcified Compact Ground Bone

1. Lamellar Systems

The lamellar organization is clearly evident as wafer-thin layers or **lamellae** constituting bone. They are then organized as **outer** and **inner circumferential lamellae, osteons,** and **interstitial lamellae.**

Osteons are cylindrical structures composed of concentric lamellae of bone. Their **lacunae** are empty, but in living bone, they contain osteocytes. **Canaliculi** radiate from **lacunae** toward the central **haversian canal,** which in living bone houses blood vessels, osteoblasts, and osteoprogenitor cells. **Cementing lines** demarcate the peripheral extent of each osteon. **Volkmann's canals** interconnect neighboring haversian canals.

C. Decalcified Cancellous Bone

1. Lamellar Systems

Lamellar organization consists of **spicules** and **trabeculae** of bone.

2. Cells

Cells are as before in that **osteocytes** are housed in lacunae. **Osteoblasts** line all trabeculae and spicules. Occasionally, multinuclear, large **osteoclasts** occupy **Howship's lacunae. Osteoid,** noncalcified bone matrix, is interposed between the cells of bone and the calcified tissue.

Bone marrow occupies the spaces among and between trabeculae.

D. Intramembranous Ossification

1. Ossification Centers

Centers of ossification are vascularized areas of **mesenchymal connective tissue** where **mesenchymal cells** probably differentiate into **osteoprogenitor cells,** which differentiate into **osteoblasts.**

2. Lamellar Systems

Lamellar organization begins when **spicules** and **trabeculae** form into primitive osteons surrounding blood vessels. The first bone formed is **primary bone (woven bone),** whose cells are larger and whose fibrillar arrangement is haphazard compared with **secondary (mature) bone.**

3. Cells

The cellular elements of intramembranous ossification are **osteoprogenitor cells, osteoblasts, osteocytes,** and **osteoclasts.** Additionally, mesenchymal and hemopoietic cells are also present.

E. Endochondral Ossification

1. Primary Ossification Center

The **perichondrium** of the **diaphysis** of the cartilage template becomes vascularized, followed by **hypertrophy** of the centrally located chondrocytes, confluence of contiguous lacunae, calcification of the cartilage remnants, and subsequent **chondrocytic death.** Concomitant with these events, the **chondrogenic cells** of the perichondrium become **osteoprogenitor cells,** which, in turn, differentiate into **osteoblasts.** The osteoblasts form the **subperiosteal bone collar,** thus converting the overlying **perichondrium** into a **periosteum.** A **periosteal bud** invades the diaphysis, entering the confluent **lacunae** left empty by the death of chondrocytes. Osteogenic cells give rise to osteoblasts, which elaborate bone on the **trabeculae of calcified cartilage.** Hemopoiesis begins in the primitive medullary cavity; **osteoclasts** (and, according to some, chondroclasts) develop, which resorb the bone-covered trabeculae of calcified cartilage as the subperiosteal bone collar becomes thicker and elongated.

2. Secondary Ossification Center

The **epiphyseal (secondary) center of ossification** is initiated somewhat after birth. It begins in the center of the epiphysis and proceeds radially from that point, leaving cartilage only at the **articular surface** and at the interface between the epiphysis and the diaphysis, the future **epiphyseal plate.**

3. Epiphyseal Plate

The **epiphyseal plate** is responsible for the future lengthening of a long bone. It is divided into five zones: (1) **zone of reserve cartilage,** a region of haphazardly arranged chondrocytes; (2) **zone of cell proliferation,** where chondrocytes are arranged in rows whose longitudinal axis parallels that of the growing bone; (3) **zone of cell maturation and hypertrophy,** where cells enlarge and the matrix between adjoining cells becomes very thin; (4) **zone of calcifying cartilage,** where lacunae become confluent and the matrix between adjacent rows of chondrocytes becomes calcified, causing subsequent chondrocytic death; and (5) **zone of provisional ossification,** where osteoblasts deposit bone on the calcified cartilage remnants between the adjacent rows. Osteoclasts (and, according to some, chondroclasts) resorb the calcified complex.

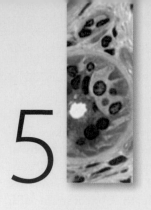

5 BLOOD AND HEMOPOIESIS

The total volume of blood in an average person is approximately 5 L; it is a **specialized type of connective tissue,** composed of cells, cell fragments, and plasma, a fluid extracellular element. Blood circulates throughout the body and is well adapted for its manifold functions in transporting nutrients, oxygen, waste products, carbon dioxide, hormones, cells, and other substances. Moreover, blood also functions in the maintenance of body temperature.

FORMED ELEMENTS OF BLOOD

The formed elements of blood are red blood cells (erythrocytes), white blood cells (leukocytes), and platelets. The nomenclature developed for these formed elements is based on their colorations with Wright's or Giemsa's modification of the Romanovsky-type stains as applied to blood and marrow smears used in hematology. (Table 5-1)

- **Red blood cells (RBCs),** the most populous, are anucleated and function entirely within the circulatory system by transporting oxygen and carbon dioxide to and from the tissues of the body (*see Chapter 12, Respiratory System*).
- **White blood cells (WBCs)** perform their functions outside the circulatory system and use the bloodstream as a mode of transportation to reach their destinations.
- There are two major categories of white blood cells, agranulocytes and granulocytes. Lymphocytes and monocytes compose the first group, whereas neutrophils, eosinophils, and basophils compose the latter and are recognizable by their distinctive specific granules.
  - **Lymphocytes** are the basic cells of the immune system and, although there are three categories (**T lymphocytes, B lymphocytes,** and **null cells**), special immunocytochemical techniques are necessary for their identification.
  - When **monocytes** leave the bloodstream and enter the connective tissue spaces, they become known as **macrophages,** cells that function in phagocytosis of particulate matter, as well as in assisting lymphocytes in their immunologic activities (*see Chapter 9, Lymphoid System*).

TABLE 5-1 • Formed Elements of Blood

Element	Diameter (μm) Smear	Section	No./μm³	% of Leukocytes	Granules	Function	Nucleus
Erythrocyte	7–8	6–7	5×10^6 (males) 4.5×10^6 (females)		None	Transport of O_2 and CO_2	None
Lymphocyte	8–10	7–8	1,500–2,500	20–25	Azurophilic only	Immunologic response	Large round acentric
Monocyte	12–15	10–12	200–800	3–8	Azurophilic only	Phagocytosis	Large, kidney-shaped
Neutrophil	9–12	8–9	3,500–7,000	60–70	Azurophilic and small specific (neutrophilic)	Phagocytosis	Polymorphous
Eosinophil	10–14	9–11	150–400	2–4	Azurophilic and large specific (eosinophilic)	Phagocytosis of antigen-antibody complexes and control of parasitic diseases	Bilobed (sausage-shaped)
Basophil	8–10	7–8	50–100	0.5–1	Azurophilic and large specific (basophilic) granules (heparin and histamine)	Perhaps phagocytosis	Large, S-shaped
Platelets	2–4	1–3	250,000–400,000		Granulomere	Agglutination and clotting	None

- Granules of **neutrophils** possess very limited affinity to stains. Neutrophils function in **phagocytosis** of bacteria, and because of that, they are frequently referred to as microphages.
- **Eosinophils** stain a reddish-orange color; they participate in antiparasitic activities and phagocytose antigen-antibody complexes.
- **Basophils** stain a dark blue color with dyes used in studying blood preparations. Although the precise function of basophils is unknown, the contents of their granules are similar to those of mast cells, and they also release the same pharmacologic agents via degranulation. Additionally, basophils also produce and release other pharmacologic agents from the arachidonic acid in their membranes.
- Circulating blood also contains cell fragments known as **platelets** (**thrombocytes**). These small, oval-to-round structures, derived from **megakaryocytes** of the bone marrow, function in hemostasis, the clotting mechanism of blood.

Lymphocytes

The three types of lymphocytes—B lymphocytes (B cells), T lymphocytes (T cells), and null cells—are morphologically indistinguishable. It is customary to speak of **T cells** as being responsible for the **cellularly mediated immune response** and **B cells** as functioning in the **humorally mediated immune response. Null cells** are few in number, possess no determinants on their cell membrane, and are of two types, **pluripotential hemopoietic stem cells (PHSCs)** and **natural killer (NK) cells.**

- **T cells** not only function in the cellularly mediated immune response but also are responsible for the formation of cytokines that facilitate the initiation of the humorally mediated immune response.
  - T cells are formed in the bone marrow and migrate to the thymic cortex to become immunocompetent cells. They recognize **epitopes** (antigenic determinants) that are displayed by cells possessing **HLA** (human leukocyte antigen; also known as major histocompatibility complex molecules).
  - There are various subtypes of T cells, each possessing a **T-cell receptor (TCR)** surface determinant and **cluster of differentiation determinants (CD molecules).** The former recognizes the epitope, whereas the latter recognizes the type of HLA on the displaying cell surface.

The various subtypes of T cells are memory T cells, T helper cells (T_H0, T_H1, T_H2, and T_H17), cytotoxic T cells (CTLs), T regulatory cell (T_{reg}), natural T killer cells, and T memory cells (see Chapter 9, Lymphoid Tissue, for additional information).

- **B cells** bear HLA type II (also known as MHC II) surface markers and **surface immunoglobulins (SIGs)** on their plasmalemma. They are formed in and become immunocompetent in the bone marrow. They are responsible for the humoral response and, under the direction of T_H2 cells and in response to an antigenic challenge, will differentiate into antibody-manufacturing **plasma cells** and **B memory cells.**
- **Null Cells** are of two types, PHSCs and NK cells.
  - **Pluripotential hemopoietic stem cells** resemble lymphocytes and are responsible for the formation of all of the formed elements of blood.
  - **NK cells** belong to the null cell population. They possess F_C receptors but no cell surface determinants and are responsible for nonspecific cytotoxicity against virus-infected and tumor cells. They also function in antibody-dependent cell-mediated cytotoxicity.

Neutrophils

Neutrophils have multilobed nuclei and possess three types of granules—specific granules, azurophilic granules, and tertiary granules.

- **Specific granules** contain pharmacologic agents and enzymes that permit the neutrophils to perform their antimicrobial roles.
- **Azurophilic granules** are lysosomes, containing the various lysosomal hydrolases, as well as myeloperoxidase, bacterial permeability increasing protein, lysozyme, and collagenase.
- **Tertiary granules** contain glycoproteins that are dedicated for insertion into the cell membrane, as well as gelatinase and cathepsins.

Neutrophils use the contents of the three types of granules to perform their antimicrobial function. When neutrophils arrive at their site of action, they exocytose the contents of their granules.

- **Gelatinase** increases the neutrophil's capability of migrating through the basal lamina, and the glycoproteins of the tertiary granules aids in the recognition and phagocytosis of bacteria into phagosomes of the neutrophil.
- Azurophilic granules and specific granules fuse with and release their hydrolytic enzymes into the phagosomes, thus initiating the enzymatic degradation of the microorganisms.

In addition to the enzymatic degradation, microorganisms are also destroyed by the capability of neutrophils to undergo a sudden increase in O_2 utilization, known as a respiratory burst.

- The O_2 is used by neutrophils to form superoxides, hydrogen peroxide, and hypochlorous acid, highly reactive compounds that destroy bacteria within the phagosomes.
- Frequently, the avid response of neutrophils results in the release of some of these highly potent compounds into the surrounding connective tissue precipitating tissue damage.
- Neutrophils also produce leukotrienes from plasmalemma arachidonic acids to aid in the initiation of an inflammatory response.
- Subsequent to the performance of these functions, the neutrophils die and become a major component of pus.

PLASMA

Plasma, the fluid component of blood, comprises approximately 55% of the total blood volume.

- Plasma contains electrolytes and ions, such as calcium, sodium, potassium, and bicarbonate; larger molecules, namely, **albumins, globulins,** and **fibrinogen;** and organic compounds as varied as amino acids, lipids, vitamins, hormones, and cofactors.
- Subsequent to clotting, a straw-colored **serum** is expressed from blood. This fluid is identical to plasma but contains no fibrinogen or other components necessary for the clotting reaction.

COAGULATION

Coagulation is the result of the exquisitely controlled interaction of a number of plasma proteins and coagulation factors. The regulatory mechanisms are in place so that coagulation typically occurs only if the endothelial lining of the vessel becomes injured.

- In the intact blood vessel, the endothelium manufactures inhibitors of platelet aggregation (NO and prostacyclins) as well as display agents, thrombomodulin and heparin-like molecule, on their luminal plasmalemmae that block coagulation.
- If the lining of a blood vessel is damaged, the endothelial cells switch from producing and displaying antiaggregation and anticoagulation agents and release **tissue factor** (tissue thromboplastin), **von Willebrand's factor** and **endothelins.**
- Tissue factor complexes with **Factor VIIa** to catalyze the conversion of Factor X to its active form, the protease **Factor Xa;**
- von Willebrand's factor activates platelets, facilitating the adhesion of platelets to the exposed laminin and collagens and induces them to release ADP and thrombospondin, which encourages their adhesion to each other; and endothelin stimulates the contraction of vascular smooth muscle cells in the region to constrict the damaged blood vessel and, thus, minimize blood loss.
- The process of coagulation ensues in one of two convergent pathways, **extrinsic** and **intrinsic,** both of which lead to the final step of converting fibrinogen to fibrin.
  - The extrinsic pathway has a faster onset and depends on the release of tissue factor.
  - The intrinsic pathway is initiated slower, is dependent on contact between vessel wall collagen and platelets (or factor XII), and requires the presence of von Willebrand's factor and **factor VIII.**
    - These two factors form a complex that not only binds to exposed collagen but also attaches to receptor sites on the platelet plasmalemma, affecting platelet aggregation and adherence to the vessel wall.
- The two pathways intersect at the conversion of Factor X to Factor Xa and from that point on the remaining steps of the coagulation pathway are referred to as the **common pathway**.

HEMOPOIESIS

Circulating blood cells have relatively short life spans and must be replaced continuously by newly formed cells. This process of blood cell replacement is known as **hemopoiesis** (hematopoiesis).

- All blood cells develop from a single pluripotential precursor cell known as the pluripotential hemopoietic stem cell (PHSC).
- These cells undergo mitotic activity, whereby they give rise to two types of **multipotential hemopoietic stem cells, CFU-GEMM** (Colony-forming unit-granulocyte, erythrocyte, monocyte, megakaryocyte, previously known as CHU-S) and **CFU-Ly (colony-forming unit-lymphocyte)**.

Most PHSCs and other hemopoietic stem cells of adults are located in the **red bone marrow** of short and flat bones. The marrow of long bones is red in young individuals, but when it becomes infiltrated by fat in the adult, it takes on a yellow appearance and is known as yellow marrow.

- Although it was once believed that adipose cells accumulated the fat, it is now known that the cells actually responsible for storing fat in the marrow are the **adventitial reticular cells**.
- Stem cells, in response to various hemopoietic growth factors, undergo cell division and maintain the population of circulating erythrocytes, leukocytes, and platelets.

As stated above, the nomenclature developed for the cells described below is based on their colorations with Wright's or Giemsa's modification of the Romanovsky-type stains as applied to blood and marrow smears used in hematology.

Erythrocytic Series

- Erythrocyte development proceeds from **CFU-S**, which, in response to elevated levels of **erythropoietin**, gives rise to cells known as BFU-E, which, in response to lower erythropoietin levels, then give rise to CFU-E.
- Later generations of **CFU-E** are recognizable histologically as **proerythroblasts.**
  - These cells give rise to **basophilic erythroblasts**, which, in turn, undergo cell division to form
  - **polychromatophilic erythroblasts** that will divide mitotically to form
  - **orthochromatophilic erythroblasts (normoblasts).** Cells of this stage no longer divide.
  - will extrude their nuclei, and differentiate into **reticulocytes** (not to be confused with reticular cells of connective tissue), which, in turn, become mature red blood cells.
    - Reticulocytes are stained with methylene blue for manual or thiazole orange for automated counting.

Granulocytic Series

The development of the granulocytic series is initiated from the multipotential **CFU-S.**

- The first histologically distinguishable member of this series is the **myeloblast,** which gives rise mitotically to
- **promyelocytes,** which also undergo cell division to yield
- **myelocytes.** Myelocytes are the first cells of this series to possess specific granules; therefore, neutrophilic, eosinophilic, and basophilic myelocytes may be recognized.
- The next cells in the series are **metamyelocytes,** which no longer divide, but differentiate into
- **band (stab)** cells, the juvenile form, which will become mature granulocytes that enter the bloodstream.

Several **hemopoietic growth factors** activate and promote hemopoiesis. These act by binding to plasma membrane receptors of their target cell, controlling their mitotic rate, as well as the number of mitotic events. Additionally, they stimulate cell differentiation and enhance the survival of the progenitor cell population (Table 5-2). The best known factors are **erythropoietin** (acts on BFU-E and CFU-E),

- **interleukin-3** (acts on PHSC, CFU-S, and myeloid progenitor cells),
- **interleukin-7** (acts on CFU-Ly),
- **granulocyte-macrophage colony-stimulating factor** (acts on granulocyte and monocyte progenitor cells),
- **granulocyte colony-stimulating factor** (acts on granulocyte progenitor cells), and
- **macrophage colony-stimulating factor** (acts on monocyte progenitor cells).

TABLE 5-2 • Hemopoietic Growth Factors

Factors	Principal Action of the Factor	Site of Origin of the Factor
Stem cell factor	Facilitates hemopoiesis	Stromal cells of bone marrow
GM-CSF	Facilitates CFU-GM mitosis, differentiation, granulocyte activity	T cells, endothelial cells
G-CSF	Induces mitosis, differentiation of CFU-G; facilitates neutrophil activity	Macrophages, endothelial cells
M-CSF	Facilitates mitosis, differentiation of CFU-M	Macrophages, endothelial cells
IL-1 (IL-3, IL-6)	Facilitates proliferation of PHSC, CFU-S, CFU-Ly; suppresses erythroid precursors	Monocytes, macrophages, endothelial cells
IL-2	Promotes proliferation of activated T cells, B cells; facilitates NK cell differentiation	Activated T cells
IL-3	Same as IL-1; also facilitates proliferation of unipotential precursors except LyB and LyT	Activated T and B cells
IL-4	Promotes activation of T cells, B cells; facilitates development of mast cells, basophils	Activated T cells
IL-5	Facilitates proliferation of CFU-Eo; activates eosinophils	T cells
IL-6	Same as IL-1; also promotes differentiation of CTLs and B cells	Monocyte, fibroblasts
IL-7	Stimulates CFU-LyB and NK cell differentiation	Adventitial reticular cells
IL-8	Promotes migration and degranulation of neutrophils	Leukocytes, endothelial cells, smooth muscle cells
IL-9	Promotes activation, proliferation of mast cells, modulates IgE synthesis, stimulates proliferation of T helper cells	T helper cells
IL-10	Inhibits synthesis of cytokines by NK cells, macrophages, T cells; promotes CTL differentiation and B-cell and mast cell proliferation	Macrophages, T cells
IL-12	Stimulates NK cells; promotes CTL and NK cell function	Macrophages
γ-Interferons	Activates monocytes, B cells; promotes CTL differentiation; enhances expression of class II HLA	T cells, NK cells
Erythropoietin	Promotes CFU-E differentiation, proliferation of BFU-E	Endothelial cells of peritubular capillary network of kidney, hepatocytes
Thrombopoietin	Enhances mitosis, differentiation of CFU-Meg and megakaryoblasts	Not known

CTL, cytotoxic lymphocyte; CFU, colony-forming unit (Eo, eosinophil; G, granulocyte; GM, granulocyte-monocyte; Ly, lymphocyte; S, spleen); CSF, colony-stimulating factor (G, granulocyte; GM, granulocyte-monocyte; M, monocyte); HLA, human leukocyte antigen; IL, interleukin.
Modified with permission from Gartner LP, Hiatt JL. Color Textbook of Histology, 2nd ed. Philadelphia: Saunders, 2001.

CLINICAL CONSIDERATIONS

NADPH Oxidase Deficiency

Certain individuals suffer from persistent bacterial infection due to a hereditary NADPH oxidase deficiency. The neutrophils of these individuals are unable to effect a respiratory burst and, therefore, are incapable of forming the highly reactive compounds, such as hypochlorous acid, hydrogen peroxide, and superoxide, that assist in the killing of bacteria within their phagosomes.

Multiple Myeloma

Multiple myeloma is a relatively uncommon malignant neoplasm with greater incidence in males than females. Its origin is the bone marrow and is characterized by the presence of large numbers of malignant plasma cells that may also be abnormal in morphology. These cells accumulate in the bone marrow of various regions of the skeletal system. Frequently, the cell proliferation is so great in the marrow that the huge number of cells place pressure on the walls of the marrow cavity causing bone pains and even fractures of bones such as the ribs. These cells also produce abnormal proteins such as Bence-Jones proteins that enter the urine where they can be detected to provide a diagnosis for multiple myeloma.

Infectious Mononucleosis

Infection with the Epstein-Barr virus causes infectious mononucleosis, also referred to as the "kissing disease," because it is common among high school and college-aged individuals and is frequently spread by saliva. The symptoms of patients suffering from infectious mononucleosis include sore throat, swollen and painful lymph nodes, low energy, and an elevated lymphocyte count. The disease can be life-threatening in immunosuppressed individuals.

Polycythemia Vera

Polycythemia vera (**primary polycythemia**) is a rare disorder of the blood that manifests itself by an excess production of red blood cells and, frequently, platelets, resulting in greater blood volume and an increase in the viscosity of blood. It mainly involves individuals who are in their early sixties, although occasionally it occurs in patients who are in their early twenties. Symptoms

may be absent for a number of years after the onset of the condition, but patients suffering from this disorder may exhibit headaches, vertigo, fatigue, shortness of breath, enlarged liver and spleen, burning sensation in the extremities, visual disorders, as well as gingival bleeding, and generalized itching. If left untreated, the patient may die within 2 years, but with proper treatment, the lifespan can be extended by 10 to 20 years.

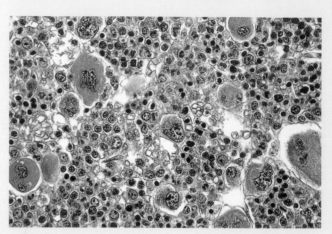

This is a bone marrow biopsy from a middle-aged woman suffering from polycythemia vera. Observe that the marrow is hypercellular exhibiting an abnormally high number of erythrocyte precursors and megakaryocytes. (Reprinted with permission from Mills SE, Carter D, Greenson JK, Reuter VE, Stoler MH eds. Sternberger's Diagnostic Surgical Pathology, 5th ed. Philadelphia: Lippincott Williams & Wilkins 2010. p. 635.)

B-Cell Prolymphocytic Leukemia

B-cell prolymphocytic leukemia is a relatively rare form of leukemia that arises relatively late in life, around 60 years of age, and affects males more frequently than females. The histopathologic picture presents bone marrow smears and blood smears with medium to large prolymphocytes. Usually, the disease is accompanied by an enlargement of the spleen. The prognosis is not good because this type of leukemia is quite aggressive and treatment modalities are not very effective; in fact, they are mostly palliative, and usually the patient succumbs in two or three years.

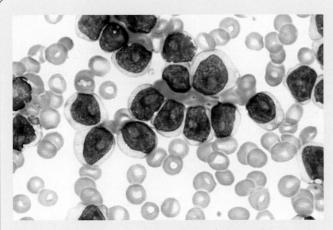

This blood smear, from a patient suffering from B-cell prolympho-cytic leukemia, displays numerous large prolymphocytes whose nucleus presents a coarse chromatin network and large vesicles. (Reprinted with permission from Mills SE, Carter D, Greenson JK, Reuter VE, Stoler MH eds. Sternberger's Diagnostic Surgical Pathology, 5th ed.., 2010. P. 644.)

Sickle Cell Anemia

Sickle cell anemia, a hereditary disease, is the result of a point mutation in the gene that codes for hemoglobin. A single amino acid substitution of alanine replacing glu-tamine occurs in some individuals who are descendants of the indigenous population of tropical and subtropi-cal regions of Africa, especially from the sub-Saharan area. Approximately 2 per 1,000 African Americans are afflicted with this disease, and 10% of that population carry one copy of the gene and, therefore, are carriers of the trait but are not afflicted by the disease. The red blood cells of patients with two copies of the gene are defective and carry a reduced amount of oxygen. These erythrocytes are fragile, do not pass easily through small capillaries, and assume a sickle shape. The abnormally shaped red blood cells have a deleterious effect on the kidneys, brain, bones, and spleen among other organs. Depending on the severity of the condition, the patient's symptoms may vary from slight to severe, and in the lat-ter case, it may result in death at an early age. Since sickle cell anemia is incurable, it is treated with avoidance of strenuous physical exertions, avoiding high altitudes, and instructing patients to seek treatment for even minor infections.

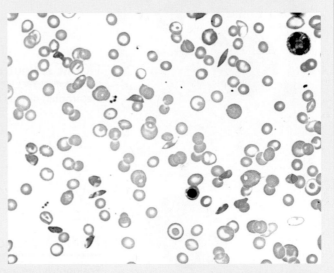

This blood smear, from a patient suffering from sickle cell anemia, displays numerous red blood cells that are distorted so that they appear spindle-shaped.

PLATE 5-1 · Circulating Blood

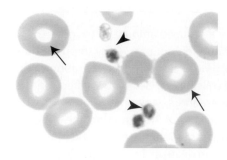

FIGURE 1. Red blood cells. Human. ×1,325.

RBCs (*arrows*) display a central clear region that represents the thinnest area of the biconcave disc. Note that the platelets (*arrowheads*) possess a central dense region, the granulomere, and a peripheral light region, the hyalomere.

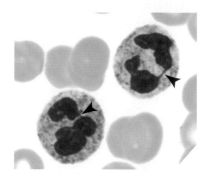

FIGURE 2. Neutrophils. Human. ×1,325.

Neutrophils display a somewhat granular cytoplasm and lobulated (*arrowheads*) nuclei.

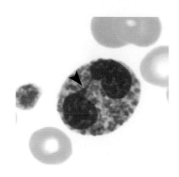

FIGURE 3. Eosinophils. Human. ×1,325.

Eosinophils are recognized by their large, pink granules and their sausage-shaped nucleus. Observe the slender connecting link (*arrowhead*) between the two lobes of the nucleus.

PLATE 5-1 · Circulating Blood

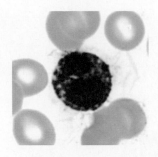

FIGURE 4. Basophils. Human. ×1,325.

Basophils are characterized by their dense, dark, large granules.

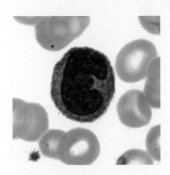

FIGURE 5. Monocytes. Human. ×1,325.

Monocytes are characterized by their large size, acentric, kidney-shaped nucleus and lack of specific granules.

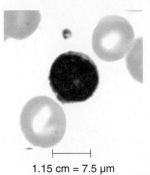

FIGURE 6. Lymphocytes. Human. ×1,325.

Lymphocytes are small cells that possess a single, large, acentrically located nucleus and a narrow rim of light blue cytoplasm.

1.15 cm = 7.5 μm

PLATE 5-2 · Circulating Blood (Drawing)

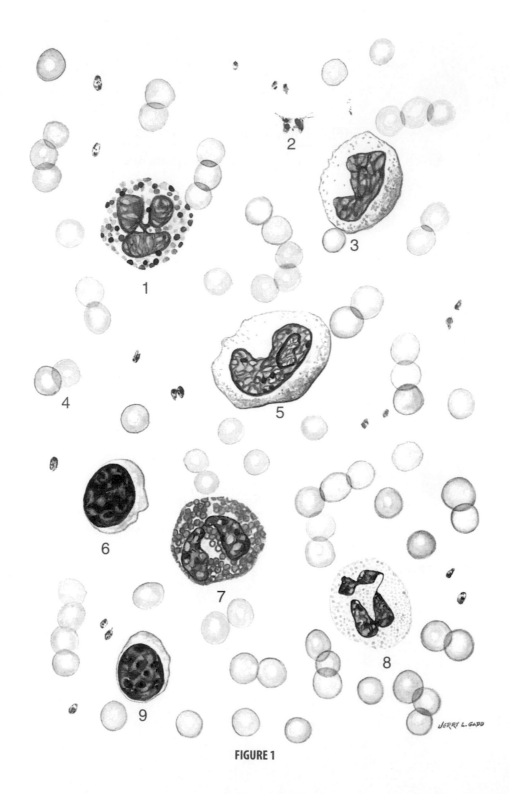

FIGURE 1

JERRY L. GADD

KEY

1. Basophil
2. Platelets
3. Monocyte

4. Erythrocytes
5. Monocyte
6. Lymphocyte

7. Eosinophil
8. Neutrophil
9. Lymphocyte

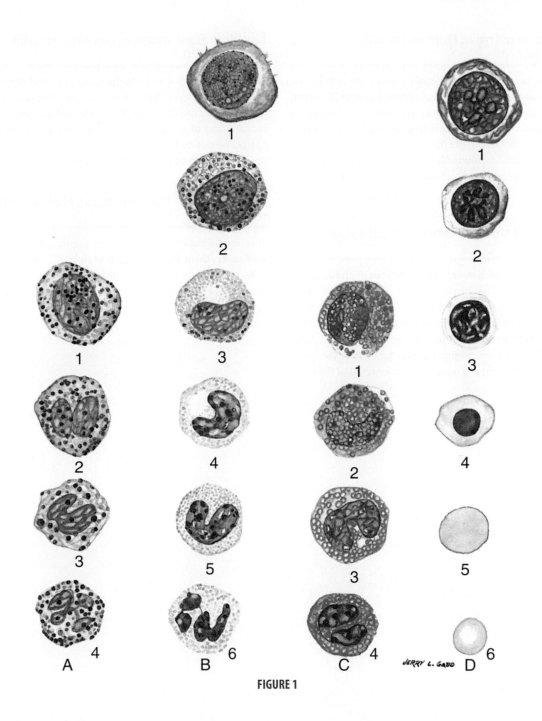

FIGURE 1

JERRY L. GADD

KEY

A
1. Basophilic myelocyte
2. Basophilic metamyelocyte
3. Basophil stab cell
4. Basophil
B
1. Myeloblast
2. Promyelocyte
3. Neutrophilic myelocyte
4. Neutrophilic metamyelocyte

5. Neutrophilic stab cell
6. Neutrophil
C
1. Eosinophilic myelocyte
2. Eosinophilic metamyelocyte
3. Eosinophil stab cell
4. Eosinophil

D
1. Proerythroblast
2. Basophilic erythroblast
3. Polychromatophilic erythroblast
4. Orthochromatophilic erythroblast
5. Reticulocyte
6. Erythrocyte

PLATE 5-4 · Bone Marrow and Circulating Blood

FIGURE 1. Bone marrow. Human. Paraffin section. ×132.

This transverse section of a decalcified human rib displays the presence of **haversian canals** (H), **Volkmann's canals** (V), **osteocytes** (O) in their lacunae, and the **endosteum** (E). The marrow presents numerous **adventitial reticular cells** (A), blood vessels, and **sinusoids** (S). Moreover, the forming blood elements are also evident as small nuclei (*arrows*). Note the large **megakaryocytes** (M), cells that are the precursors of platelets. The *boxed area* is represented in Figure 2.

FIGURE 3. Blood smear. Human. Wright's stain. ×270.

This normal blood smear presents **erythrocytes** (R), **neutrophils** (N), and **platelets** (P). The apparent holes in the centers of the erythrocytes represent the thinnest areas of the biconcave discs. Note that the erythrocytes far outnumber the platelets, and they in turn are much more numerous than the white blood cells. Since neutrophils constitute the highest percentage of white blood cells, they are the ones most frequently encountered of the white blood cell population.

FIGURE 2. Bone marrow. Human. Paraffin section. ×270.

This photomicrograph is a higher magnification of the *boxed area* of Figure 1. Observe the presence of **osteocytes** (O) in their lacunae as well as the flattened cells of the **endosteum** (E). The endothelial lining of the sinusoids (*arrows*) are clearly evident, as are the numerous cells that are in the process of hemopoiesis. Two large **megakaryocytes** (M) are also discernible.

FIGURE 4. Bone marrow smear. Human. Wright's stain. ×270.

This normal bone marrow smear presents forming blood cells as well as **erythrocytes** (R) and **platelets** (P). In comparison with a normal peripheral blood smear (Figure 3), marrow possesses many more nucleated cells. Some of these are of the erythrocytic series (*arrows*), whereas others are of the granulocytic series (*arrowheads*).

KEY

A	adventitial reticular cell	M	megakaryocyte	R	erythrocyte
BV	blood vessel	N	neutrophil	S	sinusoid
E	endosteum	O	osteocyte	V	Volkmann's canal
H	haversian canal	P	platelet		

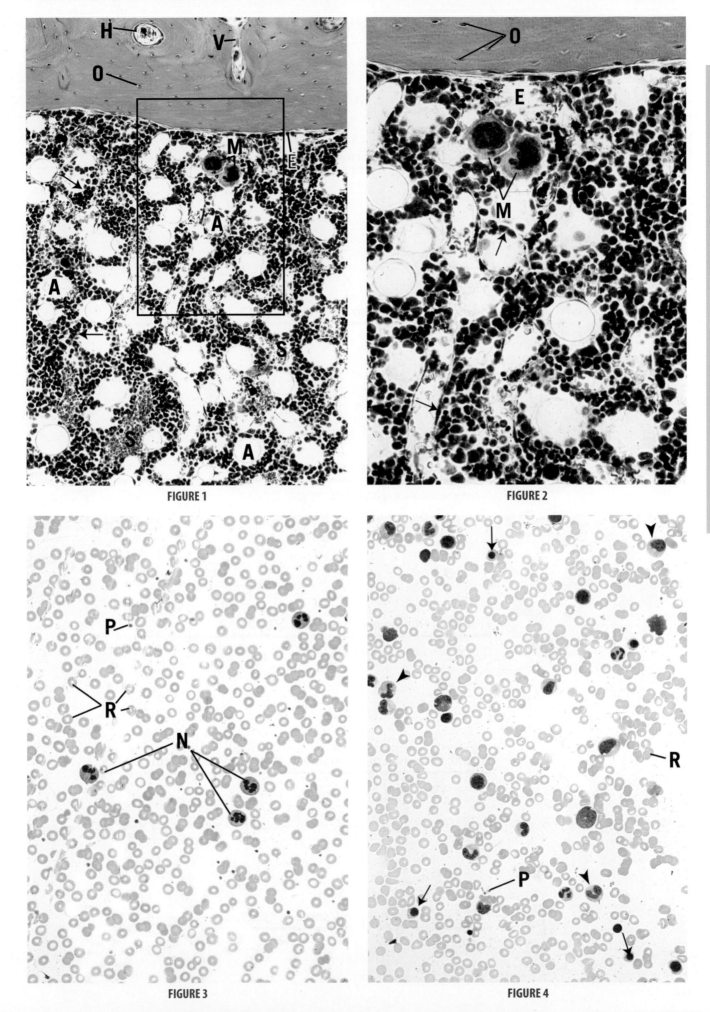

PLATE 5-4 • Bone Marrow and Circulating Blood

FIGURE 1

FIGURE 2

FIGURE 3

FIGURE 4

PLATE 5-5 · Erythropoiesis

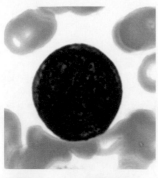

FIGURE 1. Human marrow smear. ×1,325.

Proerythroblast.

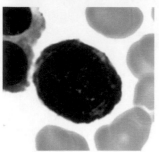

FIGURE 2. Human marrow smear. ×1,325.

Basophilic erythroblast.

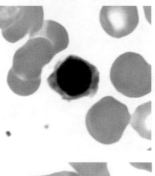

FIGURE 3. Human marrow smear. ×1,325.

Polychromatophilic erythroblast.

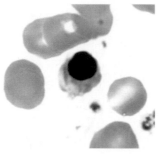

FIGURE 4. Human marrow smear. ×1,325.

Orthochromatophilic erythroblast.

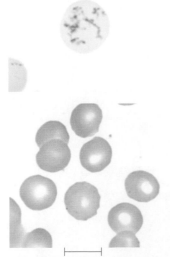

FIGURE 5. Human marrow smear. Methylene blue stain. ×1,325.

Reticulocyte.

FIGURE 6. Human marrow smear. ×1,325.

Erythrocyte.

1.15 cm = 7.5 μm

PLATE 5-6 • Granulocytopoiesis

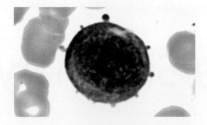

FIGURE 1. Myeloblast. Human bone marrow smear. ×1,325.

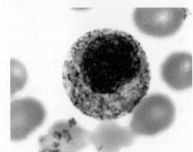

FIGURE 2. Promyelocyte. Human bone marrow smear. ×1,325.

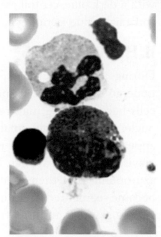

FIGURE 3a. Eosinophilic myelocyte. Human bone marrow smear. ×1,325.

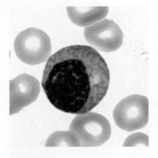

FIGURE 3b. Neutrophilic myelocyte. Human bone marrow smear. ×1,325.

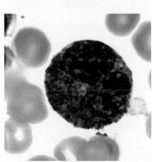

FIGURE 4a. Eosinophilic metamyelocyte. Human bone marrow smear. ×1,325.

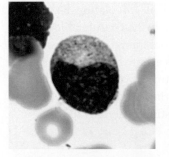

FIGURE 4b. Neutrophilic metamyelocyte. Human bone marrow smear. ×1,325.

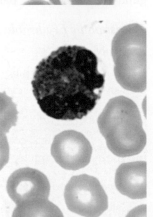

FIGURE 5a. Eosinophilic stab cell. Human bone marrow smear. ×1,325.

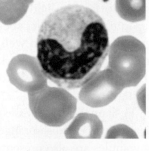

FIGURE 5b. Neutrophilic stab cell. Human bone marrow smear. ×1,325.

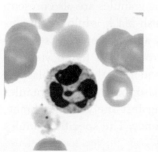

FIGURE 6. Neutrophil. Human bone marrow smear. ×1,325.

1.15 cm = 7.5 µm

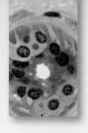

Chapter Summary

I. CIRCULATING BLOOD*

A. Erythrocytes (RBC)

RBCs are pink, biconcave discs that are 7 to 8 μm in diameter. They are filled with hemoglobin and possess no nuclei.

B. Agranulocytes

1. Lymphocytes

Histologically, **lymphocytes** may be **small, medium,** or **large** (this bears no relationship to T cells, B cells, or null cells). Most lymphocytes are small (8 to 10 μm in diameter) and possess a dense, blue, acentrically positioned nucleus that occupies most of the cell, leaving a thin rim of light blue, peripheral cytoplasm. Azurophilic granules (lysosomes) may be evident in the cytoplasm.

2. Monocytes

Monocytes are the largest of all circulating blood cells (12 to 15 μm in diameter). There is a considerable amount of **grayish-blue cytoplasm** containing numerous azurophilic granules. The **nucleus** is acentric and kidney-shaped and possesses a coarse chromatin network with clear spaces. Lobes of the nucleus are superimposed on themselves, and their outlines appear to be distinctly demarcated.

C. Granulocytes

1. **Neutrophils**, the most populous of the leukocytes, are 9 to 12 μm in diameter and display a light pink cytoplasm housing many azurophilic and smaller specific granules. The specific granules do not stain well, hence, the name of these cells. The nucleus is dark blue, coarse, and multilobed, with most being two to three lobed with thin connecting strands.
2. **Eosinophils** are 10 to 14 μm in diameter and possess numerous refractive, spherical, large, reddish-orange specific granules. Azurophilic granules are also present. The nucleus, which is brownish-black, is bilobed, resembling sausage links united by a thin connecting strand.
3. **Basophils,** the least numerous of all leukocytes, are 8 to 10 μm in diameter. Frequently, their cytoplasm is so filled with dark, large, basophilic specific granules that they appear to press against the cell membrane, giving it an angular appearance. The specific granules usually mask the azurophilic granules, as well as the S-shaped, light blue nucleus.

D. Platelets

Platelets, occasionally called **thrombocytes,** are small, round (2 to 4 μm in diameter) cell fragments. As such, they possess no nuclei, are frequently clumped together, and present with a dark blue, central granular region, the **granulomere,** and a light blue, peripheral, clear region, the **hyalomere.**

II. HEMOPOIESIS*

During the maturation process, hemopoietic cells undergo clearly evident morphologic alterations. As the cells become more mature, they decrease in size. Their nuclei also become smaller, the chromatin network appears coarser, and their nucleoli (which resemble pale grayish spaces) disappear. The granulocytes first acquire azurophilic, and then specific granules and their nuclei become segmented. Cells of the erythrocytic series never display granules and eventually lose their nuclei.

A. Erythrocytic Series

1. Proerythroblast

a. Cytoplasm

Light blue to deep blue clumps in a pale grayish-blue background.

b. Nucleus

Round with a fine chromatin network; it is a rich burgundy red with 3 to 5 pale gray nucleoli.

2. Basophilic Erythroblast

a. Cytoplasm

Bluish clumps in a pale blue cytoplasm with a hint of grayish pink in the background.

b. Nucleus

Round, somewhat coarser than the previous stage; burgundy red. A nucleolus may be present.

3. Polychromatophilic Erythroblast

a. Cytoplasm

Yellowish pink with bluish tinge.

---

*All of the colors designated in this summary are based on the Wright's or Giemsa's modification of the Romanovsky-type stains as applied to blood smears.

b. Nucleus

Small and round with a condensed, coarse chromatin network; dark, reddish black. No nucleoli are present.

4. Orthochromatophilic Erythroblast

a. Cytoplasm

Pinkish with a slight tinge of blue.

b. Nucleus

Dark, condensed, round structure that may be in the process of being extruded from the cell.

5. Reticulocyte

a. Cytoplasm

Appears just like a normal, circulating RBC; if stained with supravital dyes (e.g., methylene blue), however, a bluish reticulum—composed mostly of rough endoplasmic reticulum—is evident.

b. Nucleus

Not present.

B. Granulocytic Series

The first two stages of the granulocytic series, the myeloblast and promyelocyte, possess no specific granules. These make their appearance in the myelocyte stage, when the three types of myelocytes (neutrophilic, eosinophilic, and basophilic) may be distinguished. Since they only differ from each other in their specific granules, only the neutrophilic series is described in this summary, with the understanding that myelocytes, metamyelocytes, and stab (band) cells occur in these three varieties.

1. Myeloblast

a. Cytoplasm

Small blue clumps in a light blue background. No granules. Cytoplasmic blebs extend along the periphery of the cell.

b. Nucleus

Reddish-blue, round nucleus with fine chromatin network. Two or three pale gray nucleoli are evident.

2. Promyelocyte

a. Cytoplasm

The cytoplasm is bluish and displays numerous, small, dark, azurophilic granules.

b. Nucleus

Reddish-blue, round nucleus whose chromatin strands appear more coarse than in the previous stage. A nucleolus is usually present.

3. Neutrophilic Myelocyte

a. Cytoplasm

Pale blue cytoplasm containing dark azurophilic and smaller neutrophilic (specific) granules. A clear, paranuclear Golgi region is evident.

b. Nucleus

Round, usually somewhat flattened, acentric nucleus, with a somewhat coarse chromatin network. Nucleoli are not distinct.

4. Neutrophilic Metamyelocyte

a. Cytoplasm

Similar to the previous stage except that the cytoplasm is paler in color and the Golgi area is nestled in the indentation of the nucleus.

b. Nucleus

Kidney-shaped, acentric nucleus with a dense, dark chromatin network. Nucleoli are not present.

5. Neutrophilic Stab (Band) Cell

a. Cytoplasm

A little more blue than the cytoplasm of a mature neutrophil. Both azurophilic and neutrophilic (specific) granules are present.

b. Nucleus

The nucleus is horseshoe-shaped and dark blue, with a very coarse chromatin network. Nucleoli are not present.

The ability of animals to move is due to the presence of specific cells that have become highly differentiated, so that they function almost exclusively in contraction. The contractile process has been harnessed by the organism to permit various modes of movement and other activities for its survival. Some of these activities depend on

- quick contractions of short duration;
- long-lasting contractions without the necessity for rapid actions,
- powerful, rhythmic contractions that must be repeated in rapid sequences.

These varied needs are accommodated by three types of muscle, namely, skeletal, smooth, and cardiac. There are basic similarities among the three muscle types (see Table 6-1).

- They are all **mesodermally derived** and are elongated parallel to their axis of contraction;
- they possess numerous mitochondria to accommodate their high energy requirements, and
- all contain **contractile elements** known as **myofilaments**, in the form of **actin** and **myosin**, as well as additional contractile-associated proteins.

Myofilaments of skeletal and cardiac muscles are arranged in a specific ordered array that gives rise to a repeated sequence of uniform banding along their length—hence, their collective name, **striated muscle**.

Since muscle cells are much longer than they are wide, they are commonly referred to as **muscle fibers**. However, it must be appreciated that these fibers are living entities, unlike the nonliving fibers of connective tissue. Neither are they analogous to nerve fibers, which are living extensions of nerve cells.

- Often, certain unique terms are used to describe muscle cells; thus, the muscle cell membrane is **sarcolemma** (although earlier use of this term included the attendant basal lamina and reticular fibers), cytoplasm is **sarcoplasm**, mitochondria are **sarcosomes**, and endoplasmic reticulum is **sarcoplasmic reticulum** (SR).

SKELETAL MUSCLE

Skeletal muscle (see Graphics 6-1 and 6-2) is invested by dense collagenous connective tissue known as the

- **epimysium**, which penetrates the substance of the gross muscle, separating it into fascicles.
- Each fascicle is surrounded by **perimysium**, a looser connective tissue.
- Finally, each individual muscle fiber within a fascicle is enveloped by fine reticular fibers, the **endomysium**.

The vascular and nerve supplies of the muscle travel in these interrelated connective tissue compartments.

There are three types of skeletal muscle fibers: **red, white**, and **intermediate** depending on their contraction velocities, mitochondrial content, and types of enzymes the cell contains (see Table 6-2).

Each gross muscle, for example, biceps, usually possesses all three types of muscle cells. The innervation of a particular muscle cell determines whether it is red, white, or intermediate. Each skeletal muscle fiber is roughly cylindrical in shape, possessing numerous elongated nuclei located at the periphery of the cell, just deep to the sarcolemma.

Longitudinally sectioned muscle fibers display intracellular contractile elements, which are the parallel arrays of longitudinally disposed **myofibrils**.

- This arrangement of myofibrils produces an overall effect of **cross-banding** of alternating light and dark bands traversing each skeletal muscle cell. The dark bands are **A bands**, and the light bands are **I bands**.
- Each I band is bisected by a thin dark **Z disc**, and the region of the myofibril extending from Z disc to Z disc, the **sarcomere**, is the contractile unit of skeletal muscle cell.
- The A band is bisected by a paler **H zone**, the center of which is marked by the dark **M disc**.

During muscle contraction, the various transverse bands behave characteristically, in that the width of the A band remains constant, the two Z discs move closer to each other approaching the A band, and the I band and H zone become extinguished. Each Z disc is surrounded by intermediate filaments, known as **desmin**. The desmin filaments are bound to each other and to the Z discs by **plectin** filaments.

- Desmin filaments insert into the **costameres** which are regions of the sarcolemma that are dedicated for the attachment of these intermediate filaments.
- The heat shock protein, **αB-crystallin**, protects the desmin intermediate filaments by binding to them at their contact with the Z disc.
- The desmin-plectin-αB-crystallin complex, along with the costameres, ensures that the myofibrils of a muscle cell are aligned in the appropriate fashion so that the contraction of all of the myofibrils of each muscle cell occurs in a synchronized fashion.

Myofilaments

Electron microscopy has revealed that banding is the result of interdigitation of thick and thin myofilaments. The I band consists solely of thin filaments, whereas the A band, with the exception of its H and M components, consists of both thick and thin filaments. During contraction, the thick and thin filaments slide past each other (see below), and the Z discs are brought near the ends of the thick filaments.

TABLE 6-1 • Comparison of Skeletal, Smooth, and Cardiac Muscles

Characteristics	Skeletal Muscle	Smooth Muscle	Cardiac Muscle
Location	Generally attached to skeleton	Generally in hollow viscera, iris, blood vessels	Myocardium, major blood vessels as they enter or leave the heart.
Shape	Long, cylindrical parallel fibers	Short, spindle-shaped	Branched and blunt ended
Striations	Yes	No	Yes
Number and location of nucleus	Numerous, peripherally	Single, central	One or two, central
T tubules	Present at A-I junctions	No—but caveolae	Present at Z discs
Sarcoplasmic reticulum (SR)	Complex surrounds myofilaments forming meshwork. Forms triads with T tubules	Some smooth SR but poorly developed	Less developed than in skeletal muscle; forms diads with T tubules
Gap junctions	No	Yes	Yes—within intercalated discs
Control of contraction	Voluntary	Involuntary	Involuntary
Sarcomere	Yes	No	Yes
Regeneration	Restrictive	Extensive	Perhaps some limited
Histological distinction	Multiple striations and numerous peripherally located nuclei	No striations, central nucleus	Intercalated discs

- Thin filaments (7 nm in diameter and 1 μm in length) are composed of **F actin**, double-helical polymers of **G actin** molecules, resembling a pearl necklace twisted upon itself. Each groove of the helix houses linear **tropomyosin** molecules positioned end to end.
  - Associated with each tropomyosin molecule is a **troponin** molecule composed of three polypeptides—**troponin T (TnT)**, **troponin I (TnI)**, and **troponin C (TnC)**.
  - TnI binds to actin, masking its active site (where it is able to interact with myosin);
  - TnT binds to tropomyosin; and
  - TnC (a molecule similar to **calmodulin**) has a high affinity for calcium ions.

TABLE 6-2 • Characteristics of Muscle Fibers

Muscle Type	Myoglobin Content	Mitochondrial Population	Enzyme Content	ATP Generation	Contraction Characteristics
Red (slow)	High	Abundant	High in oxidative enzymes, low ATPase	Oxidative phosphorylation	Slow and repetitive; not easily fatigued
Intermediate	Intermediate	Intermediate	Intermediate-oxidative enzymes and ATPase	Oxidative phosphorylation and anaerobic glycolysis	Fast but not easily fatigued
White (fast)	Low	Sparse	Low oxidative enzymes; high ATPase and phosphorylases	Anaerobic glycolysis	Fast and easily fatigued

○ The **plus end** of each thin filament is bound to a Z disc by **α-actinin**.

○ Two **nebulins**, inelastic proteins that ensure that the thin filament is of the proper length, entwine along the entire extent of each thin filament and anchor it to the Z disc.

○ The **negative end** of each thin filament extends to the junction of the A and I bands and is capped by **tropomodulin**.

- Thick filaments (15 nm in diameter and 1.5 μm in length) are composed of 200 to 300 **myosin molecules** arranged in an antiparallel fashion. Each myosin molecule is composed of two pairs of light chains and two identical heavy chains.

○ Each **myosin heavy chain** resembles a golf club, with a linear tail and a globular head, where the tails are wrapped around each other in a helical fashion.

○ The enzyme **trypsin** cleaves it into a linear (most of the tail) segment (**light meromyosin**) and a globular segment with the remainder of the tail (**heavy meromyosin**).

○ Another enzyme, papain, cleaves **heavy meromyosin** into a short tail region (**S2 fragment**) and a pair of globular regions (**S1 fragments**).

○ Each pair of **myosin light chains** is associated with one of the S1 fragments. S1 fragments have **ATPase activity** but require the association with actin for this activity to be manifest.

○ Thick filaments are anchored to Z discs by the linear, elastic protein **titin** and are linked to adjacent thick filaments, at the M line, by the proteins **myomesin** and **C protein**.

○ Since titin molecules form an elastic lattice around the thick filaments, they facilitate the maintenance of the spatial relationship of these thick filaments to each other, as well as to the thin filaments.

Sliding Filament Model of Muscle Contraction

Nerve impulses, transmitted at the **myoneural junction** across the **synaptic cleft** by **acetylcholine**, cause a wave of depolarization of the sarcolemma, with the eventual result of muscle contraction. This wave of depolarization is distributed throughout the muscle fiber by transverse tubules (T tubules), tubular invaginations of the sarcolemma.

- The **T tubules** become closely associated with the terminal cisternae of the SR, so that each T tubule is flanked by two of these elements of the SR, forming a triad.

- **Voltage-sensitive** integral proteins, **dihydropyridine-sensitive receptors (DHSR)**, located in the T tubule membrane are in contact with **calcium channels** (ryanodine receptors) in the terminal cisternae of the **sarcoplasmic reticulum (SR)**.

○ This complex is visible with the electron microscope and is referred to as **junctional feet**.

- During depolarization of the skeletal muscle sarcolemma, the DHSRs of the T tubule undergo voltage-induced conformational change, causing the calcium channels of the terminal cisternae to open, permitting the influx of Ca^{2+} ions into the cytosol.

- **Troponin C** of the thin filament **binds the calcium ions** and changes its conformation, pressing the **tropomyosin** deeper into the grooves of the F actin filament, thus exposing the **active site** (myosin-binding site) on the **actin** molecule.

- **ATP**, bound to the globular head (**S1 fragment**) of the myosin molecule, is **hydrolyzed**, but both **ADP and P_i remain attached** on the S1. The myosin molecule swivels so that the myosin head approximates the active site on the actin molecule.

- The P_i moiety is released, and in the presence of **calcium**, a link is formed between the **actin** and **myosin**.

- The bound **ADP** is freed, and the **myosin head** alters its conformation, **moving the thin filament** toward the center of the sarcomere.

- A new **ATP** attaches to the globular head, and the **myosin dissociates** from the active site of the **actin**. This cycle is repeated 200 to 300 times for complete contraction of the sarcomere.

Relaxation ensues when the **calcium pump** of the **SR** transports calcium from the cytosol into the SR cisterna, where it is bound by **calsequestrin**. The decreased cytosolic Ca^{2+} induces TnC to lose its bound calcium ions, the TnC molecule returns to its previous conformational state, the tropomyosin molecule returns to its original location, and the active site of the actin molecule is once again masked.

As a protective mechanism against muscle fiber tears as a result of overstretching and to provide information concerning the position of the body in three-dimensional space, tendons and muscles are equipped with specialized receptors, **Golgi tendon organs** and **muscle spindles**, respectively.

CARDIAC MUSCLE

Cardiac muscle (see Graphic 6-2) cells are also striated, but each cell usually contains only one centrally placed nucleus. These cells form specialized junctions known as **intercalated discs** as they interdigitate with each other.

- These intercalated discs act as Z lines as well as regions of intercellular junctions.

- Intercalated discs have **transverse portions** that specialize in cell-cell attachments by forming numerous desmosomes and fasciae adherentes and **lateral**

portions that are rich in gap junctions, thus permitting cell to cell communications to occur.

Heart muscle contraction is involuntary, and the cells possess an inherent rhythm.

- The heart possesses a group of specialized cardiac muscle cells known as the **SA node** (sinoatrial node) that establishes the rate of contraction and initiates contraction of the atrial muscles.
  - The SA node receives input from the sympathetic and parasympathetic components of the autonomic nervous system; the former increase and the latter decrease the rate of contraction of the heart.
- The impulse is transmitted from the SA node to another group of specialized cardiac muscle cells, the **AV node** (atrioventricular node) that holds up the impulse for a few milliseconds and then the impulse travels along the **bundle of His** to the **Purkinje fibers** (both of which are specialized cardiac muscle cells) to cause contraction of the ventricles.

SMOOTH MUSCLE

Smooth muscle (see Graphic 6-2) is also involuntary. It may be of the **multiunit type**, where each cell possesses its own nerve supply, or of the **unitary** (visceral) smooth muscle type, where nerve impulses are transmitted via **nexus** (**gap junctions**) from one muscle cell to its neighbor.

Each fusiform smooth muscle cell houses a single, centrally placed nucleus, which becomes corkscrew-shaped during contraction of the cell. Just deep to the cell membrane, small vesicles, known as **caveolae**, which act as T tubules of cardiac muscle, housing the calcium ions necessary for smooth muscle contraction. Smooth muscle cells are rich in mitochondria, Golgi, RER, SER, glycogen, and thick and thin filaments.

- Although the **thick** and **thin filaments** of smooth muscle are not arranged into myofibrils, they are organized so that they are aligned obliquely to the longitudinal axis of the cell.
- **Myosin molecules** of smooth muscle are unusual, since the **light meromyosin moiety** is folded in such a fashion that its free terminus binds to a "sticky region" of the globular S1 portion.
- The thin filaments, composed of actin, possess tropomyosin as well as caldesmon.
  - **Caldesmon** is a protein that masks the active site of the actin monomers.
- The thin filaments are attached to **cytoplasmic densities** as well as to **dense bodies** along the cytoplasmic aspect of the sarcolemma and Z disc analogs (containing α-actinin), as are the **intermediate filaments** (**desmin** in multiunit smooth muscle and **vimentin** and **desmin** in unitary smooth muscle cells).
- The cytosol is rich in **calmodulin** and the enzyme **myosin light-chain kinase,** whereas troponin is absent.

For smooth muscle contraction to occur, calcium, released from **caveolae**, binds to calmodulin.

- The **Ca^{2+}-calmodulin complex**
  - binds to caldesmon causing it to unmask the active site of actin and
  - activates **myosin light-chain kinase,** which **phosphorylates** one of the **myosin light chains,** altering its conformation.
  - The phosphorylation causes the free terminus of the light meromyosin to be released from the S1 moiety.
  - **ATP** binds to the **S1,** and the resultant interaction between actin and myosin is similar to that of skeletal (and cardiac) muscle.
  - As long as calcium and ATP are present, the smooth muscle cell will remain contracted.
  - Smooth muscle contraction lasts longer but develops slower than cardiac or skeletal muscle contraction.

CLINICAL CONSIDERATIONS

Myasthenia Gravis

Myasthenia gravis is an autoimmune disease that is characterized by incremental weakening of skeletal muscles. Antibodies formed against acetylcholine receptors of skeletal muscle fibers bond to and, thus, block these receptors. The number of sites available for the initiation of depolarization of the muscle sarcolemma is decreased. The gradual weakening affects the most active muscles first (muscles of the face, eyes, and tongue), but eventually the muscles of respiration become compromised and the individual dies of respiratory insufficiency.

Duchenne's Muscular Dystrophy

Duchenne's muscular dystrophy is a muscle degenerative disease that is due to an X-linked genetic defect that strikes 1 in 30,000 males. The defect results in the absence of dystrophin molecules in the muscle cell membrane. Dystrophin is a protein that functions in the interconnection of the cytoskeleton to transmembrane proteins that interact with the extracellular matrix as well as in providing structural support for the muscle plasmalemma. Individuals afflicted with Duchenne's muscular dystrophy experience muscle weakness by the time they are 7 years of age and are usually wheelchair bound by the time they are 12 years old. It is very unusual to have these patients survive into their early twenties.

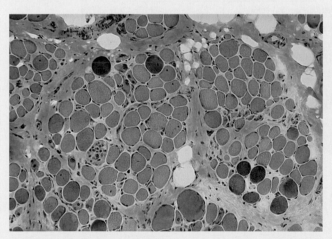

This photomicrograph of a biopsy from the vastus lateralis muscle of a patient suffering from Duchenne's muscular dystrophy was stained by a modified Gomori's trichrome stain. Note the numerous necrotic muscle cells and the presence of fibrosis evidenced by the thickened endomysium and perimysium. (Reprinted with permission from Rubin R, Strayer D, et al., eds. Rubin's Pathology. Clinicopathologic Foundations of Medicine, 5th ed. Baltimore: Lippincott Williams & Wilkins, 2008, p. 1158.)

Muscle Cramps

A sudden, powerful contraction of a muscle or muscle group is a painful event known as a muscle cramp. It may occur in people of all ages and is usually due to lowered blood flow to the muscle(s), lowered levels of potassium, or vigorous exercise without proper warm up (stretching). Cramps can also occur at night, and they usually involve the muscles of the lower leg.

Pompe's Disease

Pompe's disease is one of the inherited metabolic glycogen-storage diseases where the cells of the patient are unable to degrade glycogen due to an **acid maltase deficiency**. The inability to degrade glycogen results in the accumulation of glycogen in the lysosomes. There are two types of this disease, the early onset which occurs in the infant and the late onset that occurs either in childhood or in the adult. The early onset is fatal and children do not usually live past 2 years of age; the symptoms are enlargement of the heart and liver, generalized weakness, and lack of muscle tone. Death results from cardiac and respiratory failure. The late onset form differs from the juvenile condition in that the cardiac complications are not as assiduous but muscle weakness, especially of the legs, is more pronounced. Recent advancement in the treatment of Pompe's disease appears to decrease the mortality rate as well as the severity of the condition.

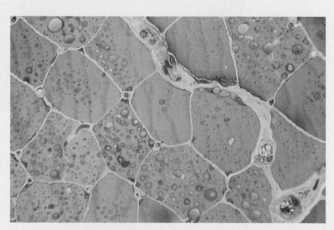

This cross section of skeletal muscle cells from a patient with adult-onset Pompe's disease, stained with toluidine blue, displays enlarged lysosomes filled with pinkish-colored glycogen. (Reprinted with permission from Rubin R, Strayer D, et al., eds. Rubin's Pathology. Clinicopathologic Foundations of Medicine, 5th ed. Baltimore: Lippincott Williams & Wilkins, 2008, p. 1164.)

Striations of skeletal muscle are resolved into **A bands** and **I bands**. I bands are divided into two equal halves by a **Z disk**, and each A band has a light zone, the **H band**. The center of each H band is a dark **M band**. Adjacent myofibrils are secured to each other by the intermediate filaments desmin and vimentin. The basic contractile unit of the skeletal muscle cell is the **sarcomere**, a precisely ordered collection of **myofilaments** (**thick** and **thin filaments**). Tubular invaginations, **T tubules** (**transverse tubules**), of the muscle cell membrane penetrate deep into the sarcoplasm and surround myofibrils in such a manner that at the junction of each A and I band these tubules become associated with the dilated **terminal cisternae** of the sarcoplasmic reticulum (smooth ER), forming triads.

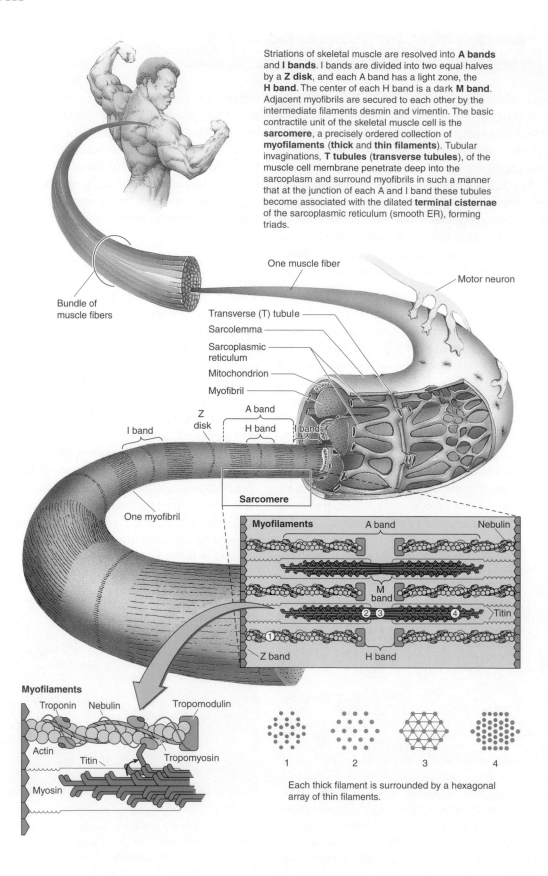

One muscle fiber

Motor neuron

Bundle of muscle fibers

Transverse (T) tubule

Sarcolemma

Sarcoplasmic reticulum

Mitochondrion

Myofibril

Z disk

A band

H band

I band

I band

One myofibril

Sarcomere

Myofilaments   A band   Nebulin

M band

Titin

Z band   H band

Myofilaments

Troponin   Nebulin   Tropomodulin

Actin

Titin   Tropomyosin

Myosin

1   2   3   4

Each thick filament is surrounded by a hexagonal array of thin filaments.

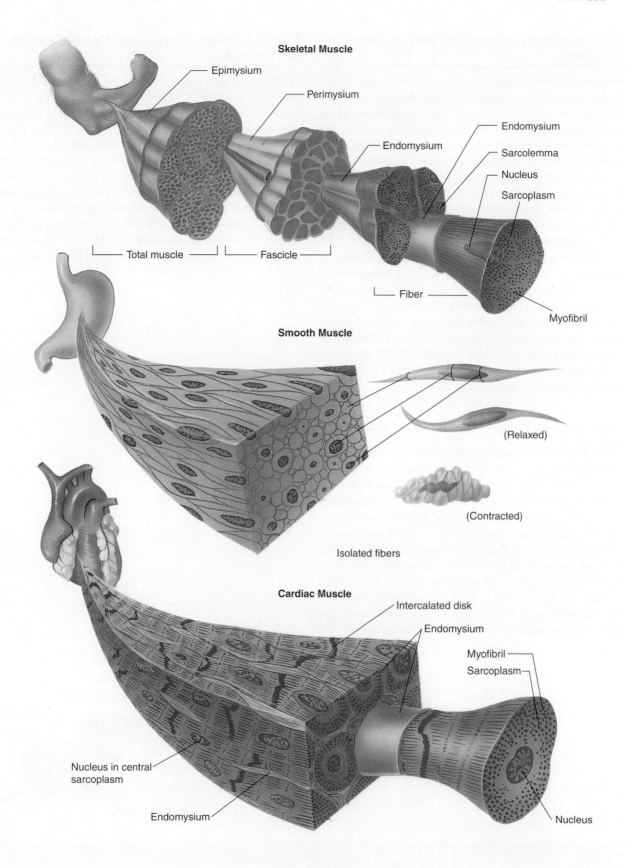

Skeletal Muscle

Epimysium

Perimysium

Endomysium

Endomysium

Sarcolemma

Nucleus

Sarcoplasm

Total muscle

Fascicle

Fiber

Myofibril

Smooth Muscle

(Relaxed)

(Contracted)

Isolated fibers

Cardiac Muscle

Intercalated disk

Endomysium

Myofibril

Sarcoplasm

Nucleus in central sarcoplasm

Endomysium

Nucleus

PLATE 6-1 · Skeletal Muscle

FIGURE 1. Skeletal muscle. l.s. Monkey. Plastic section. ×800.

This photomicrograph displays several of the characteristics of skeletal muscle in longitudinal section. The muscle fibers are extremely long and possess a uniform diameter. Their numerous **nuclei** (N) are peripherally located. The intercellular space is occupied by endomysium, with its occasional flattened **connective tissue cells** (CTs) and reticular fibers. Two types of striations are evident: longitudinal and transverse. The longitudinal striations represent **myofibrils** (M) that are arranged in almost precise register with each other. This ordered arrangement is responsible for the dark and light transverse banding that gives this type of muscle its name. Note that the **light band** (I) is bisected by a narrow, dark line, the **Z disc** (Z). The **dark band** (A) is also bisected by the clear **H zone** (H). The center of the H zone is occupied by the M disc, appearing as a faintly discernible dark line in a few regions. The basic contractile unit of skeletal muscle is the **sarcomere** (S), extending from one Z disc to its neighboring Z disc. During muscle contraction, the myofilaments of each sarcomere slide past one another, pulling Z discs closer to each other, thus shortening the length of each sarcomere. During this movement, the width of the A band remains constant, whereas the I band and H zone disappear.

FIGURE 2. Skeletal muscle. x.s. Monkey. Paraffin section. ×132.

Portions of a few fascicles are presented in this photomicrograph. Each fascicle is composed of numerous **muscle fibers** (F) that are surrounded by connective tissue elements known as the **perimysium** (P), which houses nerves and blood vessels supplying the fascicles. The nuclei of endothelial, Schwann, and connective tissue cells are evident as black dots in the perimysium. The peripherally placed **nuclei** (N) of the skeletal muscle fibers appear as black dots; however, they are all within the muscle cell. Nuclei of satellite cells are also present, just external to the muscle fibers, but their identification at low magnification is questionable. The *boxed area* is presented at a higher magnification in Figure 3.

FIGURE 3. Skeletal muscle. x.s. Monkey. Paraffin section. ×540.

This is a higher magnification of the *boxed area* of Figure 2. Transverse sections of several muscle fibers demonstrate that these cells appear to be polyhedral, that they possess peripherally placed **nuclei** (N), and that their endomysia (E) house numerous **capillaries** (C). Many of the capillaries are difficult to see because they are collapsed in a resting muscle. The pale sarcoplasm occasionally appears granular, due to the transversely sectioned myofibrils. Occasionally, nuclei that appear to belong to **satellite cells** (SC) may be observed, but definite identification cannot be expected. Moreover, the well-defined outline of each fiber was believed to be due to the sarcolemma, but now it is known to be due more to the adherent basal lamina and endomysium.

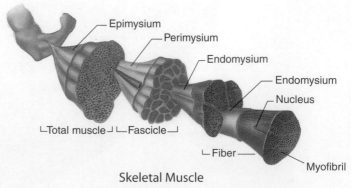

Skeletal Muscle

KEY							
A	A band		F	muscle fiber		P	perimysium
C	capillary		H	H zone		S	sarcomere
CT	connective tissue		I	I band		SC	satellite cell
E	endomysium		N	nucleus		Z	Z disc

PLATE 6-1 · Skeletal Muscle

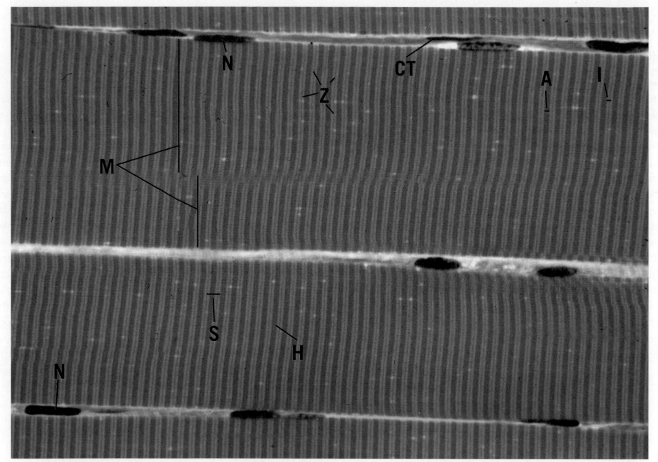

FIGURE 1

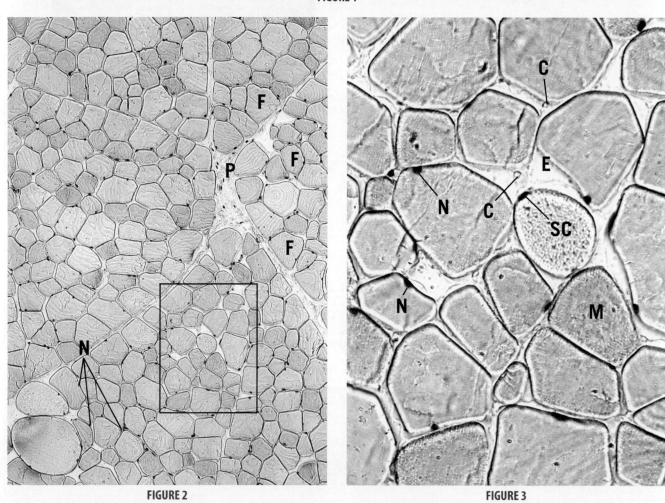

FIGURE 2

FIGURE 3

PLATE 6-2 · Skeletal Muscle, Electron Microscopy

FIGURE 1. Skeletal muscle. l.s. Rat. Electron microscopy. ×17,100.

This moderately low power electron micrograph of skeletal muscle was sectioned longitudinally. Perpendicular to its longitudinal axis, note the dark and light cross-bandings. The **A band** (A) in this view extends from the upper left-hand corner to the lower right-hand corner and is bordered by an **I band** (I) on either side. Each I band is traversed by a **Z disc** (Z). Observe that the Z disc has the appearance of a dashed line, since individual myofibrils are separated from each other by sarcoplasm. Note that the extent of a **sarcomere** (S) is from Z disc to Z disc and that an almost precise alignment of individual myofibrils ensures the specific orientation of the various bands within the sarcomere. The **H zone** (H) and the **M disc** (MD) are clearly defined in this electron micrograph. Mitochondria are preferentially located in mammalian skeletal muscle, occupying the region at the level of the I band as they wrap around the periphery of the myofibril. Several sarcomeres are presented at a higher magnification in Figure 2. (Courtesy of Dr. J. Strum.)

FIGURE 2. Skeletal muscle. l.s. Rat. Electron microscopy. ×28,800.

This is a higher power electron micrograph presenting several sarcomeres. Note that the **Z discs** (Z) possess projections (*arrows*) to which the **thin myofilaments** (tM) are attached. The **I band** (I) is composed only of thin filaments. **Thick myofilaments** (TM) interdigitate with the thin filaments from either end of the sarcomere, resulting in the **A band** (A). However, the thin filaments in a relaxed muscle do not extend all the way to the center of the A band; therefore, the **H zone** (H) is composed only of thick filaments. The center of each thick filament appears to be attached to its neighboring thick filament, resulting in localized thickenings, collectively comprising the **M disc** (MD). During muscle contraction, the thick and thin filaments slide past each other, thus pulling the Z discs toward the center of the sarcomere. Due to the resultant overlapping of thick and thin filaments, the I bands and H zones disappear, but the A bands maintain their width. The sarcoplasm houses **mitochondria** (m) preferentially located, glycogen granules (*arrowhead*), as well as a specialized system of SR and T tubules, forming **triads** (T). In mammalian skeletal muscle, triads are positioned at the junction of the I and A bands. (Courtesy of Dr. J. Strum.)

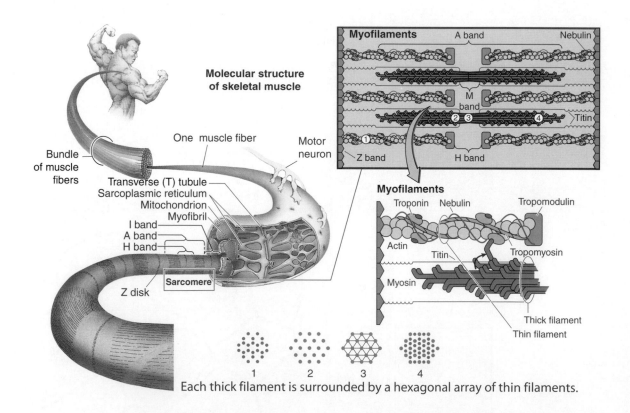

Molecular structure of skeletal muscle

Each thick filament is surrounded by a hexagonal array of thin filaments.

KEY					
A	A band	**MD**	M disc	**TM**	thick myofilament
H	H zone	**S**	sarcomere	**Z**	Z disc
I	I band	**T**	triad		
M	mitochondrion	**tM**	thin myofilament		

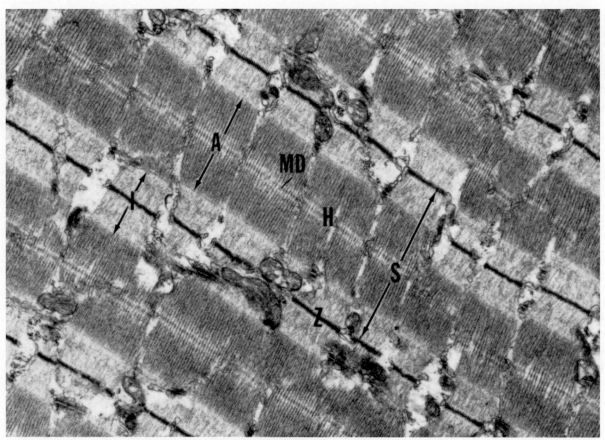

FIGURE 1

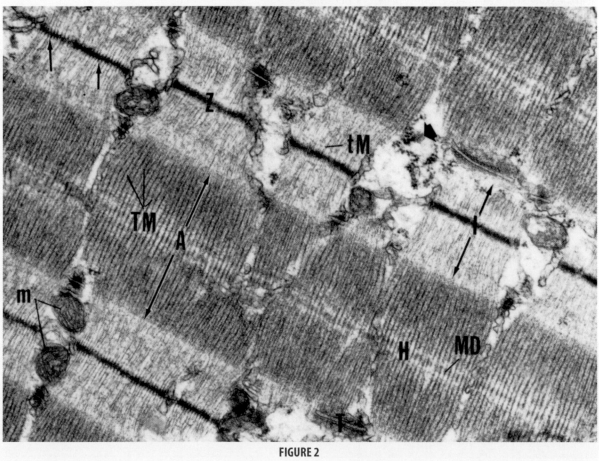

FIGURE 2

PLATE 6-3 • Myoneural Junction, Light and Electron Microscopy

FIGURE 1. Myoneural junction. Lateral view. Paraffin section. ×540.

This view of the myoneural junction clearly displays the **myelinated nerve fiber** (MN) approaching the **skeletal muscle fiber** (SM). The **A bands** (A) and **I bands** (I) are well delineated, but the Z discs are not observable in this preparation. As the axon nears the muscle cell, it loses its myelin sheath and continues on as a **nonmyelinated axon** (nMN) but retains its Schwann cell envelope. As the axon reaches the muscle cell, it terminates as a **motor end plate** (MEP), overlying the sarcolemma of the muscle fiber. Although the sarcolemma is not visible in light micrographs, such as this one, its location is clearly approximated due to its associated basal lamina and reticular fibers.

FIGURE 2. Myoneural junction. Surface view. Paraffin section. ×540.

This view of the myoneural junction demonstrates, as in the previous figure, that as the axon reaches the vicinity of the **skeletal muscle fiber** (SM), it loses its myelin sheath. The axon terminates, forming a **motor end plate** (MEP), composed of a few clusters of numerous small swellings (*arrowhead*) on the sarcolemma of the skeletal muscle fiber. Although it is not apparent in this light micrograph, the motor end plate is located in a slight depression on the skeletal muscle fiber, and the plasma membranes of the two structures do not contact each other. Figure 3 clearly demonstrates the morphology of such a synapse.

FIGURE 3. Myoneural junction. Rat. Electron microscopy. ×15,353.

This electron micrograph is of a myoneural junction taken from the diaphragm muscle of a rat. Observe that the **axon** (ax) loses its myelin sheath but the **Schwann cell** (sc) continues, providing a protective cover for the nonsynaptic surface of the **end foot** or **nerve terminal** (nt). The myelinated sheath ends in typical paranodal loops at the terminal heminode. The nerve terminal possesses **mitochondria** (m) and numerous clear synaptic vesicles. The margins of the 50-nm primary synaptic cleft are indicated by *arrowheads*. Postsynaptically, the **junctional folds** (j), many **mitochondria** (m), and portions of a **nucleus** (n) and **sarcomere** (s) are apparent in the skeletal muscle fiber. (Courtesy of Dr. C. S. Hudson.)

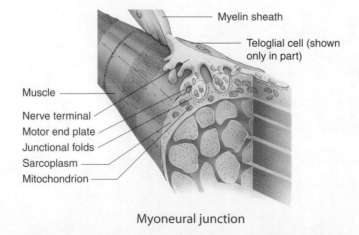

Myoneural junction

- Myelin sheath
- Teloglial cell (shown only in part)
- Muscle
- Nerve terminal
- Motor end plate
- Junctional folds
- Sarcoplasm
- Mitochondrion

KEY

A	A band	**MEP**	motor end plate	**nt**	nerve terminal
ax	axon	**MN**	myelinated nerve fiber	**s**	sarcomere
I	I band	**n**	nucleus	**sc**	Schwann cell
j	junctional fold	**nMN**	nonmyelinated axon	**SM**	skeletal muscle fiber
m	mitochondria				

PLATE 6-3 • Myoneural Junction, Light and Electron Microscopy

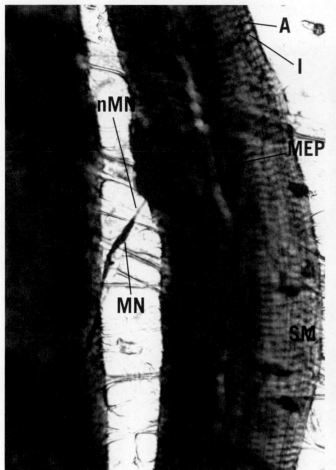

FIGURE 1

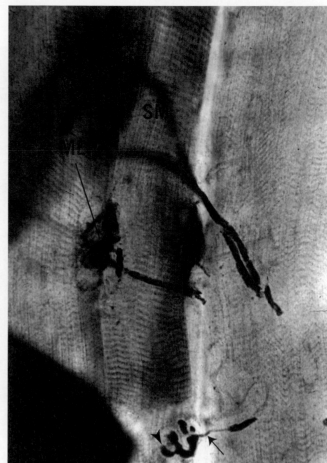

FIGURE 2

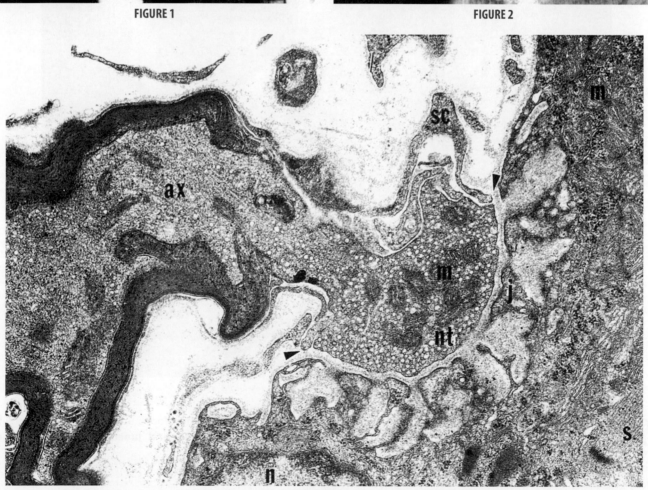

FIGURE 3

PLATE 6-4 • Myoneural Junction, Scanning Electron Microscopy

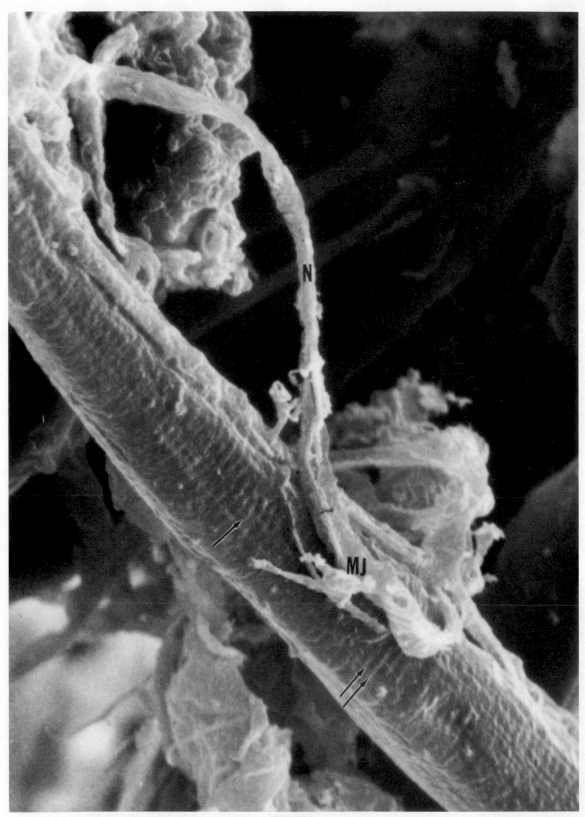

FIGURE 1

FIGURE 1. Myoneural junction. Tongue. Cat. Scanning electron microscopy. ×2,610.

The striations (*arrows*) of an isolated skeletal muscle fiber are clearly evident in this scanning electron micrograph. Note the **nerve** "twig" (N), which loops up and makes contact with the muscle at the **myoneural junction** (MJ). (Courtesy of Dr. L. Litke.)

PLATE 6-5 · Muscle Spindle, Light and Electron Microscopy

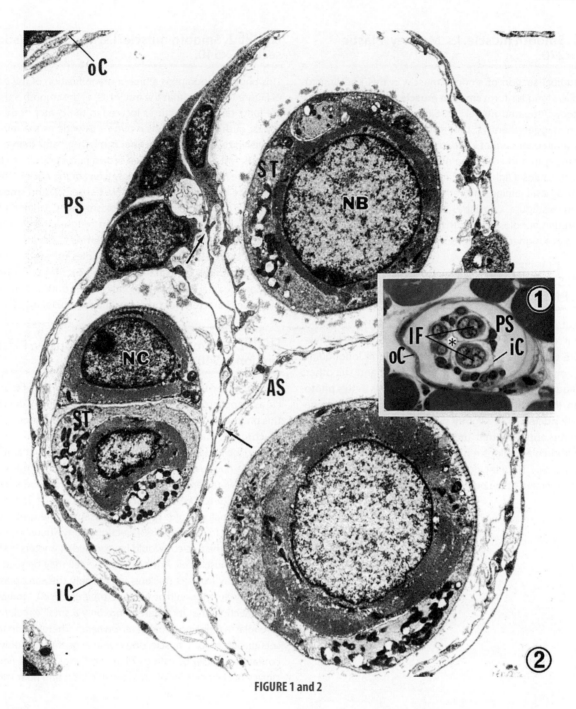

FIGURE 1 and 2

FIGURE 1. Muscle spindle. Mouse. Plastic section. ×436.

Observe that the **outer** (oC) and **inner** (iC) **capsules** of the muscle spindle define the outer **periaxial space** (PS) and the inner **axial space** (*asterisk*). The inner capsule forms an envelope around the **intrafusal fibers** (IF). (From Ovalle W, Dow P. Comparative ultrastructure of the inner capsule of the muscle spindle and the tendon organ. Am J Anat 1983;166:343–357.)

FIGURE 2. Muscle spindle. Mouse. Electron microscopy. ×6,300.

Parts of the **outer capsule** (oC) may be observed at the corners of this electron micrograph. The **periaxial space** (PS) surrounds the slender **inner capsule** (iC), whose component cells form attenuated branches, subdividing the **axial space** (AS) into several compartments for the **nuclear chain** (NC) and **nuclear bag** (NB) intrafusal fibers and their corresponding **sensory terminals** (ST). Note that the attenuated processes of the inner capsule cells establish contact with each other (*arrows*). (From Ovalle W, Dow P. Comparative ultrastructure of the inner capsule of the muscle spindle and the tendon organ. Am J Anat 1983;166:343–357.)

PLATE 6-6 • Smooth Muscle

FIGURE 1. Smooth muscle. l.s. Monkey. Plastic section. ×270.

The longitudinal section of smooth muscle in this photomicrograph displays long fusiform **smooth muscle cells** (sM) with centrally located, elongated **nuclei** (N). Since the muscle fibers are arranged in staggered arrays, they can be packed very closely, with only a limited amount of intervening **connective tissue** (CT). Using hematoxylin and eosin, the nuclei appear bluish, whereas the cytoplasm stains a light pink. Each smooth muscle cell is surrounded by a basal lamina and reticular fibers, neither of which is evident in this figure. Capillaries are housed in the connective tissue separating bundles of smooth muscle fibers. The *boxed area* is presented at a higher magnification in Figure 2.

FIGURE 3. Smooth muscle. Uterine myometrium. x.s. Monkey. Plastic section. ×270.

The myometrium of the uterus consists of interlacing bundles of smooth muscle fibers, surrounded by **connective tissue** (CT) elements. Note that some of these bundles are cut in longitudinal section (*1*), others are sectioned transversely (*2*), and still others are cut obliquely (*3*). At low magnifications, such as in this photomicrograph, the transverse sections present a haphazard arrangement of dark **nuclei** (N) in a lightly staining region. With practice, it will become apparent that these nuclei are intracellular and that the pale circular regions represent smooth muscle fibers sectioned transversely. Note the numerous **blood vessels** (BV) traveling in the connective tissue between the smooth muscle bundles.

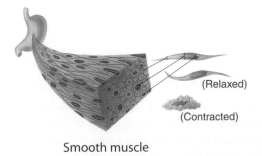

(Relaxed)

(Contracted)

Smooth muscle

FIGURE 2. Smooth muscle. l.s. Monkey. Plastic section. ×540.

This photomicrograph is a higher magnification of the *boxed area* of Figure 1. Observe that the **nuclei** (N) of the smooth muscle fibers are long, tapered structures located in the center of the cell. The widest girth of the nucleus is almost as wide as the muscle fiber. However, the length of the fiber is much greater than that of the nucleus. Note also that any line drawn perpendicular to the direction of the fibers will intersect only a few of the nuclei. Observe the difference between the **connective tissue** (CT) and **smooth muscle** (sM). The smooth muscle cytoplasm stains darker and appears smooth relative to the paleness and rough-appearing texture of the connective tissue. Observe **capillaries** (C) located in the connective tissue elements between bundles of muscle fibers. *Inset.* **Smooth muscle. Contracted. l.s. Monkey. Plastic section.** ×540. This longitudinal section of smooth muscle during contraction displays the characteristic corkscrew-shaped **nuclei** (N) of these cells.

FIGURE 4a. Smooth muscle. x.s. Monkey. Plastic section. ×540.

To understand the three-dimensional morphology of smooth muscle as it appears in two dimensions, refer to Figure 2 directly above this photomicrograph. Once again note that the muscle fibers are much longer than their nuclei and that both structures are spindle-shaped, being tapered at both ends. Recall also that at its greatest girth the nucleus is almost as wide as the cell. In transverse section, this would appear as a round nucleus surrounded by a rim of cytoplasm (*asterisk*). If the nucleus is sectioned at its tapered end, merely a small dot of it would be present in the center of a large muscle fiber (*double asterisks*). Sectioned anywhere between these two points, the nucleus would have varied diameters in the center of a large muscle cell. Additionally, the cell may be sectioned in a region away from its nucleus, where only the sarcoplasm of the large muscle cell would be evident (*triple asterisks*). Moreover, if the cell is sectioned at its tapered end, only a small circular profile of sarcoplasm is distinguishable (*arrowhead*). Therefore, in transverse sections of smooth muscle, one would expect to find only few cells containing nuclei of various diameters. Most of the field will be closely packed profiles of sarcoplasm containing no nuclei.

FIGURE 4b. Smooth muscle. Duodenum. Monkey. Plastic section. ×132.

This photomicrograph of the duodenum demonstrates the **glandular portion** (G) with its underlying **connective tissue** (CT). Deep to the connective tissue, note the two smooth muscle layers, one of which is sectioned longitudinally (*1*) and the other transversely (*2*).

KEY					
BV	blood vessel	CT	connective tissue	N	nucleus
C	capillary	G	glandular portion	sM	smooth muscle cell

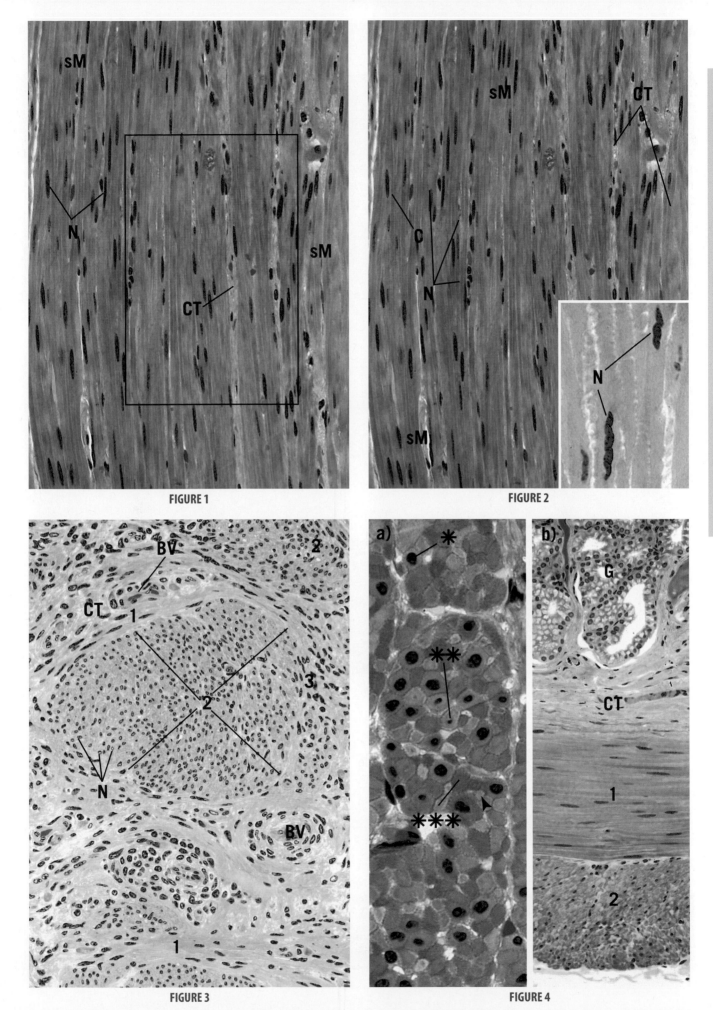

PLATE 6-6 · Smooth Muscle

FIGURE 1

FIGURE 2

FIGURE 3

FIGURE 4

PLATE 6-7 · Smooth Muscle, Electron Microscopy

FIGURE 1. Smooth muscle. l.s. Mouse. Electron microscopy. ×15,120.

Smooth muscle does not display cross-bandings, transverse tubular systems, or the regularly arranged array of myofilaments characteristic of striated muscle. However, smooth muscle does possess myofilaments that, along with a system of intermediate filaments, are responsible for its contractile capabilities. Moreover, the plasma membrane appears to possess the functional, if not the structural, aspects of the T tubule. Observe that each smooth muscle is surrounded by an **external lamina** (EL), which is similar in appearance to basal lamina of epithelial cells. The **sarcolemma** (SL) displays the presence of numerous pinocytotic-like invaginations, the **caveolae** (Ca), which are believed to act as T tubules of striated muscles in conducting impulses into the interior of the fiber. Some suggest that they may also act in concert with the SR in modulating the availability of calcium ions. The cytoplasmic aspect of the sarcolemma also displays the presence of **dense bodies** (DB), which are indicative of the attachment of **intermediate microfilaments** (IM) at that point. Dense bodies, composed of α-actinin (Z disc protein found in striated muscle), are also present in the sarcoplasm (*arrows*). The **nucleus** (N) is centrally located and, at its pole, **mitochondria** (m) are evident. Actin and myosin are also present in smooth muscle but cannot be identified with certainty in longitudinal sections. Parts of a second smooth muscle fiber may be observed to the left of the cell described. A small **capillary** (C) is evident in the lower right-hand corner. Note the **adherens junctions** (AJ) between the two epithelial cells, one of which presents a part of its **nucleus** (N).

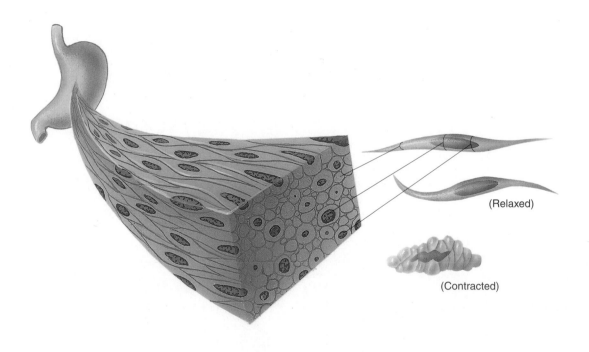

(Relaxed)

(Contracted)

Smooth muscle

KEY

AJ	adherens junction	**DB**	dense body	**m**	mitochondrion
C	capillary	**EL**	external lamina	**N**	nucleus
Ca	caveola	**IM**	intermediate filament	**SL**	sarcolemma

PLATE 6-7 • Smooth Muscle, Electron Microscopy

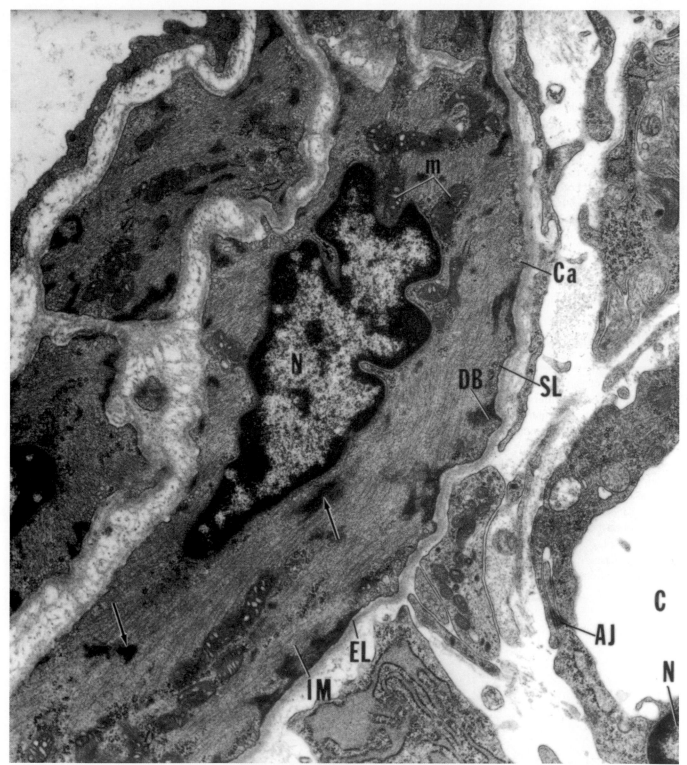

FIGURE 1

PLATE 6-8 · Cardiac Muscle

FIGURE 1. Cardiac muscle. l.s. Human. Plastic section. ×270.

This low magnification of longitudinally sectioned cardiac muscle displays many of the characteristics of this muscle type. The branching (*arrow*) of the fibers is readily apparent, as are the dark and light bands (*arrowheads*) running transversely along the length of the fibers. Each muscle cell possesses a large, centrally located, oval **nucleus** (N), although occasional muscle cells may possess two nuclei. The **intercalated discs** (ID), indicating intercellular junctions between two cardiac muscle cells, clearly delineated in this photomicrograph, are not easily demonstrable in sections stained with hematoxylin and eosin. The intercellular spaces of cardiac muscle are richly endowed by blood vessels, especially capillaries. Recall that, in contrast to cardiac muscle, the long skeletal muscle fibers do not branch, their myofilaments parallel one another, their many nuclei are peripherally located, and they possess no intercalated discs. The *boxed area* appears at a higher magnification in Figure 2.

FIGURE 3. Cardiac muscle. x.s. Human. Plastic section. ×270.

Cross sections of cardiac muscle demonstrate polygon-shaped areas of **cardiac muscle fibers** (CM) with relatively large intercellular spaces whose rich **vascular supply** (BV) is readily evident. Note that the **nucleus** (N) of each muscle cell is located in the center, but not all cells display a nucleus. The clear areas in the center of some cells (*arrows*) represent the perinuclear regions at the poles of the nucleus. These regions are rich in SR, glycogen, lipid droplets, and an occasional Golgi apparatus. The numerous smaller nuclei in the intercellular areas belong to endothelial and connective tissue cells. In contrast to cardiac muscle, cross sections of skeletal muscle fibers display a homogeneous appearance with peripherally positioned nuclei. The connective tissue spaces between skeletal muscle fibers display numerous (frequently collapsed) capillaries.

FIGURE 2. Cardiac muscle. l.s. Human. Plastic section. ×540.

This is a higher magnification of the *boxed area* of Figure 1. The branching of the fibers (*arrows*) is evident, and the cross-striations, I and A bands (*arrowheads*), are clearly distinguishable. The presence of **myofibrils** (M) within each cell is well displayed in this photomicrograph, as is the "step-like" appearance of the **intercalated discs** (ID). The oval, centrally located **nucleus** (N) is surrounded by a clear area usually occupied by mitochondria. The intercellular areas are richly supplied by **capillaries** (C) supported by slender connective tissue elements.

FIGURE 4. Cardiac muscle. x.s. Human. Plastic section. ×540.

At high magnifications of cardiac muscle in cross section, several aspects of this tissue become apparent. Numerous **capillaries** (C) and larger **blood vessels** (BV) abound in the connective tissue spaces. Note the **endothelial nuclei** (EN) of these vessels as well as the **white blood cells** (WBC) within the venule in the upper right-hand corner. **Nuclei** (N) of the muscle cells are centrally located, and the perinuclear clear areas (*arrow*) housing mitochondria are evident. The central clear zones at the nuclear poles are denoted by *asterisks*. Cross sections of myofibrils (*arrowheads*) are recognizable as numerous small dots of varying diameters within the sarcoplasm.

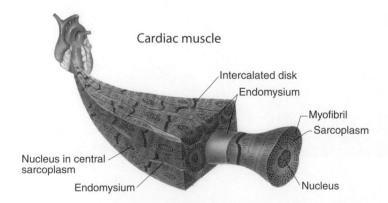

Cardiac muscle

Intercalated disk
Endomysium
Myofibril
Sarcoplasm
Nucleus in central sarcoplasm
Endomysium
Nucleus

KEY					
BV	blood vessel	**EN**	endothelial nucleus	**N**	nucleus
C	capillary	**ID**	intercalated disc	**WBC**	white blood cell
CM	cardiac muscle fiber	**M**	myofibril		

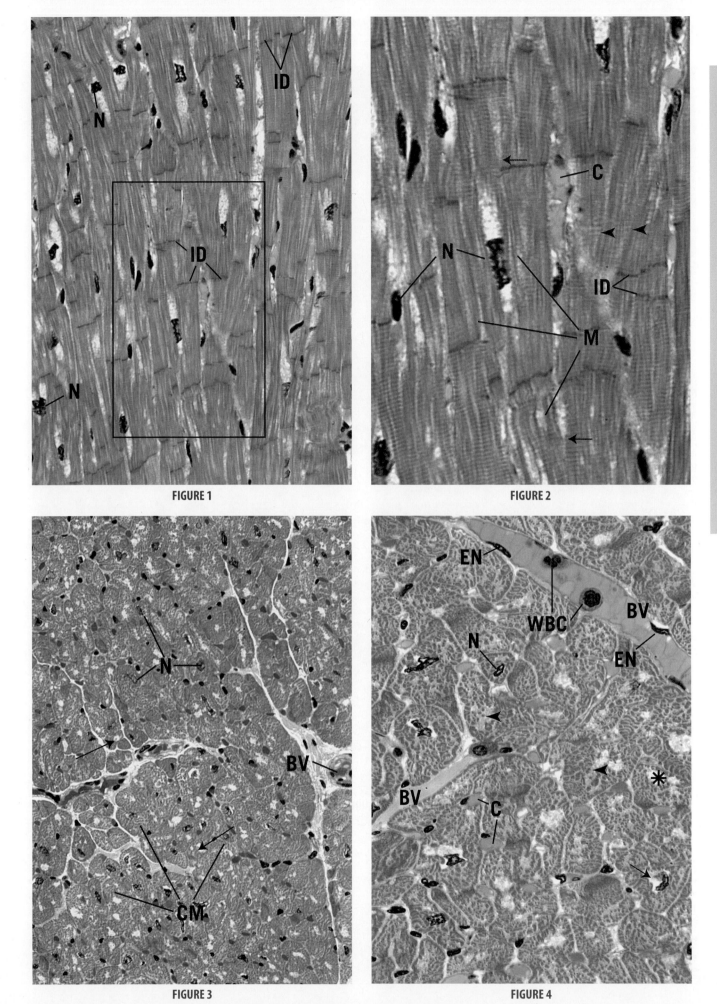

PLATE 6-8 · Cardiac Muscle

FIGURE 1

FIGURE 2

FIGURE 3

FIGURE 4

PLATE 6-9 · Cardiac Muscle, Electron Microscopy

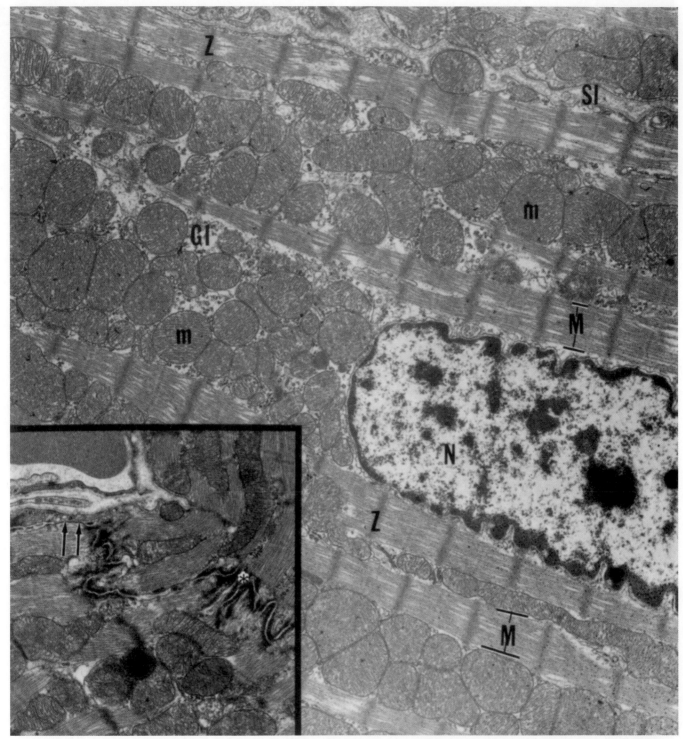

FIGURE 1

FIGURE 1. Cardiac muscle, l.s. Mouse. Electron microscopy. ×11,700.

The **nucleus** (N) of cardiac muscle cells is located in the center of the cell, as is evident from the location of the **sarcolemma** (Sl) in the upper part of the photomicrograph. The sarcoplasm is well endowed with **mitochondria** (m) and **glycogen** (Gl) deposits. Since this muscle cell is contracted, the I bands are not visible.

However, the **Z discs** (Z) are clearly evident, as are the individual **myofibrils** (M). *Inset.* **Cardiac muscle. l.s. Mouse. Electron microscopy.** ×20,700. An intercalated disc is presented in this electron micrograph. Note that this intercellular junction has two zones, the transverse portion (*asterisk*), composed mostly of desmosome-like junctions, and a longitudinal portion that displays extensive gap junctions (*arrows*).

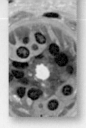

Chapter Summary

I. SKELETAL MUSCLE

A. Longitudinal Section

1. Connective tissue elements of **perimysium** contain nerves, blood vessels, collagen, fibroblasts, and occasionally other cell types. **Endomysium** is composed of fine reticular fibers and basal lamina, neither of which are normally evident with the light microscope.

2. **Skeletal muscle cells** appear as long, parallel, cylindrical fibers of almost uniform diameter. Nuclei are numerous and peripherally located. **Satellite cell** nuclei may be evident. Cross-striations, **A, I,** and **Z,** should be clearly noted at higher magnifications, and with oil immersion (or even high dry), the **H zone** and **M disc** may be distinguished in good preparations.

B. Transverse Section

1. Connective tissue elements may be noted, especially **nuclei of fibroblasts,** cross sections of **capillaries,** other small **blood vessels,** and **nerves.**

2. Muscle cells appear as irregular polygon-shaped sections of fibers of more or less uniform size. **Myofibrils** present a stippled appearance inside the fiber, frequently clustered into distinct but artifactual groups known as Cohnheim's fields. Peripherally, a **nucleus** or two may be noted in many fibers. Fasciculi are closely packed, but the delicate **endomysium** clearly outlines each cell.

II. CARDIAC MUSCLE

A. Longitudinal Section

1. Connective tissue elements are clearly identifiable because of the presence of **nuclei** that are considerably smaller than those of cardiac muscle cells. The connective tissue is rich in vascular components, especially **capillaries.** The **endomysium** is present but indistinct.

2. **Cardiac muscle cells** form long, branching, and anastomosing **muscle fibers.** Bluntly oval **nuclei** are large, are centrally located within the cell, and appear somewhat vesicular. **A** and **I bands** are present but are not as clearly defined as in skeletal muscle. **Intercalated**

discs, marking the boundaries of contiguous cardiac muscle cells, may be indistinct unless special staining techniques are used. **Purkinje fibers** are occasionally evident.

B. Transverse Section

1. Connective tissue elements separating muscle fibers from each other are obvious, since **nuclei** of these cells are much smaller than those of cardiac muscle cells.

2. Cross-sectional profiles of **muscle fibers** are irregularly shaped and vary in size. **Nuclei** are infrequent but are large and located in the center of the cell. **Myofibrils** are clumped as Cohnheim's fields (an artifact of fixation) in a radial arrangement. Occasionally, **Purkinje fibers** are noted, but they are present only in the subendocardium of the ventricles.

III. SMOOTH MUSCLE

A. Longitudinal Section

1. Connective tissue elements between individual muscle fibers are scant and consist of fine **reticular fibers.** Larger bundles or sheets of muscle fibers are separated by loose connective tissue housing blood vessels and nerves.

2. **Smooth muscle cells** are tightly packed, staggered, fusiform structures whose centrally located nuclei are oblong in shape. When the muscle fibers contract, their nuclei assume a characteristic corkscrew shape.

B. Transverse Section

1. A very limited amount of connective tissue, mostly **reticular fibers,** may be noted in the intercellular spaces. Sheets and bundles of smooth muscle are separated from each other by loose connective tissue in which neurovascular elements are evident.

2. Since **smooth muscle cells** are tightly packed, staggered, fusiform structures, transverse sections produce circular, homogeneous-appearing profiles of various diameters. Only the widest profiles contain **nuclei;** therefore, in transverse section, only a limited number of nuclei will be present.

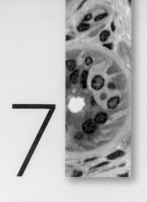

7 NERVOUS TISSUE

Nervous tissue is one of the four basic tissues of the body, and it specializes in receiving information from the external and internal milieu, integrating it, analyzing it, and comparing it with stored experiences and/or predetermined (reflex) responses, to select and effect an appropriate reaction.

- The reception of information is the function of the sensory component of the **peripheral nervous system (PNS)**.
- The processes of integration, analysis, and response are performed by the brain and spinal cord comprising the **central nervous system (CNS)** with its gray matter and white matter.
- The transmission of the response to the effector organ is relegated to the motor component of the PNS.

Therefore, it should be appreciated that the PNS is merely a physical extension of the CNS, and the separation of the two should not imply a strict dichotomy.

The nervous system may also be divided functionally into somatic and autonomic nervous systems. The **somatic nervous system** exercises conscious control over voluntary functions, whereas the **autonomic nervous system** controls involuntary functions. The autonomic nervous system is a motor system, acting on smooth muscle, cardiac muscle, and some glands. Its three components, **sympathetic**, **parasympathetic**, and **enteric nervous systems**, usually act in concert to maintain homeostasis.

- The sympathetic nervous system prepares the body for action as in a "fight or flight" mode,
- the parasympathetic system functions to calm the body and provides secretomotor innervation to most exocrine glands;
- the enteric nervous system is more or less a stand-alone system that is responsible for the process of digestion.
  - It is interesting to note that the enteric nervous system is very large, it has about the same number of neurons as those located in the spinal cord.
  - The actions of the enteric nervous system are modulated by the sympathetic and parasympathetic components of the autonomic nervous system.

The CNS is protected by a bony housing, consisting of the skull and vertebral column, and the **meninges**, a triple-layered connective tissue sheath.

- The outermost meninx is the thick fibrous **dura mater**.
- Deep to the dura mater is the **arachnoid**, a nonvascular connective tissue membrane.
- The innermost, vascular **pia mater** is the most intimate investment of the CNS.
- Located between the arachnoid and the pia mater is the **cerebrospinal fluid (CSF)**.

BLOOD-BRAIN BARRIER

The selective barrier that exists between the neural tissues of the CNS and many blood-borne substances is termed the **blood-brain barrier**. This barrier is formed by the fasciae occludentes of contiguous endothelial cells lining the continuous capillaries that course through the neural tissues.

- Certain substances (i.e., O_2, H_2O, CO_2, and selected small lipid-soluble substances and some drugs) can penetrate the barrier.
- Other substances, including glucose, certain vitamins, amino acids, and drugs, among others, access passage only by **receptor-mediated transport** and/or **facilitated diffusion**.
- Certain ions are also transported via **active transport**. It is also believed that some of the perivascular neuroglia may play a minor role in the maintenance of the blood-brain barrier.

NEURONS

The structural and functional unit of the nervous system is the **neuron**, a cell that is highly specialized to perform its two major functions of irritability and conductivity. Each neuron is composed of a **cell body (soma, perikaryon)** and processes of varied lengths, known as **axons** and **dendrites**, usually located on opposite sides of the cell body (see Graphic 7-2). A neuron possesses only a single axon. However, depending on the number of dendrites a neuron possesses, it may be

- **unipolar** (a single process but no dendrites—rare in vertebrates, but see below),
- **bipolar** (an axon and one dendrite), or
- the more common **multipolar** (an axon and several dendrites).
- An additional category exists where the single dendrite and the axon fuse during embryonic development, giving the false appearance of a unipolar neuron; therefore, it is known as a **pseudounipolar neuron**, although recently neuroanatomists began to refer to this neuron type as a **unipolar neuron**.

Neurons also may be classified according to their function. **Sensory neurons** receive stimuli from either the internal or external environment then transmit these impulses toward the CNS for processing. **Interneurons** act as connectors between neurons in a chain or typically between sensory and motor neurons within the CNS. **Motor neurons** conduct impulses from the CNS to the targets cells (muscles, glands, and other neurons).

Information is transferred from one neuron to another across an intercellular space or gap, the **synapse**. Depending on the regions of the neurons participating in the formation of the synapse, it could be axodendritic, axosomatic, axoaxonic, or dendrodendritic.

- Most synapses are axodendritic and involve one of many **neurotransmitter substances** (such as **acetylcholine**) that is released by the axon of the first neuron into the synaptic cleft.
- The chemical momentarily destabilizes the plasma membrane of the dendrite, and a wave of depolarization passes along the second neuron, which will cause the release of a neurotransmitter substance at the terminus of its axon.
  - This type of a chemical synapse is an **excitatory synapse**, which results in the transmission of an impulse.
  - Another type of synapse may stop the transmission of an impulse by stabilizing the plasma membrane of the second neuron; it is called an **inhibitory synapse**.

Membrane Resting Potential

The normal concentration of K^+ is about 20 times greater inside the cell than outside, whereas the concentration of Na^+ is 10 times greater outside the cell than inside. The **resting potential** across the neuron cell membrane is maintained by the presence of **potassium leak channels** in the plasmalemma.

- These potassium leak channels are always open, and it is through these channels that K^+ ions diffuse from inside the cell to the outside, thus establishing a **positive charge on the outer** aspect and a **negative (less positive) charge on the internal** aspect of the cell membrane, with a total differential of about 40 to 100 mV.
- Na^+ ions can also traverse this channel, but at a 100-fold slower rate than potassium ions.
- Although the majority of the establishment of the membrane potential is due to the potassium leak channel, the action of the **Na^+-K^+ pump** does contribute to it to a certain extent.

Action Potential

The **action potential** is an electrical activity where charges move along the membrane surface. It is an **all-or-none response** whose duration and amplitude are constant. Some axons are capable of sustaining up to 1,000 impulses/second.

- **Generation of an action potential** begins when a region of the plasma membrane is **depolarized**.
- As the resting potential diminishes, a **threshold level** is reached, voltage-gated Na^+ channels open, Na^+ rushes

into the cell, and at that point, the **resting potential is reversed**, so that the inside becomes positive with respect to the outside.

- In response to this reversal of the resting potential, the Na^+ channel closes and for the next 1 to 2 ms cannot be opened (the **refractory period**).
- Depolarization also causes the **opening** of voltage-gated K^+ channels (note that these are different from the potassium leak channels) through which potassium ions exit the cell, thus repolarizing the membrane and ending not only the refractory period of the Na^+ channel but also the closure of the voltage-gated potassium channel.

The movement of Na^+ ions that enter the cell causes depolarization of the cell membrane toward the axon terminal (**orthodromic spread**). Although sodium ions also move away from the axon terminal (**antidromic spread**), they are unable to affect sodium channels in the antidromic direction, since those channels are in their refractory period.

Myoneural Junctions

Neurons also communicate with other effector cells at synapses. A special type of synapse, between skeletal muscle cells and neurons is known as a myoneural junction. The axon forms a terminal swelling, known as the **axon terminal** (**end-foot**), that comes close to but does not contact the muscle cell's sarcolemma.

- Mitochondria, synaptic vesicles, and elements of smooth endoplasmic reticulum are present in the axon terminal.
- The axolemma involved in the formation of the synapse is known as the **presynaptic membrane**, whereas
- the sarcolemmal counterpart is known as the **postsynaptic membrane**.
  - The presynaptic membrane has **sodium channels, voltage-gated calcium channels**, and **carrier proteins** for the cotransport of Na^+ and choline.
  - The postsynaptic membrane has **acetylcholine receptors** as well as slight invaginations known as **junctional folds**.
  - A basal lamina containing the enzyme **acetylcholinesterase** is also associated with the postsynaptic membrane.
- As the impulse reaches the end-foot, sodium channels open, and the presynaptic membrane becomes depolarized, resulting in the opening of the voltage-gated calcium channels and the influx of Ca^+ into the end-foot.
- The high intracellular calcium concentration causes the synaptic vesicles, containing **acetylcholine**,

TABLE 7-1 • Common Neurotransmitters

Neurotransmitter	Location	Function
Acetylcholine	Myoneural junctions; all parasympathetic synapses; preganglionic sympathetic synapses	Activates skeletal muscle, autonomic nerves, brain functions
Norepinephrine	Postganglionic sympathetic synapses	Increases cardiac output
Glutamate	CNS; presynaptic sensory and cortex	Most common excitatory neurotransmitter of CNS
GABA	CNS	Most common inhibitory neurotransmitter of CNS
Dopamine	CNS	Inhibitory and excitatory, depending on receptor
Glycine	Brainstem and spinal cord	Inhibitory
Serotonin	CNS	Pain inhibitor; mood control; sleep
Aspartate	CNS	Excitatory
Enkephalins	CNS	Analgesic; inhibits pain transmission
Endorphins	CNS	Analgesic; inhibits pain transmission

proteoglycans, and ATP, to fuse with the presynaptic membrane and release their contents into the synaptic cleft.

- The process of fusion depends on receptor molecules in both vesicles and the presynaptic membranes.
  - These receptor molecules are known as **vesicular docking proteins** and **presynaptic membrane docking proteins**.
- After the contents of the synaptic vesicle are released, the presynaptic membrane is larger than prior to fusion, and this excess membrane will be recycled via the formation of clathrin-coated vesicles, thus maintaining the morphology and requisite surface area of the presynaptic membrane.
- The released acetylcholine binds to **acetylcholine receptors** of the sarcolemma, thus opening **sodium channels**, resulting in sodium influx into the muscle cell, depolarization of the postsynaptic membrane, and the subsequent generation of an action potential and muscle cell contraction.
- **Acetylcholinesterase** of the basal lamina cleaves acetylcholine into **choline** and **acetate**, ensuring that a single release of the neurotransmitter substance will not continue to generate excess action potentials.
  - The choline is returned to the end-foot via carrier proteins that are powered by a sodium gradient, where it is combined with activated acetate (derived from mitochondria), a reaction catalyzed by **acetylcholine transferase**, to form acetylcholine.
  - The newly formed acetylcholine is transported into forming synaptic vesicles by a proton pump-driven, antiport carrier protein.

Neurotransmitter Substances

Neurotransmitter substances are signaling molecules (chemical messengers) that are released at the presynaptic membrane and effect a response by binding to receptor molecules (integral proteins) of the postsynaptic membrane. Neurotransmitter substances are varied in chemical composition and are categorized according to their chemical construction as cholinergic, monoaminergic, peptidergic, nonpeptidergic, GABAergic, glutamatergic, and glycinergic (Table 7-1).

SUPPORTING CELLS

Neuroglial cells function in the metabolism and the support of neurons. To prevent spontaneous or accidental depolarization of the neuron's cell membrane, specialized neuroglial cells provide a physical covering over its entire surface. In the CNS, these cells are known as **astrocytes** and **oligodendroglia**, whereas in the PNS they are **capsule** and **Schwann cells**.

- Oligodendroglia and Schwann cells have the capability of forming **myelin sheaths** around axons (Graphic 7-2), which increases the conduction velocity of the impulse along the axon (Table 7-2). The region where the myelin sheath of one Schwann cell (or oligodendroglion) ends and the next one begins is referred to as the **node of Ranvier**.
- Additionally, the CNS possesses **microglia**, which are **macrophages** derived from monocytes, and **ependymal cells**, which line brain ventricles and the central canal of the spinal cord.

TABLE 7-2 • Nerve Fiber Classification and Conduction Velocities

Fiber Group	Diameter (μm)	Conduction Velocity (m/s)	Function
A fibers—highly myelinated	1–20	15–120	High velocity—motor to skeletal muscles. Most sensory: pain, touch, proprioception, temperature
B fibers—less highly myelinated	1–3	3–15	Moderate velocity—mostly visceral afferents, preganglionic to ganglion soma, nocioceptive, pressure,
C fibers—nonmyelinated	0.5–1.5	0.5–2	Slow velocity—chronic pain fibers, postganglionic autonomic fibers

PERIPHERAL NERVES

- **Peripheral nerves** are composed of numerous nerve fibers collected into several fascicles (bundles). These bundles possess a thick connective tissue sheath, the **epineurium** (see Graphic 7-1).
- Each fascicle within the epineurium is surrounded by a **perineurium** consisting of an outer connective tissue layer and an inner layer of flattened epithelioid cells.
- Each nerve fiber and associated Schwann cell has its own slender connective tissue sheath, the **endoneurium**, whose components include fibroblasts, an occasional macrophage, and collagenous and reticular fibers.

Certain terms must be defined to facilitate understanding of the nervous system. A **ganglion** is a collection of nerve cell bodies in the PNS, whereas a similar collection of soma in the CNS is called a **nucleus**. A bundle of axons traveling together in the CNS is known as a **tract** (or **fasciculus** or **column**), whereas a similar bundle in the PNS is known as a **peripheral nerve** (nerve).

 CLINICAL CONSIDERATIONS

Neuroglial Tumors
Almost 50% of the intracranial tumors are due to proliferation of neuroglial cells. Some of the neuroglial tumors, such as **oligodendroglioma**, are of mild severity, whereas others, such as **glioblastoma** that are neoplastic cells derived from astrocytes, are highly invasive and usually fatal.

Huntington's Chorea
Huntington's chorea is a hereditary condition that becomes evident in the third and fourth decade of life. Initially, this condition affects only the joints but later is responsible for motor dysfunction and dementia. It is thought to be caused by the loss of neurons of the CNS that produce the neurotransmitter **GABA** (**gamma-aminobutyric acid**). The advent of dementia is thought to be related to the loss of acetylcholine-secreting cells.

Parkinson's Disease
Parkinson's disease is related to the loss of the neurotransmitter **dopamine** in the brain. This crippling disease causes muscular rigidity, tremor, slow movement, and progressively difficult voluntary movement.

Therapeutic Circumvention of the Blood-Brain Barrier
The selective nature of the blood-brain barrier prevents certain therapeutic drugs and neurotransmitters conveyed by the bloodstream from entering the CNS. For example, the perfusion of **mannitol** into the blood stream changes the capillary permeability by altering the tight junctions, thus permitting administration of therapeutic drugs. Other therapeutic drugs can be attached to antibodies developed against **transferrin receptors** located on the luminal aspect of the plasma membranes of these endothelial cells that will permit transport into the CNS.

Guillain-Barré Syndrome
Guillain-Barré syndrome is a form of immune-mediated condition resulting in rapidly progressing weakness with possible paralysis of the extremities and,

occasionally, even of the respiratory and facial muscles. This demyelinating disease is often associated with a recent respiratory or gastrointestinal infection; the muscle weakness reaches its greatest point within 3 weeks of the initial symptoms, and 5% of the afflicted individuals die of the disease. Early recognition of the disease is imperative for complete (or nearly complete) recovery.

Ischemic Injury

Ischemia, the reduction of blood supply to an organ, such as the brain, results in hypoxia and subsequent cell death. The cause of ischemia could be blockage of a blood vessel that serves the particular area, or of another vessel farther away whose responsibility is to supply blood flow to the particular vessels in question. Other causes of diminished blood supply could be lowered blood pressure, cardiac insufficiency, accidental injury to a vessel, as well as a myriad of other factors. Ischemia in the brain is evidenced by the presence of necrotic neurons (different from apoptotic neurons) whose cytoplasm displays a high degree of eosinophilia. These necrotic neurons are known as **red neurons**.

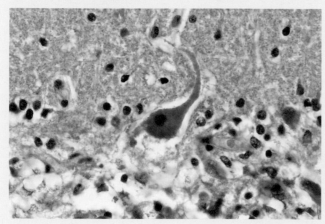

This Purkinje cell from the cerebellum of a patient displays a high degree of eosinophilia and is considered to be a red neuron. The presence of such cells indicates that the patient had an ischemic injury of a region of the cerebellum. Note that the cell is reduced in size, its nucleus is pyknotic, and the nucleolus is not evident. If this cell had died because of an apoptotic event, its cytoplasm would be basophilic. (Reprinted with permission from Mills SE, ed. Histology for Pathologists, 3rd ed., Philadelphia: Lippincott, Williams & Wilkins, 2007. p. 287.)

Alzheimer's Disease

Alzheimer's disease (**AD**) is one of the most common forms of dementia that affects approximately 5 million people in the United States and more than 30 million globally.

This devastating condition begins, on the average, around the age of 65 but may affect individuals at a much younger age. The early onset of AD is often masked as symptoms of stress or "senior moments"; however, it progresses to include the incapacity to remember newly acquired information. Additional symptoms develop as the disease continues its progress, namely, personality changes to a more hostile and petulant behavior accompanied by uncertainty and language difficulty. Moreover, the patient experiences an inability to remember previously known personal and general information and the patient eventually becomes unable to take care of bodily functions, resulting in immobility and muscle loss. Individuals diagnosed with AD usually die within 7 to 10 years. Although the cause of the disease is not known, it has been suggested that the intraneuron presence of neurofibrillary tangles, formed by coalescence of modified tau proteins, and the deposition of beta-amyloid-like protein interfere with neuronal function.

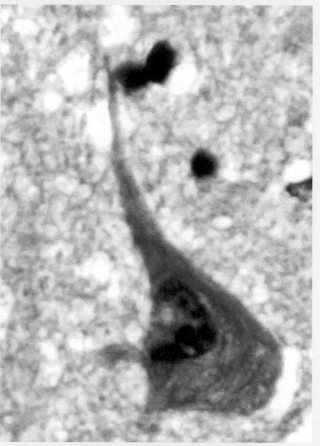

The neuron depicted in this photomicrographs is from a patient who died as a result of AD. Note the presence of neurofibrillary tangles in its cytoplasm. (Reprinted with permission from Mills SE, Carter D, et al., eds. Sternberg's Diagnostic Surgical Pathology, 5th ed. Philadelphia: Lippincott, Williams & Wilkins, 2010. p. 441.)

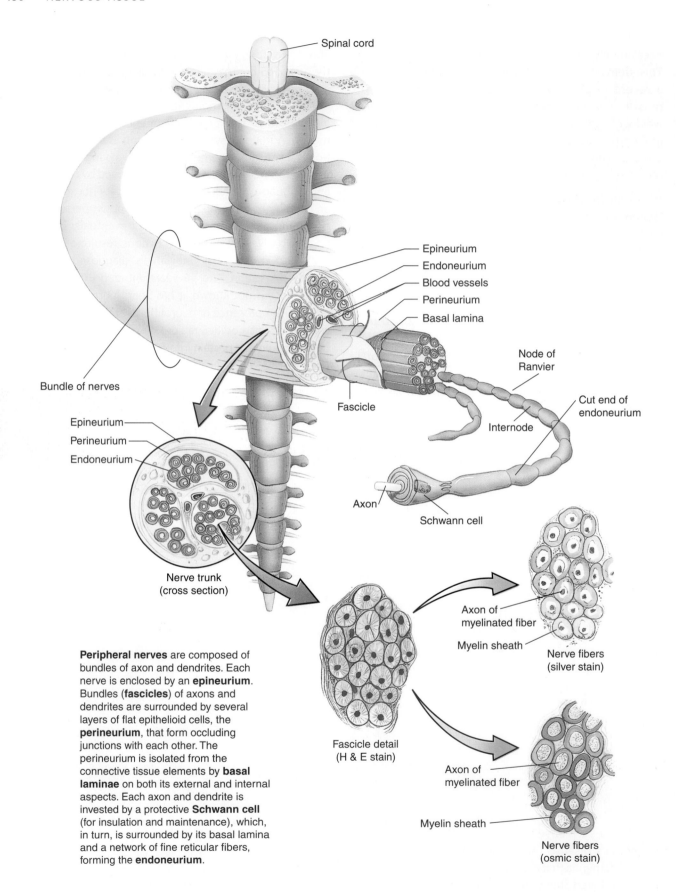

Spinal cord

Epineurium
Endoneurium
Blood vessels
Perineurium
Basal lamina

Node of Ranvier

Cut end of endoneurium

Internode

Fascicle

Bundle of nerves

Axon

Schwann cell

Epineurium
Perineurium
Endoneurium

Nerve trunk
(cross section)

Axon of
myelinated fiber

Myelin sheath

Nerve fibers
(silver stain)

Fascicle detail
(H & E stain)

Axon of
myelinated fiber

Myelin sheath

Nerve fibers
(osmic stain)

Peripheral nerves are composed of bundles of axon and dendrites. Each nerve is enclosed by an **epineurium**. Bundles (**fascicles**) of axons and dendrites are surrounded by several layers of flat epithelioid cells, the **perineurium**, that form occluding junctions with each other. The perineurium is isolated from the connective tissue elements by **basal laminae** on both its external and internal aspects. Each axon and dendrite is invested by a protective **Schwann cell** (for insulation and maintenance), which, in turn, is surrounded by its basal lamina and a network of fine reticular fibers, forming the **endoneurium**.

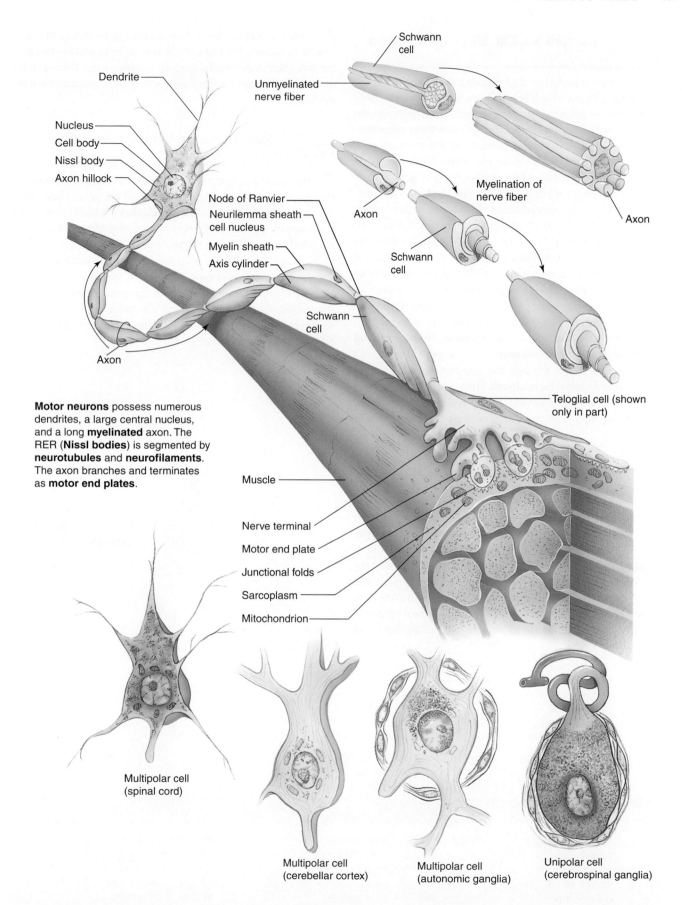

Dendrite

Nucleus
Cell body
Nissl body
Axon hillock

Schwann cell

Unmyelinated nerve fiber

Axon

Myelination of nerve fiber

Schwann cell

Axon

Node of Ranvier
Neurilemma sheath cell nucleus
Myelin sheath
Axis cylinder

Schwann cell

Axon

Teloglial cell (shown only in part)

Motor neurons possess numerous dendrites, a large central nucleus, and a long **myelinated** axon. The RER (**Nissl bodies**) is segmented by **neurotubules** and **neurofilaments**. The axon branches and terminates as **motor end plates**.

Muscle

Nerve terminal

Motor end plate

Junctional folds

Sarcoplasm

Mitochondrion

Multipolar cell
(spinal cord)

Multipolar cell
(cerebellar cortex)

Multipolar cell
(autonomic ganglia)

Unipolar cell
(cerebrospinal ganglia)

PLATE 7-1 • Spinal Cord

FIGURE 1. Spinal cord. x.s. Cat. Silver stain. Paraffin section. ×21.

The spinal cord is invested by a protective coating, the three-layered meninges. Its outermost fibrous layer, the **dura mater** (DM), is surrounded by epidural fat, not present in this photomicrograph. Deep to the dura is the **arachnoid** (A) with its **subarachnoid space** (SS), which is closely applied to the most intimate layer of the meninges, the vascular **pia mater** (PM). The spinal cord itself is organized into **white matter** (W) and **gray matter** (G). The former, which is peripherally located and does not contain nerve cell bodies, is composed of nerve fibers, most of which are myelinated, that travel up and down the cord. It is cellular, however, since it houses various types of glial cells. The centrally positioned gray matter contains the cell bodies of the neurons as well as the initial and terminal ends of their processes, many of which are not usually myelinated. These nerve cell processes and those of the numerous glial cells form an intertwined network of fibers that is referred to as the neuropil. The gray matter is subdivided into regions, namely, the **dorsal horn** (DH), the **ventral horn** (VH), and the **gray commissure** (Gc). The **central canal** (CC) of the spinal cord passes through the gray commissure, dividing it into dorsal and ventral components. Processes of neurons leave and enter the spinal cord as **ventral** (VR) and **dorsal** (DR) **roots**, respectively. A region similar to the *boxed area* is represented in Figure 2.

FIGURE 2. Spinal cord. x.s. White and gray matter. Human. Paraffin section. ×132.

This photomicrograph represents the *boxed region* of Figure 1. Observe that the interface between **white matter** (W) and **gray matter** (G) is readily evident (*asterisks*). The numerous nuclei (*arrowheads*) present in white matter belong to the various neuroglia, which support the axons and dendrites traveling up and down the spinal cord. The large **nerve cell bodies** (CB) in the ventral horn of the gray matter possess vesicular-appearing nuclei with dense, dark nucleoli. **Blood vessels** (BV), which penetrate deep into the gray matter, are surrounded by processes of neuroglial cells, forming the blood-brain barrier, not visible in this photomicrograph. Small nuclei (*arrows*) in gray matter belong to the neuroglial cells, whose cytoplasm and cellular processes are not evident.

FIGURE 3. Spinal cord. x.s. Ventral horn. Human. Paraffin section. ×270.

The multipolar neurons and their various processes (*arrows*) are clearly evident in this photomicrograph of the ventral horn. Note the large **nucleus** (N) and dense **nucleolus** (n), both of which are characteristic of neurons. Observe the clumps of basophilic material, **Nissl bodies** (NB), that electron microscopy has demonstrated to be rough endoplasmic reticulum. The small nuclei belong to the various **neuroglial cells** (Ng), which, along with their processes and processes of the neurons, compose the **neuropil** (Np), the matted-appearing background substance of gray matter. The white spaces (*asterisks*) surrounding the soma and blood vessels are due to shrinkage artifacts.

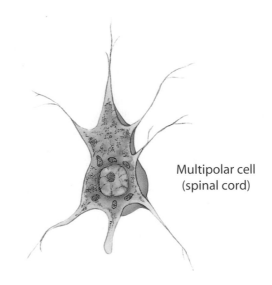

Multipolar cell
(spinal cord)

KEY							
A	arachnoid	G	gray matter	PM	pia mater
BV	blood vessel	Gc	gray commissure	SS	subarachnoid space
CB	nerve cell body	N	nucleus	VH	ventral horn
CC	central canal	N	nucleolus	VR	ventral root
DH	dorsal horn	NB	Nissl body	W	white matter
DM	dura mater	Ng	neuroglial cell		
DR	dorsal root	Np	neuropil		

PLATE 7-1 • Spinal Cord

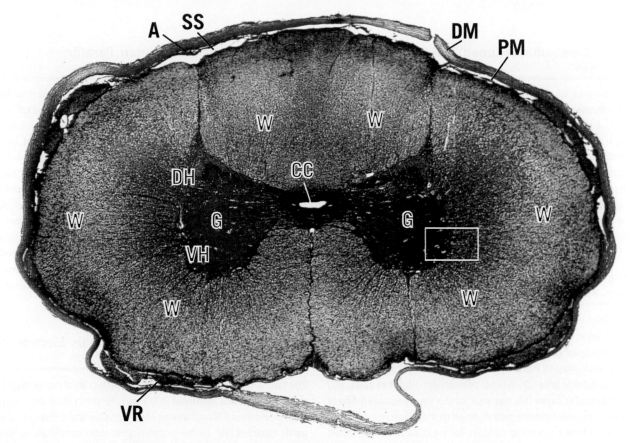

FIGURE 1

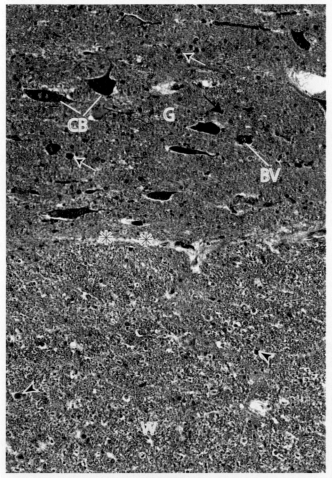

FIGURE 2

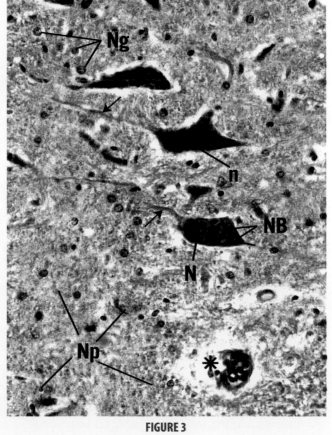

FIGURE 3

PLATE 7-2 • Cerebellum, Synapse, Electron Microscopy

FIGURE 1. Cerebellum. Human. Paraffin section. ×14.

The cerebellum, in contrast to the spinal cord, consists of a core of **white matter** (W) and the superficially located **gray matter** (G). Although it is difficult to tell from this low-magnification photomicrograph, the gray matter is subdivided into three layers: the outer **molecular layer** (ML), a middle **Purkinje cell layer** (PL), and the inner **granular layer** (GL). The less dense appearance of the molecular layer is due to the sparse arrangement of nerve cell bodies, whereas the darker appearance of the granular layer is a function of the great number of darkly staining nuclei packed closely together. A region similar to the *boxed area* is represented in Figure 2.

FIGURE 3. Purkinje cell. Human cerebellum. Paraffin section. ×540.

This is a higher magnification of the *boxed area* of Figure 2. The **granular layer** (GL) of the cerebellum is composed of two cell types, the smaller **granule cells** (GC) and larger **Golgi type II cells** (G2). The flask-shaped **Purkinje cell** (PC) displays its large **nucleus** (N) and **dendritic tree** (D). Nuclei of numerous **basket cells** (BC) of the **molecular layer** (ML) as well as the **unmyelinated fibers** (UF) of the granule cells are well defined in this photomicrograph. These fibers make synaptic contact (*arrows*) with the dendritic processes of the Purkinje cells. *Inset.* **Astrocyte. Human cerebellum. Golgi stain. Paraffin section.** ×132. Note the numerous processes of this **fibrous astrocyte** (A) in the white matter of the cerebellum.

FIGURE 2. Cerebellum. Human. Paraffin section. ×132.

This photomicrograph is taken from a region similar to the *boxed area* in Figure 1. The **granular layer** (GL) is composed of closely packed **granule cells** (GC), which, at first glance, resemble lymphocytes due to their dark, round nuclei. Interspersed among these cells are clear spaces called glomeruli or **cerebellar islands** (CI), where synapses occur between axons entering the cerebellum from outside and dendrites of granule cells. The **Purkinje cells** (PC) send their axons into the granular layer; their dendrites arborize in the **molecular layer** (ML). This layer also contains unmyelinated fibers from the granular layer as well as two types of cells, **basket cells** (BC) and the more superficially located **stellate cells** (SC). The surface of the cerebellum is invested by **pia matter** (PM), just barely evident in this photomicrograph. The *boxed area* is presented at a higher magnification in Figure 3.

FIGURE 4. Synapse. Afferent terminals. Electron microscopy. ×16,200.

The lateral descending nucleus of the fifth cranial nerve displays a **primary afferent terminal** (AT) that is forming multiple synapses with **dendrites** (D) and **axons** (Ax). Observe the presence of **synaptic vesicles** (SV) in the postsynaptic axon terminals as well as the thickening of the membrane of the primary afferent terminal (*arrows*). This terminal also houses **mitochondria** (m) and **cisternae** (Ci) for the synaptic vesicles. (From Meszler RM. Fine structure and organization of the infrared receptor relays: lateral descending nucleus of V in Boidae and nucleus reticularis caloris in the rattlesnake. *J Comp Neurol* 1983;220:299–309.)

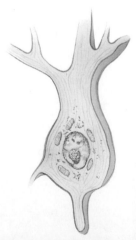

Multipolar cell
(cerebellar cortex)

KEY					
A	fibrous astrocyte	**G**	gray matter	**PC**	Purkinje cell
AT	primary afferent terminal	**G2**	Golgi type II cell	**PL**	Purkinje cell layer
Ax	axons	**GC**	granule cell	**PM**	pia mater
BC	basket cell	**GL**	granular layer	**SC**	stellate cell
CI	cerebellar island	**M**	mitochondrion	**SV**	synaptic vesicle
Ci	cistern	**ML**	molecular layer	**UF**	unmyelinated fiber
D	dendrite	**N**	nucleus	**W**	white matter

PLATE 7-2 · Cerebellum, Synapse, Electron Microscopy

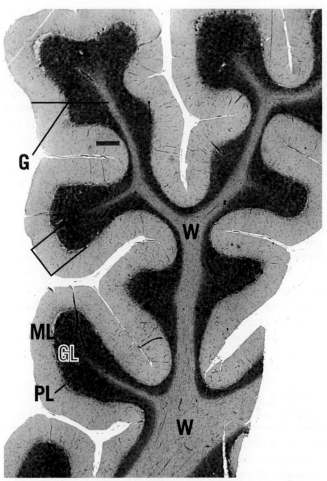

FIGURE 1

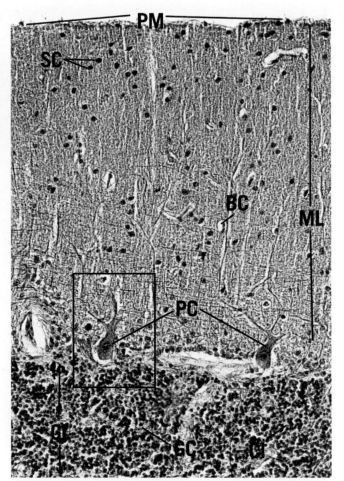

FIGURE 2

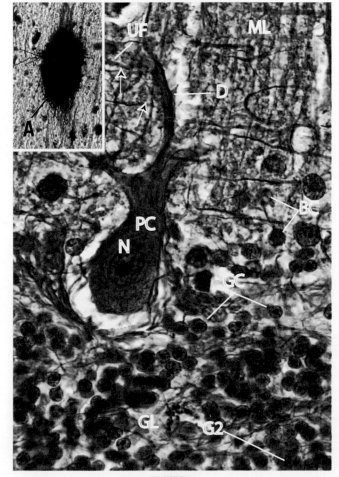

FIGURE 3

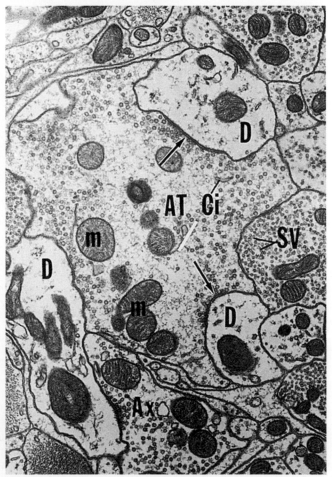

FIGURE 4

PLATE 7-3 · Cerebrum, Neuroglial Cells

FIGURES 1 and 2. Cerebrum. Human. Paraffin section. ×132.

These figures represent a montage of the entire human cerebral cortex and some of the underlying **white matter** (W) at a low magnification. Observe that the numerous **blood vessels** (BV) that penetrate the entire cortex are surrounded by a clear area (*arrow*), which is due to shrinkage artifact. The six layers of the cortex are not clearly defined but are approximated by brackets. The **pia mater** (PM), covering the surface of the cortex, is a vascular tissue that provides larger blood vessels as well as **capillaries** (Ca) that penetrate the brain tissue. Layer one of the cortex is known as the **molecular layer** (1), which contains numerous fibers and only a few neuron cell bodies. It is difficult to distinguish these somata from the neuroglial cells at this magnification. The second, **external granular layer** (2) is composed of small **granule cells** (GC) as well as many **neuroglial cells** (Ng). The third layer is known as the **external pyramidal layer** (3), which is the thickest layer in this section of the cerebral cortex. It consists of **pyramidal cells** (Py) and some **granule cells** (GC) as well as numerous **neuroglia** (Ng) interspersed among the soma and fibers. The fourth layer, the **internal granular layer** (4), is a relatively narrow band whose cell population consists mostly of small and a few large **granule cells** (GC) and the ever-present **neuroglial cells** (Ng). The **internal pyramidal layer** (5) houses medium and large **pyramidal cells** (Py) as well as the ubiquitous **neuroglia** (Ng), whose nuclei appear as small dots. Although not evident in this preparation, nerve fibers of the internal band of Baillarger pass horizontally through this layer,

whereas those of the external band of Baillarger traverse the internal granular layer. The deepest layer of the cerebral cortex is the **multiform layer** (6), which contains cells of various shapes, many of which are fusiform in morphology. Neuroglial cells and Martinotti cells are also present in this layer but cannot be distinguished from each other at this magnification. The **white matter** (W) appears very cellular, due to the nuclei of the numerous neuroglial cells supporting the cell processes derived from and traveling to the cortex.

FIGURE 3. Astrocytes. Silver stain. Paraffin section. ×132.

This photomicrograph of the white matter of the cerebrum presents a matted appearance due to the interweaving of various nerve cell and glial cell processes. Note also the presence of two **blood vessels** (BV) passing horizontally across the field. The long processes of the **fibrous astrocytes** (FA) approach the blood vessels (*arrows*) and assist in the formation of the blood-brain barrier.

FIGURE 4. Microglia. Silver stain. Paraffin section. ×540.

This photomicrograph is of a section of the cerebral cortex, demonstrating **nuclei** (N) of nerve cells as well as the presence of **microglia** (Mi). Note that microglia are very small and possess a dense **nucleus** (N) as well as numerous cell processes (*arrows*).

KEY

BV	blood vessel	Ng	neurological cell	3	external pyramidal layer
Ca	capillary	PM	pia mater	4	internal granular layer
FA	fibrous astrocyte	Py	pyramidal cell	5	internal pyramidal layer
GC	granule cell	W	white matter	6	multiform layer
Mi	microglia	1	molecular layer		
N	nucleus	2	external granular layer		

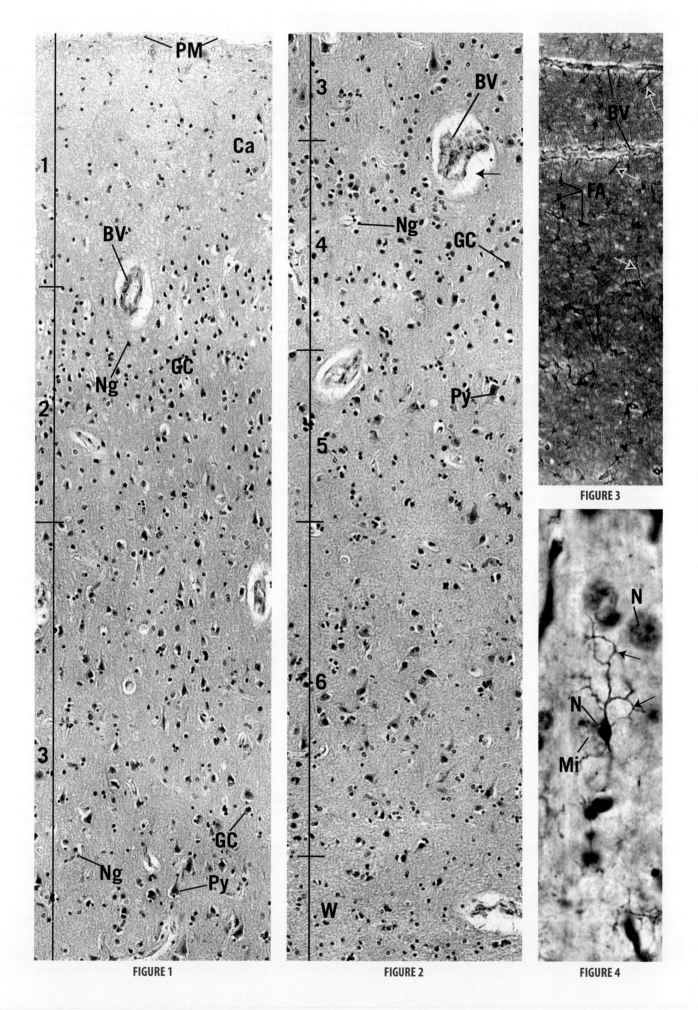

PLATE 7-3 · Cerebrum, Neuroglial Cells

FIGURE 1

FIGURE 2

FIGURE 3

FIGURE 4

PLATE 7-4 · Sympathetic Ganglia, Sensory Ganglia

FIGURE 1. Sympathetic ganglion. l.s. Paraffin section. ×132.

Sympathetic ganglia are structures that receive axons of presynaptic cells, whose soma is within the CNS. Located within the ganglion are somata of postsynaptic neurons upon which the presynaptic cell axons synapse. These ganglia are enveloped by a collagenous connective tissue **capsule** (C), which sends **septa** (S) containing **blood vessels** (BV) within the substance of the ganglion. The arrangement of the cell bodies of the **multipolar neurons** (MN) within the ganglion appears to be haphazard. This very vascular structure contains numerous nuclei that belong to **endothelial cells** (E), intravascular **leukocytes** (L), **fibroblasts** (F), **Schwann cells** (ScC), and those of the **supporting cells** (SS) surrounding the nerve cell bodies. A region similar to the *boxed area* is presented in Figure 2.

FIGURE 3. Sensory ganglion. l.s. Human. Paraffin section. ×132.

The dorsal root ganglion provides a good representative example of a sensory ganglion. It possesses a **vascular** (BV) connective tissue **capsule** (C), which also envelops its sensory root. The neurons of the dorsal root ganglion are pseudounipolar in morphology; therefore, their **somata** (So) appear spherical in shape. The **fibers** (f), many of which are myelinated, alternate with rows of cell bodies. Note that some somata are large (*arrow*), whereas others are small (*arrowhead*). Each soma is surrounded by neuroectodermally derived **capsule cells** (Cc). A region similar to the *boxed area* is presented at a high magnification in Figure 4.

FIGURE 2. Sympathetic ganglion. l.s. Paraffin section. ×540.

This photomicrograph presents a higher magnification of a region similar to the *boxed area* of Figure 1. Although neurons of the sympathetic ganglion are multipolar, their processes are not evident in this specimen stained with hematoxylin and eosin. The **nucleus** (N), with its prominent **nucleolus** (n), is clearly visible. The cytoplasm contains **lipofuscin** (Li) a yellowish pigment that is prevalent in neurons of older individuals. The clear space between the soma and the **supporting cells** (SS) is a shrinkage artifact. Note the numerous **blood vessels** (BV) containing red blood cells (*arrows*) and a **neutrophil** (Ne).

FIGURE 4. Sensory ganglion. l.s. Human. Paraffin section. ×270.

This photomicrograph is a higher magnification of a region similar to the *boxed area* of Figure 3. The spherical cell bodies display their centrally located **nuclei** (N) and **nucleoli** (n). Observe that both small (*arrowheads*) and large (*arrows*) somata are present in the field and that the nuclei are not always in the plane of section. Hematoxylin and eosin stain the somata a more or less homogeneous pink, so that organelles such as Nissl substance are not visible. However, the nuclei and cytoplasm of **capsule cells** (Cc) are clearly evident. Moreover, the small, elongated, densely staining nuclei of **fibroblasts** (F) are also noted to surround somata, just peripheral to the capsule cells. **Axons** (Ax) of myelinated nerve fibers belong to the large pseudounipolar neurons.

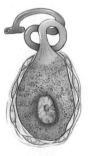
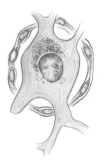
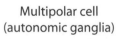

Multipolar cell
(autonomic ganglia)

Unipolar cell
(pseudounipolar
cell from dorsal
root ganglion)

KEY

Ax	axon	F	nerve fiber	Ne	neutrophil
BV	blood vessel	L	leukocyte	S	septum
C	capsule	Li	lipofuscin	ScC	Schwann cell
Cc	capsule cell	N	nucleolus	So	soma
E	endothelial cell	MN	multipolar neuron	SS	supporting cell
F	fibroblast	N	nucleus		

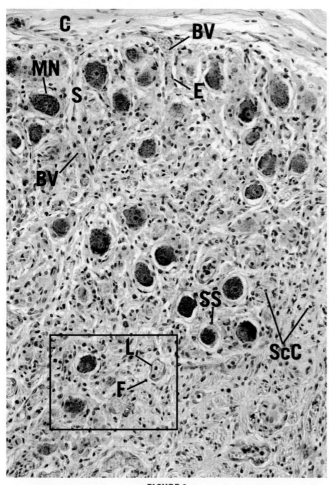

FIGURE 1

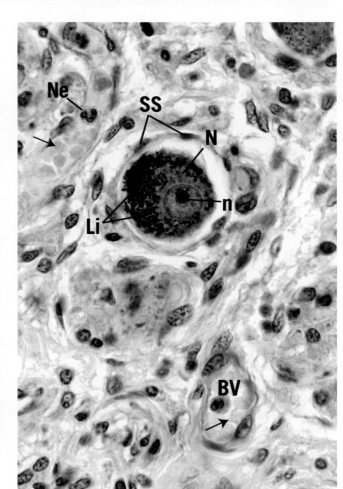

FIGURE 2

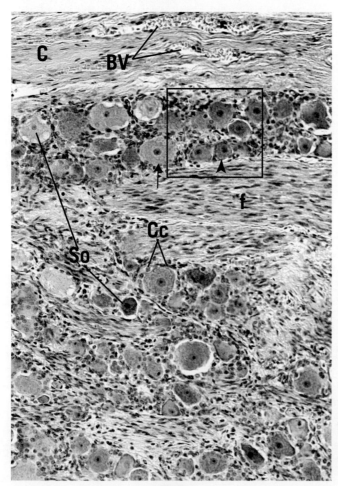

FIGURE 3

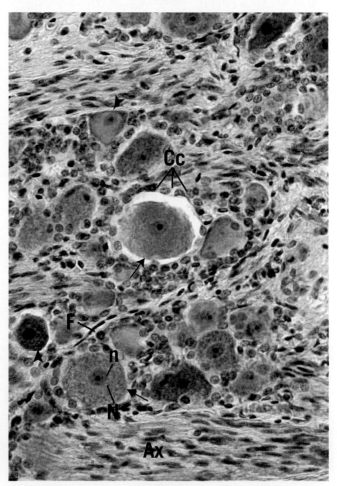

FIGURE 4

PLATE 7-4 · Sympathetic Ganglia, Sensory Ganglia

PLATE 7-5 • Peripheral Nerve, Choroid Plexus

FIGURE 1a. Peripheral nerve. l.s. Monkey. Plastic section. ×132.

The longitudinal section of the peripheral nerve fascicle presented in this photomicrograph is enveloped by its **perineurium** (P), composed of an outer **connective tissue layer** (CT) and an inner layer of flattened **epithelioid cells** (E). The perineurium conducts small **blood vessels** (BV), which are branches of larger vessels traveling in the surrounding epineurium, a structure composed of loose connective tissue with numerous fat cells. The peripheral nerve is composed of numerous nonmyelinated and myelinated nerve fibers, an example of which is presented in **Figure 1b**. The dense nuclei (*arrows*) within the nerve fascicle belong to Schwann cells and endoneurial cells. A region similar to the *boxed area* is presented in Figure 2.

FIGURE 1b. Teased, myelinated nerve fiber. Paraffin section. l.s. ×540.

This longitudinal section of a single myelinated nerve fiber displays its **axon** (Ax) and the neurokeratin network, the remnants of the dissolved **myelin** (M). Note the **node of Ranvier** (NR), a region where two Schwann cells meet. It is here, where the axon is not covered by myelin, that saltatory conduction of impulses occurs. Observe that **Schmidt-Lanterman incisures** (SL) are clearly evident. These are regions where the cytoplasm of Schwann cells is trapped in the myelin sheath.

FIGURE 3. Peripheral nerve. x.s. Paraffin section. ×132.

This transverse section presents portions of two fascicles, each surrounded by **perineurium** (P). The intervening loose connective tissue of the **epineurium** (Ep) with its **blood vessels** (BV) is clearly evident. The perineurium forms a **septum** (S), which subdivides this fascicle into two compartments. Note that the **axons** (Ax) are in the center of the **myelin sheath** (MS) and occasionally a crescent-shaped nucleus of a **Schwann cell** (ScC) is evident. The denser, smaller nuclei (*arrows*) belong to endoneurial cells. *Inset.* **Peripheral nerve. x.s. Silver stain. Paraffin section.** ×540. Silver-stained sections of myelinated nerve fibers have the large, clear spaces (*arrow*) that indicate the dissolved myelin. The **axons** (Ax) stain well as dark, dense structures, and the delicate **endoneurium** (En) is also evident.

FIGURE 2. Peripheral nerve. l.s. Paraffin section. ×270.

This is a higher magnification of a region similar to the *boxed area* of Figure 1a. A distinguishing characteristic of longitudinal sections of peripheral nerves is that they appear to follow a zigzag course, particularly evident in this photomicrograph. The sinuous course of these fibers is accentuated by the presence of nuclei of **Schwann cells** (ScC), **fibroblasts** (F), and endothelial cells of capillaries belonging to the endoneurium. Many of these nerve fibers are **myelinated** (M) as corroborated by the presence of the **nodes of Ranvier** (NR) and myelin proteins around the **axons** (Ax).

FIGURE 4. Choroid plexus. Paraffin section. ×270.

The choroid plexus, located within the ventricles of the brain, is responsible for the formation of CSF. This structure is composed of tufts of **capillaries** (Ca) whose tortuous course is followed by **villi** (Vi) of the simple cuboidal **choroid plexus epithelium** (cp). The **connective tissue core** (CT) of the choroid plexus is contributed by pia-arachnoid, whereas the simple cuboidal epithelium is modified ependymal lining of the ventricle. The clear spaces surrounding the choroid plexus belong to the ventricle of the brain.

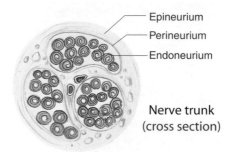

Epineurium
Perineurium
Endoneurium

Nerve trunk
(cross section)

KEY

Ax	axon	**En**	endoneurium	**P**	perineurium
BV	blood vessel	**Ep**	epineurium	**S**	septum
Ca	capillary	**F**	fibroblast	**ScC**	Schwann cell
Cp	choroid plexus epithelium	**M**	myelin	**SL**	Schmidt-Lanterman incisure
CT	connective tissue	**MS**	myelin sheath	**Vi**	villus
E	epithelioid cell	**NR**	node of Ranvier		

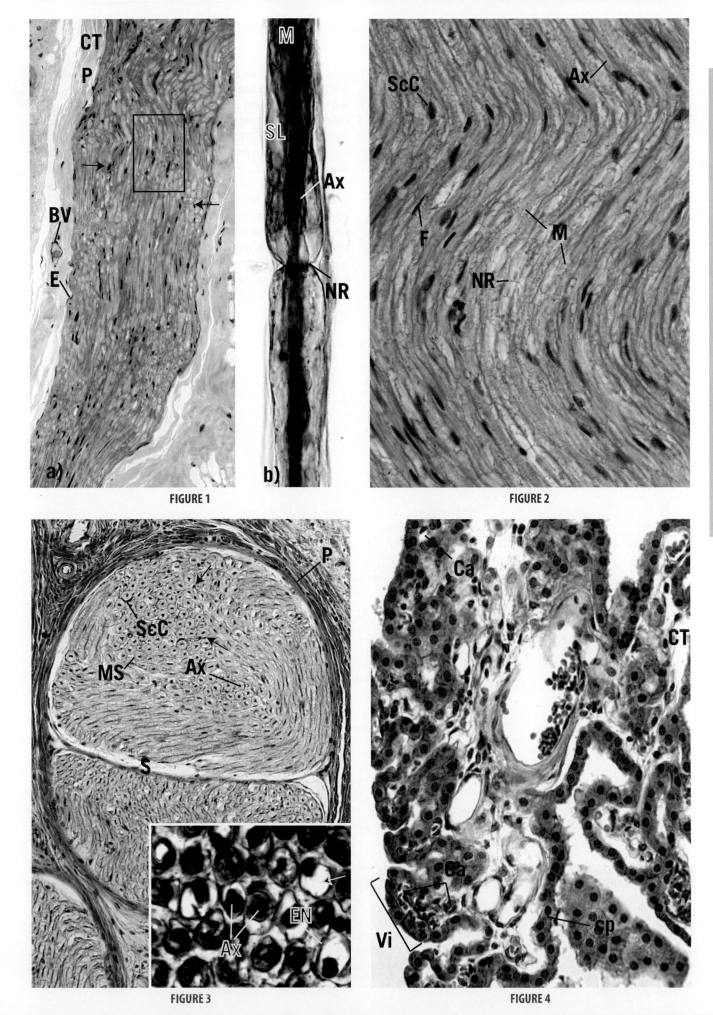

PLATE 7-5 • Peripheral Nerve, Choroid Plexus

FIGURE 1

FIGURE 2

FIGURE 3

FIGURE 4

PLATE 7-6 · Peripheral Nerve, Electron Microscopy

FIGURE 1. Peripheral nerve. x.s. Mouse. Electron microscopy. ×33,300.

This electron micrograph presents a cross section of three myelinated and several unmyelinated nerve fibers. Note that the **axons** (Ax) (although they may be the afferent fibers of pseudounipolar neurons) are surrounded by a thick **myelin sheath** (MS), peripheral to which is the bulk of the **Schwann cell cytoplasm** (ScC) housing **mitochondria** (m), **rough endoplasmic reticulum** (rER), and **pinocytotic vesicles** (PV). The Schwann cell is surrounded by a **basal lamina** (BL) isolating this cell from the **endoneurial connective tissue** (CT). The myelin sheath is derived from the plasma membrane of the Schwann cell, which presumably wraps spirally around the axon, resulting in the formation of an **external** (EM) and **internal** (IM) **mesaxon**. The **axolemma** (Al) is separated from the Schwann cell membrane by a narrow cleft,

the periaxonal space. The axoplasm houses **mitochondria** (m) as well as **neurofilaments** (Nf) and **neurotubules** (Nt). Occasionally, the myelin wrapping is surrounded by Schwann cell cytoplasm on its outer and inner aspects, as in the nerve fiber in the upper right-hand corner. The **unmyelinated nerve fibers** (f) in the top of this electron micrograph display their relationship to the **Schwann cell** (ScC). The fibers are positioned in such a fashion that each lies in a complicated membrane-lined groove within the Schwann cell. Some fibers are situated superficially, whereas others are positioned more deeply within the grooves. However, a periaxonal (or peridendritic) space (*arrows*) is always present. **Mitochondria** (m), **neurofilaments** (Nf), and **neurotubules** (Nt) are also present. Note that the entire structure is surrounded by a **basal lamina** (BL), which covers but does not extend into the grooves (*arrowheads*) housing the nerve fibers. (Courtesy of Dr. J. Strum.)

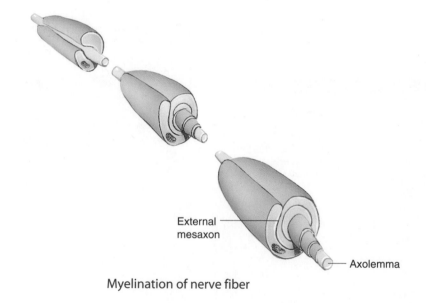

External mesaxon

Axolemma

Myelination of nerve fiber

KEY

Al	axolemma	**EM**	external mesaxon	**Nf**	neurofilament
Ax	axon	**F**	nerve fiber	**Nt**	neurotubule
BL	basal lamina	**IM**	internal mesaxon	**PV**	pinocytotic vesicle
CT	endoneurial connective tissue	**M**	mitochondrion	**rER**	rough ER
		MS	myelin sheath	**ScC**	Schwann cell cytoplasm

PLATE 7-6 • Peripheral Nerve, Electron Microscopy

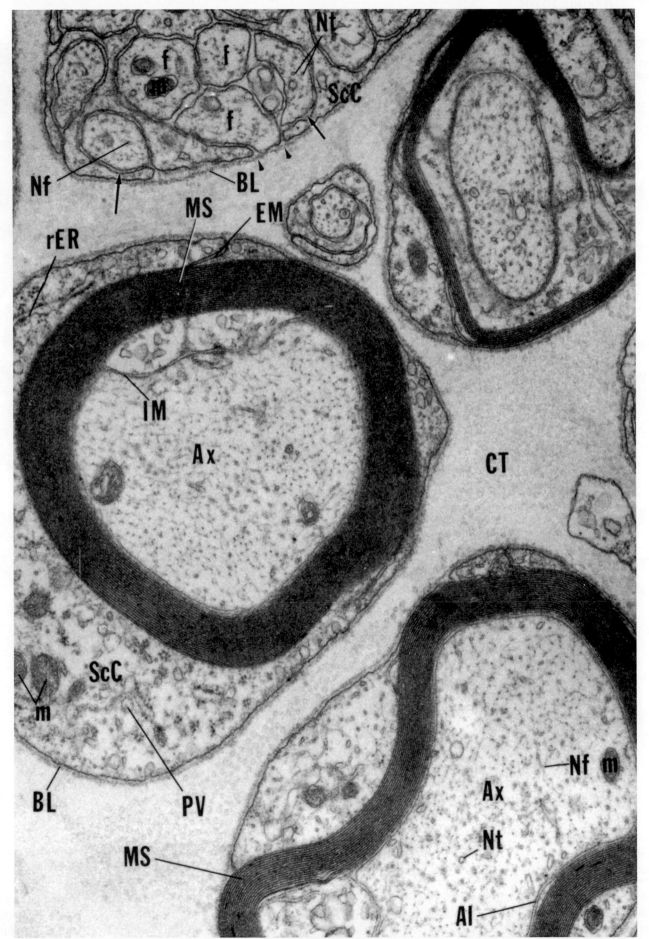

FIGURE 1

PLATE 7-7 · Neuron Cell Body, Electron Microscopy

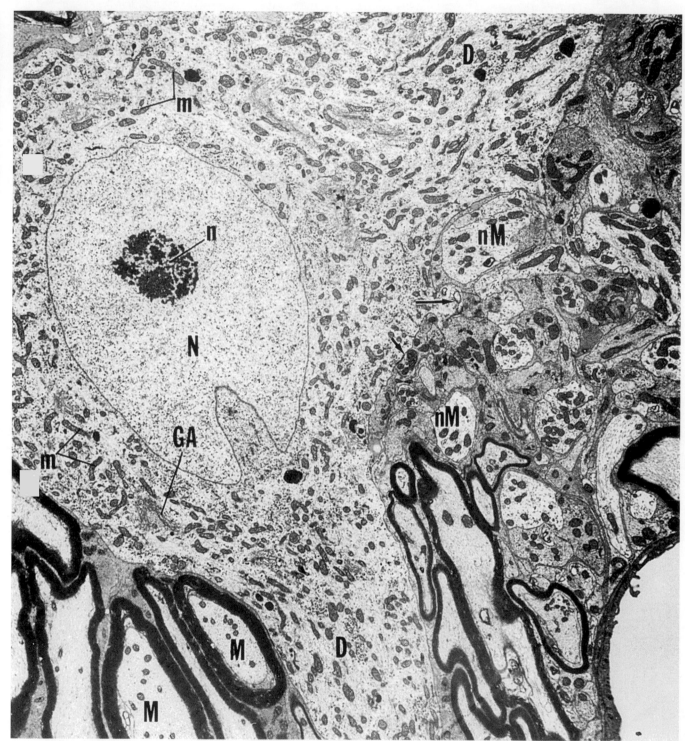

FIGURE 1

FIGURE 1. Neuron. Lateral descending nucleus. Electron microscopy. ×3,589.

The soma of this neuron presents a typical appearance. Note the large **nucleus** (N) and **nucleolus** (n) surrounded by a considerable amount of cytoplasm rich in organelles. Observe the extensive **Golgi apparatus** (GA), numerous **mitochondria** (m), and elements of rough endoplasmic reticulum, which extend into the **dendrites** (D). **Myelinated** (M) and **nonmyelinated** (nM) fibers are also present, as are synapses (*arrows*) along the cell surface. (From Meszler R, Auker C, Carpenter D. Fine structure and organization of the infrared receptor relay, the lateral descending nucleus of the trigeminal nerve in pit vipers. *J Comp Neurol* 1981;196:571–584.)

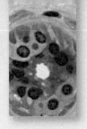

Chapter Summary

I. SPINAL CORD

A. Gray Matter

The **gray matter**, centrally located and more or less in the shape of an H, has two **dorsal horns** and two **ventral horns**. Ventral horns display numerous **multipolar (motor) cell bodies**. The perikaryon possesses a large, clear **nucleus** and a dense **nucleolus**. Its cytoplasm is filled with clumps of basophilic **Nissl substance** (rough endoplasmic reticulum) that extends into **dendrites** but not into the **axon**. The origin of the axon is indicated by the **axon hillock** of the **soma**. Numerous small nuclei abound in the gray matter; they belong to the various **neuroglia**. The nerve fibers and neuroglial processes in the gray matter are referred to as the **neuropil**. The right and left halves of the gray matter are connected to each other by the **gray commissure**, which houses the **central canal** lined by simple cuboidal **ependymal cells**.

B. White Matter

The **white matter** of the spinal cord is peripherally located and consists of **ascending** and **descending fibers**. These fibers are mostly **myelinated** (by **oligodendroglia**), accounting for the coloration in live tissue. **Nuclei** noted in white matter belong to the various **neuroglia**.

C. Meninges

The **meninges** of the spinal cord form three layers. The most intimate layer is the **pia mater**, surrounded by the **arachnoid**, which, in turn, is invested by the thick, collagenous **dura mater**.

II. CEREBELLUM

A. Cortex

The **cortex** of the cerebellum consists of an outer **molecular layer** and an inner **granular layer** with a single layer of **Purkinje cells** interposed between them. The **perikaryons** of the molecular layer are small and relatively few in number. Most of the fibers are unmyelinated. **Purkinje cells** are easily distinguished by their location, large size, and extensive **dendritic arborization**. The **granular layer** displays crowded arrays of nuclei belonging to **granule cells** and intervening clear regions known as **glomeruli** (or **cerebellar islands**). These mainly represent areas of synapses on granule cell dendrites.

B. Medullary Substance

The **medullary substance** (internal white mass) is the region of **white matter** deep to the granular layer of the cerebellum, composed mostly of myelinated fibers and associated **neuroglial cells**.

III. CEREBRUM

A. Cortex

The **cerebral cortex** is composed of **gray matter**, mostly subdivided into six layers, with each housing neurons whose morphology is characteristic of that particular layer. The major neuronal types are **pyramidal cells**, **stellate (granule) cells**, **horizontal cells**, and **inverted (Martinotti) cells**. The following description refers to the **neocortex** and is presented from superficial to deep order. The first layer is just deep to the pia mater, whereas the sixth level is the deepest cortical layer, bordering the central white matter of the cerebrum.

1. Molecular Layer

Composed of **horizontal cells** and cell processes.

2. External Granular Layer

Consists mostly of **granule (stellate) cells**, tightly packed.

3. External Pyramidal Layer

Large **pyramidal cells** and **granule (stellate) cells**.

4. Internal Granular Layer

Closely packed **granule (stellate) cells**, most of which are small, although some are larger.

5. Internal Pyramidal Layer

Medium and large **pyramidal cells** constitute this layer.

6. Multiform Layer

Consisting of various cell shapes, many of which are fusiform. This layer also houses **Martinotti cells**.

B. White Matter

Deep to the cerebral cortex is the **subcortical white matter**, composed mostly of myelinated fibers and associated **neuroglial cells**.

IV. CHOROID PLEXUS

The **choroid plexus** consists of tufts of small vascular elements (derived from the pia-arachnoid) that are covered by **modified ependymal cells** (simple cuboidal in shape). These structures, located in the ventricles of the brain, are responsible for the formation of the **cerebrospinal fluid**.

V. DORSAL ROOT GANGLION (DRG)

A. Neurons

The **somata** of these cells are **pseudounipolar**, with large nuclei and nucleoli. Surrounding each soma are **capsule cells**, recognized by their small, round nuclei. **Fibroblasts** (satellite cells) are also evident. Synapses do not occur in the DRG.

B. Fibers

Fibers are mostly myelinated and travel in bundles through the DRG.

C. Connective Tissue

The DRG is surrounded by collagenous **connective tissue**, whose septa penetrate the substance of the ganglion.

VI. PERIPHERAL NERVE

A. Longitudinal Section

The parallel fibers stain a pale pink with hematoxylin and eosin, although **Schwann cells** and occasional **fibroblast nuclei** are clearly evident. The most characteristic feature is the apparent wavy, zigzag course of the nerve fibers. At low magnification, the **perineurium** is clearly distinguishable, whereas at high magnification the **nodes of Ranvier** may be recognizable.

B. Transverse Section

The most characteristic feature of transverse sections of nerve fibers is the numerous, small, irregular circles with a centrally located dot. Thin spokes appear to traverse the empty-looking space between the dot and the circumference of the circle. These represent the **neurolemma**, the extracted **myelin** (myelin proteins), and the central **axon**. Occasionally, crescent-shaped nuclei hug the myelin; these belong to **Schwann cells**. The **endoneurium** may show evidence of **nuclei of fibroblasts** also. At lower magnification, the **perineuria** of several fascicles of nerve fibers are clearly distinguishable. When stained with OsO_4, the **myelin sheath** stands out as dark, round structures with lightly staining centers.

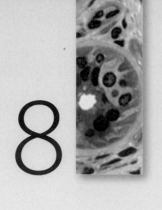

8 | CIRCULATORY SYSTEM

The circulatory system is composed of two separate but connected components: the blood vascular system (**cardiovascular system**) that transports blood and the **lymphatic vascular system** that collects and returns excess extracellular fluid (lymph) to the blood vascular system. Lymphoid tissue is presented in Chapter 9.

BLOOD VASCULAR SYSTEM

The **blood vascular system**, consisting of the heart and blood vessels, functions in propelling and transporting blood and its various constituents throughout the body.

- The **heart**, acting as a pump, forces blood at high pressure into large, elastic arteries that carry the blood away from the heart.
- **Arteries** give way to increasingly smaller muscular arteries.
- Eventually, blood reaches extremely thin-walled vessels, capillaries, and small venules (postcapillary venules), where exchange of materials occurs. It is mostly here that certain cells, oxygen, nutrients, hormones, certain proteins, and additional materials leave the bloodstream, whereas carbon dioxide, waste products, certain cells, and various secretory products enter the bloodstream.
- Capillary beds, except those of the glomerulus (in the kidney), which are drained by arterioles, are drained by the **venous components** of the circulatory system, which return blood to the heart.

Blood vessels are composed of three concentric layers: tunica intima, tunica media, and tunica adventitia (see Graphic 8-1).

- The **tunica intima** is composed of a continuous sheet of simple squamous endothelial cells lining the lumen and of various amounts of subendothelial connective tissue.
- The **tunica media**, usually the thickest of the three layers in the arterial leg of the circulatory system, is composed of circularly arranged smooth muscle cells and fibroelastic connective tissue, whose elastic content increases greatly with the size of the vessel.
- The **tunica adventitia** is the outermost layer of the vessel wall, consisting of fibroelastic connective tissue. In larger vessels, the tunica adventitia houses **vasa vasorum**, small blood vessels that supply the tunica adventitia and media of that vessel. In the venous leg of the circulatory system, it is the tunica adventitia that is the thickest of the three layers.

The blood vascular system is subdivided into the pulmonary and systemic circuits, which originate from the right and left sides of the heart, respectively.

- The **pulmonary circuit** takes oxygen-poor blood to the lungs to become oxygenated and returns it to the left side of the heart.
- The oxygen-rich blood is propelled via the **systemic circuit** to the remainder of the body to be returned to the right side of the heart, completing the cycle.

HEART

The heart is a four-chambered organ composed of two atria and two ventricles. The atria, subsequent to receiving blood from the pulmonary veins, venae cavae, and coronary sinus, discharge it into the ventricles. Contractions of the ventricles then propel the blood either from the right ventricle into the pulmonary trunk for distribution to the lungs or from the left ventricle into the aorta for distribution to the remainder of the body. Although the walls of the ventricles are thicker than those of the atria, these chambers possess common characteristics in that they are composed of three layers: epicardium, myocardium, and endocardium.

- **Epicardium**, the outermost layer, is covered by a simple squamous mesothelium deep to which is a fibroelastic connective tissue. The deepest aspect of the epicardium is composed of adipose tissue that houses nerves and the coronary vessels.
- Most of the wall of the heart is composed of **myocardium**, consisting of bundles of cardiac muscle that are attached to the thick collagenous connective tissue skeleton of the heart.
- The **endocardium** forms the lining of the atria and ventricles and is composed of a simple squamous endothelium as well as a subendothelial fibroelastic connective tissue.
  - The endocardium participates in the formation of the heart valves, which control the direction of blood flow through the heart.
    - **Atrioventricular valves** between the atria and ventricles prevent regurgitation of blood into the atria.
    - Similarly, **semilunar valves** located in the pulmonary trunk and the aorta prevent regurgitation of blood from these vessels back into their respective ventricles. The closing of these valves is responsible for the sounds associated with the heartbeat.

Additionally, some cardiac muscle fibers are modified and specialized to regulate the sequence of atrial and ventricular contractions. These are the sinoatrial and atrioventricular nodes and the bundle of His and Purkinje fibers.

- The **sinoatrial node (SA node)**, the pacemaker of the heart, is located at the junction of the superior vena cava and the right atrium. The SA node generates impulses that result in the contraction of the atrial muscles; blood from the atria then enters the ventricles.
- Impulses generated at the SA node are then conducted to the **atrioventricular node (AV node)**, which is located on the medial wall of the right ventricle near the tricuspid valve, as well as to the atrial myocardium.
- Arising from the AV node is the **bundle of His**, which bifurcates in the septum membranaceum to serve both ventricles.
- As these fibers reach the subendocardium, they ramify and are known as **Purkinje fibers**, which deliver the impulse to the cardiac muscle cells of the ventricles that contract to pump the blood from the right ventricle into the pulmonary trunk and from the left ventricle into the aorta.

The arrangement of the cardiac myocytes as well as the atrioventricular bundle permits the contraction of the atria first, followed, after a time lag, by contraction of the ventricles. In this fashion, blood from the atria can enter the ventricles, and once the ventricles are filled, they contract and propel the blood into the systemic and pulmonary circuits.

The inherent rhythm of the SA node is modulated by the autonomic nervous system, in that parasympathetic fibers derived from the vagus nerve decrease the rate of the heartbeat, whereas fibers derived from sympathetic ganglia increase it.

ARTERIES

Arteries, by definition, conduct blood away from the heart; they are classified into three categories: elastic (also known as conducting or large), muscular (also known as distributing or medium), and arterioles (see Graphic 8-1 and Table 8-1).

- **Elastic arteries**, such as the aorta, receive blood directly from the heart and consequently are the largest of the arteries.
  - Since they arise directly from the heart, they are subject to cyclic changes of blood pressure, high as the ventricles pump blood into their lumina and low between the emptying of these chambers.
  - To compensate for these intermittent pressure alterations, an abundance of elastic fibers are located in the walls of these vessels.
  - These elastic fibers not only provide structural stability and permit distention of the elastic arteries but they also assist in the maintenance of blood pressure in between heartbeats.
- **Muscular arteries** comprise most of the named arteries of the body and supply blood to various organs. Their tunica media is composed mostly of many layers of smooth muscle cells. Both elastic and muscular arteries are supplied by **vasa vasorum** (see Graphic 8-1) and nerve fibers.
- **Arterioles** regulate blood pressure and the distribution of blood to capillary beds via vasoconstriction and vasodilatation of vessel walls.

TABLE 8-1 • Characteristics of the Different Types of Arteries

Artery	Tunica Intima	Tunica Media	Tunica Adventitia
Elastic arteries (**conducting**) (e.g., aorta, pulmonary trunk)	Endothelium (containing Weibel-Palade bodies), basal lamina, subendothelial layer, incomplete internal elastic lamina	Layers of smooth muscle cells interspersed with 40–70 fenestrated elastic membranes, thin incomplete external elastic lamina, vasa vasorum	Thin layer of fibroelastic CT, limited vasa vasorum, lymphatic vessels, nerve fibers
Muscular arteries (**distributing**) (e.g., carotid and femoral arteries)	Endothelium (containing Weibel-Palade bodies), basal lamina, subendothelial layer, thick internal elastic lamina	~40 layers of smooth muscle cells, thick external elastic lamina, relatively little additional elastic tissue	Thin layer of fibroelastic CT, limited vasa vasorum, lymphatic vessels, nerve fibers
Arterioles	Endothelium (containing Weibel-Palade bodies), basal lamina, subendothelial layer, internal elastic lamina mostly replaced by elastic fibers	1–2 layers of smooth muscle cells	Ill-defined sheath of loose connective tissue, nerve fibers
Metarterioles	Endothelium and basal lamina	Precapillary sphincter formed by smooth muscle cells	Sparse loose connective tissue

- Metarterioles are the terminal ends of the arterioles, and they are characterized by the presence of incomplete rings of smooth muscle cells (precapillary sphincters) that encircle the origins of the capillaries.
  - Metarterioles form the arterial (proximal) end of a central channel, and they are responsible for delivering blood into the capillary bed. The venous (distal) end of the central channel, known as a thoroughfare channel, is responsible for draining blood from the capillary bed and delivering it into venules.
  - Contraction of precapillary sphincters of the metarteriole shunts the blood into the thoroughfare channel and from there into the venule; this way, the blood bypasses the capillary bed (see Graphic 8-2).
  - Arteriovenous anastomoses are direct connections between arteries and venules, and they also function in having blood bypass the capillary bed. These shunts function in thermoregulation and blood pressure control.
- **Capillaries** are very small vessels that consist of a single layer of endothelial cells surrounded by a basal lamina and occasional **pericytes** (see Graphic 8-2), but these vessels possess no smooth muscle cells; therefore, they do not exhibit vasomotor activities. Capillaries exhibit **selective permeability**, and they, along with venules, are responsible for the exchange of gases, metabolites, and other substances between the bloodstream and the tissues of the body. Capillaries are composed of highly attenuated **endothelial cells** that form narrow vascular channels 8 to 10 μm in diameter and are usually less than 1 mm long. There are three types of capillaries: continuous, fenestrated, and sinusoidal (Table 8-2).
  - **Continuous capillaries** lack fenestrae, display only occasional pinocytotic vesicles, and possess a continuous basal lamina. They are present in regions such as peripheral nerve fibers, skeletal muscle, lungs, and thymus.
  - **Fenestrated capillaries** are penetrated by relatively large diaphragm-covered pores. These cells also possess pinocytotic vesicles and are enveloped by a continuous basal lamina. Fenestrated capillaries are located in endocrine glands, pancreas, and lamina propria of the intestines, and they also constitute the glomeruli of the kidneys, although their fenestrae are not covered by a diaphragm.
  - **Sinusoidal capillaries** (also known as **sinusoids, discontinuous capillaries**) are much larger than their fenestrated or continuous counterparts. They are enveloped by a discontinuous basal lamina, and their endothelial cells do not possess pinocytotic vesicles. The intercellular junctions of their endothelial cells display gaps, thus permitting leakage of material into and out of these vessels. Frequently, macrophages are associated with sinusoidal capillaries. Sinusoidal capillaries are located in the liver, spleen, lymph nodes, bone marrow, and the suprarenal cortex.

Capillary Permeability

Capillary permeability is dependent not only on the endothelial cells comprising the capillary but also on the (physico)-chemical characteristics, such as size, charge, and shape, of the traversing substance.

- Some molecules, such as H_2O, diffuse through, whereas others are actively transported by carrier proteins across the endothelial cell plasma membrane.
- Other molecules move through fenestrae or through gaps in the intercellular junctions.
  - Certain pharmacological agents, such as **bradykinin** and **histamine**, have the ability to alter capillary permeability.
  - Leukocytes leave the bloodstream by passing through intercellular junctions of the endothelial cells (**diapedesis**) to enter the extracellular spaces of tissues and organs.

TABLE 8-2 • Characteristics of the Different types of Capillaries

Characteristics	Continuous Capillaries	Fenestrated Capillaries	Sinusoidal Capillaries
Location	CT, muscle, nerve tissue; modified in brain tissue	Endocrine glands, pancreas, intestines	Bone marrow, spleen, liver, lymph nodes, certain endocrine glands
Diameter	Smallest diameter	Intermediate diameter	Largest diameter
Endothelium	Forms tight junctions at marginal fold with itself or adjacent cells	Forms tight junctions at marginal fold with itself or adjacent cells	Frequently the endothelium and basal lamina are discontinuous
Fenestrae	Not present	Present	Present in addition to gaps

Endothelial Cell Functions

Endothelial cells function in formation of a selectively permeable membrane, vasoconstriction, vasodilation, initiation of coagulation, facilitation of transepithelial migration of inflammatory cells, angiogenesis, synthesis of growth factors, modifying angiotensin I, and oxidation of lipoproteins.

- **Vasoconstriction** is due not only to the action of sympathetic nerve fibers that act on the smooth muscles of the tunica media but also to the pharmacologic agent **endothelin 1**, produced and released by endothelial cells of blood vessels.
- **Vasodilation** is accomplished by parasympathetic nerve fibers in an indirect fashion. Instead of acting on smooth muscle cells, acetylcholine, released by the nerve end-foot, is bound to receptors on the endothelial cells, inducing them to release **nitric oxide (NO)**, previously known as endothelial-derived relaxing factor. NO acts on the cGMP system of the smooth muscle cells, causing their relaxation. Additionally, endothelial cells can produce **prostacyclins**, pharmacologic agents that induce the cAMP second messenger pathway in smooth muscle cells, effecting their relaxation.
- Endothelial cells also release **tissue factor** (also known as **thromboplastin**), an agent that facilitates entry into the common pathway of **blood coagulation**, and **von Willebrand's factor**, which activates and facilitates the adhesion of platelets to the exposed laminin and collagens and induces them to release adenosine diphosphate and thrombospondin, which encourages their adhesion to each other.
- When inflammatory cells have to leave the bloodstream to enter the connective tissue spaces, endothelial cells express on their luminal plasma membranes **E-selectins**. These signaling molecules are recognized by carbohydrate ligands on the surface of the inflammatory cells, triggering their **epithelial transmigration**.
- **Angiogenesis** occurs in adult tissues in response to repair of damaged vessels, establishment of new vessels in repairing injuries, formation of new vessels subsequent to menstruation, formation of the corpus luteum, as well as in response to tumor formation. New vessels arise from existing vessels due to the interactions of various signaling molecules, such as angiopoietins 1 and 2, with specific receptors on endothelial cells that induce mitotic activity in preexisting endothelial cells and recruit smooth muscle cells to form the tunica media of the developing vessels.
- Endothelial cells also **synthesize growth factors** such as various colony-stimulating factors, which induce cells of blood lineage to undergo mitosis and produce various blood cells, and growth inhibitors, such as transforming growth factor-B
- Additionally, endothelial cells convert angiotensin I to angiotensin II, a powerful smooth muscle contractant and inducer of aldosterone release by the suprarenal cortex.
- Endothelial cells also oxidize high-cholesterol–containing low-density lipoproteins and very low-density lipoproteins, so that the oxidized by-product can be phagocytosed by macrophages.

VEINS

Veins conduct blood away from body tissues and back to the heart (see Graphic 8-1). Generally, the diameters of veins are larger than those of corresponding arteries; however, veins are thinner walled, since they do not bear high blood pressures. Veins also possess three concentric, more or less definite layers: **tunica intima**, **tunica media**, and **tunica adventitia**. Furthermore, veins have fewer layers of smooth muscle cells in their tunica media than do arteries. Finally, many veins possess valves that act to prevent regurgitation of blood. Three categories of veins exist: **small**, **medium**, and **large** (see Table 8-3).

- The smallest of the **veins**, **venules**, especially **postcapillary venules**, are also responsible for the exchange of materials.
  - Postcapillary venules have **pericytes** instead of a tunica media, and their walls are more permeable than those of venules and even of capillaries.
  - **Vasodilator substances**, such as **serotonin** and **histamine**, appear to act on small venules, causing them to become "leaky" by increasing the intercellular distances between the membranes of contiguous endothelial cells.
    - Most such intercellular gaps occur in postcapillary venules rather than in capillaries.
    - Leukocytes preferentially leave the vascular system at the postcapillary venules to enter the connective tissue spaces via diapedesis.
- **Medium veins** receive blood from most of the body, including the upper and lower extremities. They also possess three layers.
  - Tunica intima frequently forms valves, especially in the lower extremities, to counteract the gravitational forces and avert the backflow of blood.
  - Tunica media is slender and houses only a loosely organized network of smooth muscle cells interspersed with fibroblasts and type I collagen fibers.

TABLE 8-3 • Characteristics of Veins

Type of Vein	Tunica Intima	Tunica Media	Tunica Adventitia
Large veins	Endothelium, basal lamina, subendothelial CT, some veins possess valves	Connective tissue and a few layers of smooth muscle cells	Bundles of smooth muscle cells are oriented longitudinally. Cardiac muscle cells located where veins enter into the heart; layers of collagen fiber bundles with fibroblasts
Medium and small veins	Endothelium, basal lamina, subendothelial CT, some veins possess valves	Reticular and elastic fibers and some smooth muscle cells	Layers of collagen fiber bundles containing fibroblasts
Venules	Endothelium, basal lamina (pericytes are associated with some postcapillary venules)	Some connective tissue, along with a few smooth muscle cells	Some collagen fiber bundles and a few fibroblasts

- ○ Tunica adventitia is the thickest of the three layers consisting mostly of elastic fibers and type I collagen bundles arranged parallel to the longitudinal axis of the vein. Occasional smooth muscle cells are also present in the adventitia.
- **Large veins**, such as the venae cavae, pulmonary, and renal veins, are more than 1 cm in diameter.
  - ○ As the venae cavae and pulmonary veins approach the heart, they exhibit the presence of cardiac muscle cells in their adventitia.
  - ○ Most of the large veins (except for those in the lower extremities) possess no smooth muscle cells in their tunica media instead those cells are located in their tunica adventitia.
  - ○ The tunica intima of large veins are rich in elastic fibers and fibroblasts.
  - ○ The walls of these large veins are supplied by slender vessels derived from the vasa vasorum located in their adventitia.

LYMPH VASCULAR SYSTEM

Excess extracellular fluid, which does not enter the venous return system at the level of the capillary bed or venule, gains entry into **lymphatic capillaries**, blindly ending thin vessels of the lymph vascular system. Subsequent to passing through chains of lymph nodes and larger lymph vessels, the fluid known as lymph enters the blood vascular system at the root of the neck.

CLINICAL CONSIDERATIONS

Valve Defects

Children who have had rheumatic fever may develop valve defects. These valve defects may be related to improper closing (**incompetency**) or improper opening (**stenosis**). Fortunately, most of these defects can be repaired surgically.

Aneurysm

A damaged vessel wall may, over time, become weakened and begin to enlarge and form a bulging defect known as an aneurysm. This condition occurs most often in large vessels such as the aorta and renal artery. If undetected or left untreated, it may rupture without warning and cause internal bleeding with fatal consequences. Surgical repair is possible, depending on the health of the individual.

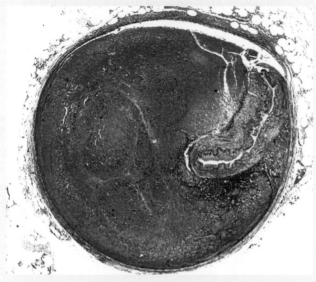

This is a photomicrograph of an aneurysm of the renal artery. The blood escaping from the lumen dissected the vessel wall and pooled between the tunica media and the tunica adventitia. (Reprinted with permission from Mills SE, Carter D, et al., eds. Sternberg's Diagnostic Surgical Pathology, 5th ed. Philadelphia: Lippincott Williams & Wilkins, 2010, p. 1231.)

Atherosclerosis

Atherosclerosis, the deposition of plaque within the walls of large- and medium-sized arteries, results in reduced blood flow within that vessel. If this condition involves the coronary arteries, the decreased blood flow to the myocardium causes coronary heart disease. The consequences of this disease may be angina pectoris, myocardial infarct, chronic ischemic cardiopathy, or sudden death.

Raynaud's Disease

Raynaud's disease is an idiopathic condition in which the arterioles of the fingers and toes go into sudden spasms lasting minutes to hours, cutting off blood supply to the digits with a resultant cyanosis and loss of sensation. This condition, affecting mostly younger women, is believed to be due to exposure to cold as well as to the patient's emotional state. Other causes include atherosclerosis, scleroderma, injury, and reaction to certain medications.

Von Willebrand's Disease

Von Willebrand's disease is a genetic disorder in which the individual is either incapable of producing a normal quantity of von Willebrand's factor or the factor that they produce is deficient. Most individuals have a mild form of the condition that is not life-threatening. These individuals have problems with the process of blood clotting and display symptoms such as bruising easily, longer bleeding time, excessive bleeding from tooth extraction, excessive menstrual bleeding, and bloody mucous membranes.

Stroke

Stroke is a condition in which blood flow to a part of the brain is interrupted either due to a blockage of blood vessels or because of hemorrhage of blood vessels. The lack of blood causes anoxia of the affected region with a consequent death of the neurons of that region, resulting in weakness, paralysis, sensory loss, or the inability to speak. If stroke victims can reach a health facility equipped with dealing with the problem and depending on the extent of the injury, they can be rehabilitated to recover some or all of the lost function.

Acute Rheumatic Fever

Rheumatic fever, a frequent sequelae of **group A β-hemolytic streptococcal pharyngitis**, is an inflammatory response to the bacterial insult. Although many body organs may be affected, most patients recover, although in some cases the heart bears permanent injury. In first world countries, where the streptococcal infection is aggressively treated by antibiotics, the occurrence of rheumatic fever is much less than in underdeveloped nations. In affected children, usually between 5 and 15 years of age, the symptoms appear a few weeks after an untreated strep throat infection has been resolved, and these patients may exhibit painful, swollen joints; skin rash; chest pain; fever; and small nodules deep to the skin. The symptoms disappear in less than a month; however, a number of years later, a small percentage of these children develop damaged **mitral valves** (left atrioventricular valve).

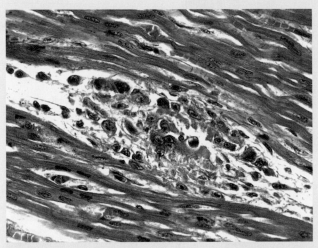

The myocardium of a patient who died from acute rheumatic fever displays the presence of Aschoff bodies, composed of plasma cells, lymphocytes, macrophages, and multinucleated giant Aschoff cells. (Reprinted with permission from Mills SE, Carter D, et al., eds. Sternberg's Diagnostic Surgical Pathology, 5th ed. Philadelphia: Lippincott Williams & Wilkins, 2010, p. 1197.)

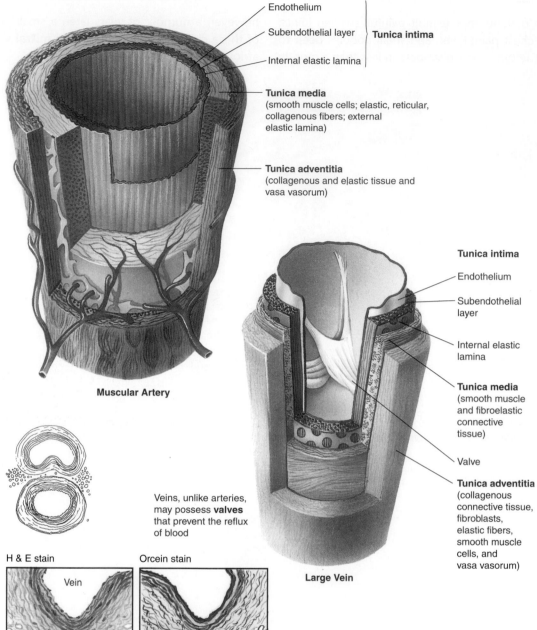

Endothelium
Subendothelial layer — **Tunica intima**
Internal elastic lamina

Tunica media
(smooth muscle cells; elastic, reticular, collagenous fibers; external elastic lamina)

Tunica adventitia
(collagenous and elastic tissue and vasa vasorum)

Muscular Artery

Tunica intima

Endothelium

Subendothelial layer

Internal elastic lamina

Tunica media
(smooth muscle and fibroelastic connective tissue)

Valve

Tunica adventitia
(collagenous connective tissue, fibroblasts, elastic fibers, smooth muscle cells, and vasa vasorum)

Large Vein

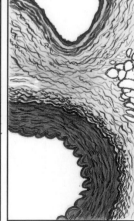

Veins, unlike arteries, may possess **valves** that prevent the reflux of blood

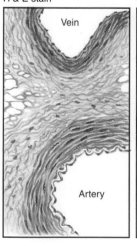

H & E stain

Vein

Artery

Orcein stain

Arteries have a more muscular wall, thus a much thicker tunica media than the veins, and they have a greater amount of elastic tissue. Conversely, the tunica adventitia of veins are much thicker than those of the arteries.

The outermost layer is the **tunica adventitia**, composed of fibroelastic connective tissue, whose vessels, the **vasa vasorum**, penetrate the outer regions of the tunica media, supplying its cells with nutrients.

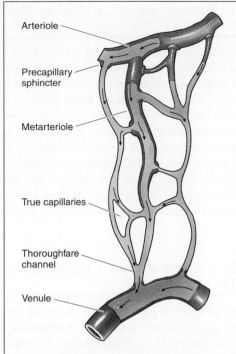

Arteriole

Precapillary
sphincter

Metarteriole

True capillaries

Thoroughfare
channel

Venule

Some capillary beds, such as those of the skin,
are designed so that they may be bypassed
under certain circumstances. One method
whereby blood flow may be controlled is the use
of **central channels** that convey blood from and
arteriole to a venule. The proximal half of the
central channel is a **metarteriole**, a vessel with
an incomplete smooth muscle coat. Flow of
blood into each capillary that arises from the
metarteriole is controlled by a smooth muscle
cell, the **precapillary sphincter**. The distal half
of the central channel is the **thoroughfare
channel**, which possesses no smooth muscle
cells and accepts blood from the capillary bed.
If the capillary bed is to be bypassed, the
precapillary sphincters contract, preventing blood
flow into the capillary bed, and the blood goes
directly into the venule.

Capillaries consists of a simple squamousv
epithelium rolled into a narrow cylinder 8–10 μm
in diameter. **Continuous (somatic) capillaries**
have no fenestrae: material transverses the
endothelial cell in either direction via **pinocytotic
vesicles**. **Fenestrated (visceral) capillaries** are
characterized by the presence of perforations,
fenestrae, 60–80 μm in diameter, which may or
may not be bridged by a diaphraga. **Sinusoidal
capillaries** have a large lumen (30–40 μm in
diameter), possess numerous fenestrae, have
discontinuous basal lamina, and lack pinocytotic
vesicles. Frequently, adjacent endothelial cells of
sinusoidal capillaries overlap one another in an
incomplete fashion

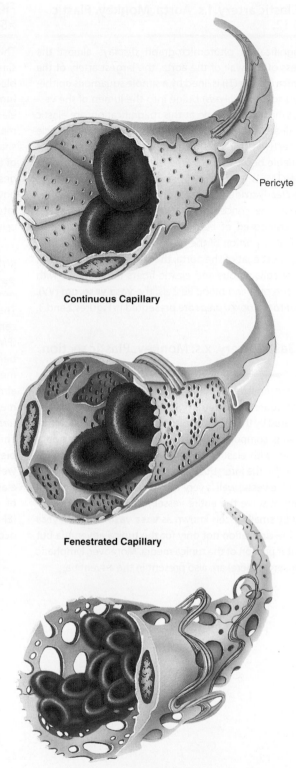

Pericyte

Continuous Capillary

Fenestrated Capillary

Sinusoidal (Discontinuous) Capillary

PLATE 8-1 • Elastic Artery

FIGURE 1. Elastic artery. l.s. Aorta. Monkey. Plastic section. ×132.

This low magnification photomicrograph displays almost the entire thickness of the wall of the aorta, the largest artery of the body. The **tunica intima** (TI) is lined by a simple squamous epithelium whose nuclei (*arrowheads*) bulge into the lumen of the vessel. The lines, which appear pale at this magnification, are elastic fibers and laminae, whereas the nuclei belong to smooth muscle cells and connective tissue cells. The internal elastic lamina is not readily identifiable because the intima is rich in elastic fibers. The **tunica media** (TM) is composed of smooth muscle cells whose **nuclei** (N) are clearly evident. These smooth muscle cells lie in the spaces between the concentrically layered **fenestrated membranes** (FM), composed of elastic tissue. The **external elastic lamina** (xEL) is that portion of the media that adjoins the adventitia. The outermost coat of the aorta, the **tunica adventitia** (TA), is composed of collagenous and elastic fibers interspersed with connective tissue cells and blood vessels, the **vasa vasorum** (VV). Regions similar to the *boxed areas* are presented in Figures 2 and 3.

FIGURE 3. Elastic artery. x.s. Monkey. Plastic section. ×540.

This is a higher magnification of the tunica adventitia similar to the *boxed region* of Figure 1. The outermost region of the **tunica media** (TM) is demarcated by the **external elastic lamina** (xEL). The **tunica adventitia** (TA) is composed of thick bundles of **collagen fibers** (CF) interspersed with elastic fibers. Observe the nuclei of **fibroblasts** (F) located in the interstitial spaces among the collagen fiber bundles. Since the vessel wall is very thick, nutrients diffusing from the lumen cannot serve the entire vessel; therefore, the adventitia is supplied by small vessels known as **vasa vasorum** (VV). Vasa vasorum provide circulation not only for the tunica adventitia but also for the outer portion of the tunica media. Moreover, lymphatic vessels (not observed here) are also present in the adventitia.

FIGURE 2. Elastic artery. x.s. Monkey. Plastic section. ×540.

This is a higher magnification of a region of the tunica intima, similar to the *boxed area* of Figure 1. The endothelial lining of the blood vessel presents **nuclei** (*arrowhead*), which bulge into the **lumen** (L). The numerous **elastic fibers** (EF) form an incomplete elastic lamina. Note that the interstices of the tunica intima house many **smooth muscle cells** (SM), whose nuclei are corkscrew-shaped (*arrows*), indicative of muscle contraction. Although most of the cellular elements are smooth muscle cells, it has been suggested that fibroblasts and macrophages may also be present; however, it is believed that the elastic fibers and the amorphous intercellular substances are synthesized by the smooth muscle cells.

FIGURE 4. Elastic artery. x.s. Human. Elastic stain. Paraffin section. ×132.

The use of a special stain to demonstrate the presence of concentric elastic sheets, known as **fenestrated membranes** (FM), displays the highly elastic quality of the aorta. The number of fenestrated membranes, as well as the thickness of each membrane, increases with age, so that the adult will possess almost twice as many of these structures as an infant. These membranes are called fenestrated, since they possess spaces (*arrows*) through which nutrients and waste materials diffuse. The interstices between the fenestrated membranes are occupied by smooth muscle cells, whose **nuclei** (N) are evident, as well as amorphous intercellular materials, collagen, and fine elastic fibers. The **tunica adventitia** (TA) is composed mostly of **collagenous fiber bundles** (CF) and some **elastic fibers** (EF). Numerous **fibroblasts** (F) and other connective tissue cells occupy the adventitia.

KEY

CF	collagen fiber	L	lumen	TI	tunica intima
EF	elastic fiber	N	nucleus	TM	tunica media
F	fibroblast	SM	smooth muscle cell	VV	vasa vasorum
FM	fenestrated membrane	TA	tunica adventitia	xEL	external elastic lamina

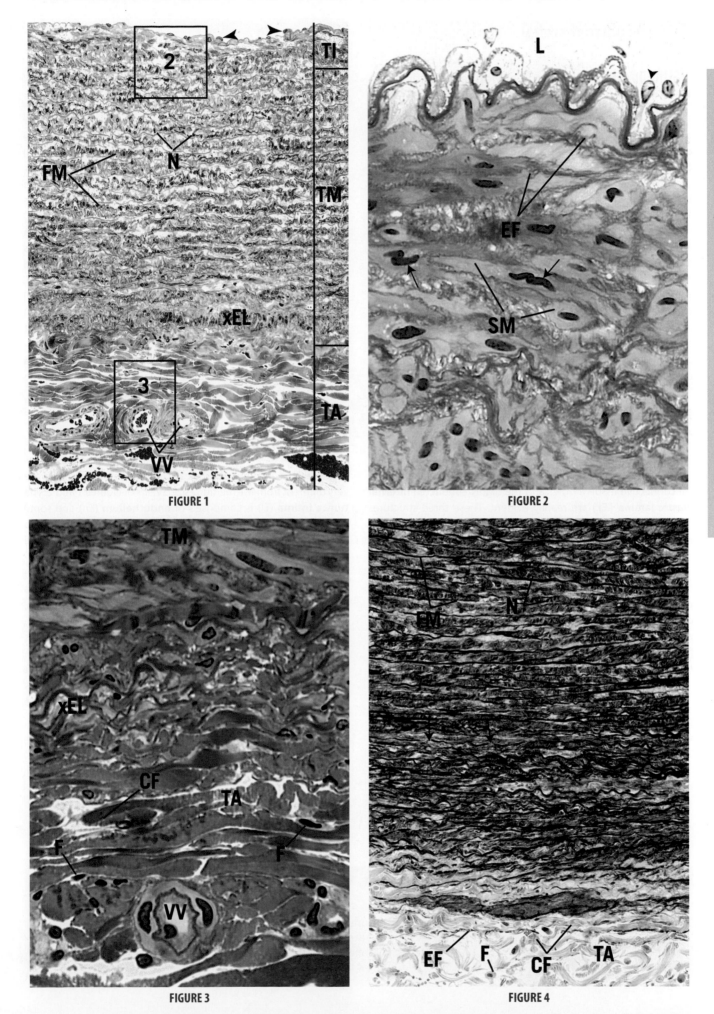

PLATE 8-1 • Elastic Artery

FIGURE 1

FIGURE 2

FIGURE 3

FIGURE 4

PLATE 8-2 • Muscular Artery, Vein

FIGURE 1. Artery and vein. x.s. Monkey. Plastic section. ×132.

This low magnification photomicrograph presents a **muscular artery** (MA) and corresponding **vein** (V). Observe that the wall of the artery is much thicker than that of the vein and contains considerably more muscle fibers. The three concentric tunicae of the artery are evident. The **tunica intima** (TI), with its **endothelial layer** (En) and **internal elastic lamina** (iEL), is readily apparent. The thick **tunica media** (TM) is identified by the circularly or spirally displayed **smooth muscle cells** (SM) that are embedded in an elastic type of intercellular material. These elastic fibers, as well as the external elastic lamina—the outermost layer of the tunica media—are not apparent with hematoxylin and eosin stain. The **tunica adventitia** (TA), which is almost as thick as the media, contains no smooth muscle cells. It is composed chiefly of **collagen** (CF) and **elastic** (EF) fibers as well as fibroblasts and other connective tissue cells. The wall of the companion vein presents the same three tunicae: **intima** (TI), **media** (TM), and **adventitia** (TA); however, all three (but especially the media) are reduced in thickness.

FIGURE 3. Artery. x.s. Elastic stain. Paraffin section. ×132.

This photomicrograph is a higher magnification of a region similar to the *boxed area* of Figure 2. The **endothelium** (En), subendothelial connective tissue (*arrow*), and the highly contracted **internal elastic lamina** (iEL) are readily evident. These three structures constitute the tunica intima of the muscular artery. The **tunica media** (TM) is very thick and consists of many layers of spirally or circularly disposed **smooth muscle cells** (SM), whose **nuclei** (N) are readily identifiable with this stain. Numerous **elastic fibers** (EF) ramify through the intercellular spaces between smooth muscle cells. The **external elastic lamina** (xEL), which comprises the outermost layer of the tunica media, is seen to advantage in this preparation. Finally, note the **collagenous** (CF) and **elastic** (EF) fibers of the **tunica adventitia** (TA), as well as the nuclei (*arrowhead*) of the various connective tissue cells.

FIGURE 2. Artery and vein. x.s. Elastic stain. Paraffin section. ×132.

The elastic stain used in this transverse section of a **muscular artery** (MA) and corresponding **vein** (V) clearly demonstrates the differences between arteries and veins. The **tunica intima** (TI) of the artery stains dark, due to the thick internal elastic lamina, whereas that of the vein does not stain nearly as intensely. The thick **tunica media** (TM) of the artery is composed of numerous layers of circularly or spirally disposed **smooth muscle cells** (SM) with many elastic fibers ramifying through this tunic. The **tunica media** (TM) of the vein has only a few smooth muscle cell layers with little intervening elastic fibers. The **external elastic lamina** (xEL) of the artery is much better developed than that of the vein. Finally, the **tunica adventitia** (TA) constitutes the bulk of the wall of the vein and is composed of **collagenous** (CF) and **elastic** (EF) fibers. The **tunica adventitia** (TA) of the artery is also thick, but it comprises only about half the thickness of its wall. It is also composed of collagenous and EF. Both vessels possess their own **vasa vasorum** (VV) in their tunicae adventitia. A region similar to the *boxed area* is presented at a higher magnification in Figure 3.

FIGURE 4. Large vein. Vena cava. x.s. Human. Paraffin section. ×270.

Large veins, as the inferior vena cava in this photomicrograph, are very different from the medium-sized veins of Figures 1 and 2. The **tunica intima** (TI) is composed of **endothelium** (En) and some subendothelial connective tissue, whereas the **tunica media** (TM) is greatly reduced in thickness and contains only occasional smooth muscle cells. The bulk of the wall of the vena cava is composed of the greatly thickened **tunica adventitia** (TA), consisting of three concentric regions. The innermost layer (1) displays thick collagen bundles (*arrows*) arrayed in a spiral configuration, which permits it to become elongated or shortened with respiratory excursion of the diaphragm. The middle layer (2) presents smooth muscle (or cardiac muscle) cells, longitudinally disposed. The outer layer (3) is characterized by thick bundles of **collagen fibers** (CF) interspersed with elastic fibers. This region contains **vasa vasorum** (VV), which supply nourishment to the wall of the vena cava.

KEY

CF	collagen fiber	N	nucleus	V	vein
EF	elastic fiber	SM	smooth muscle cell	VV	vasa vasorum
En	endothelial layer	TA	tunica adventitia	xEL	external elastic lamina
iEL	internal elastic lamina	TI	tunica intima		
MA	muscular artery	M	tunica media		

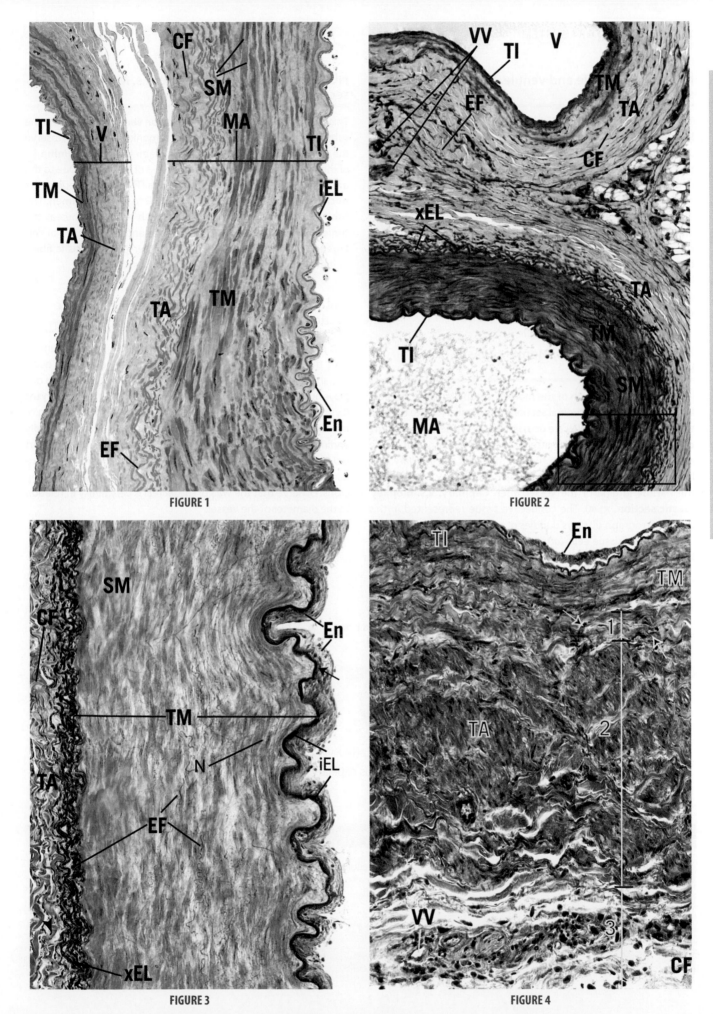

PLATE 8-2 • Muscular Artery.Vein

FIGURE 1

FIGURE 2

FIGURE 3

FIGURE 4

PLATE 8-3 · Arterioles, Venules, Capillaries, and Lymph Vessels

FIGURE 1. Arteriole and venule. l.s. Monkey. Plastic section. ×270.

This longitudinal section of a large **arteriole** (A) and companion **venule** (Ve) from the connective tissue septum of a monkey submandibular gland displays a **duct** (D) of the gland between the two vessels. Observe that the thickness of the arteriole wall approximates the diameter of the **lumen** (L). The endothelial cell **nuclei** (N) are readily evident in both vessels, as are the **smooth muscle cells** (SM) of the tunica media. The arteriole also presents an **internal elastic lamina** (iEL) between the tunica media and the endothelial cells. The **tunica adventitia** (TA) of the arteriole displays nuclei of fibroblasts, whereas those of the venule merge imperceptibly with the surrounding connective tissue. Glandular acini are evident in this field as are **serous units** (SU) and **serous demilunes** (SD).

FIGURE 3. Capillary. l.s. Monkey. Plastic section. ×540.

In this photomicrograph of the monkey cerebellum, the molecular layer displays longitudinal sections of a capillary. Note that the endothelial cell **nuclei** (N) are occasionally in the field of view. The **cytoplasm** (Cy) of the highly attenuated endothelial cells is visible as thin, dark lines, bordering the **lumina** (L) of the capillary. Red blood cells (*arrows*) are noted to be distorted as they pass through the narrow lumina of the vessel. *Inset.* **Capillary. x.s. Monkey. Plastic section.** ×540. The connective tissue represented in this photomicrograph displays bundles of **collagen fibers** (CF), nuclei of connective tissue cells (*arrow*), and a cross-section of a **capillary** (C), whose endothelial cell **nucleus** (N) is clearly evident.

FIGURE 2. Arteriole and venule. x.s. Monkey. Plastic section. ×540.

This small **arteriole** (A) and its companion **venule** (Ve) are from the submucosa of the fundic region of a monkey stomach. Observe the obvious difference between the diameters of the **lumina** (L) of the two vessels as well as the thickness of their walls. Due to the greater muscularity of the **tunica media** (TM) of the arteriole, the **nuclei** (N) of its endothelial cells bulge into its round lumen. The **tunica media** (TM) of the venule is much reduced, whereas the **tunica adventitia** (TA) is well developed and is composed of **collagenous connective tissue** (CT) interspersed with elastic fibers (not evident in this hematoxylin and eosin section).

FIGURE 4. Lymphatic vessel. l.s. Monkey. Plastic section. ×270.

This photomicrograph presents a villus from monkey duodenum. Note the simple columnar **epithelium** (E) interspersed with occasional **goblet cells** (GC). The connective tissue lamina propria displays numerous **plasma cells** (PC), **mast cells** (MC), **lymphocytes** (Ly), and **smooth muscle fibers** (SM). The longitudinal section of the **lumen** (L) lined with **endothelium** (En) is a lacteal, a blindly ending lymphatic channel. Since lymph vessels do not transport red blood cells, the lacteal appears to be empty, but in fact it contains lymph. Subsequent to a fatty meal, lacteals contain chylomicrons. Observe that the wall of the lacteal is very flimsy in relation to the diameter of the vessel.

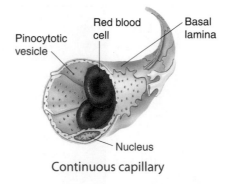

Pinocytotic vesicle   Red blood cell   Basal lamina

Nucleus

Continuous capillary

KEY					
A	arteriole	**En**	endothelium	**SD**	serous demilune
C	capillary	**GC**	goblet cell	**SM**	smooth muscle cell
CF	collagen fiber	**iEL**	internal elastic lamina	**SU**	serous unit
CT	collagenous connective tissue	**L**	lumen	**TA**	tunica adventitia
Cy	cytoplasm	**Ly**	lymphocyte	**TM**	tunica media
D	duct	**MC**	mast cell	**Ve**	venule
E	epithelium	**N**	nucleus		
		PC	plasma cell		

PLATE 8-3 • Arterioles, Venules, Capillaries, and Lymph Vessels

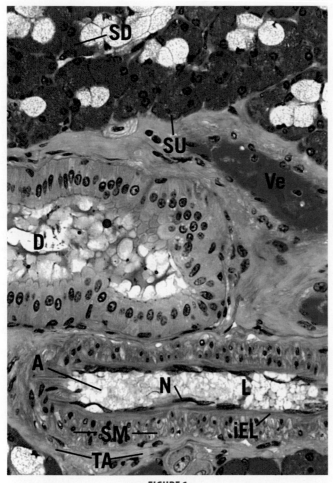

FIGURE 1

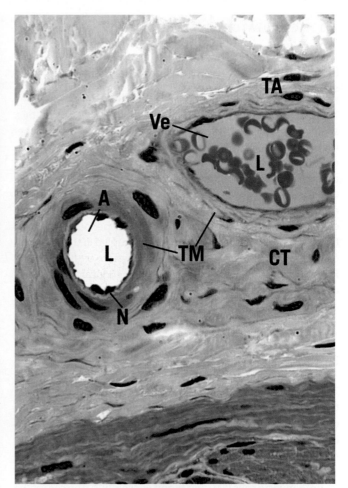

FIGURE 2

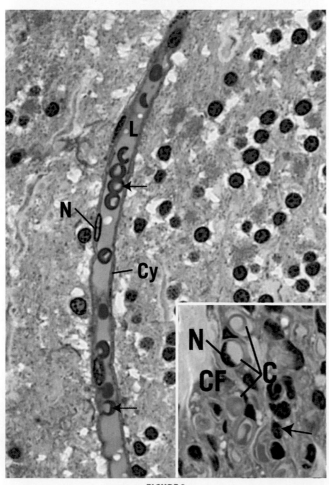

FIGURE 3

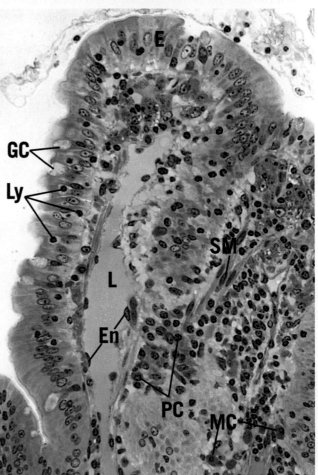

FIGURE 4

PLATE 8-4 · Heart

FIGURE 1. Endocardium. Human. Paraffin section. ×132.

The endocardium, the innermost layer of the heart, is lined by a simple squamous epithelium that is continuous with the endothelial of the various blood vessels entering or exiting the heart. The endocardium is composed of three layers, the innermost of which consists of the **endothelium** (En) and the subendothelial **connective tissue** (CT), whose collagenous fibers and connective tissue cell **nuclei** (N) are readily evident. The middle layer of the endocardium, although composed of dense collagenous and elastic fibers and some smooth muscle cells, is occupied in this photomicrograph by branches of the conducting system of the heart, the **Purkinje fibers** (PF). The third layer of the endocardium borders the thick **myocardium** (My) and is composed of looser connective tissue elements housing blood vessels, occasional adipocytes, and additional connective tissue cells.

FIGURE 3. Heart valve. l.s. Paraffin section. ×132.

This figure is a montage, displaying a **valve leaflet** (Le) as well as the **endocardium** (EC) of the heart. The leaflet is in the **lumen** (L) of the ventricle, as evidenced by the numerous trapped **red blood cells** (RBC). The **endothelial** (En) lining of the endocardium is continuous with the endothelial lining of the leaflet. The three layers of the endocardium are clearly evident, as are the occasional **smooth muscle cells** (SM) and **blood vessels** (BV). The core of the leaflet is composed of dense collagenous and elastic connective tissue, housing numerous cells whose nuclei are readily observed. Since the core of these leaflets is devoid of blood vessels, the connective tissue cells receive their nutrients directly from the blood in the lumen of the heart via simple diffusion. The connective tissue core of the leaflet is continuous with the skeleton of the heart, which forms a fibrous ring around the opening of the valves.

FIGURE 2. Purkinje fibers. Iron hematoxylin. Paraffin section. ×132.

The stain utilized in preparing this section of the ventricular myocardium intensively stains **red blood cells** (RBC) and **cardiac muscle cells** (CM). Therefore, the thick bundle of **Purkinje fibers** (PF) is shown to advantage, due to its less dense staining quality. The **connective tissue** (CT) surrounding these fibers is highly vascularized, as evidenced by the red blood cell–filled capillaries. Purkinje fibers are composed of individual cells, each with a centrally placed single **nucleus** (N). These fibers form numerous gap junctions with each other and with cardiac muscle cells. The *boxed area* is presented at a higher magnification in the inset. *Inset.* **Purkinje fibers. Iron hematoxylin. Paraffin section.** ×270. Individual cells of Purkinje fibers are much larger than cardiac muscle cells. However, the presence of peripherally displaced **myofibrils** (m) displaying A and I bands (*arrow*) clearly demonstrates that they are modified cardiac muscle cells. The **nucleus** (N) is surrounded by a clear area, housing glycogen and mitochondria.

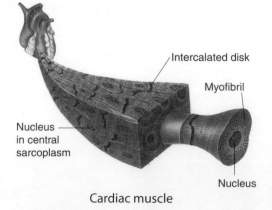

Intercalated disk

Myofibril

Nucleus in central sarcoplasm

Nucleus

Cardiac muscle

KEY

BV	blood vessel	**En**	endothelium	**My**	myocardium
CM	cardiac muscle cell	**L**	lumen	**N**	nucleus
CT	connective tissue	**Le**	valve leaflet	**PF**	Purkinje fiber
EC	endocardium	**m**	myofibril	**RBC**	red blood cell

PLATE 8-4 · Heart

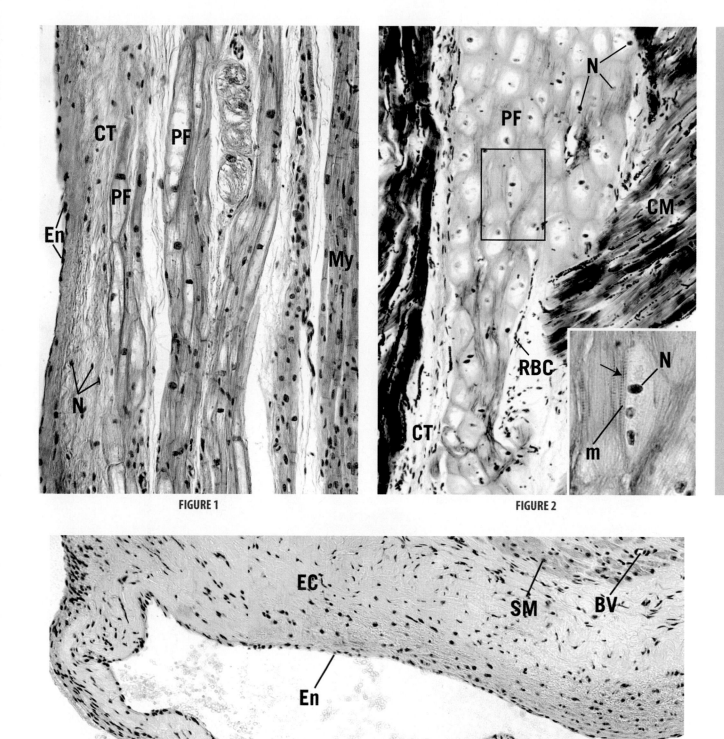

FIGURE 1

FIGURE 2

FIGURE 3

PLATE 8-5 · Capillary, Electron Microscopy

FIGURE 1. Continuous capillary. x.s. Cardiac muscle. Mouse. Electron microscopy. ×29,330.

This electron micrograph of a continuous capillary in cross-section was taken from mouse heart tissue. Observe that the section passes through the **nucleus** (N) of one of the endothelial cells constituting the wall of the vessel and that the lumen contains **red blood cells** (RBC). Note that the endothelial cells are highly attenuated and that they form tight junctions (*arrows*) with each other. *Arrowheads* point to pinocytotic vesicles that traverse the endothelial cell. The **lamina densa** (LD) and **lamina lucida** (LL) of the basal lamina are clearly evident.

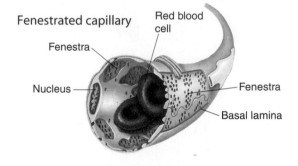

Fenestrated capillary
Red blood cell
Fenestra
Nucleus
Fenestra
Basal lamina

PLATE 8-5 • Capillary, Electron Microscopy

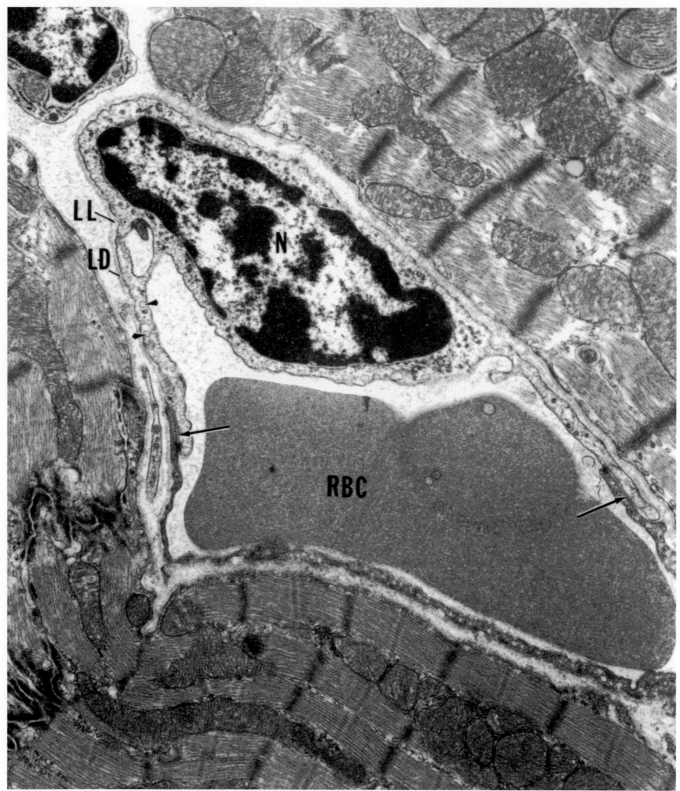

FIGURE 1

PLATE 8-6 · Freeze Etch, Fenestrated Capillary, Electron Microscopy

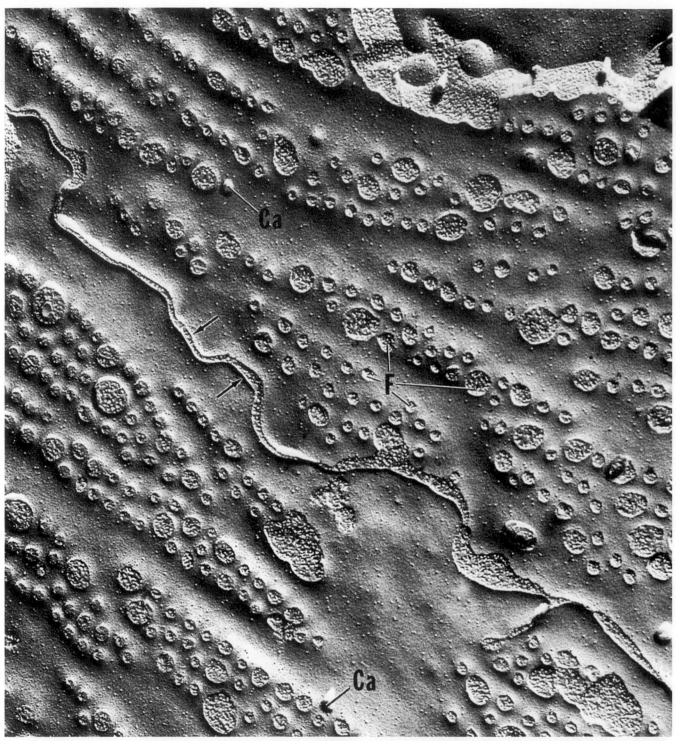

FIGURE 1

FIGURE 1. Fenestrated capillary. Hamster. Electron microscopy. Freeze fracture. ×205,200.

This electron micrograph is a representative example of fenestrated capillaries from the hamster adrenal cortex, as revealed by the freeze fracture replica technique. The parallel lines (*arrows*) running diagonally across the field represent the line of junction between two endothelial cells, which are presented in a surface view. Note that the numerous **fenestrae** (F), whose diameters range from 57 to 166 nm, are arranged in tracts, with the regions between tracts nonfenestrated. Occasional **caveolae** (Ca) are also present. (From Ryan U, Ryan J, Smith D, Winkler H. Fenestrated endothelium of the adrenal gland: freeze fracture studies. Tissue Cell 1975;7:181–190.)

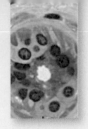

Chapter Summary

I. ELASTIC ARTERY (CONDUCTING ARTERY)

Among these are the **aorta**, **common carotid**, and **subclavian arteries**.

A. Tunica Intima

Lined by short, polygonal **endothelial cells**. The **subendothelial connective tissue** is fibroelastic and houses some longitudinally disposed smooth muscle cells. **Internal elastic lamina** is not clearly defined.

B. Tunica Media

Characterized by numerous **fenestrated membranes** (spiral to concentric sheets of fenestrated elastic membranes). Enmeshed among the elastic material are circularly disposed **smooth muscle cells** and associated **collagenous**, **reticular**, and **elastic fibers**.

C. Tunica Adventitia

Thin, **collagenous connective tissue** containing some **elastic fibers** and a few longitudinally oriented **smooth muscle cells**. **Vasa vasorum** (vessels of vessels) are also present.

II. MUSCULAR ARTERY (DISTRIBUTING ARTERY)

Among these are the named arteries, with the exception of the elastic arteries.

A. Tunica Intima

These are lined by polygonal-shaped, flattened **endothelial cells** that bulge into the lumen during vasoconstriction. The **subendothelial connective tissue** houses fine **collagenous fibers** and few longitudinally disposed **smooth muscle cells**. The **internal elastic lamina**, clearly evident, is frequently split into two membranes.

B. Tunica Media

Characterized by many layers of circularly disposed **smooth muscle cells**, with some **elastic**, **reticular**, and **collagenous fibers** among the muscle cells. The **external elastic lamina** is well defined.

C. Tunica Adventitia

Usually a very thick **collagenous** and **elastic tissue**, with some longitudinally oriented **smooth muscle fibers**. **Vasa vasorum** are also present.

III. ARTERIOLES

These are arterial vessels whose diameter is less than 100 μm.

A. Tunica Intima

Endothelium and a variable amount of **subendothelial connective tissue** are always present. The **internal elastic lamina** is present in larger arterioles but absent in smaller arterioles.

B. Tunica Media

The spirally arranged **smooth muscle fibers** may be up to three layers thick. An **external elastic lamina** is present in larger arterioles but absent in smaller arterioles.

C. Tunica Adventitia

This is composed of **collagenous** and **elastic connective tissues**, whose thickness approaches that of the tunica media.

IV. CAPILLARIES

Most **capillaries** in cross-section appear as thin, circular profiles 8 to 10 μm in diameter. Occasionally, a fortuitous section will display an **endothelial cell nucleus**, a red blood cell, or, very infrequently, a white blood cell. Frequently, capillaries will be collapsed and not evident with the light microscope. **Pericytes** are usually associated with capillaries.

V. VENULES

Venules possess much larger lumina and thinner walls than corresponding arterioles.

A. Tunica Intima

Endothelium lies on a very thin **subendothelial connective tissue** layer, which increases with the size of the vessel. **Pericytes** are frequently associated with smaller venules.

B. Tunica Media

Absent in smaller venules, whereas in larger venules one or two layers of **smooth muscle cells** may be observed.

C. Tunica Adventitia

Consists of **collagenous connective tissue** with **fibroblasts** and some **elastic fibers**.

VI. MEDIUM-SIZED VEINS

A. Tunica Intima

The **endothelium** and a scant amount of **subendothelial connective tissue** are always present. Occasionally, a thin **internal elastic lamina** is observed. **Valves** may be evident.

B. Tunica Media

Much thinner than that of the corresponding artery but does possess a few layers of **smooth muscle cells**. Occasionally, some of the muscle fibers, instead of being circularly disposed, are longitudinally disposed. Bundles of **collagen fibers** interspersed with a few **elastic fibers** are also present.

C. Tunica Adventitia

Composed of **collagen** and some **elastic fibers**, which constitute the bulk of the vessel wall. Occasionally, longitudinally oriented **smooth muscle cells** may be present. **Vasa vasorum** are noted to penetrate even the **tunica media**.

VII. LARGE VEINS

A. Tunica Intima

Same as that of medium-sized veins but displays thicker **subendothelial connective tissue**. Some large veins have well-defined **valves**.

B. Tunica Media

Not very well defined, although it may present some **smooth muscle cells** interspersed among **collagenous** and **elastic fibers**.

C. Tunica Adventitia

Thickest of the three layers and accounts for most of the vessel wall. May contain longitudinally oriented **smooth muscle fiber bundles** among the thick layers of **collagen** and **elastic fibers**. **Vasa vasorum** are commonly present.

VIII. HEART

An extremely thick, muscular organ composed of three layers: **endocardium**, **myocardium**, and **epicardium**. The presence of **cardiac muscle** is characteristic of this organ. Additional structural parameters may include **Purkinje fibers**, thick **valves**, **atrioventricular** and **sinoatrial nodes**, as well as the **chordae tendineae** and the thick, connective tissue **cardiac skeleton**.

IX. LYMPHATIC VESSELS

Lymphatic vessels are either collapsed and therefore not discernible, or they are filled with lymph. In the latter case, they present the appearance of a clear, endothelial-lined space resembling a blood vessel. However, the lumina contain no **red blood cells**, though **lymphocytes** may be present. The **endothelium** may display **valves**.

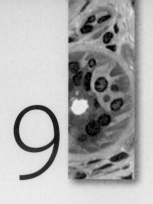

9 LYMPHOID TISSUE

CHAPTER OUTLINE

ymphoid tissue forms the basis of the immune system of the body and is organized into diffuse and nodular lymphatic tissues (see Graphics 9-1 and 9-2). The immune system relies on the interactions of its primary cell components, lymphocytes, and antigen-presenting cells (APCs), to effect a **cell-mediated immune response** against microorganisms, foreign cells, and virally altered cells and **humoral immune response**, release of **antibodies** against **antigens**.

- **Antibodies (immunoglobulins)**, glycoproteins produced by plasma cells, form the principal armamentarium of the humoral immune response. These glycoproteins bind to those antigens for which they are specific, forming antibody-antigen complexes. Each antibody
  - is composed of two **heavy chains** and two **light chains**
  - possesses a constant region and a variable region
    - **constant regions** are the same for all antibodies of the same class (isotype)
    - **variable regions** that are identical in all antibodies against a specific antigen but differ from all other antibodies that are specific for different antigens.
  - There are five classes (isotypes) of immunoglobulins: IgA, IgD, IgE, IgG, and IgM (see Table 9-1). The heavy chains of these isotypes differ from one another in their amino acid composition.

COMPONENTS OF THE IMMUNE SYSTEM

There are two components of the immune system, namely, the innate (nonspecific) immune system and the adaptive (specific) immune system.

TABLE 9-1 • Immunoglobulin Isotypes and Their Characteristics

Class	Cytokines*	Binding to Cells	Biological Characteristics
IgA Secretory immunoglobulin	TgF-β	Forms temporary attachment to epithelial cells as it is being secreted	Secreted as dimers, which are protected by its secretory component, into saliva, tears, bile, gut lumen, nasal discharge, and milk (providing passive immunity for infants). Provides protection against pathogens and invading antigens
IgD Reaginic antibody		B-cell plasmalemma	The presence of IgD on B-cell plasma membranes permits them to recognize antigens and initiate an immune response by inducing B cells to differentiate into plasma cells.
IgE Reaginic antibody	IL-4 and IL-5	Plasmalemmae of mast cells and basophils	When antigens bind to IgE antibodies attached to mast cell and basophil plasma membranes, the binding prompts the release of pharmacological agents from these cells initiating the immediate hypersensitivity response.
IgG Serum immunoglobulin	IFN-γ, IL-4, and IL-6	Neutrophils and macrophages	IgG is a serum antibody that crosses the placental barrier protecting the fetus (passive immunity). In the blood stream, IgG binds to antigenic sites on invading microorganisms, opsonizing these pathogens, so that neutrophils and macrophages can phagocytose them. Natural killer cells are activated by IgG, thereby initiating antibody-dependent cell-mediated cytotoxicity.
IgM First to be formed in immune response		IgM is a pentamer; however, its monomeric form binds to B cells.	The pentameric form activates the complement system.

*Cytokines responsible for switching to this isotype.
IFN, interferon; IL, interleukin; NK, natural killer.

TABLE 9-2 • Components of the Innate Immune System

Component	Function
Complement	A series of blood-associated macromolecules that combine in a predetermined order to form a membrane-attack complex on the plasmalemmae of intravascular pathogens.
Toll-like receptors (TLR)	A family of 15 or more integral proteins located on the plasmalemmae of dendritic cells, macrophages, and mast cells as well as in endosomal membranes. TLRs recognize extracellular pathogens as well as intracellular ligands formed due to cell injury and initiate responses to combat them. TLRs activate not only cells of the innate immune system but also those of the adaptive immune system. See Table 9-3 for some of their functions.
Mast cells	See Chapter 3
Eosinophils	See Chapter 5
Neutrophils	See Chapter 5
Macrophages	Phagocytose foreign substances, breaking them down to epitopes (antigenic determinants). They present these epitopes on their cell surface in conjunction with major histocompatibility complex molecules (MHC molecules) and other membrane-associated markers.
Natural killer cells	Kill virally altered cells and tumor cells in a nonspecific and not MHC-restricted manner. These cells become activated by the Fc portions of those antibodies that are bound to cell surface epitopes and thus kill these decorated cells by a procedure known as antibody-dependent cell-mediated cytotoxicity.

PROPERTY OF LIBRARY
SOUTH UNIVERSITY CLEVELAND CAMPUS
WARRENSVILLE HEIGHTS, OH 44128

- The **innate immune system** is nonspecific in that it is not designed to combat a particular (i.e., a specific) antigen. It is an evolutionarily older system than its adaptive counterpart; it possesses no immunologic memory but acts in a rapid fashion in response to **pathogen-associated molecular patterns** that are shared by most pathogenic invaders. The components of the innate immune system are listed in Table 9-2, and toll-like receptors are also presented in Table 9-3.

- The **adaptive immune system** is distinguished by four primary characteristics: immunological memory, immunological specificity, immunological diversity, and the capability to differentiate between self and nonself.

TABLE 9-3 • Toll-Like Receptors

Location	Receptor Pair	Function
Extracellular and intracellular	TLR1-TLR2	Binds to parasite proteins and bacterial lipoproteins
	TLR2-TLR6	In gram-positive bacteria, it binds to lipoteichoic acid; in fungi, it binds to zymosan.
	TLR4-TLR4	In gram-negative bacteria, it binds to lipopolysaccharides (lipoglycans) of the outer membranes.
	TLR5-?*	Binds to the protein flagellin (principal constituent of bacterial flagella)
	TLR11-?*	Host recognition of *Toxoplasmosis gondii*
Intracellular only	TLR3-?*	Binds to double-stranded RNA of viruses
	TLR7-?*	Binds to single-stranded RNA of viruses
	TLR8-?*	Binds to single-stranded RNA of viruses
	TLR9-?*	Binds to viral and bacterial DNA
Unknown	TLR10-?*	Unknown
	TLR12-?*	Unknown
	TLR13-?*	Unknown
	TLR15-?*	Unknown

*Currently, TLR partner is unknown.
TLR, toll-like receptor.

CELLS OF THE IMMUNE SYSTEM

The cells of the immune system exchange information by releasing cytokines (signaling molecules) and by physically contacting each other to recognize membrane-bounded molecules. These cells may be subdivided into four major categories: antigen presenting cells (APCs), natural killer cells (NK cells), clones of T lymphocytes (T cells), and clones of B lymphocytes (B cells). A **clone** is a small population of identical cells, each of which is capable of recognizing and responding to one specific (or very closely related) **epitope**.

Antigen-Presenting Cells

Antigen-presenting cells (APCs), macrophages, and B lymphocytes possess class II major histocompatibility complex molecules (**MHC II molecules**), whereas all other nucleated cells possess **MHC I molecules**. In humans, MHC molecules are also referred to as **human leukocyte antigen molecules (HLA molecules)**.

- **Macrophages** and some other **APCs** can degrade antigens into **epitopes**, small highly antigenic peptides 7 to 11 amino acids long.
  - Each epitope is attached to an MHC II molecule, and this complex is placed on the external aspect of its cell membrane.
  - The MHC II-epitope complex is recognized by the T-cell receptor (**TCR**) in conjunction with the **CD4 molecule** of the T_H1 or T_H2 cells, a process known as **MHC II restriction**.
- **B cells** have the capability of acting as APCs and present their MHC II-epitope complex to T_H1 cells (discussed below).

APCs, specifically **macrophages**, produce and release a variety of cytokines that modulate the immune response. These include

  - **interleukin 1**, which stimulates T helper cells and self-activated macrophages, as well as
  - **prostaglandin E_2**, which attenuates some immune responses.
  - Cytokines, such as **interferon-γ**, released by other lymphoid cells as well as by macrophages, enhance the phagocytic and cytolytic avidity of macrophages.

Lymphocytes

The **lymphocyte**, the principal cell of lymphoid tissue, is a key controller responsible for the proper functioning of the immune system. Lymphocytes may be subdivided, according to function, into three categories: null cells, T lymphocytes, and B lymphocytes.

Null Cells

Null cells are composed of two categories of cells, namely, stem cells and NK cells (although some immunologists prefer not to use this classification system and avoid the null cell category).

- **Stem cells** are undifferentiated cells that will give rise to the various cellular elements of blood cell lineage,
- **NK cells** are cytotoxic cells that are responsible for the destruction of certain categories of foreign cells. NK cells resemble cytotoxic T cells, but they do not have to enter the thymus to become mature killer cells; instead, they are immunocompetent as soon as they leave the bone marrow.
  - These cells kill virally altered cells and tumor cells in a **nonspecific** manner, and they are not MHC restricted.
  - NK cells also recognize and become activated by the Fc portions of those antibodies that are bound to cell surface epitopes.
  - Once activated, NK cells release **perforins** and **fragmentins** to kill these decorated cells by a procedure known as **antibody-dependent cell-mediated cytotoxicity**.
  - Perforins assemble as pores within the plasmalemma of target cells, contributing to **necrotic cell death**, whereas fragmentins drive the target cell into apoptosis, **directed cell death**.
  - NK cells also possess integral proteins known as **killer activating receptors** that have an affinity to specific proteins on the cell membranes of nucleated cells.
  - To protect self cells from this response, NK cells also possess additional transmembrane proteins, known as **killer-inhibitor receptors**, that avoid the killing of healthy cells.

T Lymphocytes (T cells)

T cells are immunoincompetent until they enter the cortex of the thymus. Here, under the influence of the cortical environment, they express their **T cell receptors (TCRs)** and **cluster of differentiation markers** (CD2, CD3, CD4, CD8, and CD28) and become immunocompetent.

- Once immunocompetent, the T cells enter the medulla of the thymus or are killed if they are committed against the self.
- In the medulla, they will lose either their CD4 or their CD8 markers and thus develop into **CD8⁺** or **CD4⁺** cells, respectively.
- These cells enter into blood vessels of the medulla to become members of the circulating population of lymphocytes. They do not produce antibodies; instead, they function in the cell-mediated immune response.

- There are several categories of T cells that are responsible not only for the **cell-mediated immune response** but also for facilitating the **humorally mediated response** of B cells to **thymic-dependent antigens**.
- To be able to perform their functions, T cells possess characteristic integral membrane proteins on their cell surfaces.
  - One of these is the **T-cell receptor** (TCR), which has the capability of recognizing that particular epitope for which the cell is genetically programmed.
  - T cells can recognize only those epitopes that are bound to **MHC molecules** present on the surface of antigen-presenting cells.
  - Thus, T cells are said to be **MHC restricted**. There are three general categories of T cells: naïve T cells, memory T cells, and effector T cells.

It is the T lymphocytes that participate in the graft rejection phenomenon and in the elimination of virally transformed cells. There are three general categories of T cells: naïve T cells, memory T cells, and effector T cells.

- **Naïve T cells** are immunologically competent and possess CD45RA molecules on their plasma membrane, but they have to become activated before they can function as T cells.
  - Activation involves the interaction of the naïve T cell's TCR-CD3 complex with the MHC-epitope complex of APCs, as well as the interaction of the T cell's CD28 molecule with the antigen-presenting cell's B7 molecule.
  - The activated naïve T cell enters the cell cycle and forms memory T cells and effector T cells.
- **Memory T cells** are immunocompetent cells that are the progeny of activated T cells that undergo mitotic activity during an antigenic challenge. These cells are long-lived, circulating cells that are added to and increase the number of cells of the original clone. It is this increase in the size of the clone that is responsible for the **anamnestic response** (a more rapid and more intense secondary response) against another encounter with the same antigen.
- **Effector T cells**. The categories of effector T cells are T helper cells (T_H cells), cytotoxic T lymphocytes (CTLs, T killer cells), regulatory T cells (T reg cells), and natural T killer cells.
  - **T Helper cells** are all CD4+ cells and are subdivided into four categories: T_H0, T_H1, T_H2, and T_H17 cells.
    - **T_H0 cells** enter the cell cycle and can give rise to T_H1 and T_H2 cells.
    - **T_H1 cells** produce and release the cytokines interleukin 2, interferon-γ, and tumor necrosis factor-α. T_H1 cells have an essential role in the initiation of the cell-mediated immune response and in the destruction of intracellular pathogens.
    - **T_H2 cells** produce and release interleukins 4, 5, 6, 9, 10, and 13, which, among other roles, induce B cells to proliferate and differentiate into **plasma cells** that produce antibodies. Additionally, T_H2 cells initiate the reaction against parasites and mucosal infections.
    - **T_H17 cells** are proinflammatory cells that are responsible for some autoimmune diseases, such as rheumatoid arthritis and multiple sclerosis. T_H17 cells produce
      - interleukin 17 (IL-17), which acts on stromal and other cells to initiate the inflammatory process, and
      - interleukin 21 (IL-21), which acts in an autocrine fashion to induce the proliferation of T_H17 cells.
  - **Cytotoxic T lymphocytes** are CD8+ cells. Upon contacting the proper MHC-epitope complex displayed by APCs and having been activated by interleukin 2, these cells undergo mitosis to form numerous **cytotoxic T lymphocytes** (CTLs).
    - These newly formed cells kill foreign and virally transformed self cells by secreting **perforins** and **fragmentins** and by expressing CD95L (the death ligand) on their plasmalemma, which activates CD95 (death receptor) on the target cell's plasma membrane, which drives the target cell into apoptosis.
  - **T reg cells** are CD4+ cells that function in the suppression of the immune response. There are two types of T regulatory cells:
    - **natural T reg cells**, whose TCR binds to APCs and thus suppresses the immune response, and
    - **inducible T reg cells** that release cytokines that inhibit the formation of T_H1 cells.
  - **Natural T killer** cells are similar to NK cells, but they have to enter the cortex of the thymus to be immunocompetent. They are unusual because they have the ability to recognize lipid antigens.

Once a T lymphocyte becomes activated by the presence of an antigen, it releases cytokines, substances that activate macrophages, attract them to the site of antigenic invasion, and enhance their phagocytic capabilities. Frequently, T lymphocytes also assist B lymphocytes to amplify and modulate their immune response. The major interactions among T cells, B cells, and antigen-presenting cells are illustrated in Graphics 9-3 to 9-5.

B Lymphocytes (B Cells)

B lymphocytes (B cells) are formed and become immunocompetent in the bone marrow (bursa of Fabricius in birds). They enter the general circulation, establish clones whose members seed various lymphoid organs, and are responsible for the **humoral immune response**.

- As the **B cell** is becoming immunocompetent, it manufactures **IgM** or **IgD** and places them on their cell membrane in such a fashion that the epitope binding sites are located in the extracellular space and the Fc moiety of the **surface immunoglobulins (SIGs)** is embedded in the plasmalemma in association with two pairs of integral proteins, **Igβ** and **Igα**.
- The **SIGs** of a particular B cell target the same epitope. Unlike T cells, B cells have the capability of acting as APCs and present their MHC II-epitope complex to T_H1 cells.
- When the newly formed B cell binds to its epitope, the Igβ and the Igα transduce the information with the resultant **activation** of the B cell. Once activated, B cells manufacture and release IL-12, a cytokine that promotes the formation of T_H1 cells. B cells proliferate during a humoral immune response to form plasma cells and B memory cells.

Plasma cells are differentiated cells that do not possess SIGs but are "antibody factories" that synthesize and release an enormous number of identical copies of the same antibody that is specific against a particular epitope (although it may cross-react with similar epitopes).

- Antibodies, once released, bind to a specific antigen. In some instances,
  - binding inactivates the antigen, whereas in others
  - the attachment of antibodies to antigens may enhance phagocytosis (opsonization) or activate the complement cascade, resulting in chemotaxis of neutrophils and, frequently, lysis of the invader.

B memory cells are similar to T memory cells in that they are long-lived, circulating cells that are added to and increase the number of cells of the original clone. They possess SIGs so that they can be activated by an appropriate antigen during a secondary immune response. Thus, it is this increase in the size of the clone that is responsible for the **anamnestic response** against a subsequent encounter with the same antigen.

DIFFUSE LYMPHOID TISSUE

Diffuse lymphoid tissue occurs throughout the body, especially under moist epithelial membranes, where the loose connective tissue is infiltrated by lymphoid cells, such as lymphocytes, plasma cells, macrophages, and reticular cells. Therefore, these are referred to as **mucosa-associated lymphoid tissue (MALT)**.

- MALT is particularly evident in the lamina propria of the digestive tract and in the subepithelial connective tissue of the respiratory tract, where they are known as

  - **gut-associated lymphoid tissue (GALT)** and
  - **bronchus-associated lymphoid tissue (BALT)**, respectively.

It may be noted that the lymphoid cells are not arranged in any particular pattern but are scattered in a haphazard manner. Frequently, lymphoid nodules, transitory structures that are a denser aggregation of lymphoid tissue composed mainly of lymphocytes, may be observed. Lymphoid nodules may be primary or secondary, where the secondary lymphoid nodules present the characteristic appearance of a lighter **germinal center** and a darker, peripherally located **corona**, indicating activation by antigen. The germinal centers are sites of plasma cell production, whereas the corona is produced by mitosis from existing B lymphocytes.

LYMPH NODES

Lymph nodes are ovoid- to kidney-shaped organs through which lymph is filtered by exposure to large numbers of lymphoid cells (see Graphic 9-2).

- They possess a **convex surface**, which receives afferent lymph vessels, and
- a **hilum**, where blood vessels leave and enter and efferent lymph vessels leave and drain lymph from the organ.
- Lymphocytes enter lymph nodes via the **afferent lymph vessels** as well as via arterioles that penetrate the lymph node at the hilum, travel to the paracortex within connective tissue trabeculae, and form **high endothelial vessels** (postcapillary venules).

Each lymph node has a dense, irregular, collagenous connective tissue **capsule** and septa, derived from the capsule, subdividing the cortex into incomplete compartments. Attached to the septa and the internal aspect of the capsule is a network of reticular tissue and associated reticular cells that act as a framework for housing the numerous free and migratory cells, mostly lymphocytes, antigen-presenting cells, and macrophages, occupying the organ.

- The **cortex** of the lymph node houses the capsular and cortical sinuses, as well as lymphoid nodules, composed mainly of **B lymphocytes, APCs, macrophages,** and **reticular cells**.
- Between the cortex and the medulla is the **paracortex**, populated by **T lymphocytes, APCs, and macrophages**.
- The **medulla** consists of **medullary cords** and **medullary sinusoids**.
  - The **medullary cords** are composed mainly of **T cells, B cells,** and **plasma cells** that arise in the cortex and paracortex and migrate into the medulla.

○ The **medullary sinusoids** are continuous with the capsular and cortical sinuses.
  ■ T cells and B cells enter the sinusoids and leave the lymph node via efferent lymph vessels.

Additional cell components of lymph nodes are **macrophages, antigen-presenting cells**, and some **granulocytes**. Aside from functioning in the maintenance and production of immunocompetent cells, lymph nodes also filter lymph.

• The **filtering procedure** is facilitated by the elongated processes of **reticular cells** that span the sinuses of the node and thus disturb and retard lymph flow, providing more time for the resident macrophages to phagocytose antigens and other debris.

TONSILS

Tonsils are aggregates of incompletely **encapsulated lymphoid tissue** situated at the entrances to the oral pharynx and to the nasal pharynx. Participating in the formation of the **tonsillar ring** are the

• **palatine**,
• **pharyngeal**, and
• **lingual tonsils**.

The tonsils produce antibodies against the numerous antigens and microorganisms that abound in their vicinity. There are additional, smaller tonsils, such as the tubal and lingual tonsils, that function in the same manner.

SPLEEN

The **spleen** is the largest lymphoid organ of the body (see Graphic 9-2). Its principal functions are to filter blood, phagocytose senescent red blood cells and invading microorganisms, supply immunocompetent **T** and **B** lymphocytes, and manufacture **antibodies**. Unlike lymph nodes, the spleen is not divided into cortical and medullary regions, nor is it supplied by afferent lymphatic vessels. Blood vessels enter and leave the spleen at its hilum and travel within the parenchyma via trabeculae derived from its connective tissue capsule.

• The spleen is subdivided into **white** and **red pulps**.
  ○ **White pulp** is composed of lymphoid tissue that is arranged in a specific fashion, either as **periarterial lymphatic sheaths (PALS)** composed of T lymphocytes or as **lymphoid nodules** consisting of B lymphocytes.
  ○ The **red pulp** consists of **pulp cords (of Billroth)** interposed between a spongy network of **sinusoids** lined by unusual elongated endothelial cells displaying large intercellular spaces, supported by a

thick, discontinuous, hoop-like basement membrane. Reticular cells and reticular fibers associated with these sinusoids extend into the pulp cords to contribute to the cell population that consists of **macrophages, plasma cells**, and extravasated blood cells.
  ○ A region of smaller sinusoids forms the interface between the white and red pulps, and this interface is known as the **marginal zone**. Capillaries arising from the central arteries deliver their blood to sinusoids of the marginal zone, which is rich in arterial vessels and avidly phagocytic macrophages. APCs of the marginal zone monitor this blood for the presence of antigens and foreign substances.

Understanding splenic organization depends on knowing the vascular supply of the spleen.

• The **splenic artery** entering at the hilum is distributed to the interior of the organ via trabeculae as trabecular arteries.
• On leaving a trabecula, the vessel enters the parenchyma to be surrounded by the periarterial lymphatic sheaths (PALS) and occasional lymphoid nodules and is termed the central artery.
• **Central arteries** enter the red pulp by losing their PALS and subdivide into numerous small, straight vessels known as **penicillar arteries**.
• Penicillar arteries possess three regions: **pulp arterioles, sheathed arterioles**, and **terminal arterial capillaries**. Whether these terminal arterial capillaries drain directly into the sinusoids (closed circulation) or terminate as open-ended vessels in the pulp cords (open circulation) has not been determined conclusively; however, in humans, the open circulation is believed to predominate.
• It is during this passage of red blood cells from the splenic cords into the sinusoids that damaged and aging red blood cells are eliminated.
• Sinusoids are drained by pulp veins, which lead to trabecular veins and eventually join the splenic vein.

THYMUS

The **thymus** is an endodermally derived, bilobed, encapsulated lymphoid organ located in the mediastinum, overlying the great vessels of the heart (see Graphic 9-2). The thymus attains its greatest development shortly after birth, but subsequent to puberty, it begins to **involute** and becomes infiltrated by adipose tissue; however, even in the adult, the thymus retains its ability to form a reduced number of T lymphocytes. The thin connective tissue capsule of the thymus sends septa deep into the organ, incompletely subdividing it into lobules.

The thymus possesses no lymphoid nodules; instead, it is divided into an

- outer darker staining **cortex**, composed of **epithelial reticular cells**, **macrophages**, and **small T lymphocytes (thymocytes)**, and an
- inner lighter staining **medulla** consisting of **large T lymphocytes**, **epithelial reticular cells**, and **thymic (Hassall's) corpuscles** (see Table 9-4).

The major functions of the thymus are the formation, potentiation, and destruction of T lymphocytes.

- Immunoincompetent (immature) **T-lymphocyte precursors** enter the corticomedullary junction of the thymus, where they become known as **thymocytes**, and migrate to the **outer cortex** where they are activated by cytokines released by epithelial reticular cells to express certain **T-cell markers**.
- The markers that thymocytes express do *not* include CD4, CD8, or the CD3-TCR complex and become known as **double negative thymocytes**. These cells migrate into the inner cortex and express **pre-TCRs (pre–T-cell receptors)** that trigger their propagation.
- The progeny of the pre–TCR-bearing thymocytes express *both* CD4 and CD8 molecules as well as a limited number of CD3-TCR molecules and are known as **double-positive thymocytes**.
- Cortical epithelial reticular cells assess if double-positive thymocytes are able to recognize **self-MHC-self-epitope complexes**. About 90% of double-positive thymocytes are unable to recognize these complexes, and they undergo apoptosis. The remaining 10% of these double-positive thymocytes that do recognize the self-MHC-self-epitope complexes mature, express many more TCRs, and lose either CD8 or CD4 molecules from their cell surface.

- Thymocytes that express many TCRs and either CD4 or CD8 molecules are known as **single-positive thymocytes**, which pass through the corticomedullary border to enter the **medulla**.
- **Dendritic cells** and **epithelial reticular cells** of the medulla assess the abilities of single-positive thymocytes to initiate an immune response against the self.
  - Single-positive thymocytes that can initiate an immune response against the self undergo apoptosis (**clonal deletion**) due to the effect of **thymic stromal lymphopoietin**, released by epithelial reticular cells of Hassall's corpuscles.
  - Single-positive thymocytes that are unable to attack the self are released from the thymus as **naïve T lymphocytes**. These naïve T cells migrate to the secondary lymphoid organs to set up clones of T cells.

Blood vessels gain entrance to the medulla by traveling in the connective tissue septa, which they exit at the corticomedullary junction, where they provide capillary loops to the cortex.

- The **capillaries** that enter the cortex are the continuous type and are surrounded by epithelial reticular cells that isolate them from the cortical lymphocytes, thus establishing a **blood-thymus barrier**, providing an antigen-free environment for the potentiation of the immunocompetent T lymphocytes.
- The blood vessels of the medulla are not unusual and present no blood-thymus barrier.
- The thymus is drained by **venules** in the medulla, which also receives blood from the cortical capillaries.
- **Epithelial reticular cells** form a specialized barrier between the cortex and medulla to prevent medullary material from gaining access to the cortex.

TABLE 9-4 • Thymic Epithelial Reticular Cells

Cell Type	Location	Function
Type I	Cortex	Surround blood vessels and isolate cortex from capsule and septa
Type II	Midcortex	Form a boundary around and present MHC I, MHC II, and self-antigen molecules to thymocytes
Type III	Corticomedullary junction	Present MHC I, MHC II, and self-antigen molecules to thymocytes
Type IV	Corticomedullary junction	Isolate type III epithelial reticular cells from the medulla
Type V	Medulla	Form the cellular scaffolding of the medulla
Type VI	Medulla	Form Hassall's corpuscles; release the cytokine thymic stromal lymphopoietin responsible for clonal deletion

CLINICAL CONSIDERATIONS

Hodgkin's Disease

Hodgkin's disease is a neoplastic transformation of lymphocytes that is prevalent mostly in young males. Its clinical signs are asymptomatic initially because the swelling of the liver, spleen, and lymph nodes are not accompanied by pain. Other manifestations include the loss of weight, elevated temperature, diminished appetite, and generalized weakness. Histopathologic characteristics include the presence of Reed-Sternberg cells, easily recognizable by their large size, and the presence of two large, pale, oval nuclei in each cell.

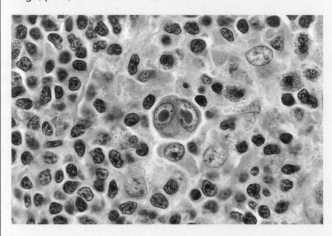

This photomicrograph is from the lymph node of a patient with Hodgkin's lymphoma displaying the characteristic binucleate Reed-Sternberg cell in the center of the field. Note the distinguishing eosinophilic nuclei that resemble nuclear inclusions. (Reprinted with permission from Mills SE, Carter D, et al., eds. Sternberg's Diagnostic Surgical Pathology, 5th ed. Philadelphia: Lippincott Williams & Wilkins, 2010, p. 701.)

Wiskott-Aldrich Syndrome

Wiskott-Aldrich syndrome is an immunodeficiency disorder occurring only in boys and is characterized by eczema (dermatitis), lowered platelet count, and lymphocytopenia (abnormally low levels of lymphocytes, both B- and T-cell populations). The immunosuppressed state of these children leads to recurring bacterial infections, hemorrhage, and death at an early age. Most children who survive the first decade of life are stricken with leukemia or lymphoma.

DiGeorge's Syndrome

DiGeorge's syndrome is the name of the congenital disorder when the thymus fails to develop and the patient is unable to produce T lymphocytes. These patients cannot mount a cellularly mediated immune response, and some of their humorally mediated responses are also disabled or curtailed. Most individuals with this syndrome die in early childhood as a result of uncontrollable infections.

Lymph Nodes During Infection

In a healthy patient with a normal amount of adipose tissue, the lymph nodes are small, soft structures that cannot be palpated easily. However, during an infection, the regional lymph nodes become enlarged and hard to the touch due to the large number of lymphocytes that are being formed within the node.

Burkitt's Lymphoma

Burkitt's lymphoma is a very rapidly growing non–Hodgkin's lymphoma that has its origins in B cells. It is relatively rare in the United States but is more common in Central Africa, where it affects young males infected with the Epstein-Barr virus. It is also prevalent in people afflicted with the HIV. The lymphoma cells proliferate quickly and spread to the lymph nodes and the small intestine. In more severe cases, the lymphoma cells can invade the central nervous system, bone marrow, and blood. If untreated, the disease is fatal, but treatment, especially in the early stages of the disease, has a very good prognosis.

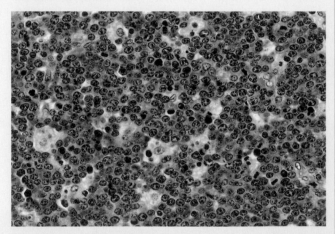

This photomicrograph is from a lymph node of a patient with Burkitt's lymphoma. Note the presence of several mitotic figures in the field. The image resembles a "starry sky" due to the presence of an abundance of tingible-body macrophages. (Reprinted with permission from Mills SE, Carter D, et al., eds. Sternberg's Diagnostic Surgical Pathology, 5th ed. Philadelphia: Lippincott Williams & Wilkins, 2010, p. 722.)

Peripheral T-cell Lymphoma in the Spleen

A relatively rare disease, peripheral T-cell lymphomas in the spleen are derived from T cells and T-cell precursors that proliferate and invade various organs, including the skin and the spleen. When the spleen is affected, the cells are large and aggressive with clear cytoplasms. They congregate in the vicinity of the periarterial lymphatic sheaths (PALSs). The prognosis of patients with peripheral T-cell lymphomas depends on whether or not the invading cells express the protein anaplastic lymphoma kinase (ALK). Patients whose cells express ALK respond to treatment much better than patients whose cells do not express this protein.

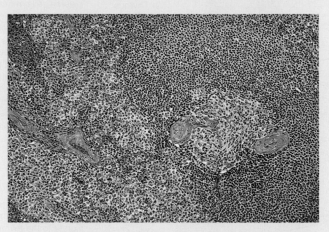

This photomicrograph is of the spleen of a patient with peripheral T-cell lymphoma. The large, clear cells surround the PALS and the B-cell–rich germinal center appears unaffected. (Reprinted with permission from Mills SE, Carter D, et al., eds. Sternberg's Diagnostic Surgical Pathology, 5th ed. Philadelphia: Lippincott Williams & Wilkins, 2010, p. 755 Fig. 18-17.)

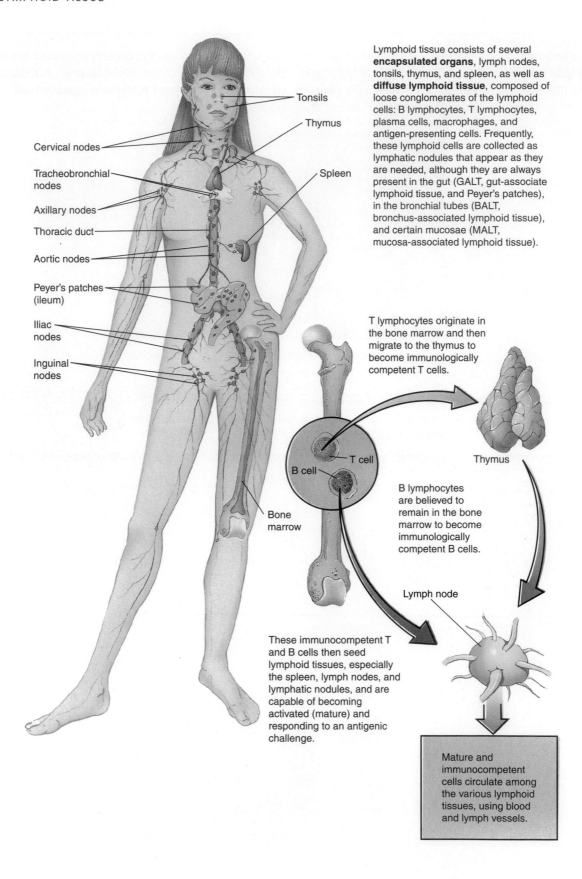

Tonsils

Thymus

Cervical nodes

Tracheobronchial nodes

Spleen

Axillary nodes

Thoracic duct

Aortic nodes

Peyer's patches (ileum)

Iliac nodes

Inguinal nodes

Bone marrow

T cell

B cell

Thymus

Lymph node

Lymphoid tissue consists of several **encapsulated organs**, lymph nodes, tonsils, thymus, and spleen, as well as **diffuse lymphoid tissue**, composed of loose conglomerates of the lymphoid cells: B lymphocytes, T lymphocytes, plasma cells, macrophages, and antigen-presenting cells. Frequently, these lymphoid cells are collected as lymphatic nodules that appear as they are needed, although they are always present in the gut (GALT, gut-associate lymphoid tissue, and Peyer's patches), in the bronchial tubes (BALT, bronchus-associated lymphoid tissue), and certain mucosae (MALT, mucosa-associated lymphoid tissue).

T lymphocytes originate in the bone marrow and then migrate to the thymus to become immunologically competent T cells.

B lymphocytes are believed to remain in the bone marrow to become immunologically competent B cells.

These immunocompetent T and B cells then seed lymphoid tissues, especially the spleen, lymph nodes, and lymphatic nodules, and are capable of becoming activated (mature) and responding to an antigenic challenge.

Mature and immunocompetent cells circulate among the various lymphoid tissues, using blood and lymph vessels.

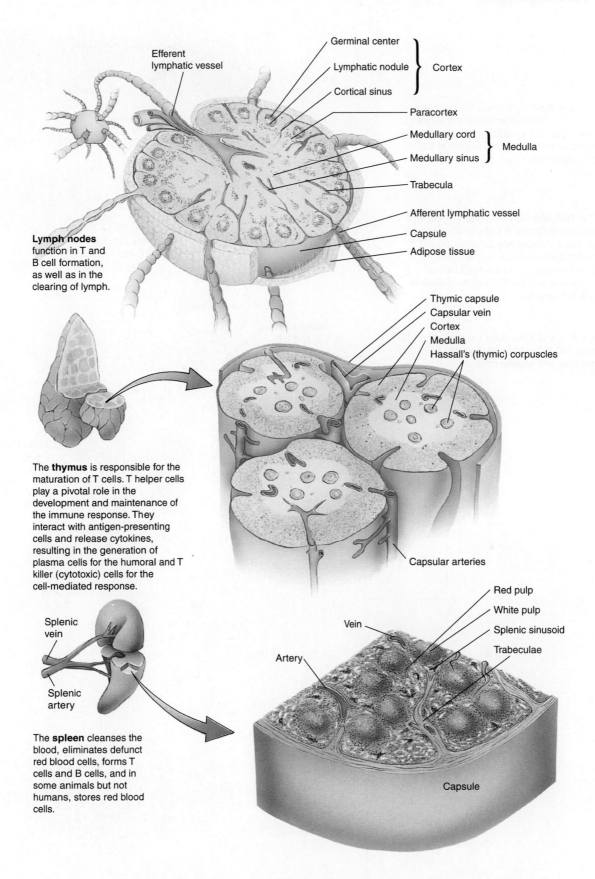

Efferent lymphatic vessel

Germinal center
Lymphatic nodule } Cortex
Cortical sinus

Paracortex

Medullary cord } Medulla
Medullary sinus

Trabecula

Afferent lymphatic vessel

Capsule

Adipose tissue

Lymph nodes function in T and B cell formation, as well as in the clearing of lymph.

Thymic capsule
Capsular vein
Cortex
Medulla
Hassall's (thymic) corpuscles

The **thymus** is responsible for the maturation of T cells. T helper cells play a pivotal role in the development and maintenance of the immune response. They interact with antigen-presenting cells and release cytokines, resulting in the generation of plasma cells for the humoral and T killer (cytotoxic) cells for the cell-mediated response.

Capsular arteries

Splenic vein

Splenic artery

The **spleen** cleanses the blood, eliminates defunct red blood cells, forms T cells and B cells, and in some animals but not humans, stores red blood cells.

Vein

Artery

Red pulp
White pulp
Splenic sinusoid
Trabeculae

Capsule

Antigen-dependent cross linking of the surface antibodies activates the B cell which places the epitope-MHC II complex on the external aspect of its plasmalemma.

The TCR and CD4 molecules of the T$_H$2 cell recognize the B cell's MHC II-epitope complex. Additionally, binding of the B cell's CD40 molecule to the T$_H$2 cell's CD40 receptor induces the B cell to proliferate and the T$_H$2 cell to release of IL4, IL5, and IL6.

IL4, IL5, and IL6 induce the activation of B cells and their differentiation into B memory and plasma cells.

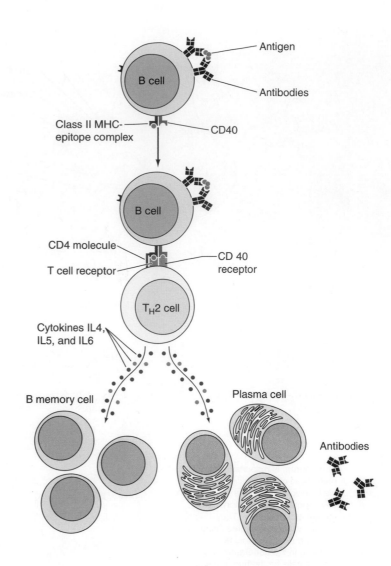

The T cell receptor (TCR) and CD4 molecule of the T$_H$1 cell binds to the epitope and the MHC II of the antigen-presenting cell (APC), respectively. The binding induces the APC to express B7 molecules on its plasmalemma, which then binds to the CD28 molecule of the T$_H$1 cell, inducing that cell to release IL2.

The same APC expresses the MHC I-epitope complex, which is recognized by the CD8 molecule and the TCR of the cytotoxic T lymphocyte (CTL). Additionally, the CD28 molecule of the CTL binds with the B7 molecule on the APC plasmalemma. These interactions induce the expression of IL2 receptors on the CTL plasma membrane. Binding of IL2 (released by the T$_H$1 cell) to the IL2 receptors of the CTL induces that cell to proliferate.

The plasmalemma of virally transformed cells expresses MHC I-epitope complex, which is recognized by the CD8 molecule and TCR of the newly formed cytotoxic T lymphocytes. The binding of the CTL induces these cells to secrete perforins and fragmentins. The former assemble to form pores in the plasma membrane of the transformed cell, and framentin drives the transformed cell into apoptosis.

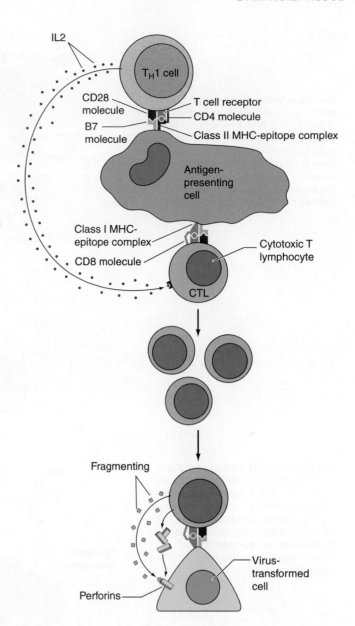

IL2

T$_H$1 cell

CD28 molecule

B7 molecule

T cell receptor

CD4 molecule

Class II MHC-epitope complex

Antigen-presenting cell

Class I MHC-epitope complex

CD8 molecule

Cytotoxic T lymphocyte

CTL

Fragmenting

Perforins

Virus-transformed cell

Bacteria-infected macrophages bear MHC II-epitope complexes on their plasmalemma that, if recognized by the CD4 molecule and TCR of T$_H$1 cells, activates these T cells, causing them to release IL2 and to express IL2 receptors on their plasma membrane. Binding of IL2 to the IL2 receptors induces proliferation of the T$_H$1 cells.

The TCR and CD4 molecules of the newly formed T$_H$1 cells recognize and bind to the MHC II-epitope complexes of bacteria-infected macrophages. The binding causes activation of these T$_H$1 cells so that they release γ-interferon, a cytokine that encourages the macrophages to destroy their endocytosed bacteria.

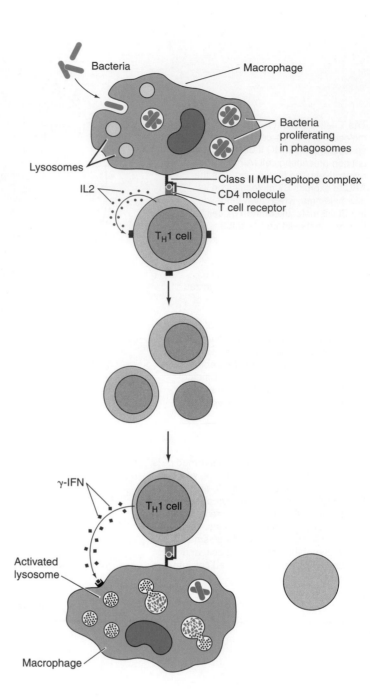

Bacteria

Macrophage

Bacteria proliferating in phagosomes

Lysosomes

Class II MHC-epitope complex

CD4 molecule

T cell receptor

IL2

T$_H$1 cell

γ-IFN

T$_H$1 cell

Activated lysosome

Macrophage

PLATE 9-1 • Lymphatic Infiltration, Lymphatic Nodule

FIGURE 1. Lymphatic infiltration. Monkey duodenum. Plastic section. ×540.

The **connective tissue** (CT) deep to moist epithelia is usually infiltrated by loosely aggregated **lymphocytes** (Ly) and **plasma cells** (PC), evident from their clockface nuclei. Observe that the simple columnar **epithelium** (E) contains not only the **nuclei** (N) of epithelial cells but also dark, dense nuclei of lymphocytes (*arrows*), some of which are in the process of migrating from the lamina propria (connective tissue) into the lumen of the duodenum. Note also the presence of a **lacteal** (La), a blindly ending, lymph-filled lymphatic channel unique to the small intestine. These vessels can be recognized by the absence of red blood cells, although nucleated white blood cells may frequently occupy their lumen.

FIGURE 3. Lymphatic nodule. Monkey. Plastic section. ×270.

This is a higher magnification of a lymphatic nodule from Peyer's patches in the monkey ileum. Note that the lighter staining **germinal center** (Gc) is surrounded by the **corona** (Co) of darker staining cells possessing only a limited amount of cytoplasm around a dense nucleus. These cells are small **lymphocytes** (Ly). Germinal centers form in response to an antigenic challenge and are composed of lymphoblasts and plasmablasts, whose nuclei stain much lighter than those of small lymphocytes. The *boxed area* is presented at a higher magnification in the following figure.

FIGURE 2. Lymphatic nodule. Monkey. Plastic section. ×132.

The gut-associated lymphatic nodule in this photomicrograph is part of a cluster of nodules known as **Peyer's patches** (PP) and is taken from the monkey ileum. The **lumen** (L) of the small intestine is lined by a simple columnar **epithelium** (E) with numerous **goblet cells** (GC). However, note that the epithelium is modified over the lymphoid tissue into a **follicle-associated epithelium** (FAE), whose cells are shorter, infiltrated by lymphocytes, and display no goblet cells. Observe that this particular lymphatic nodule presents no germinal center but is composed of several cell types, as recognized by nuclei of various sizes and densities. These are described in Figures 3 and 4. Although this lymphatic nodule is unencapsulated, the **connective tissue** (CT) between the **smooth muscle** (SM) and the lymphatic nodule is free of infiltrate.

FIGURE 4. Lymphatic nodule. Monkey. Plastic section. ×540.

This is a higher magnification of the *boxed area* of the previous figure. Observe the **small lymphocytes** (Ly) at the periphery of the **germinal center** (Gc). The activity of this center is evidenced by the presence of mitotic figures (*arrows*) as well as the **lymphoblasts** (LB) and **plasmablasts** (PB). The germinal center is the site of production of small lymphocytes that then migrate to the periphery of the lymphatic nodule to form the corona.

KEY

Co	corona	GC	goblet cell	N	nucleus
CT	connective tissue	L	lumen	PB	plasmablast
E	epithelium	La	lacteal	PC	plasma cell
FAE	follicle-associated epithelium	LB	lymphoblast	PP	Peyer's patch
Gc	germinal center	Ly	small lymphocyte	SM	smooth muscle

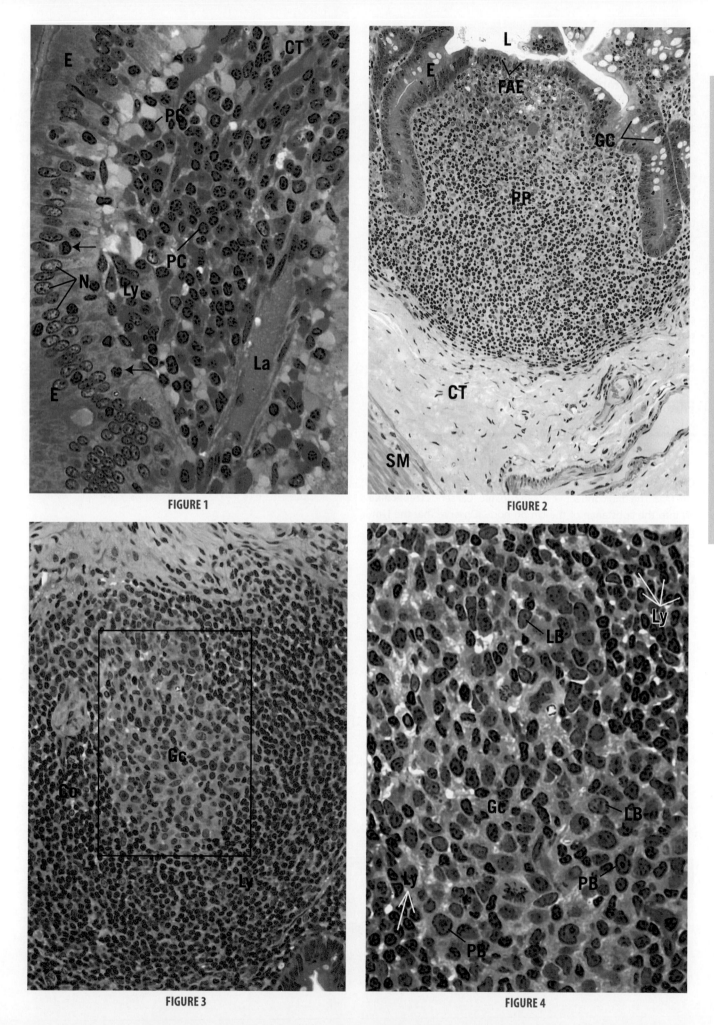

PLATE 9-1 · Lymphatic Infiltration, Lymphatic Nodule

FIGURE 1

FIGURE 2

FIGURE 3

FIGURE 4

PLATE 9-2 · Lymph Node

FIGURE 1. Lymph node. Paraffin section. ×14.

Lymph nodes are kidney-shaped structures possessing a convex and a concave (hilar) surface. They are invested by a connective tissue **capsule** (Ca) that sends **trabeculae** (T) into the substance of the node, thereby subdividing it into incomplete compartments. The compartmentalization is particularly prominent in the **cortex** (C), the peripheral aspect of the lymph node. The lighter staining central region is the **medulla** (M). The zone between the medulla and cortex is the **paracortex** (PC). Observe that the cortex displays numerous **lymphatic nodules** (LN), many with **germinal centers** (Gc). This is the region of B lymphocytes, whereas the paracortex is particularly rich in T lymphocytes. Note that the medulla is composed of **sinusoids** (S), **trabeculae** (T) of connective tissue conducting blood vessels, and **medullary cords** (MC). The medullary cords are composed of lymphocytes, macrophages, reticular cells, and plasma cells. Lymph enters the lymph node, and as it percolates through sinuses and sinusoids, foreign substances and nonself antigenic elements are removed from it by phagocytic activity of macrophages.

FIGURE 3. Lymph node. Monkey. Plastic section. ×132.

The cortex of the lymph node is composed of numerous lymphatic nodules, one of which is presented in this photomicrograph. Observe that the lymph node is usually surrounded by **adipose tissue** (AT). The thin connective tissue **capsule** (Ca) sends **trabeculae** (T) into the substance of the lymph node. Observe that the lymphatic nodule possesses a dark staining **corona** (Co), composed mainly of **small lymphocytes** (Ly) whose heterochromatic nuclei are responsible for their staining characteristics. The **germinal center** (Gc) displays numerous cells with lightly staining nuclei, belonging to dendritic reticular cells, plasmablasts, and lymphoblasts.

FIGURE 2. Lymph node. Monkey. Plastic section. ×270.

Afferent lymphatic vessels (AV) enter the lymph node at its convex surface. These vessels bear **valves** (V) that regulate the direction of flow. Lymph enters the **subcapsular sinus** (SS), which contains numerous **macrophages** (Ma), **lymphocytes** (Ly), and antigen-transporting cells. These sinuses are lined by **endothelial cells** (EC), which also cover the fine collagen fibers that frequently span the sinus to create a turbulence in lymph flow. Lymph from the subcapsular sinus enters the cortical sinus and then moves into the medullary sinusoids. It is here that lymphocytes also migrate into the sinusoids, leaving the lymph node via the efferent lymph vessels eventually to enter the general circulation.

FIGURE 4. Lymph node. Human. Silver stain. Paraffin section. ×132.

The hilum of the human lymph node displays the collagenous connective tissue **capsule** (Ca), from which numerous **trabeculae** (T) enter into the substance of the lymph node. Observe that the region of the hilum is devoid of lymphatic nodules but is particularly rich in **medullary cords** (MC). Note that the basic framework of these medullary cords, as well as of the lymph node, is composed of thin reticular fibers (*arrows*), which are connected to the collagen fiber bundles of the trabeculae and capsule.

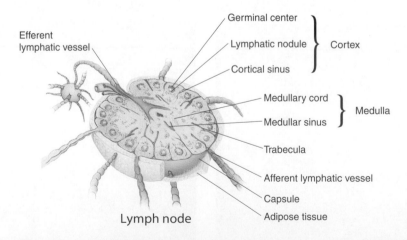

Lymph node

KEY							
AT	adipose tissue	**Gc**	germinal center	**PC**	paracortex
AV	afferent lymphatic vessel	**LN**	lymphatic nodule	**S**	sinusoid
C	cortex	**Ly**	small lymphocyte	**SS**	subcapsular sinus
Ca	capsule	**M**	medulla	**T**	trabeculae
Co	corona	**Ma**	macrophage	**V**	valve
EC	endothelial cell	**MC**	medullary cord		

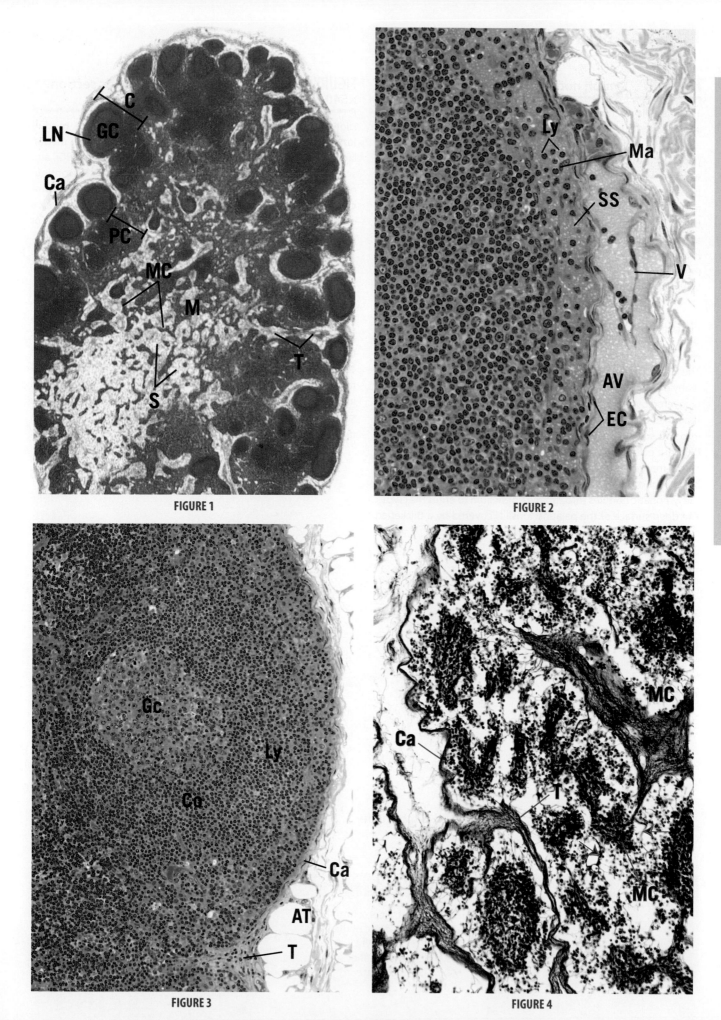

PLATE 9-2 · Lymph Node

FIGURE 1

FIGURE 2

FIGURE 3

FIGURE 4

PLATE 9-3 · Lymph Node, Tonsils

FIGURE 1.   Lymph node. Paraffin section. ×132.

The medulla of the lymph node is rich in endothelially lined **sinusoids** (S), which receive lymph from the cortical sinuses. Surrounding the sinusoids are many **medullary cords** (MC), packed with macrophages, small lymphocytes, and plasma cells, whose nuclei (*arrows*) stain intensely. Both T and B lymphocytes populate the medullary cords, since they are in the process of migrating from the paracortex and cortex, respectively. Some of these lymphocytes will leave the lymph node using the sinusoids and efferent lymphatic vessels at the hilum. The medulla also displays connective tissue **trabeculae** (T), connective tissue elements that are conduits for **blood vessels** (BV), which enter and leave the lymph node at the hilum.

FIGURE 3.   Palatine tonsil. Human. Paraffin section. ×14.

The palatine tonsil is an aggregate of **lymphatic nodules** (LN), many of which possess **germinal centers** (Gc). The palatine tonsil is covered by a stratified squamous nonkeratinized **epithelium** (E) that lines the deep **primary crypts** (PCr) that invaginate deeply into the substance of the tonsil. Frequently, **secondary crypts** (SCr) are evident, also lined by the same type of epithelium. The crypts frequently contain debris (*arrow*) that consists of decomposing food particles as well as lymphocytes that migrate from the lymphatic nodules through the epithelium to enter the crypts. The deep surface of the palatine tonsil is covered by a thickened connective tissue **capsule** (Ca).

FIGURE 2.   Lymph node. Monkey. Plastic section. ×540.

High magnification of a **sinusoid** (S) and surrounding **medullary cords** (MC) of a lymph node medulla. Note that the medullary cords are populated by macrophages, **plasma cells** (PC), and small **lymphocytes** (Ly). The sinusoids are lined by a discontinuous **endothelium** (EC). The lumen contains lymph, small **lymphocytes** (Ly), and **macrophages** (Ma). The vacuolated appearance of these macrophages is indicative of their active phagocytosis of particulate matter.

FIGURE 4.   Pharyngeal tonsil. Human. Paraffin section. ×132.

The pharyngeal tonsil, located in the nasopharynx, is a loose aggregate of lymphatic nodules, often displaying **germinal centers** (Gc). The **epithelial lining** (E) is pseudostratified ciliated columnar with occasional patches of stratified squamous nonkeratinized epithelium (*asterisk*). The lymphatic nodules are located in a loose, collagenous **connective tissue** (CT) that is infiltrated by small **lymphocytes** (Ly). Note that lymphocytes migrate through the epithelium (*arrows*) to gain access to the nasopharynx.

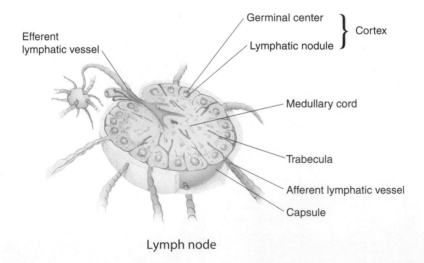

Lymph node

KEY							
BV	blood vessel	Gc	germinal center	PC	plasma cell
Ca	capsule	LN	lymphatic nodule	PCr	primary crypt
CT	connective tissue	Ly	lymphocyte	S	sinusoid
E	epithelium	Ma	macrophage	T	trabeculae
EC	endothelial cell	MC	medullary cord	SCr	secondary crypt

PLATE 9-3 • Lymph Node, Tonsils

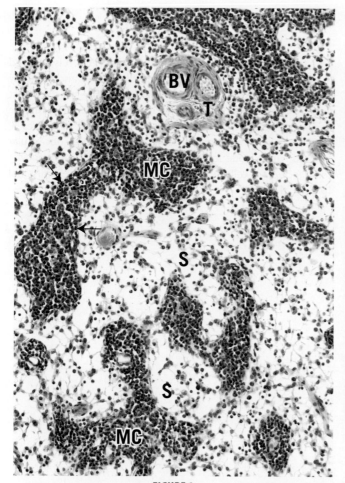

FIGURE 1

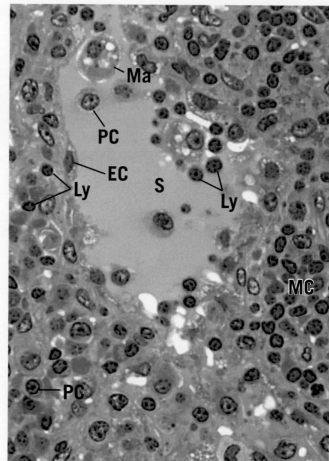

FIGURE 2

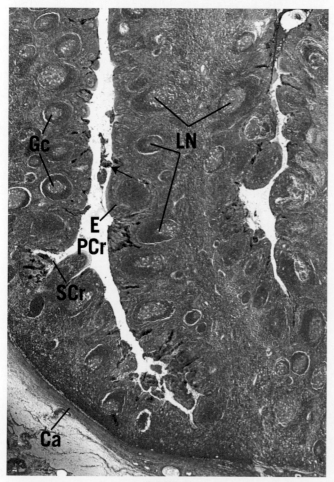

FIGURE 3

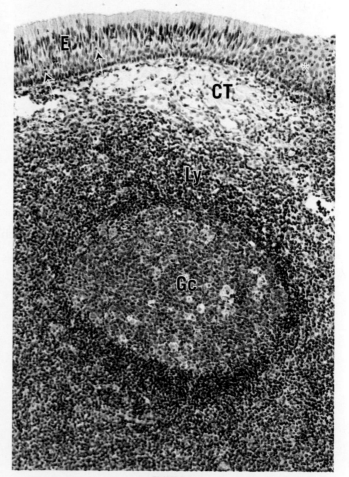

FIGURE 4

PLATE 9-4 · Lymph Node, Electron Microscopy

FIGURE 1.   Popliteal lymph node. Mouse. Electron microscopy. ×8,608.

Electron micrograph of a mouse lymph node. Immediately deep to the **capsule** (Ca) lies the subcapsular sinus occupied by three **lymphocytes**, one of which is labeled (L), as well as the **process** (P) of an antigen-transporting (antigen-presenting) cell, whose cell body (*arrowheads*) and nucleus are in the cortex, deep to the sinus. The process enters the lumen of the subcapsular sinus via a pore (*arrows*) in the epithelial lining of its floor (FL). It is believed that antigen-transporting cells are nonphagocytic and that they trap antigens at the site of antigenic invasion and transport them to lymphatic nodules of lymph nodes, where they mature to become dendritic reticular cells. (From Szakal A, Homes K, Tew J. Transport of immune complexes from the subcapsular sinus to lymph node follicles on the surface of nonphagocytic cells, including cells with dendritic morphology. J Immunol 1983;131:1714–1717.)

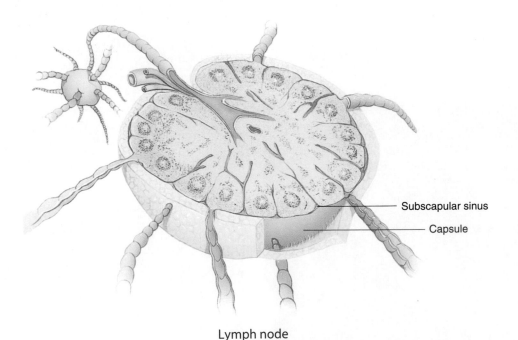

Subscapular sinus

Capsule

Lymph node

PLATE 9-4 • Lymph Node, Electron Microscopy

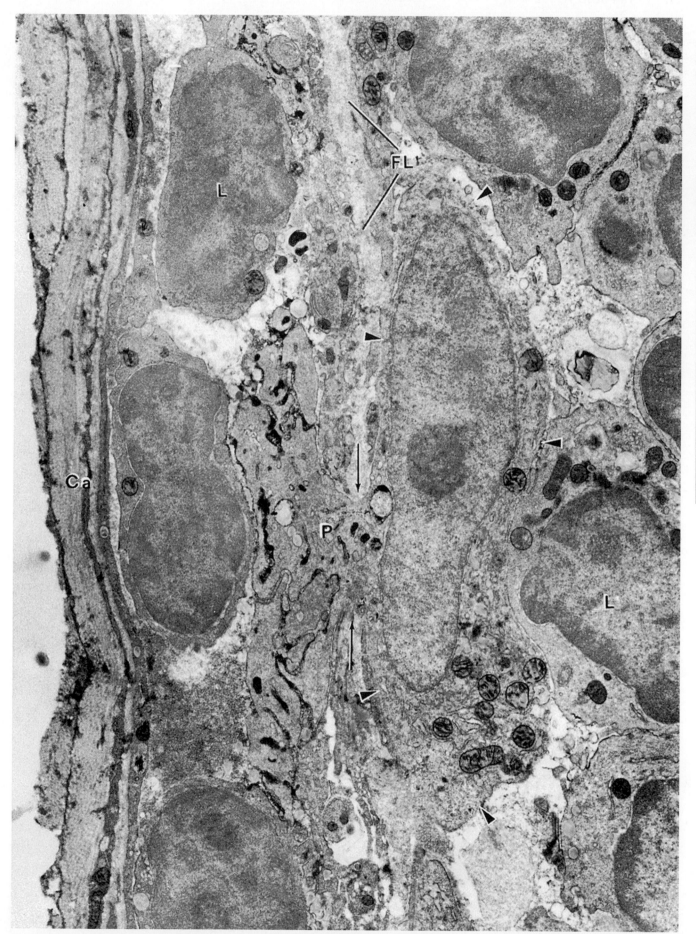

FIGURE 1

PLATE 9-5 · Thymus

FIGURE 1. Thymus. Human infant. Paraffin section. ×14.

The thymus of a prepubescent individual is a well-developed organ that displays its many characteristics to advantage. This photomicrograph presents a part of one lobe. It is invested by a thin connective tissue **capsule** (Ca) that incompletely subdivides the thymus into **lobules** (Lo) by connective tissue **septa** (Se). Each lobule possesses a darker staining peripheral **cortex** (C) and a lighter staining **medulla** (M). The medulla of one lobule, however, is continuous with that of other lobules. The connective tissue capsule and septa convey blood vessels into the medulla of the thymus. The thymus begins to involute in the postpubescent individual, and the connective tissue septa become infiltrated with adipocytes.

FIGURE 3. Thymus. Monkey. Plastic section. ×270.

The center of this photomicrograph is occupied by the **medulla** (M) of the thymus, presenting a large **thymic (Hassall's) corpuscle** (TC), composed of concentrically arranged **epithelial reticular cells** (ERC). The function, if any, of this structure is not known. The thymic medulla houses numerous **blood vessels** (BV), macrophages, **lymphocytes** (Ly), and occasional plasma cells.

FIGURE 2. Thymus. Monkey. Plastic section. ×132.

The lobule of the thymus presented in this photomicrograph appears to be completely surrounded by connective tissue **septa** (Se); three-dimensional reconstruction would reveal this lobule to be continuous with surrounding **lobules** (Lo). Observe the numerous **blood vessels** (BV) in the septa as well as the darker staining **cortex** (C) and the lighter staining **medulla** (M). The characteristic light patches of the cortex correspond to the high density of epithelial reticular cells and macrophages (*arrows*). The darker staining structures are nuclei of the T-lymphocyte series. The medulla contains the characteristic **thymic corpuscles** (TC) as well as blood vessels, macrophages, and epithelial reticular cells.

FIGURE 4. Thymus. Monkey. Plastic section. ×540.

The cortex of the thymus is bounded externally by collagenous connective tissue **septa** (Se). The substance of the cortex is separated from the septa by a zone of **epithelial reticular cells** (ERC), recognizable by their pale nuclei. Additional ERC form a cellular reticulum; in whose interstices, **lymphocytes** (Ly) develop into mature T lymphocytes. Numerous **macrophages** (Ma) are also evident in the cortex. These cells phagocytose lymphocytes destroyed in the thymus.

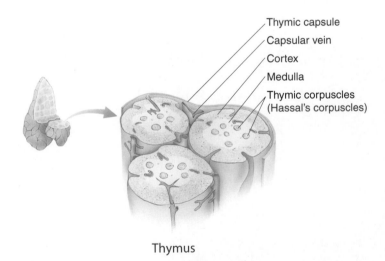

Thymic capsule
Capsular vein
Cortex
Medulla
Thymic corpuscles
(Hassall's corpuscles)

Thymus

KEY					
BV	blood vessel	Lo	lobule	Ma	macrophage
C	cortex	Ly	lymphocyte	Se	septum
Ca	capsule	M	medulla	TC	thymic corpuscle
ERC	epithelial reticular cell				

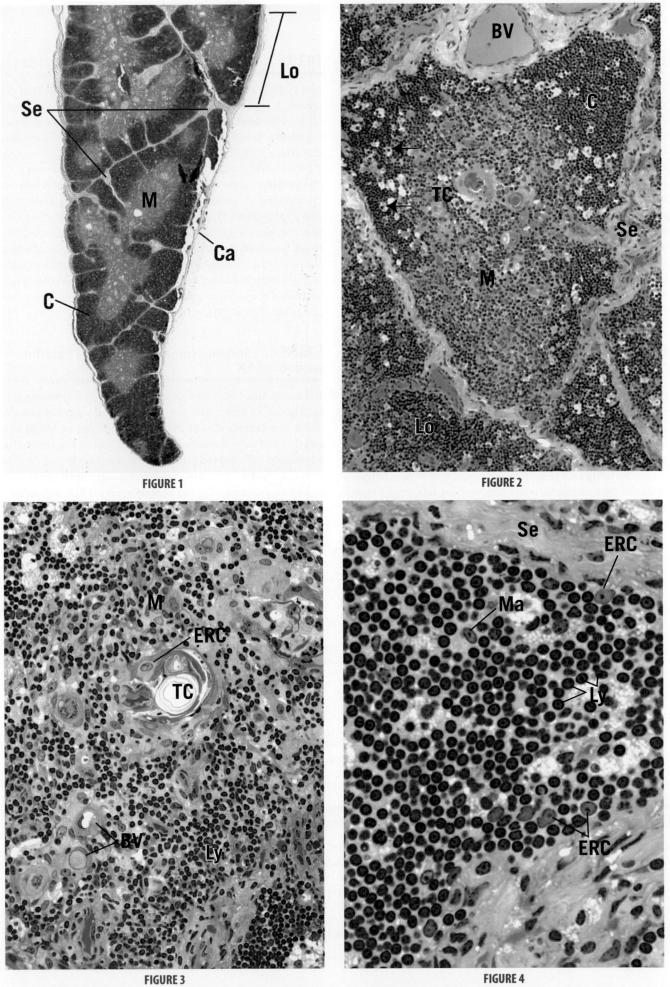

PLATE 9-5 · Thymus

FIGURE 1

FIGURE 2

FIGURE 3

FIGURE 4

PLATE 9-6 · Spleen

FIGURE 1. Spleen. Human. Paraffin section. ×132.

The spleen, the largest lymphoid organ, possesses a thick collagenous connective tissue **capsule** (Ca). Since it lies within the abdominal cavity, it is surrounded by a simple squamous **epithelium** (E). Connective tissue **septa** (SE), derived from the capsule, penetrate the substance of the spleen, conveying **blood vessels** (BV) into the interior of the organ. Histologically, the spleen is composed of **white pulp** (WP) and **red pulp** (RP). White pulp is arranged as a cylindrical, multilayered sheath of **lymphocytes** (Ly) surrounding a blood vessel known as the **central artery** (CA). The red pulp consists of **sinusoids** (S) meandering through a cellular tissue known as **pulp cords** (PC). The white pulp of the spleen is found in two different arrangements. The one represented in this photomicrograph is known as a **periarterial lymphatic sheath** (PALS), composed mostly of T lymphocytes. The zone of lymphocytes at the junction of the PALS and the red pulp is known as the **marginal zone** (MZ).

FIGURE 2. Spleen. Monkey. Plastic section. ×132.

Lying within the **periarterial lymphatic sheaths** (PALS) of the spleen, a second arrangement of white pulp may be noted, namely, **lymphatic nodules** (LN) bearing a **germinal center** (Gc). Lymphatic nodules frequently occur at the branching of the **central artery** (CA). Nodules are populated mostly by B lymphocytes (*arrows*), which account for the dark staining of the **corona** (CO). The germinal center is the site of active production of B lymphocytes during an antigenic challenge. The **marginal zone** (MZ), also present around lymphatic nodules, is the region where lymphocytes leave the small capillaries and first enter the connective tissue spaces of the spleen. It is from here that T lymphocytes migrate to the PALSs, whereas B lymphocytes seek out lymphatic nodules. Both the marginal zone and the white pulp are populated with numerous macrophages and antigen-presenting cells (*arrowheads*), in addition to lymphocytes.

FIGURE 3. Spleen. Monkey. Plastic section. ×540.

The red pulp of the spleen, presented in this photomicrograph, is composed of **splenic sinusoids** (S) and **pulp cords** (PC). The splenic sinusoids are lined by a discontinuous type of epithelium, surrounded by an unusual arrangement of **basement membrane** (BM) that encircles the sinusoids in a discontinuous fashion. Sinusoids contain numerous **blood cells** (BC). **Nuclei** (N) of the sinusoidal lining cells bulge into the lumen. The regions between sinusoids are occupied by pulp cords, rich in macrophages, reticular cells, and plasma cells. The vascular supply of the red pulp is derived from penicillar arteries, which give rise to **arterioles** (AR), whose **endothelial cells** (EC) and **smooth muscle** (SM) cells are evident in the center of this field.

FIGURE 4. Spleen. Human. Silver stain. Paraffin section. ×132.

The connective tissue framework of the spleen is demonstrated by the use of silver stain, which precipitates around reticular fibers. The **capsule** (Ca) of the spleen is pierced by **blood vessels** (BV) that enter the substance of the organ via trabeculae. The **white pulp** (WP) and **red pulp** (RP) are clearly evident. In fact, the lymphatic nodule presents a well-defined **germinal center** (Gc) as well as a **corona** (CO). The **central artery** (CA) is also evident in this preparation. **Reticular fibers** (RF), which form an extensive network throughout the substance of the spleen, are attached to the capsule and to the trabeculae.

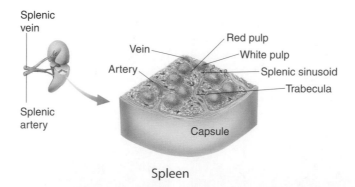

Spleen

KEY

AR	arteriole	EC	endothelial cell	PC	pulp cord
BC	blood cell	Gc	germinal center	RF	reticular fiber
BM	basement membrane	LN	lymphatic nodule	RP	red pulp
BV	blood vessel	Ly	lymphocyte	S	sinusoid
Ca	capsule	MZ	marginal zone	SE	septum
CA	central artery	N	nucleus	SM	smooth muscle
CO	corona	PALS	periarterial lymphatic	T	trabeculae
E	epithelium		sheath	WP	white pulp

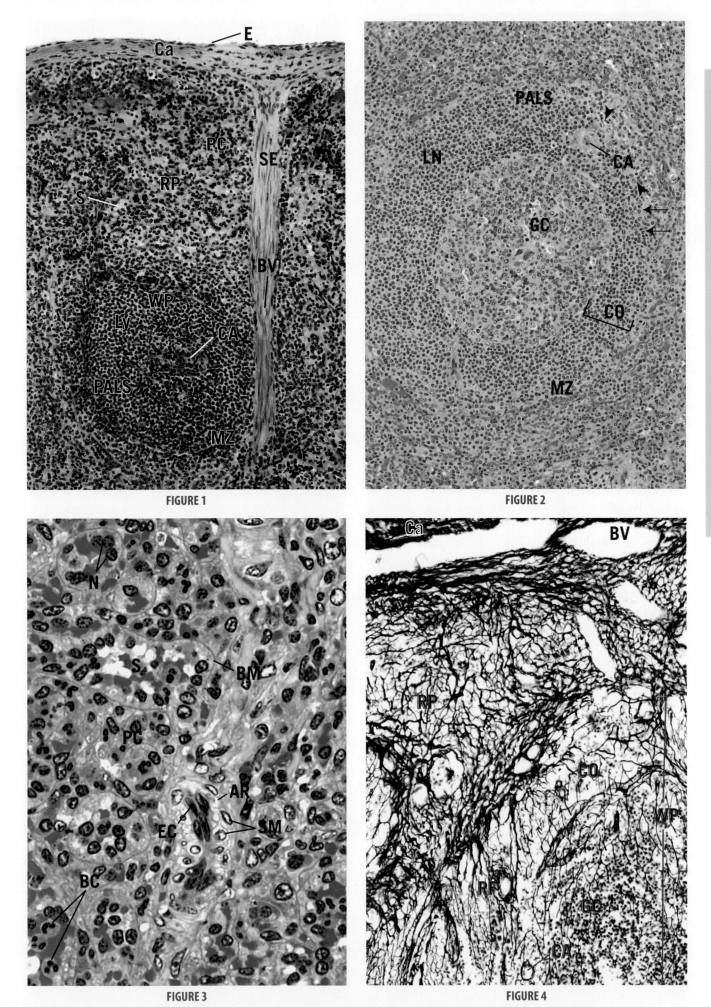

PLATE 9-6 • Spleen

FIGURE 1

FIGURE 2

FIGURE 3

FIGURE 4

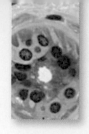

Chapter Summary

Lymphoid tissue consists of **diffuse** and **dense lymphoid tissue**. The principal cell of lymphoid tissue is the **lymphocyte**, of which there are three categories: **null cells**, **B lymphocytes** and **T lymphocytes**. Additionally, **macrophages**, **reticular cells**, **plasma cells**, **dendritic cells**, and **antigen-presenting cells** perform important functions in lymphatic tissue.

I. LYMPH NODE

A. Capsule

The **capsule**, usually surrounded by **adipose tissue**, is composed of dense irregular **collagenous connective tissue** containing some **elastic fibers** and **smooth muscle**. **Afferent lymphatic vessels** enter the convex aspect; **efferent lymphatics** and **blood vessels** pierce the **hilum**.

B. Cortex

The **cortex** of a lymph node is characterized by the presence of **lymphatic nodules**, which have a dark **corona**, predominantly occupied by **B lymphocytes**, and lighter staining **germinal centers**, housing activated **B lymphoblasts**, **macrophages**, and **dendritic reticular cells**. Connective tissue **trabeculae** subdivide the cortex into incomplete compartments. **Subcapsular** and **cortical sinuses** possess **lymphocytes**, **reticular cells**, and **macrophages**.

C. Paracortex

The **paracortex** is the zone between the cortex and medulla, composed of **T lymphocytes**. **Postcapillary venules**, with their characteristic **cuboidal endothelium**, are present.

D. Medulla

The **medulla** displays connective tissue **trabeculae**, **medullary cords** (composed of macrophages, plasma cells, and lymphocytes), and **medullary sinusoids** lined by discontinuous **endothelial cells**. **Lymphocytes**, **plasma cells**, and **macrophages** are the common cell types in the lumina of sinusoids. The region of the **hilum** is distinguished by the thickened capsule and lack of lymphatic nodules.

E. Reticular Fibers

With the use of special stains, such as silver stains, an extensive network of **reticular fibers** may be demonstrated to constitute the framework of lymph nodes.

II. TONSILS

A. Palatine Tonsils

1. Epithelium

Covered by **stratified squamous nonkeratinized epithelium** that extends into the **tonsillar crypts**. Lymphocytes may migrate through the epithelium.

2. Lymphatic Nodules

Surround **crypts** and frequently display **germinal centers**.

3. Capsule

Dense, irregular collagenous connective tissue **capsule** separates the tonsil from the underlying pharyngeal wall musculature. **Septa**, derived from the capsule, extend into the tonsil.

4. Glands

Not present.

B. Pharyngeal Tonsils

1. Epithelium

For the most part, **pseudostratified ciliated columnar epithelium** (infiltrated by lymphocytes) covers the free surface as well as the folds that resemble crypts.

2. Lymphatic Nodules

Most **lymphatic nodules** possess **germinal centers**.

3. Capsule

The thin **capsule**, situated deep to the tonsil, provides **septa** for the tonsil.

4. Glands

Ducts of the **seromucous glands**, beneath the capsule, pierce the tonsil to open onto the epithelially covered surface.

C. Lingual Tonsils

1. Epithelium

Stratified squamous nonkeratinized epithelium covers the tonsil and extends into the shallow **crypts**.

2. Lymphatic Nodules

Most **lymphatic nodules** present **germinal centers**.

3. Capsule

The **capsule** is thin and ill defined.

4. Glands

Seromucous glands open into the base of **crypts**.

III. SPLEEN

A. Capsule

The **capsule**, composed predominantly of **dense irregular collagenous connective tissue**, is significantly thickened at the **hilum**. The capsule also possesses a small amount of **elastic fibers** and some **smooth muscle cells**. It is covered by **mesothelium** (simple squamous epithelium) but is not surrounded by adipose tissue. **Trabeculae**, bearing blood vessels, extend from the capsule into the substance of the spleen.

B. White Pulp

White pulp is composed of **periarterial lymphatic sheaths** and **lymphatic nodules** with germinal centers. Both periarterial lymphatic sheaths (predominantly **T lymphocytes**) and lymphatic nodules (predominantly **B lymphocytes**) surround the acentrically located **central artery**.

C. Marginal Zone

A looser accumulation of **lymphocytes, macrophages,** and **plasma cells** are located between white and red pulps. The vascular supply of this zone is provided by **capillary loops** derived from the **central artery**.

D. Red Pulp

Red pulp is composed of **pulp cords** and **sinusoids**. Pulp cords are composed of delicate reticular fibers, stellate-shaped **reticular cells, plasma cells, macrophages,** and **cells of the circulating blood**. Sinusoids are lined by elongated discontinuous **endothelial cells** surrounded by thickened hoop-like **basement membrane** in association with **reticular fibers**. The various regions of **penicilli** are evident in the red pulp. These are **pulp arterioles, sheathed arterioles,** and **terminal arterial capillaries**. Convincing evidence to determine whether circulation in the red pulp is open or closed is not available, although, in humans, the open circulation is believed to be the most prevalent.

E. Reticular Fibers

With the use of special stains, an extensive network of **reticular fibers**, which constitute the framework of the spleen, can be demonstrated.

IV. THYMUS

A. Capsule

The thin **capsule** is composed of **dense irregular collagenous connective tissue** (with some elastic fibers). **Interlobular trabeculae** extending from the capsule incompletely subdivide the thymus into **lobules**.

B. Cortex

Typically, the **cortex** is devoid of lymphatic nodules or plasma cells. It is composed of lightly staining **epithelial reticular cells, macrophages,** and densely packed, darkly staining, small **T lymphocytes (thymocytes)** responsible for the dark appearance of the cortex. Epithelial reticular cells also surround **capillaries**, the only blood vessels present in the cortex.

C. Medulla

The lightly staining **medulla** is continuous from lobule to lobule. It is occupied by **plasma cells, lymphocytes, macrophages,** and **epithelial reticular cells**. Moreover, **thymic (Hassall's) corpuscles**, concentrically arranged epithelial reticular cells, are characteristic features of the thymic medulla.

D. Involution

The thymus begins to involute subsequent to puberty. The **cortex** becomes less dense because its population of lymphocytes and epithelial reticular cells is, to some extent, replaced by fat. In the medulla, **thymic corpuscles** increase in number and size.

E. Reticular Fibers and Sinusoids

The thymus possesses neither reticular fibers nor sinusoids.

10 ENDOCRINE SYSTEM

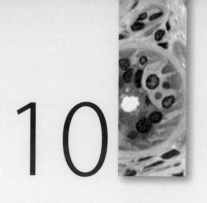

The endocrine system, in cooperation with the nervous system, orchestrates homeostasis by influencing, coordinating, and integrating the physiological functions of the body. The endocrine system consists of several glands, isolated groups of cells within certain organs, and individual cells scattered among parenchymal cells of the body. This chapter considers only that part of the endocrine system that is composed of glands. Islets of Langerhans, interstitial cells of Leydig, cells responsible for ovarian hormone production, and DNES (diffuse neuroendocrine) cells are treated in more appropriate chapters.

The **endocrine glands** to be discussed here are the

- pituitary,
- thyroid,
- parathyroid,
- suprarenal glands, and
- pineal body.

All of these glands produce **hormones** that they secrete into the connective tissue spaces. There are three types of hormones, depending on how far they act from their site of secretion:

- those that act on the cell, which releases them (**autocrine hormones**)
- those that act in the immediate vicinity of their secretion (**paracrine hormones**), and
- those that enter the vascular system and find their target cells at a distance from their site of origin (**endocrine hormones**).

This chapter details endocrine hormones (see Tables 10-1 and 10-2), whereas other chapters (nervous tissue, respiratory system, and digestive system) discuss autocrine and paracrine hormones.

Some hormones (e.g., **thyroid hormone**) have a generalized effect, in that most cells are affected by them; other hormones (e.g., **aldosterone**) affect only certain cells.

- **Receptors** located either on the cell membrane or within the cell are specific for a particular hormone.
- The binding of a hormone initiates a sequence of reactions that results in a particular response.
- Because of the specificity of the reaction, only a minute quantity of the hormone is required.
- Some hormones elicit and others inhibit a particular response.

Hormones, based on their chemical nature, are of three types, nonsteroid, steroid based, and amino acid derivatives. **Nonsteroid-based hormones (proteins and polypeptides)** are small peptides (antidiuretic hormone [ADH] and oxytocin) or small proteins (glucagon, insulin, anterior pituitary proteins, and parathormone). **Amino acid derivatives** include insulin, norepinephrine, and thyroid hormone. **Steroid-based hormones and those of fatty acid derivates** are cholesterol derivatives (aldosterone, cortisol, estrogen, progesterone, and testosterone).

Nonsteroid-Based Hormones and Amino Acid Derivatives

Nonsteroid-based endocrine hormones and amino acid derivatives bind to **receptors** (some are G protein linked, and some are catalytic) located on the target cell membrane, activate them, and thus initiate a sequence of intracellular reactions. These may act by

- altering the state of an **ion channel** (opening or closing) or
- by activating (or inhibiting) an **enzyme** or group of enzymes associated with the cytoplasmic aspect of the cell membrane.

Opening or closing an ion channel will permit the particular ion to traverse or inhibit the particular ion from traversing the cell membrane, thus altering the membrane potential. Neurotransmitters and **catecholamines** act on ion channels.

- The binding of most hormones to their receptor will have only a single effect, which is the activation of **adenylate cyclase**.
- This enzyme functions in the transformation of ATP to **cAMP (cyclic adenosine monophosphate)**, the major **second messenger** of the cell. cAMP then activates a specific sequence of enzymes that are necessary to accomplish the desired result.
- There are a few hormones that activate a similar compound, **cyclic guanosine monophosphate (cGMP)**, which functions in a comparable fashion.

Some hormones facilitate the opening of **calcium channels**;

- calcium enters the cell, and three or four calcium ions bind to the protein **calmodulin**, altering its conformation.
- The altered calmodulin is a **second messenger** that activates a sequence of enzymes, causing a specific response.

Thyroid hormones are unusual among the amino acid derivative and nonsteroid-based hormones, in that they directly enter the nucleus, where they bind with **receptor molecules**. The hormone-receptor complexes control the activities of **operators** and/or **promoters**, resulting in mRNA transcription. The newly formed mRNAs enter the cytoplasm, where they are translated into proteins that elevate the cell's metabolic activity.

Steroid-Based Hormones

Steroid-based endocrine hormones diffuse into the target cell through the plasma membrane and, once inside the cell, bind to a **receptor molecule**.

TABLE 10-1 • Pituitary Gland Hormones

	Pituitary Gland			
Region	Hormone Produced	Releasing Hormone	Inhibiting Hormone	Principal Functions
Pars distalis	Somatotropin (growth hormone [GH])	SRH	Somatostatin	Generally increases cellular metabolism; stimulates liver to release insulin-like growth factors I and II resulting in cartilage proliferation and long bone growth
	Prolactin	PRH	PIF	Stimulates mammary gland development during pregnancy and production of milk after parturition
	Adrenocorticotropic hormone (ACTH, corticotropin)	CRH		Induces the zona fasciculata to synthesize and secrete cortisol and corticosterone and cells of the zona reticularis to synthesize and release androgens
	Follicle-stimulating hormone (FSH)	LHRH	Inhibin (in males)	Promotes secondary and graafian follicle development as well as estrogen secretion in females; stimulates Sertoli cells to produce androgen binding protein in males
	Luteinizing hormone (LH)	LHRH		Promotes ovulation, corpus luteum formation, secretion of estrogen and progesterone in females
	Interstitial cell-stimulating hormone (ICSH)			Promotes secretion of testosterone by Leydig cells in men
	Thyroid-stimulating hormone (TSH; thyrotropin)	TRH		Stimulates secretion and release of triiodothyronine and thyroxine by thyroid follicular cells
Pars nervosa	Oxytocin			Stimulates uterine smooth muscle contraction during parturition. Stimulates contractions of mammary gland myoepithelial cells during suckling
	Vasopressin (antidiuretic hormone; ADH)			Elevates blood pressure by inducing vascular smooth muscle contraction, causes water resorption in collecting tubules of the kidney

- The receptor molecule-hormone complex enters the nucleus, seeks out a specific region of the DNA molecule, and initiates the synthesis of mRNA.
- The newly formed mRNA codes for the formation of specific enzymes that will accomplish the desired result.

The presence of most hormones also elicits a vascularly mediated negative feedback response, in that subsequent to a desired response, the further production and/or release of that particular hormone is inhibited.

PITUITARY GLAND

The **pituitary gland** (hypophysis) is composed of several regions, namely, pars anterior (pars distalis), pars tuberalis, infundibular stalk, pars intermedia, and pars nervosa (the last two are known as the pars posterior) (see Table 10-1 and Graphic 10-1).

Since the pituitary gland develops from two separate embryonic origins, the epithelium of the pharyngeal roof and the floor of the diencephalon, it is frequently discussed as being subdivided into two parts:

- the **adenohypophysis** (**pars anterior, pars tuberalis,** and **pars intermedia**) and the
- **neurohypophysis** (**pars nervosa** and **infundibular stalk**).
  - The pars nervosa is continuous with the **median eminence of the hypothalamus** via the thin neural stalk (**infundibular stalk**).

The pituitary gland receives its **blood supply** from the right and left **superior hypophyseal arteries**, serving the median eminence, pars tuberalis, and the infundibulum, and from the right and left **inferior hypophyseal arteries**, which serve the pars nervosa.

Hypophyseal Portal System: The two superior hypophyseal arteries give rise to the

- **primary capillary plexus** located in the region of the median eminence.
- **Hypophyseal portal veins** drain the primary capillary plexus and deliver the blood into the **secondary capillary plexus**, located in the pars distalis.
- Both capillary plexuses are composed of **fenestrated capillaries**.

Pars Anterior

The **pars anterior** is composed of numerous parenchymal cells arranged in thick cords, with large capillaries known as sinusoids, richly vascularizing the intervening regions. The parenchymal cells are classified into two main categories: those whose granules readily take up stain, chromophils, and those cells that do not possess a strong affinity for stains, chromophobes.

- **Chromophils** are of two types: **acidophils** and **basophils**. Although considerable controversy surrounds the classification of these cells vis-à-vis their function, it is probable that at least six of the seven hormones manufactured by the pars anterior are made by separate cells (see Table 10-1).
  - Hormones that modulate the secretory functions of the pituitary-dependent endocrine glands are **somatotropin, thyrotropin (TSH), follicle-stimulating hormone (FSH), luteinizing hormone (LH), interstitial cell stimulating hormone (ICSH), prolactin, adrenocorticotropin hormone (ACTH),** and **melanocyte-stimulating hormone (MSH)**.
  - It is believed that two types of acidophils produce somatotropin and prolactin, whereas various populations of basophils produce the remaining five hormones.
- **Chromophobes**, however, probably do not produce hormones. They are believed to be acidophils and basophils that have released their granules.

Control of Anterior Pituitary Hormone Release:

- The axons of parvicellular, hypophyseotropic neurons whose soma are located in the paraventricular and arcuate nuclei of the hypothalamus terminate at the primary capillary bed.
  - These axons store releasing hormones (somatotropin-releasing hormone, prolactin-releasing hormone, corticotropin-releasing hormone, thyrotropin-releasing hormone, and gonadotropin-releasing hormone) and inhibitory hormones (prolactin-inhibiting hormone, inhibin, and somatostatin).
  - The hormones are released by these axons into the primary capillary plexus and are conveyed to the secondary capillary plexus by the hypophyseal portal veins.
  - The hormones then activate (or inhibit) chromophils of the adenohypophysis, causing them to release or prevent them from releasing their hormones.
- An additional control is the mechanism of negative feedback, so that the presence of specific plasma levels of the pituitary hormones prevents the chromophils from releasing additional quantities of their hormones.

Pars Intermedia

The **pars intermedia** is not well developed. It is believed that the cell population of this region may have migrated into the pars anterior to produce **melanocyte-stimulating hormone (MSH)** and **adrenocorticotropin**. It is quite probable that a single **basophil** can produce both of these hormones.

Pars Nervosa and Infundibular Stalk

- The **pars nervosa** does not present a very organized appearance. It is composed of **pituicytes**, cells believed to be neuroglial in nature that may fulfill a supporting function for the numerous **unmyelinated axons** of the pars nervosa.

- These axons, whose cell bodies are located in the **supraoptic** and **paraventricular nuclei** of the hypothalamus, enter the pars nervosa via the **hypothalamo-hypophyseal tract**.

- Their axons possess expanded axon terminals, referred to as **Herring bodies**, within the pars nervosa.
  - Herring bodies contain **oxytocin** and **antidiuretic hormone (ADH, vasopressin)**, two neurosecretory hormones that are stored in the pars nervosa but are manufactured in the cell bodies in the **hypothalamus**.
  - The release of these neurosecretory hormones (**neurosecretion**) is mediated by nerve impulses and occurs at the interface between the axon terminals and the fenestrated capillaries.
  - When the axon is ready to release its secretory products, the pituicytes withdraw their processes and permit the secretory product a clear access to the capillaries.

Pars Tuberalis

The **pars tuberalis** is composed of numerous cuboidal cells whose function is not known.

THYROID GLAND

The **thyroid gland** consists of right and left lobes that are interconnected by a narrow isthmus across the thyroid cartilage and upper trachea (see Table 10-2 and Graphic 10-2). It is enveloped by a connective tissue capsule whose septa penetrate the substance of the gland, forming not only its supporting framework but also its conduit for its rich vascular supply.

The parenchymal cells of the gland are arranged in numerous follicles, composed of a **simple cuboidal epithelium** lining a central **colloid-filled lumen**. The colloid, secreted and resorbed by the **follicular cells**, is composed of thyroid hormone that is bound to a large protein, and the complex is known as **thyroglobulin**.

To synthesize thyroid hormone

- **Iodide** from the bloodstream is actively transported into follicular cells at their basal aspect via **iodide pumps**.

- Iodide is oxidized by **thyroid peroxidase** on the apical cell membrane and is bound to tyrosine residues of thyroglobulin molecules.

- Within the colloid, the iodinated tyrosine residues become rearranged to form **triiodothyronine (T_3)** and **thyroxine (T_4)**.

To release thyroid hormone

- The binding of **thyroid-stimulating hormone (TSH)** released by the pituitary, to receptors on the basal aspect of their plasmalemma induces follicular cells to become tall cuboidal cells.

- They form **pseudopods** on their apical cell membrane that engulf and endocytose colloid.

- The colloid-filled vesicles fuse with **lysosomes**, and T_3 and T_4 **residues** are removed from thyroglobulin, liberated into the cytosol, and are released at the basal aspect of the cell into the perifollicular capillary network.

- Thyroid hormone (see Table 10-2) is essential for regulating basal metabolism and for influencing growth rate and mental processes and generally stimulates endocrine gland functioning.

An additional secretory cell type, **parafollicular cells (clear cells)**, is present in the thyroid. These cells have no contact with the colloidal material. They manufacture the hormone **calcitonin**, which is released directly into the connective tissue in the immediate vicinity of capillaries. Calcitonin (see Table 10-2) helps control calcium concentrations in the blood by inhibiting bone resorption by osteoclasts (i.e., when blood calcium levels are high, calcitonin is released).

Parathyroid Glands

The **parathyroid glands**, usually four in number, are embedded in the fascial sheath of the posterior aspect of the thyroid gland. They possess slender connective tissue capsules from which septa are derived to penetrate the glands and convey a vascular supply to the interior. In the adult, two types of parenchymal cells are present in the parathyroid glands:

- numerous small **chief cells** and a smaller number of
- large **acidophilic cells**, the **oxyphils**.

Fatty infiltration of the glands is common in older individuals. Although there is no known function of oxyphils, chief cells produce **parathyroid hormone (PTH** see Table 10-2).

- **Parathyroid hormone (PTH)** is responsible for maintaining proper calcium ion balance.

- The concentration of calcium ions is extremely important in the normal function of muscle and nerve cells and as a release mechanism for neurotransmitter substance.

- A drop in blood calcium concentration activates a feedback mechanism that stimulates chief cell secretion.

- PTH binds to receptors on osteoblasts that release osteoclast-stimulating factor followed by bone resorption and a consequent increase in blood calcium ion concentration.

- In the kidneys, PTH prevents urinary calcium loss; thus, ions are returned to the bloodstream.
- PTH also controls calcium uptake in the intestines indirectly by modulating kidney production of vitamin D, which is essential for calcium absorption.

Increased levels of PTH cause an elevation in plasma calcium concentration; however, it takes several hours for this level to peak. The concentration of PTH in the blood is also controlled by plasma calcium levels.

- **Calcitonin** acts as an antagonist to PTH.
- Unlike PTH, calcitonin is fast acting, and since it binds directly to receptors on osteoclasts, it elicits a peak reduction in blood calcium levels within one hour.
- Calcitonin inhibits bone resorption, thus reducing calcium ion levels in the blood. High levels of calcium ions in the blood stimulate calcitonin release.

Absence of parathyroid glands is not compatible with life.

Suprarenal Glands

The **suprarenal glands** (adrenal glands in some animals) are invested by a connective tissue capsule (see Table 10-2 and Graphics 10-2 and 10-3). The glands are derived from two different embryonic origins, namely, **mesodermal epithelium**, which gives rise to the **cortex**, and **neuroectoderm**, from which the **medulla** originates. The rich vascular supply of the gland is conveyed to the interior in connective tissue elements derived from the capsule.

Cortex

The **cortex** is subdivided into three concentric regions or zones that secrete specific hormones (see Table 10-2). Control of these hormonal secretions is mostly regulated by ACTH from the pituitary gland.

- The outermost region, just beneath the capsule, is the **zona glomerulosa**, where the cells are arranged in arches and spherical clusters with numerous capillaries surrounding them.
  - Cells of the zona glomerulosa secrete **aldosterone**, a mineralocorticoid that acts on cells of the distal convoluted tubules of the kidney to modulate water and electrolyte balance.
- The second region, the **zona fasciculata**, is the most extensive. Its parenchymal cells, usually known as **spongiocytes**, are arranged in long cords, with numerous capillaries between the cords.
- Zona fasciculata cells secrete **cortisol** and **corticosterone**.

- These glucocorticoids regulate carbohydrate metabolism, facilitate the catabolism of fats and proteins, exhibit anti-inflammatory activity, and suppress the immune response.
- The innermost region of the cortex, the **zona reticularis**, is arranged in anastomosing cords of cells with a rich intervening capillary network.
  - Zona reticularis cells secrete weak **androgens** that promote masculine characteristics.

Medulla

Parenchymal cells of the **medulla**, derived from neural crest material, are disposed in irregularly arranged short cords surrounded by capillary networks. They contain numerous granules that stain intensely when the freshly cut tissue is exposed to chromium salts. This is referred to as the **chromaffin reaction**, and the cells are called **chromaffin cells**. There are two populations of chromaffin cells that secrete the two hormones (see Table 10-2) of the suprarenal medulla, mainly

- **epinephrine** (adrenaline) or
- **norepinephrine** (noradrenaline).

Secretion of these two catecholamines is directly regulated by preganglionic fibers of the sympathetic nervous system that impinge on the postganglionic sympathetic neuron-like chromaffin cells, which are considered to be related to postganglionic sympathetic neurons (see Graphic 10-3). Catecholamine release occurs in physical and psychological stress. Moreover, scattered, large **postganglionic sympathetic ganglion cells** in the medulla act on smooth muscle cells of the medullary veins, thus controlling blood flow in the cortex.

Pineal Body

The **pineal body (epiphysis)** is a projection of the roof of the diencephalon (see Table 10-2 and Graphic 10-2). The connective tissue covering of the pineal body is pia mater, which sends trabeculae and septa into the substance of the pineal body, subdividing it into incomplete lobules. Blood vessels, along with postganglionic sympathetic nerve fibers from the superior cervical ganglia, travel in these connective tissue elements. As the nerve fibers enter the pineal body, they lose their myelin sheath. The parenchyma of the pineal body is composed of pinealocytes and neuroglial cells.

- The **pinealocytes** form communicating junctions with each other and manufacture **melatonin**. Interestingly, melatonin is manufactured only at night.
- **Neuroglial cells** provide physical and nutritional support to pinealocytes.
- The pineal body receives indirect input from the **retina**, which allows the pineal to differentiate between

TABLE 10-2 • Hormones of the Thyroid, Parathyroid, Adrenal, and Pineal Glands

Gland	Hormone	Stimulating Hormone	Principal Functions
Thyroid gland	Thyroxine (T_4) and triiodothyronine (T_3)	Thyroid-stimulating hormone	Promotes gene transcription and stimulates carbohydrate and fat metabolism. Increases basal metabolism, growth rates, endocrine gland secretion, heart rate, and respiration. Decreases cholesterol, phospholipid, and triglyceride levels and lowers body weight
	Calcitonin (thyrocalcitonin)		Lowers blood calcium levels by suppressing osteoclastic activity
Parathyroid gland	Parathyroid hormone		Increases blood calcium levels
Suprarenal (adrenal) gland			
Cortex			
Zona glomerulosa	Mineralocorticoids (aldosterone and deoxycorticosterone)	Angiotensin II and adrenocorticotropic hormone (ACTH)	Stimulates distal convoluted tubules of the kidney to resorb sodium and excrete potassium
Zona fasciculata	Glucocorticoids (cortisol and corticosterone)	ACTH	Controls carbohydrate, lipid, and protein metabolism. Stimulates gluconeogenesis. Reduces inflammation and suppresses the immune system
Zona reticularis	Androgens (dehydroepiandrosterone and androstenedione)	ACTH	No significant effect in a healthy individual
Medulla	Catecholamines (epinephrine and norepinephrine)	Preganglionic sympathetic and splanchnic nerves	Epinephrine—increases blood pressure and heart rate, promotes glucose release by the liver. Norepinephrine—elevates blood pressure via vasoconstriction
Pineal body (pineal gland)	Melatonin	Norepinephrine	Influences the individual's diurnal rhythm

day and night, and, in that manner, assists in the establishment of the circadian rhythm.

- The extracellular spaces of the pineal body contain calcified granular material known as **brain sand (corpora arenacea)**, whose significance, if any, is not known.

It is unclear how the pineal gland functions in humans, but it does exert an affect on the control of the circadian rhythm. Nonetheless, melatonin is used to treat jet lag and in regulating emotional responses related to shortened daylight during winter, a condition called **seasonal affective disorder (SAD)**.

CLINICAL CONSIDERATIONS

Pituitary Gland

Galactorrhea is a condition in which a male produces breast milk or a woman who is not breast-feeding produces breast milk. In men, it is often accompanied by impotence, headache, and loss of peripheral vision and in women by hot flashes, vaginal dryness, and an abnormal menstrual cycle. This rather uncommon condition is usually a result of prolactinoma, a tumor of prolactin-producing cells of the pituitary gland. The condition is usually treated by drug intervention or surgery, or both.

Postpartum pituitary infarct is a condition due the pregnancy-induced enlarging of the pituitary gland and its concomitant increase in its vascularity. The high vascularity of the pituitary increases the chances of a vascular accident, such as hemorrhage, which results in the partial destruction of the pituitary gland. The condition may be severe enough to produce Sheehan's syndrome, which is recognized by the lack of milk production, the loss of pubic and axillary hair, and fatigue.

Pituitary Somatotrope Adenoma

Pituitary somatotrope adenoma is one of the pituitary adenomas, benign tumors, that are more common in adults than in children. Somatotrope adenomas involve proliferation of acidophils, which produce an excess of growth hormones which, in children, result in **gigantism**, whereas in adults it results in **acromegaly**. These acidophils grow slowly and usually do not grow outside the sella turcica. Individuals afflicted with untreated

acromegaly frequently suffer from complications that increase their chance of succumbing to cardiovascular, cerebrovascular, and respiratory problems. These individuals also present with hypertension.

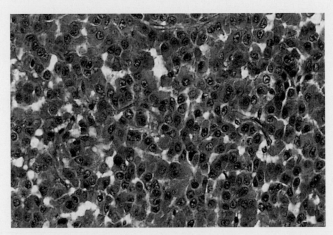

This is a photomicrograph from the pituitary gland of a patient with pituitary somatotrope adenoma. Note that the adenoma cells are arranged in ribbons and cords. (Reprinted with permission from Rubin R, Strayer D, et al., eds. Rubin's Pathology. Clinicopathologic Foundations of Medicine, 5th ed. Baltimore: Lippincott Williams & Wilkins, 2008, p. 938.)

Thyroid Gland

Graves' disease is caused by binding of autoimmune IgG antibodies to TSH receptors thus stimulating increased thyroid hormone production (**hyperthyroidism**). Clinically, the thyroid gland becomes enlarged, and there is evidence of exophthalmic goiter (protrusion of the eyeballs).

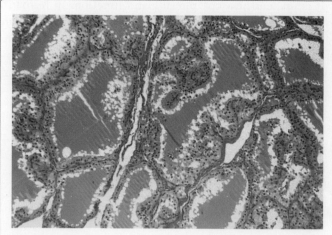

This photomicrograph is from the thyroid gland of a patient with Graves' disease. Note that the follicular cells are high columnar hyperplastic cells enclosing pinkish colloid that is scalloped along its periphery. (Reprinted with permission from Rubin R, Strayer D, et al., eds. Rubin's Pathology. Clinicopathologic Foundations of Medicine, 5th ed. Baltimore: Lippincott Williams & Wilkins, 2008, p. 946.)

Parathyroid Gland

Hyperparathyroidism may be due to the presence of a benign tumor causing the excess production of parathyroid hormone (PTH). The high levels of circulating PTH cause increased bone resorption with a resultant greatly elevated blood calcium. The excess calcium may become deposited in arterial walls and in the kidneys, creating kidney stones.

Suprarenal Gland

Addison's disease is an autoimmune disease, although it may also be the aftermath of tuberculosis. It is characterized by decreased production of adrenocortical hormones due to the destruction of the suprarenal cortex, and without the administration of steroid treatment, it may have fatal consequences.

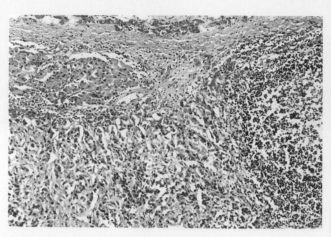

This photomicrograph of the adrenal gland of a patient with Addison's disease displays cortical fibrosis and inflammation, as well as a mass of atrophic cortical cells. (Reprinted with permission from Rubin R, Strayer D, et al., eds. Rubin's Pathology. Clinicopathologic Foundations of Medicine, 5th ed. Baltimore: Lippincott Williams & Wilkins, 2008, p. 962.)

Type 2 polyglandular syndrome, a hereditary disorder, affects the thyroid and suprarenal glands in such a fashion that they are underactive (although the thyroid may become overactive). Frequently, patients with this disorder also develop diabetes.

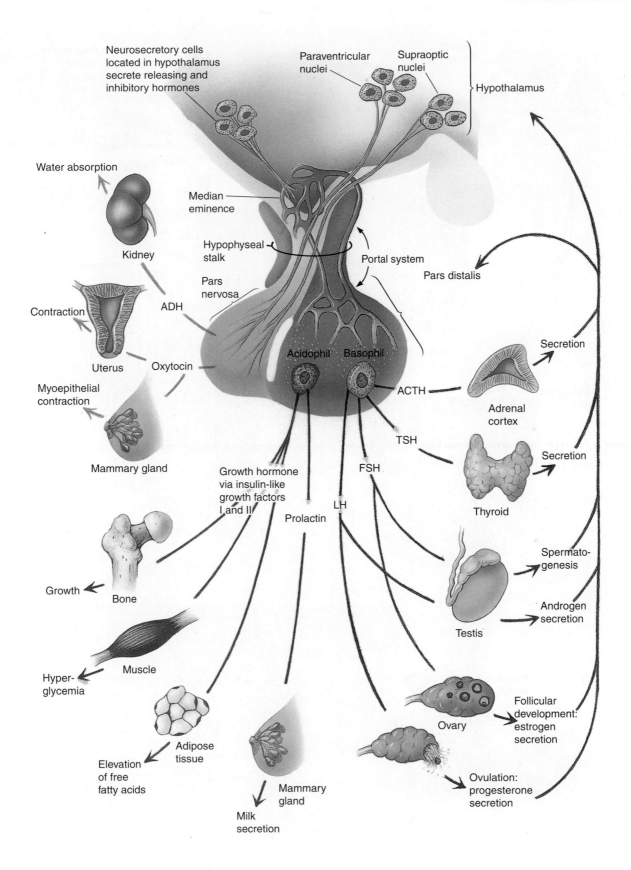

Neurosecretory cells located in hypothalamus secrete releasing and inhibitory hormones

Paraventricular nuclei

Supraoptic nuclei

Hypothalamus

Water absorption

Kidney

Median eminence

Hypophyseal stalk

Portal system

Pars distalis

Pars nervosa

ADH

Contraction

Uterus

Oxytocin

Acidophil

Basophil

Secretion

ACTH

Adrenal cortex

Myoepithelial contraction

Mammary gland

Growth hormone via insulin-like growth factors I and II

Prolactin

FSH

LH

TSH

Secretion

Thyroid

Spermato-genesis

Growth

Bone

Hyper-glycemia

Muscle

Adipose tissue

Elevation of free fatty acids

Mammary gland

Milk secretion

Testis

Androgen secretion

Ovary

Follicular development: estrogen secretion

Ovulation: progesterone secretion

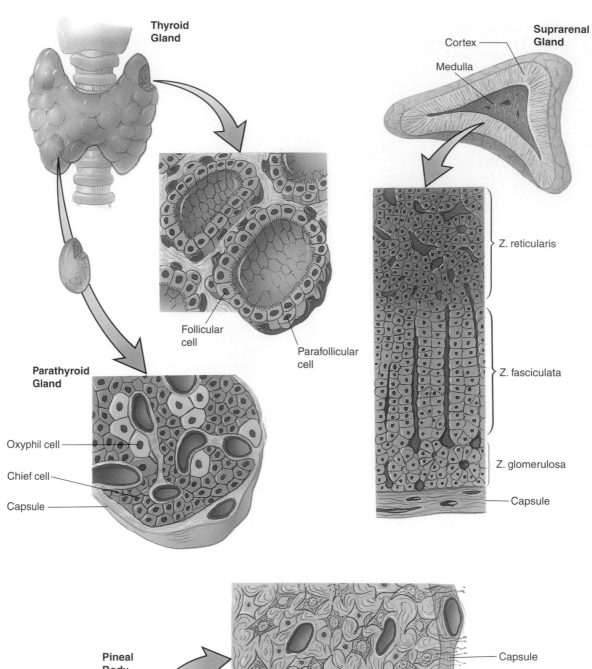

Thyroid Gland

Follicular cell

Parafollicular cell

Suprarenal Gland

Cortex

Medulla

Z. reticularis

Z. fasciculata

Z. glomerulosa

Capsule

Parathyroid Gland

Oxyphil cell

Chief cell

Capsule

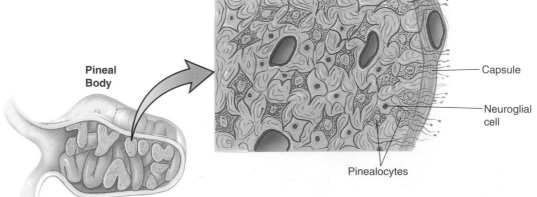

Pineal Body

Capsule

Neuroglial cell

Pinealocytes

Preganglionic sympathetic neuron and fiber ●▬▬▬
Postganglionic sympathetic neuron and fiber ●▬▬▬

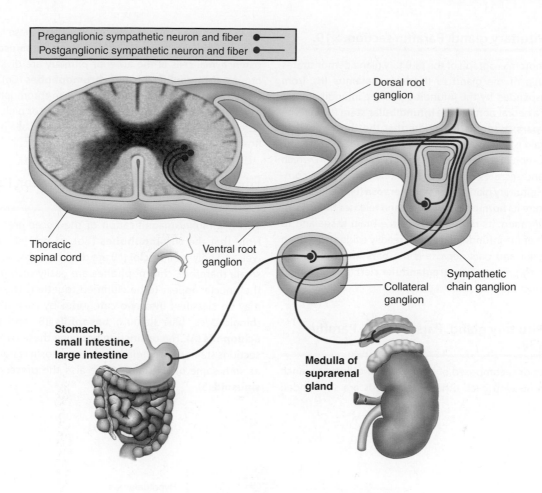

Dorsal root ganglion

Thoracic spinal cord

Ventral root ganglion

Collateral ganglion

Sympathetic chain ganglion

Stomach, small intestine, large intestine

Medulla of suprarenal gland

PLATE 10-1 · Pituitary Gland

FIGURE 1. Pituitary gland. Paraffin section. ×19.

This survey photomicrograph of the pituitary gland demonstrates the relationship of the gland to the **hypothalamus** (H), from which it is suspended by the infundibulum. The infundibulum is composed of a neural portion, the **infundibular stem** (IS) and the surrounding **pars tuberalis** (PT). Note that the **third ventricle** (3V) of the brain is continuous with the **infundibular recess** (IR). The largest portion of the pituitary is the **pars anterior** (PA), which is glandular and secretes numerous hormones. The neural component of the pituitary gland is the **pars nervosa** (PN), which does not manufacture its hormones but stores and releases them. Even at this magnification, its resemblance to the brain tissue and to the substance of the infundibular stalk is readily evident. Between the pars anterior and pars nervosa is the **pars intermedia** (PI), which frequently presents an **intraglandular cleft** (IC), a remnant of Rathke's pouch.

FIGURE 2. Pituitary gland. Pars anterior. Paraffin section. ×132.

The pars anterior is composed of large cords of cells that branch and anastomose with each other. These cords are surrounded by an extensive capillary network. However, these capillaries are wide, endothelially lined vessels known as **sinusoids** (S). The parenchymal cells of the anterior pituitary are divided into two groups: **chromophils** (Ci) and **chromophobes** (Co). With hematoxylin and eosin, the distinction between chromophils and chromophobes is obvious. The former stain blue or pink, whereas the latter stain poorly. The *boxed area* is presented at a higher magnification in Figure 3.

FIGURE 3. Pituitary gland. Pars anterior. Paraffin section. ×270.

This is a higher magnification of the *boxed area* of Figure 2. Note that the **chromophobes** (Co) do not take up the stain well and only their **nuclei** (N) are demonstrable. These cells are small; therefore, chromophobes are easily recognizable since their nuclei appear to be clumped together. The chromophils may be classified into two categories by their affinity to histologic dyes: blue-staining **basophils** (B) and pink-colored **acidophils** (A). The distinction between these two cell types in sections stained with hematoxylin and eosin is not as apparent as with some other stains. Note also the presence of a large **sinusoid** (S).

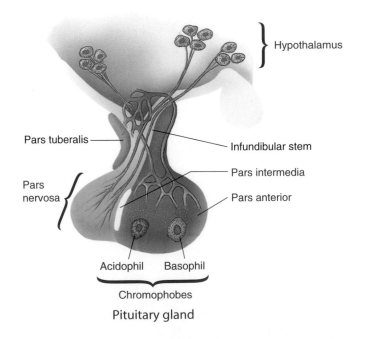

Pars tuberalis

Infundibular stem

Pars intermedia

Pars anterior

Pars nervosa

Acidophil Basophil

Chromophobes

Hypothalamus

Pituitary gland

KEY					
A	acidophils	**IC**	intraglandular cleft	**PI**	pars intermedia
B	basophils	**IR**	infundibular recess	**PN**	pars nervosa
Ci	chromophils	**IS**	infundibular stem	**PT**	pars tuberalis
Co	chromophobes	**N**	nucleus	**S**	sinusoids
H	hypothalamus	**PA**	pars anterior	**3V**	third ventricle

PLATE 10-1 • Pituitary Gland

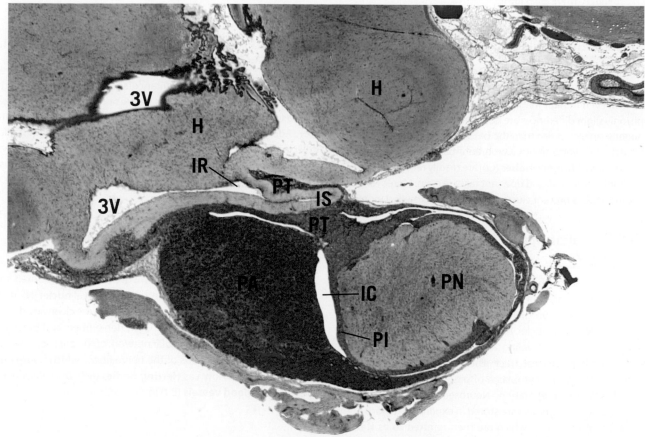

FIGURE 1

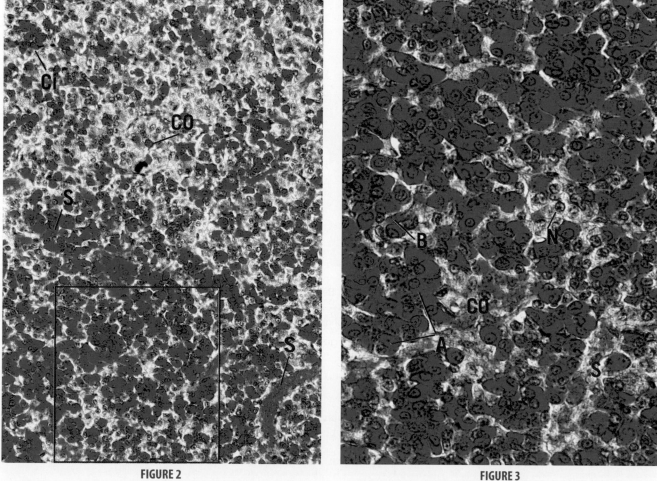

FIGURE 2

FIGURE 3

FIGURE 1. Pituitary gland. Paraffin section. ×540.

It is somewhat difficult to discriminate between the **acidophils** (A) and **basophils** (B) of the pituitary gland stained with hematoxylin and eosin. Even at high magnification, such as in this photomicrograph, only slight differences are noted. Acidophils stain pinkish and are slightly smaller in size than the basophils, which stain pale blue. In a black and white photomicrograph, basophils appear darker than acidophils. **Chromophobes** (Co) are readily recognizable, since their cytoplasm is small and does not take up stain. Moreover, cords of chromophobes present clusters of **nuclei** (N) crowded together.

FIGURE 3. Pituitary gland. Pars nervosa. Paraffin section. ×132.

The pars nervosa of the pituitary gland is composed of elongated cells with long processes known as **pituicytes** (P), which are thought to be neuroglial in nature. These cells, which possess more or less oval nuclei, appear to support numerous unmyelinated nerve fibers traveling from the hypothalamus via the hypothalamo-hypophyseal tract. These nerve fibers cannot be distinguished from the cytoplasm of pituicytes in a hematoxylin and eosin–stained preparation. Neurosecretory materials pass along these nerve fibers and are stored in expanded regions at the termination of the fibers, which are then referred to as **Herring bodies** (HB). Note that the pars nervosa resembles neural tissue. The *boxed area* is presented at a higher magnification in Figure 4.

FIGURE 2. Pituitary gland. Pars intermedia. Human. Paraffin section. ×270.

The pars intermedia of the pituitary gland is situated between the **pars anterior** (PA) and the **pars nervosa** (PN). It is characterized by **basophils** (B), which are smaller than those of the pars anterior. Additionally, the pars intermedia contains **colloid** (Cl)-filled follicles, lined by pale, small, low cuboidal-shaped cells (*arrows*). Note that some of the basophils extend into the pars nervosa. Numerous **blood vessels** (BV) and **pituicytes** (P) are evident in this area of the pars nervosa.

FIGURE 4. Pituitary gland. Pars nervosa. Paraffin section. ×540.

This photomicrograph is a higher magnification of the *boxed area* of Figure 3. Note the numerous more or less oval **nuclei** (N) of the pituicytes, some of whose processes (*arrows*) are clearly evident at this magnification. The unmyelinated nerve fibers and processes of pituicytes make up the cellular network of the pars nervosa. The expanded terminal regions of the nerve fibers, which house neurosecretions, are known as **Herring bodies** (HB). Also observe the presence of **blood vessels** (BV) in the pars nervosa.

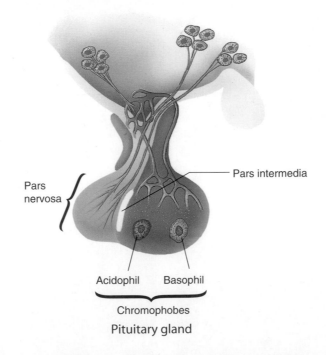

Pars nervosa

Pars intermedia

Acidophil   Basophil

Chromophobes

Pituitary gland

KEY					
A	acidophils	**Co**	chromophobes	**PA**	pars anterior
B	basophils	**HB**	Herring bodies	**PN**	pars nervosa
BV	blood vessels	**N**	nucleus		
CL	colloid	**P**	pituicytes		

PLATE 10-2 · Pituitary Gland

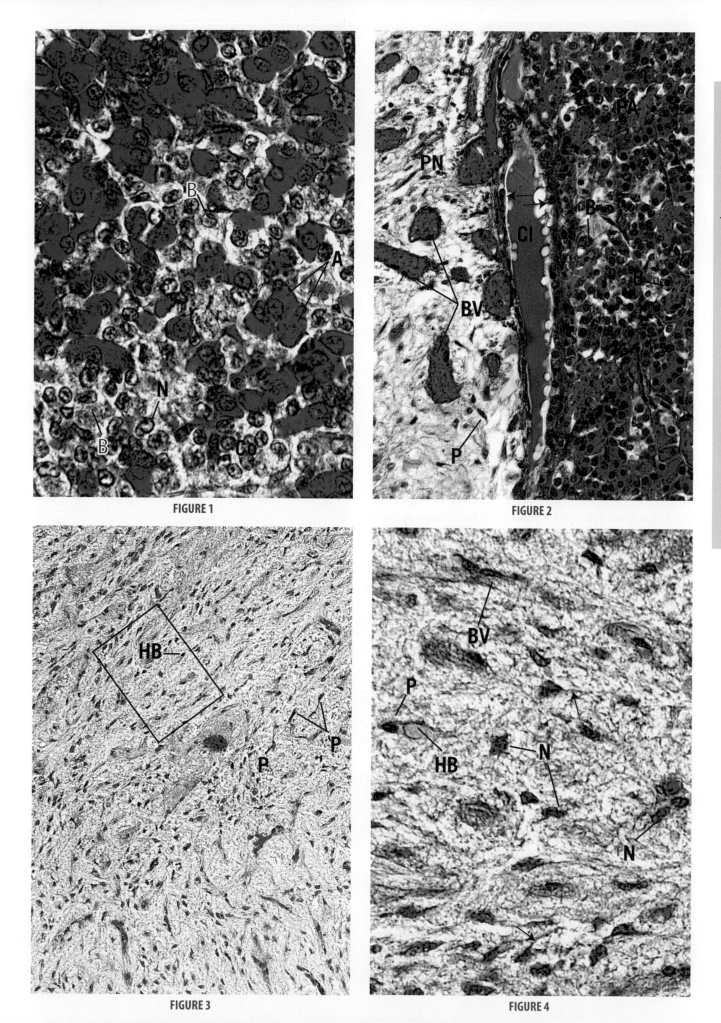

FIGURE 1

FIGURE 2

FIGURE 3

FIGURE 4

PLATE 10-3 · Thyroid Gland, Parathyroid Gland

FIGURE 1. Thyroid gland. Monkey. Plastic section. ×132.

The capsule of the thyroid gland sends septa of connective tissue into the substance of the gland, subdividing it into incomplete lobules. This photomicrograph presents part of a lobule displaying many **follicles** (F) of varied sizes. Each follicle is surrounded by slender **connective tissue** (CT), which supports the follicles and brings **blood vessels** (BV) in close approximation. The follicles are composed of **follicular cells** (FC), whose low cuboidal morphology indicates that the cells are not producing secretory product. During the active secretory cycle, these cells become taller in morphology. In addition to the follicular cells, another parenchymal cell type is found in the thyroid gland. These cells do not border the colloid, are located on the periphery of the follicles, and are known as **parafollicular cells** (PF) or C cells. They are large and possess centrally placed round nuclei, and their cytoplasm appears paler.

FIGURE 3. Thyroid and parathyroid glands. Monkey. Plastic section. ×132.

Although the **parathyroid** (PG) and **thyroid glands** (TG) are separated by their respective **capsules** (Ca), they are extremely close to each other. The capsule of the parathyroid gland sends **trabeculae** (T) of connective tissue carrying **blood vessels** (BV) into the substance of the gland. The parenchyma of the gland consists of two types of cells, namely, **chief cells** (CC), also known as principal cells, and **oxyphil cells** (OC). Chief cells are more numerous and possess darker staining cytoplasm. Oxyphil cells stain lighter and are usually larger than chief cells, and their cell membranes are evident. A region similar to the *boxed area* is presented at a higher magnification in Figure 4.

FIGURE 2. Thyroid gland. Monkey. Plastic section. ×540.

The thyroid **follicle** (F) presented in this photomicrograph is surrounded by several other follicles and intervening **connective tissue** (CT). **Nuclei** (N) in the connective tissue may belong either to endothelial cells or to connective tissue cells. Since most capillaries are collapsed in excised thyroid tissue, it is often difficult to identify endothelial cells with any degree of certainty. The **follicular cells** (FC) are flattened, indicating that these cells are not actively secreting thyroglobulin. Note that the follicles are filled with a **colloid** (Cl) material. Observe the presence of a **parafollicular cell** (PF), which may be distinguished from the surrounding cells by its pale cytoplasm (*arrow*) and larger nucleus.

FIGURE 4. Parathyroid gland. Monkey. Plastic section. ×540.

This photomicrograph is a region similar to the *boxed area* of Figure 3. The **chief cells** (CC) of the parathyroid gland form small cords surrounded by slender **connective tissue** (CT) elements and **blood vessels** (BV). The **nuclei** (N) of connective tissue cells may be easily recognized due to their elongated appearance. **Oxyphil cells** (OC) possess a paler cytoplasm, and frequently, the cell membranes are evident (*arrows*). The glands of older individuals may become infiltrated by adipocytes.

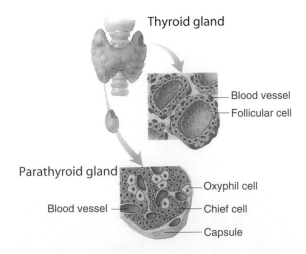

Thyroid gland

Blood vessel
Follicular cell

Parathyroid gland

Oxyphil cell
Blood vessel
Chief cell
Capsule

KEY					
BV	blood vessels	F	follicle	PG	parathyroid gland
Ca	capsule	FC	follicular cells	T	trabeculae
CC	chief cells	N	nucleus	TG	thyroid gland
CL	colloid	OC	oxyphil cells		
CT	connective tissue	PF	parafollicular cells		

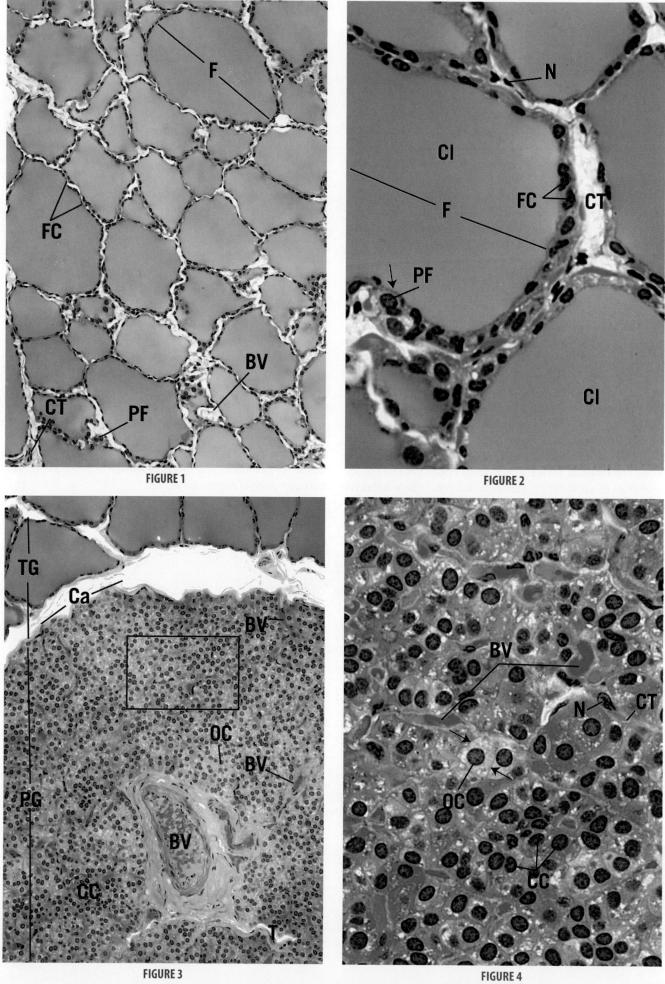

PLATE 10-3 · Thyroid Gland, Parathyroid Gland

FIGURE 1

FIGURE 2

FIGURE 3

FIGURE 4

PLATE 10-4 · Suprarenal Gland

FIGURE 1. Suprarenal gland. Paraffin section. ×14.

The suprarenal gland, usually embedded in **adipose tissue** (AT), is invested by a collagenous connective tissue **capsule** (Ca) that provides thin connective tissue elements that carry blood vessels and nerves into the substance of the gland. Since the **cortex** (Co) of the suprarenal gland completely surrounds the flattened **medulla** (M), it appears duplicated in any section that completely transects the gland. The cortex is divided into three concentric regions: the outermost **zona glomerulosa** (ZG), middle **zona fasciculata** (ZF), and the innermost **zona reticularis** (ZR). The medulla, which is always bounded by the zona reticularis, possesses several large **veins** (V), which are always accompanied by a considerable amount of connective tissue.

FIGURE 3. Suprarenal gland. Monkey. Plastic section. ×132.

The columnar arrangement of the cords of the **zona fasciculata** (ZF) is readily evident by viewing the architecture of the blood vessels indicated by the *arrows*. The cells in the deeper region of the ZF are smaller and appear denser than the more superficially located **spongiocytes** (Sp). Cells of the **zona reticularis** (ZR) are arranged in irregular, anastomosing cords whose interstices contain wide capillaries. The cords of the ZR merge almost imperceptibly with those of the ZF. This is a relatively narrow region of the cortex. The **medulla** (M) is clearly evident since its cells are much larger than those of the ZR. Moreover, numerous large **veins** (V) are characteristic of the medulla.

FIGURE 2. Suprarenal gland. Cortex. Monkey. Plastic section. ×132.

The collagenous connective tissue **capsule** (Ca) of the suprarenal gland is surrounded by adipose tissue through which **blood vessels** (BV) and **nerves** (Ne) reach the gland. The parenchymal cells of the cortex, immediately deep to the capsule, are arranged in an irregular array, forming the more or less oval to round clusters or arch-like cords of the **zona glomerulosa** (ZG). The cells of the **zona fasciculata** (ZF) form long, straight columns of cords oriented radially, each being one to two cells in width. These cells are larger than those of the ZG. They present a vacuolated appearance due to the numerous lipid droplets that were extracted during processing and are often referred to as **spongiocytes** (Sp). The interstitium is richly vascularized by **blood vessels** (BV).

FIGURE 4. Suprarenal gland. Monkey. Plastic section. ×540.

The **capsule** (Ca) of the suprarenal gland displays its **collagen fibers** (Cf) and the **nuclei** (N) of the fibroblasts. The **zona glomerulosa** (ZG), which occupies the upper part of the photomicrograph, displays relatively small cells with few vacuoles (*arrows*). The lower part of the photomicrograph demonstrates the **zona fasciculata** (ZF), whose cells are larger and display a more vacuolated (*arrowheads*) appearance. Note the presence of **connective tissue** (CT) elements and **blood vessels** (BV) in the interstitium between cords of parenchymal cells.

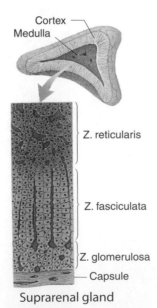

Cortex
Medulla

Z. reticularis

Z. fasciculata

Z. glomerulosa

Capsule

Suprarenal gland

KEY

AT	adipose tissue	**CT**	connective tissue	**V**	veins
BV	blood vessels	**M**	medulla	**ZF**	zona fasciculata
Ca	capsule	**N**	nuclei	**ZG**	zona glomerulosa
Cf	collagen fibers	**Ne**	nerves	**ZR**	zona reticularis
Co	cortex	**Sp**	spongiocytes		

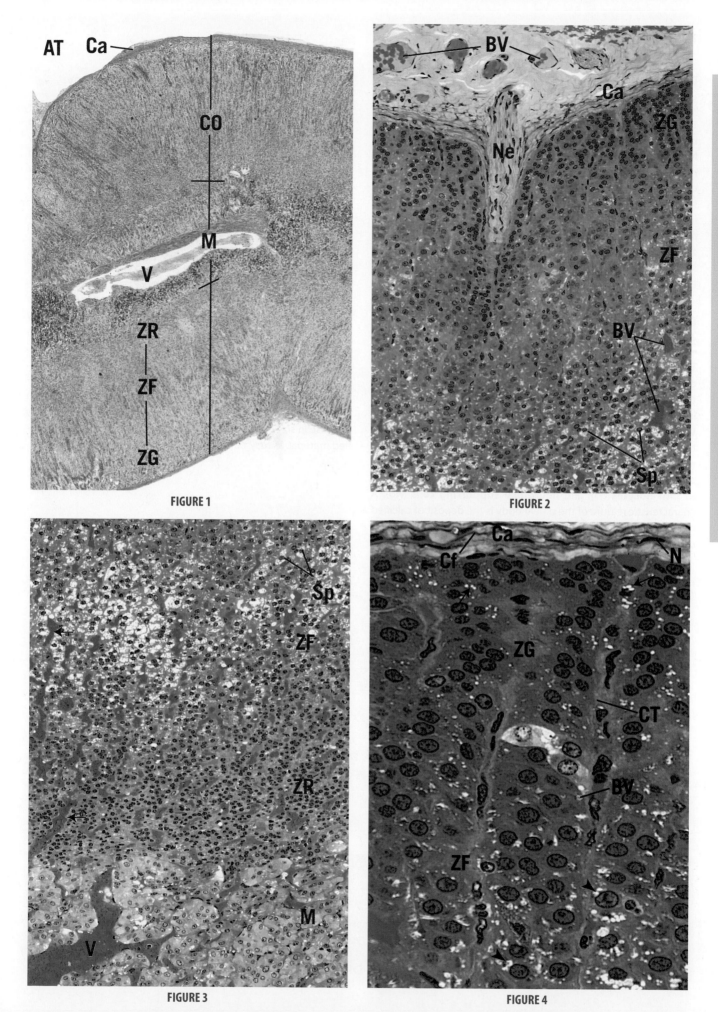

PLATE 10-4 · Suprarenal Gland

FIGURE 1

FIGURE 2

FIGURE 3

FIGURE 4

PLATE 10-5 · Suprarenal Gland, Pineal Body

FIGURE 1. Suprarenal gland. Cortex. Monkey. Plastic section. ×540.

The upper part of this photomicrograph presents the border between the **zona fasciculata** (ZF) and the **zona reticularis** (ZR). Note that the **spongiocytes** (Sp) of the fasciculata are larger and more vacuolated than the cells of the reticularis. The parenchymal cells of the zona reticularis are arranged in haphazardly anastomosing cords. The interstitium of both regions houses large capillaries containing **red blood cells** (RBC). *Inset.* **Zona fasciculata. Monkey. Plastic section**. ×540. The **spongiocytes** (Sp) of the zona fasciculata are of two different sizes. Those positioned more superficially in the cortex, as in this inset, are larger and more vacuolated (*arrows*) than spongiocytes close to the zona reticularis.

FIGURE 3. Pineal body. Human. Paraffin section. ×132.

The pineal body is covered by a capsule of connective tissue derived from the pia mater. From this capsule, connective tissue **trabeculae** (T) enter the substance of the pineal body, subdividing it into numerous incomplete **lobules** (Lo). Nerves and **blood vessels** (BV) travel in the trabeculae to be distributed throughout the pineal, providing it with a rich vascular supply. In addition to endothelial and connective tissue cells, two other types of cells are present in the pineal, namely, the parenchymal cells, known as **pinealocytes** (Pi), and **neuroglial supporting cells** (Ng). A characteristic feature of the pineal body is the deposit of calcified material known as corpora arenacea or **brain sand** (BS). The *boxed area* is presented at a higher magnification in Figure 4.

FIGURE 2. Suprarenal gland. Medulla. Monkey. Plastic section. ×270.

The cells of the adrenal medulla, often referred to as **chromaffin cells** (ChC), are arranged in round to ovoid clusters or in irregularly arranged short cords. The cells are large and more or less round to polyhedral in shape with a pale **cytoplasm** (Cy) and vesicular appearing **nucleus** (N), displaying a single, large **nucleolus** (n). The interstitium presents large **veins** (V) and an extensive **capillary** (Cp) network. Large ganglion cells are occasionally noted.

FIGURE 4. Pineal body. Human. Paraffin section. ×540.

This photomicrograph is a higher magnification of the *boxed area* of Figure 3. With the use of hematoxylin and eosin stain, only the nuclei of the two cell types are clearly evident. The larger, paler, more numerous nuclei belong to the **pinealocytes** (Pi). The smaller, denser nuclei are those of the **neuroglial cells** (Ng). The pale background is composed of the long, intertwining processes of these two cell types. The center of the photomicrograph is occupied by **brain sand** (BS). Observe that these concretions increase in size by apposition of layers on the surface of the calcified material, as may be noted at the *arrow*.

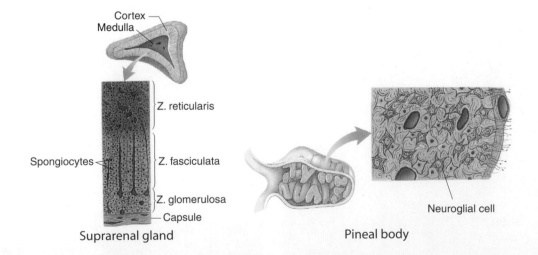

Cortex
Medulla

Z. reticularis

Spongiocytes

Z. fasciculata

Z. glomerulosa

Capsule

Suprarenal gland

Neuroglial cell

Pineal body

KEY							
BS	brain sand	**N**	nucleus	**T**	trabeculate
BV	blood vessels	**n**	nucleolus	**V**	veins
ChC	chromaffin cells	**Ng**	neuroglial cells	**ZF**	zona fasciculata
Cp	capillaries	**Pi**	pinealocytes	**ZR**	zona reticularis
Cy	cytoplasm	**RBC**	red blood cells		
Lo	lobules	**Sp**	spongiocytes		

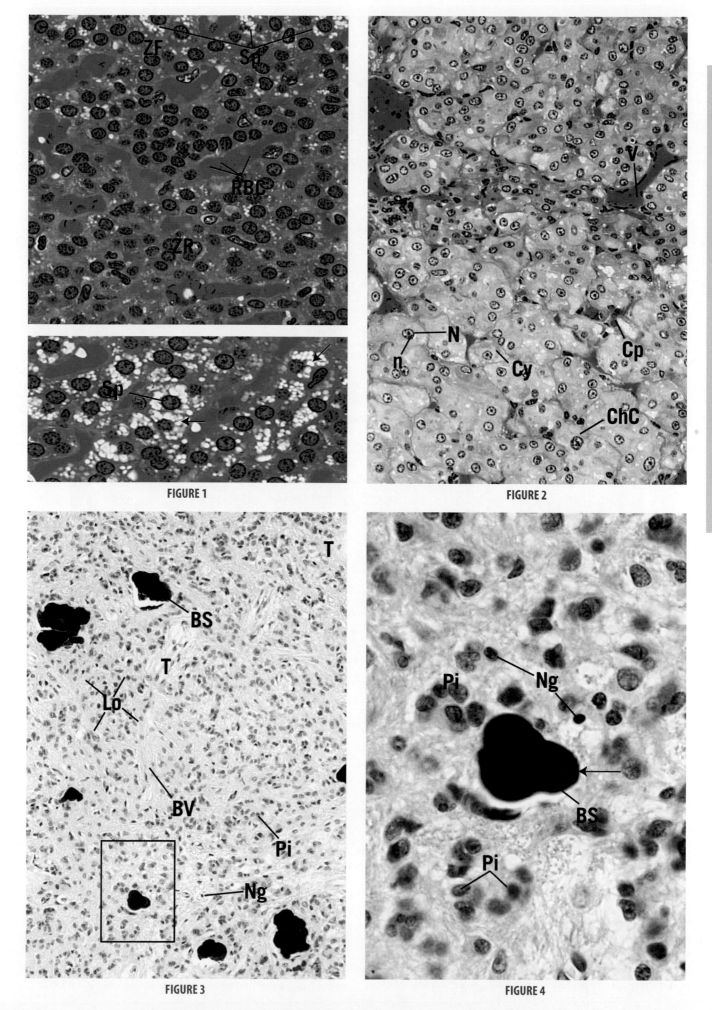

PLATE 10-5 · Suprarenal Gland, Pineal Body

FIGURE 1

FIGURE 2

FIGURE 3

FIGURE 4

PLATE 10-6 · Pituitary Gland, Electron Microscopy

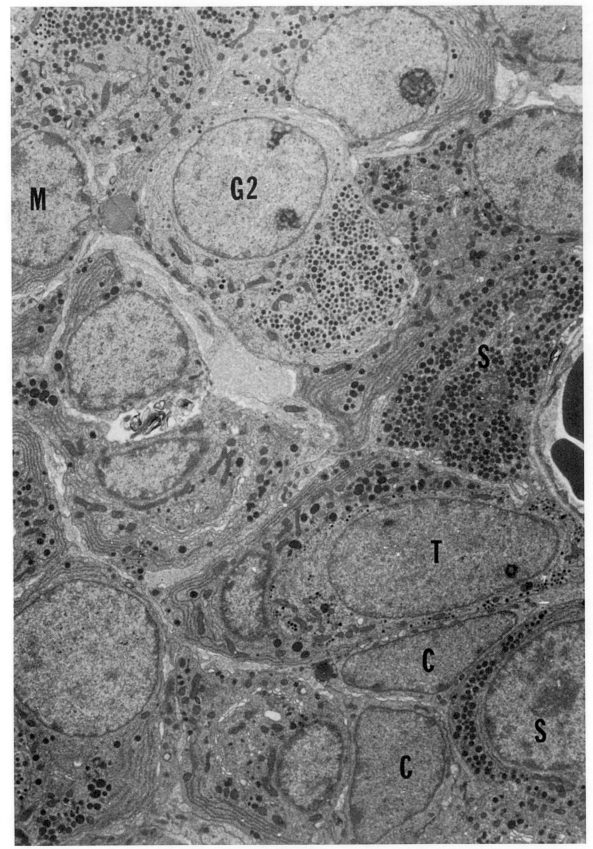

FIGURE 1

FIGURE 1. Pituitary gland. Pars anterior. Electron microscopy. ×4,950.

Although considerable controversy surrounds the precise fine structural identification of the cells of the pars anterior, it is reasonably certain that the several cell types presented in this electron micrograph are acidophils, basophils, and chromophobes, as observed by light microscopy. The acidophils are **somatotropes** (S) and **mammotropes** (M), whereas only two types of basophils are included in this electron micrograph, namely, **type II gonadotropes** (G2) and **thyrotropes** (T). The **chromophobes** (C) may be recognized by the absence of secretory granules in their cytoplasm. (From Poole M. Cellular distribution within the rat adenohypophysis: a morphometric study. Anat Rec 1982;204:45–53.)

PLATE 10-7 · Pituitary Gland, Electron Microscopy

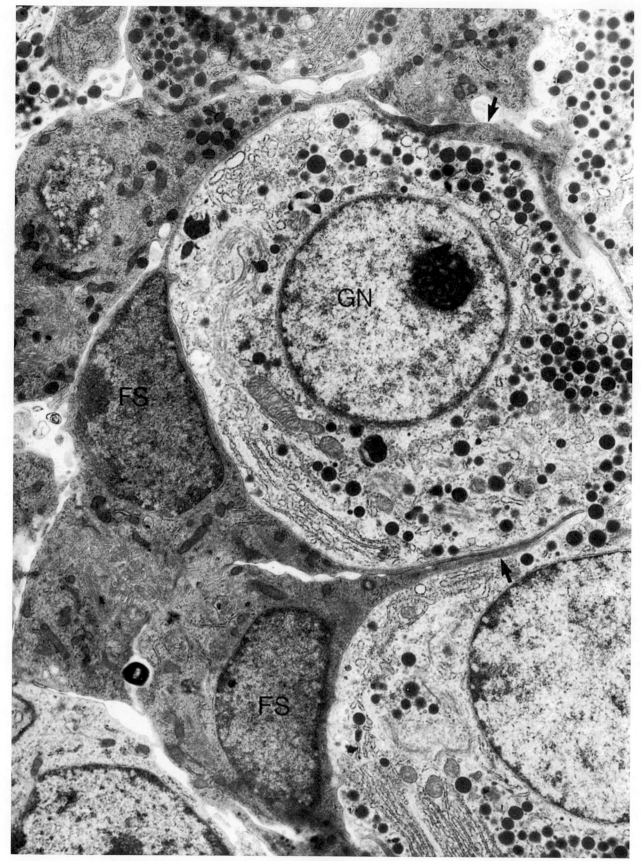

FIGURE 1

FIGURE 1. Pituitary gland. Rat. Electron microscopy. ×8,936.

The pars distalis of the rat pituitary houses various cell types, two of which are represented here. The granule-containing **gonadotrophs** (GN) are surrounded by nongranular **folliculostellate cells** (FS), whose processes are demarcated by *arrows*. The functions of folliculostellate cells are in question, although some believe them to be supportive, phagocytic, regenerative, or secretory in nature. (From Strokreef JC, Reifel CW, Shin SH. A possible phagocytic role for folliculo-stellate cells of anterior pituitary following estrogen withdrawal from primed male rats. Cell Tissue Res 1986;243:255–261.)

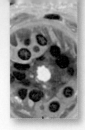

Chapter Summary

Endocrine glands are characterized by the absence of ducts and the presence of a rich vascular network. The parenchymal cells of endocrine glands are usually arranged in **short cords**, **follicles**, or **clusters**, although other arrangements are also common.

I. PITUITARY GLAND

The **pituitary gland** is invested by a **connective tissue capsule**. The gland is subdivided into four component parts.

A. Pars Anterior

1. Cell Types

a. Chromophils

1. Acidophils

Stain pink with hematoxylin and eosin. They are found mostly in the center of the pars anterior.

2. Basophils

Stain darker than acidophils with hematoxylin and eosin. They are more frequently found at the periphery of the pars anterior.

b. Chromophobes

Chromophobes are smaller cells whose cytoplasm is not granular and has very little affinity for stain. They may be recognized as clusters of nuclei throughout the pars anterior.

B. Pars Intermedia

The **pars intermedia** is rudimentary in man. Small basophils are present as well as **colloid-filled follicles**.

C. Pars Nervosa and Infundibular Stalk

These have the appearance of nervous tissue. The cells of the **pars nervosa** are **pituicytes**, resembling neuroglial cells. They probably support the **unmyelinated nerve fibers**, whose terminal portions are expanded, since they store **neurosecretions** within the pars nervosa. These expanded terminal regions are known as **Herring bodies**.

D. Pars Tuberalis

The **pars tuberalis** is composed of **cuboidal cells** arranged in cords. They may form small colloid-filled **follicles**.

II. THYROID GLAND

A. Capsule

The **capsule** of the thyroid gland consists of a thin **collagenous connective tissue** from which **septa** extend into the substance of the gland, subdividing it into lobules.

B. Parenchymal Cells

The **parenchymal cells** of the thyroid gland form **colloid-filled follicles** composed of

1. *Follicular Cells* (simple cuboidal epithelium)
2. *Parafollicular Cells* (clear cells) located at the periphery of the follicles

C. Connective Tissue

Slender connective tissue elements support a rich vascular supply.

III. PARATHYROID GLAND

A. Capsule

The gland is invested by a slender collagenous connective tissue **capsule** from which **septa** arise to penetrate the substance of the gland.

B. Parenchymal Cells

1. Chief Cells

Chief cells are numerous, small cells with large nuclei that form cords.

2. Oxyphils

Oxyphils are larger, acidophilic, and much fewer in number than chief cells.

C. Connective Tissue

Collagenous connective tissue **septa** as well as slender **reticular fibers** support a rich vascular supply. **Fatty infiltration** is common in older individuals.

IV. SUPRARENAL GLAND

The **suprarenal gland** is invested by a collagenous connective tissue **capsule**. The gland is subdivided into a **cortex** and a **medulla**.

A. Cortex

The **cortex** is divided into three concentric zones: **zona glomerulosa**, **zona fasciculata**, and **zona reticularis**.

1. Zona Glomerulosa

The **zona glomerulosa** is immediately deep to the capsule. It consists of columnar cells arranged in arches and spherical clusters.

2. Zona Fasciculata

The thickest zone of the cortex is the **zona fasciculata**. The more or less cuboidal cells (**spongiocytes**) are arranged in long, parallel cords. **Spongiocytes** appear highly vacuolated except for those of the deepest region, which are smaller and much less vacuolated.

3. Zona Reticularis

The innermost zone of the cortex is the **zona reticularis**. It is composed of small, dark cells arranged in irregularly anastomosing cords. The intervening capillaries are enlarged.

B. Medulla

The **medulla** is small in humans and is composed of large, granule-containing **chromaffin cells** arranged in short cords. Additionally, large **autonomic ganglion cells** are also present. A characteristic of the medulla is the presence of large veins.

V. PINEAL BODY

A. Capsule

The **capsule**, derived from **pia mater**, is thin collagenous connective tissue. **Septa** derived from the capsule divide the pineal body into incomplete lobules.

B. Parenchymal Cells

1. Pinealocytes

Pinealocytes are recognized by the large size of their nuclei.

2. Neuroglial Cells

Neuroglial cells possess smaller, denser nuclei than the pinealocytes.

C. Brain Sand

Characteristic of the pineal body are the calcified accretions in the extracellular spaces, known as **brain sand** or **corpora arenacea**.

11 INTEGUMENT

CHAPTER OUTLINE

The integument, the largest and heaviest organ of the body, is composed of skin and its various derivatives, including sebaceous glands, sweat glands, hair, and nails. The skin covers the entire body and is continuous with the mucous membranes at the lips, at the anus, in the nose, at the leading edges of the eyelids, and at the external orifices of the urogenital system. Some of the many functions of skin include

- protection against physical, chemical, and biologic assaults;
- providing a waterproof barrier;
- absorbing ultraviolet radiation for both vitamin D synthesis and protection;
- excretion (i.e., sweat) and thermoregulation;
- monitoring the external milieu via its various nerve endings;
- and immunologic defense of the body.

SKIN

Skin is composed of a superficial **stratified squamous keratinized epithelium** known as the **epidermis** and of a deeper connective tissue layer, the **dermis** (see Graphic 11-1—please note that free nerve endings are not depicted in this diagram).

- The epidermis and dermis interdigitate with each other by the formation of **epidermal ridges** and **dermal ridges (dermal papillae)**, where the two are separated by a basement membrane.
  - Frequently, a dermal ridge is subdivided into two secondary dermal ridges with an intervening interpapillary peg from the epidermis.
- The ridges on the fingertips that imprint as fingerprints are evidence of this interdigitation.

Interposed between skin and deeper structures is a fascial sheath known as the hypodermis, which is not a part of skin.

Skin can be classified as thick or thin depending on the thickness of its epidermis and of its dermis. Since it is the thickness of the epidermis that is usually obvious when viewed with the microscope, the epidermis of thick skin is presented here. The epidermis of skin can be thick, as on the sole of the foot and the palm of the hand, or thin, as over the remainder of the body (see Table 11-1).

The **epidermis** of

- **thick skin** has five well-developed layers: stratum basale, stratum spinosum, stratum granulosum, stratum lucidum, and stratum corneum.
- **thin skin** has three layers since the stratum granulosum and stratum lucidum are absent as well-defined layers. However, individual cells of the two absent layers are present even in thin skin.

Epidermis of Thick Skin

The epidermis is composed of four cell types, keratinocytes, melanocytes, Langerhans cells, and Merkel cells. Approximately 95% of the cells of the epidermis are keratinocytes, and it is their morphology that is responsible for the characteristics of the five layers.

Keratinocytes and the Five Layers of the Epidermis

The deepest layer of the epidermis, the **stratum basale** (formerly known as stratum germinativum), is a single layer of cuboidal to columnar cells. These cells are responsible for cell renewal, via mitosis (usually at night), and the newly formed cells are pushed surfaceward, giving rise to the thickest layer, the stratum spinosum.

- The cuboidal/columnar cells sit on a **basement membrane**, separating them from the connective tissue dermis, and form **hemidesmosomes** with the basal lamina and **desmosomal** contacts with each other and with the basal-most cells of the stratum spinosum.
- These cells of the stratum basale form **keratin 5** and **keratin 14**.
- The **stratum spinosum** is a number of cells in thickness and is composed of polyhedral **prickle cells** characterized by numerous processes (intercellular bridges) that form desmosomes with processes of surrounding prickle cells.
  - Cells, mostly in the deeper layer of the stratum spinosum, also display mitotic activity (usually at night).
    - These prickle cells form **keratin 1** and **keratin 10** that replace keratins 5 and 14 formed by the stratum basale. The keratins are **intermediate filaments** that begin to form bundles known as **tonofilaments**.
    - These prickle cells in the superficial layers of the stratum spinosum also form
      - **keratohyalin granules**, non–membrane-bound structures that are composed of **trichohyalin** and **filaggrin**. These two proteins, associated with intermediate filaments, promote **the aggregation of keratin** by cross-linking the keratin filaments into thick bundles of tonofilaments.
      - **membrane-coating granules (Odland bodies, lamellar bodies)**, whose lipid-rich contents are composed of **ceramides, phospholipids, and glycosphingolipids**.
- Continuous migration of the cells of the stratum spinosum forms the next layer, the **stratum granulosum**.
  - Cells of this layer accumulate more **keratohyalin granules**, which eventually overfill the cells, destroying their nuclei and organelles.

TABLE 11-1 • Characteristics of Thick and Thin Skin

Cellular Strata (Superficial to deepest)	Thick Skin	Thin Skin
Epidermis	Is a stratified squamous keratinized epithelium derived from ectoderm. Cells of the epidermis consist of four cell types: keratinocytes, melanocytes, Langerhans cells, and Merkel cells.	
Stratum corneum (*Cornified cell layer*)	Composed of several layers of dead, anucleated, flattened keratinocytes (squames) that are being sloughed from the surface. As many as 50 layers of keratinocytes are located in the thickest skin (e.g., sole of the foot).	Only about five or so layers of keratinocytes (squames) comprise this layer in the thinnest skin (e.g., eyelids).
Stratum lucidum (*Clear cell layer*)	Poorly stained keratinocytes filled with keratin compose this thin, well-defined layer. Organelles and nuclei are absent.	Layer is absent but individual cells of the layer are probably present.
Stratum granulosum (*Granular cell layer*)	Only three to five layers thick with polygonal-shaped nucleated keratinocytes with a normal complement of organelles as well as keratohyalin and membrane-coating granules	Layer is absent but individual cells of the layer are probably present.
Stratum spinosum (*prickle cell layer*)	This thickest layer is composed of mitotically active and maturing polygonal keratinocytes (prickle cells) that interdigitate with one another via projections (intercellular bridges) that are attached to each other by desmosomes. The cytoplasm is rich in tonofilaments, organelles, and membrane-coating granules. Langerhans cells are present in this layer.	This stratum is the same as in thick skin but the number of layers is reduced.
Stratum basale (*stratum germinativum*)	This deepest stratum is composed of a single layer of mitotically active tall cuboidal keratinocytes that are in contact with the basal lamina. Keratinocytes of the more superficial strata originate from this layer and eventually migrate to the surface where they are sloughed. Melanocytes and Merkel cells are also present in this layer.	This layer is the same in thin skin as in thick skin.
Dermis	Located deep to the epidermis, and separated from it by a basement membrane, the dermis is derived from mesoderm and is composed mostly of dense irregular collagenous connective tissue. It contains capillaries, nerves, sensory organs, hair follicles, sweat and sebaceous glands, as well as arrector pili muscles It is divided into two layers: a superficial papillary layer and a deeper reticular layer.	
Papillary layer	Is comprised of loose connective tissue containing capillary loops and terminals of mechanoreceptors. These dermal papillae interdigitate with the epidermal ridges of the epidermis. These interdigitations are very prominent in thick skin.	The papillary layer is comprised of the same loose connective tissue as in thick skin. However, its volume is much reduced. The depth of the dermal/epidermal interdigitations is also greatly reduced.
Reticular layer	Is composed of dense irregular collagenous connective tissue containing the usual array of connective tissue elements, including cells, blood, and lymphatic vessels. Sweat glands and cutaneous nerves are also present and their branches extend into the papillary layer and into the epidermis.	Same as in thick skin with the addition of. Sebaceous glands and hair follicles along with their arrector pili muscles are observed.

○ Cells of the stratum granulosum also continue to manufacture **membrane-coating granules.**

○ Cells of the stratum granulosum contact each other via desmosomes and, in their superficial layers, also form claudin-containing **occluding junctions** with each other as well as with cells of the stratum lucidum (or, in the absence of the stratum lucidum, with the stratum corneum).

○ In the superficial layers, cells of the stratum granulosum release the contents of their membrane-coating granules into the extracellular space. These cells no longer contain organelles or a nucleus and are considered to be dead having undergone **apoptosis.**

○ The stratum spinosum and stratum granulosum together are frequently referred to as the **stratum Malpighii.**

• The fourth layer, the **stratum lucidum**, is relatively thin and is usually absent in thin skin. When evident in thick skin, palmar and plantar skin, it usually appears as a thin, translucent region, interposed between the strata granulosum and the corneum.

○ The cells of the stratum lucidum have no nuclei or organelles but contain a large amount of tonofibrils embedded in keratohyalin.

• The surface-most layer is the **stratum corneum**, composed of preferentially arranged stacks of dead hulls known as **squames.**

○ The squames, similar to the cells of the stratum lucidum, are filled with the keratohyalin-keratin complex, which deposits on the internal aspect of the cell membrane, forming a **cornified cell envelope.**

○ The cornified cell envelope is further buttressed by at least three proteins, **involucrin, loricrin,** and **small proline-rich protein.**

○ The contents of the Odland bodies, released by cells of the strata spinosum and granulosum, form a **lipid envelope** that provides a waterproof barrier.

○ The cornified cell envelope and the lipid envelope form a structure known as the **compound cornified cell envelope.**

○ The superficial layers of the stratum corneum are desquamated at the same rate as they are being replaced by the mitotic activity of the strata basale and spinosum while maintaining the integrity of the compound cornified cell envelope.

Recent investigations indicate that keratinocytes produce immunogenic molecules and are probably active in the immune process. Evidence also shows that these cells are capable of producing several interleukins, colony-stimulating factors, interferons, tumor necrosis factors, as well as platelet- and fibroblast-stimulating growth factors.

Nonkeratinocytes of the Epidermis

There are three types of nonkeratinocytes in the epidermis: melanocytes, Langerhans cells, and Merkel cells (see Table 11-2).

Melanocytes

Melanoblasts, derived from neural crest cells, differentiate into **melanocytes** under the influence of the signaling molecule **stem cell factor.** Melanocytes manufacture a dark **melanin pigment.**

• **Melanocytes** and **premelanocytes** migrate into the epidermis during embryonic development and establish residence in the forming stratum basale and may establish hemidesmosomes with the basal lamina. Some of the premelanocytes differentiate into melanocytes, whereas other remain in an undifferentiated state even in the adult.

• Once there, they do *not* make desmosomal contact with other cells in their vicinity but form long processes, **dendrites**, that penetrate the stratum spinosum.

• Each melanocyte forms an association, via its dendrites, with a number of keratinocytes, referred to as **epidermal-melanin unit.**

• The number of keratinocytes per melanocyte varies with regions of the body but is relatively constant across the races, and approximately 3% of the cells of the epidermis consist of melanocytes.

In the adult premelanocytes enter into the cell cycle to maintain their population as well as to differentiate into melanocytes.

• The hormone α-MSH binds to **melanocortin receptors** on the melanocyte cell membrane that activates a cAMP pathway prompting the melanocyte to express **microphthalmia-associated transcription factor (MITF)**.

○ MITF not only regulates the mitotic activity of the premelanocytes but also induces the formation of melanin, in specialized organelles of melanocytes known as **melanosomes.**

There are two types of melanin, **eumelanin**, a dark brown to black pigment composed of polymers of **hydroxyindole**, and **pheomelanin**, a red to rust-colored compound composed of **cysteinyl dopa** polymers.

• Eumelanin is present in individuals with dark hair.
• Pheomelanin is found in individuals with red and blond hair.

Both types of melanin are derived from the amino acid **tyrosine**, which is transported into specialized **tyrosinase**-containing vesicles derived from the *trans*-Golgi network, known as **premelanosomes.**

- Within these oval (1.0 by 0.5 µm) premelanosomes, **tyrosinase** converts tyrosine into **3,4-dihydroxy-phenylalanine (DOPA)**, which is transformed into **dopaquinone** and, eventually, into filamentous **melanin (melanofilaments)**.
- As the amount of melanin increases within the premelanosomes, its filamentous structure is no longer evident, and the organelles mature into much darker structures known as **melanosomes**.
- Melanosomes possess the transmembrane protein **Rab27a** in their membranes.
- Melanosomes travel, along **microtubules** powered by **kinesin**, into the dendrites of melanocytes.
- The Rab27a binds a cytoplasmic molecule, **melanophilin**, which
  - permits a detachment of the melanosome from the kinesin and
  - facilitates its attachment to **myosin Va,** which transfers the melanosome to **F-actin**
  - melanosomes are **transported** to the immediate vicinity of the dendrite plasmalemma along the F-actin pathway.
  - Myosin Va detaches from the F-actin and permits the exocytosis of the melanosome into the extracellular space.

Once melanosomes enter the extracellular space, keratinocytes of the stratum spinosum **phagocytose** them. The melanosomes migrate to the nuclear region of the keratinocyte and form a protective umbrella, shielding the nucleus (and its chromosomes) from the ultraviolet rays of the sun. Soon thereafter, **lysosomes** attack and destroy the melanosomes.

- Ultraviolet rays not only increase the rates of darkening of melanin and endocytosis of the melanosomes but also enhance tyrosinase activity and thus melanin production.
- Fewer melanocytes are located on the insides of the thighs and undersides of the arms and face. Skin pigmentation is related to the location of melanin rather than to the numbers of melanocytes.
- Melanosomes are fewer and congregate around the keratinocyte nucleus in Caucasians, whereas in dark-skinned individuals they are larger and are more dispersed throughout the keratinocyte cytoplasm. The destruction of the melanosomes occurs at a slower rate in darker than in lighter skin.

Langerhans Cells

Langerhans cells (also known as dendritic cells because of their long processes) are derived from bone marrow and located mostly in the stratum spinosum. They function as **antigen-presenting cells** in immune responses. The nucleus of these cells possesses numerous indentations, and their cytoplasm contain, in addition to the usual organelles, **Birbeck granules**, elongated vesicles whose end is ballooned. Langerhans cells:

- do not make desmosomal contact with the cells of the stratum spinosum.
- express **CD1a** surface marker and **MHC I**, **MHC II, Fc receptors for IgG**, **C3b receptors,** and the transmembrane protein **langerin** that is associated with Birbeck granules. Langerin and CD1a facilitate the immune defense against *Mycobacterium leprae*, the microorganism responsible for **leprosy**
- **phagocytose antigens** entering the epidermis, including nonprotein antigens.

When a Langerhans cell phagocytoses an antigen, the cell migrates into a lymph vessel of the dermis to enter the paracortex of a nearby lymph node. Here, the Langerhans cell presents its antigen to T cells to activate a **delayed-type hypersensitivity response**.

Merkel Cells

Merkel cells, whose origin is uncertain, although most authors believe them to be a modified type of keratinocyte, are interspersed among the cells of the stratum basale and are most abundant in the fingertips. Afferent nerve terminals approximate these cells, forming complexes, known as Merkel discs that are believed to function as **mechanoreceptors** (touch receptors). There is some evidence that Merkel cells may also have a neurosecretory function.

Dermis

The **dermis** of the skin, lying directly deep to the epidermis, is derived from mesoderm. It is composed of **dense**, **irregular collagenous connective tissue** containing mostly type I collagen and numerous elastic fibers that assist in securing the skin to the underlying **hypodermis**.

- The dermis is subdivided into a loosely woven **papillary layer** (composed of primary and secondary dermal ridges), a superficial region that interdigitates with the epidermal ridges (and interpapillary pegs) of the epidermis, and
- a deeper, coarser, and denser **reticular layer**. The interface between the papillary and reticular layers is indistinct.
- **Dermal ridges** (as well as secondary dermal ridges) display encapsulated nerve endings, such as **Meissner's corpuscles**, as well as capillary loops that bring nourishment to the avascular epidermis.

TABLE 11-2 • Nonkeratinocytes of the Epidermis

Nonepithelial Cells	Origin	Location	Features	Function
Melanocytes	Derived from neural crest	Migrate into stratum basale during embryonic development. Some remain undifferentiated even in adulthood (reserved to maintain melanocyte population). Do not form desmosomal contact with keratinocytes but some may form hemidesmosomes with basal lamina.	Form long processes (dendrites) that pass into the stratum spinosum. Melanocytes possess melanosomes within their cytoplasm where melanin is manufactured. Melanocytes form associations with several keratinocytes (epidermal-melanin unit). Population = to about 3% of epidermal population.	Manufacture melanin pigment. Melanosomes located in the cytoplasm are activated to produce melanin (eumelanin in dark hair and pheomelanin in red and blond hair). Once melanosomes are filled with melanin, they travel up the dendrites and are released into the extracellular space. Keratinocytes of the stratum spinosum phagocytose these melanin-laden melanosomes. The melanosomes migrate to the nuclear region of the keratinocyte and form a protective umbrella, shielding the nucleus (and its chromosomes) from the ultraviolet rays of the sun. Soon, the melanosomes are destroyed by keratinocyte lysosomes. UV rays increase melanin production, its darkening, and its endocytosis. Caucasians possess fewer melanosomes, which congregate around the nucleus, whereas in dark-skinned individuals, they are larger and dispersed throughout the cytoplasm. Melanosome destruction is at a slower pace in darker skin.
Langerhans cells	Derived from bone marrow	Mostly located in the stratum spinosum	Possess long processes; thus, they are known as dendritic cells. Nucleus possesses many indentations. Cytoplasm contains Birbeck granules, elongated vesicles exhibiting a ballooned out terminus. Do not form desmosomal contact with keratinocytes	Are antigen-presenting cells. These cells possess surface markers and receptors as well as langerin, a transmembrane protein associated with Birbeck granules. Some of these elements facilitate an immune response against the organism responsible for leprosy. Additionally, Langerhans cells phagocytose antigens that enter the epidermis and migrate to lymph vessels located in the dermis and from there into the paracortex of a lymph node to present these antigens to T cells, thereby activating a delayed-type hypersensitivity response.
Merkel cells	Believed to be a modified keratinocyte although origin is uncertain	Interspersed with keratinocytes of the stratum basale. They are most abundant in the fingertips.	Merkel cells form complexes, known as Merkel discs, with terminals of afferent nerves.	Merkel cells function as mechanoreceptors (touch receptors). There is some evidence that Merkel cells may also function as neurosecretory cells.

DERIVATIVES OF SKIN

Derivatives of skin include hair, sebaceous glands, sweat glands, and nails (see Graphic 11-2). These structures originate from epidermal downgrowths into the dermis and hypodermis, while maintaining their connection to the outside.

- Each **hair** is composed of a shaft of cornified cells and a root contained within a hair follicle
  - is associated with a **sebaceous gland** that secretes an oily **sebum** into the neck of the hair follicle.
  - A small bundle of smooth muscle cells, the **arrector pili muscle**, attaches to the hair follicle and, cradling the sebaceous gland, inserts into the superficial aspects of the skin.

- **Sweat glands** do not develop in association with hair follicles. These are simple, coiled, tubular glands whose secretory units produce sweat, which is delivered to the surface of the skin by long ducts.
  - **Myoepithelial cells** surround the secretory portion of these glands.
- **Nails** are cornified structures on the distal phalanx of each finger and toe. These horny plates lie on a nail bed and are bounded laterally by a nail wall.
  - The **cuticle** (**eponychium**) lies over the **lunula**, an opaque, crescent-shaped area of the nail plate.
  - The **hyponychium** is located beneath the free edge of the nail plate.

CLINICAL CONSIDERATIONS

Itching (Pruritis)

The sensation of itching is accompanied by an instinctive, almost irrepressible urge to scratch. There are many different causes of itching, some as simple as a fly walking on one's skin and moving the hair follicles, or as serious as debilitating systemic conditions such as kidney failure or liver disease. If the itching is accompanied by a rash, then the probable cause is not the kidney or the liver. Parasitic infestations (mites, scabies, etc.), insect bites, plant toxins (such as poison oak and poison ivy), and drug allergies are usually accompanied by a rash and require medical intervention. If the itching is long-term, the patient should seek the assistance of a physician. Pregnancy and cold, dry weather may also be contributing factors to itching.

Psoriasis Vulgaris

Psoriasis vulgaris is a commonly occurring condition characterized by reddish patchy lesions on the skin with grayish sheen, located especially around joints, sacral region, the navel, and the scalp. This condition is produced by increased proliferation of keratinocytes and an acceleration of the cell cycle, resulting in an accumulation of cells in the stratum corneum but with an absence of a stratum granulosum and, frequently, the presence of lymphocytic infiltrates in the papillary layer. The condition is cyclic and is of unknown etiology.

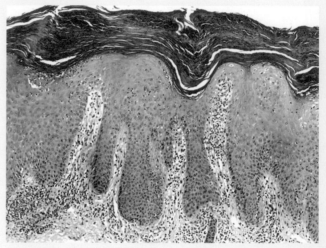

This photomicrograph is of a patient suffering from psoriasis vulgaris. Note that the stratum spinosum and stratum corneum are thickened and that the stratum granulosum is absent. The papillary layer of the dermis displays an infiltration by lymphocytes. (Reprinted with permission from Mills SE, Carter D, et al., eds. Sternberg's Diagnostic Surgical Pathology, 5th ed., Philadelphia, Lippincott, Williams & Wilkins, 2010, p. 6.)

Erythema Multiforme

Patches of elevated red skin, frequently resembling a target, displaying a symmetrical distribution over the face and extremities, that occurs periodically indicate the disorder erythema multiforme. It is most frequently due

CLINICAL CONSIDERATIONS

to herpes simplex infection. The condition is not usually accompanied by itching, although painful lesions (blisters) on the lips and buccal cavity are common occurrences. Usually the condition resolves itself, but in more severe cases, medical intervention is indicated.

Warts

Warts are benign epidermal growths on the skin caused by papilloma viral infection of the keratinocytes. Warts are common in young children, in young adults, and in immunosuppressed patients.

Vitiligo

A condition in which the skin has patches of white areas due to the lack of pigmentation is known as vitiligo. The melanocytes of the affected region are destroyed in an autoimmune response. The condition may appear suddenly after a physical injury or as a consequence of sunburn. If the area affected has hair, as the hair grows it will be white. Although there are no physical consequences to vitiligo, there may be psychological sequelae.

Malignancies of Skin

The three most common malignancies of skin are basal cell carcinoma, squamous cell carcinoma, and malignant melanoma.

Basal cell carcinoma, the most common human malignancy, develops in the stratum basale from damage caused by ultraviolet radiation. The foremost type of basal cell carcinoma is the **nodulocystic type** where small hyperchromatic cells form spherical nodules that are separated from the surrounding connective tissue elements of the dermis by narrow spaces. The most frequent site of basal cell carcinoma is on the nose, occurring as papules or nodules, which eventually craters. Surgery is usually 90% effective with no recurrence.

Squamous cell carcinoma, the second most frequent skin malignancy, is invasive and metastatic. Its probable etiology is environmental factors, such as ultraviolet radiation and x-irradiation, as well as a variety of chemical carcinogens, including arsenic. The carcinoma originates in cells of the stratum spinosum and appears clinically as a hyperkeratotic, scaly plaque with deep invasion of underlying tissues, often accompanied by bleeding. Surgery is the treatment of choice.

Malignant melanoma may be a life-threatening malignancy. It develops in the epidermis where melanocytes become mitotically active and form a dysplastic nevus. It may then enter a **radial-growth phase** where individual melanocytes invade the dermis, then enter the **vertical growth phase** where they begin to form tumors in the dermis, and eventually become a full-fledged, **metastatic melanoma** whose cells eventually enter the lymphatic and circulatory system to metastasize to other organ systems.

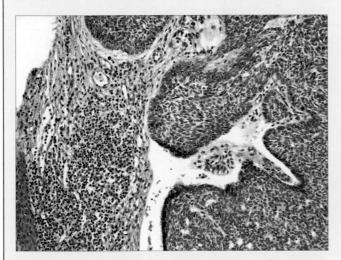

This photomicrograph is of a patient with basal cell carcinoma. Note that the lesion is composed of dark, dense basal cells that form rounded nodules that are separated from the dermal connective tissue by narrowed spaces. (Reprinted with permission from Mills SE, Carter D, et al., eds. Sternberg's Diagnostic Surgical Pathology, 5th ed., Philadelphia, Lippincott, Williams & Wilkins, 2010. p. 49.)

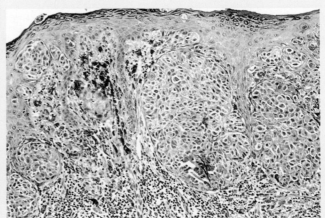

This photomicrograph is of a patient suffering from malignant melanoma. Note that the melanocytes are invading the dermis in large numbers, indicating that the melanoma is in the vertical growth phase. (Reprinted with permission from Mills SE, Carter D, et al., eds. Sternberg's Diagnostic Surgical Pathology, 5th ed., Philadelphia, Lippincott, Williams & Wilkins, 2010. p. 92.)

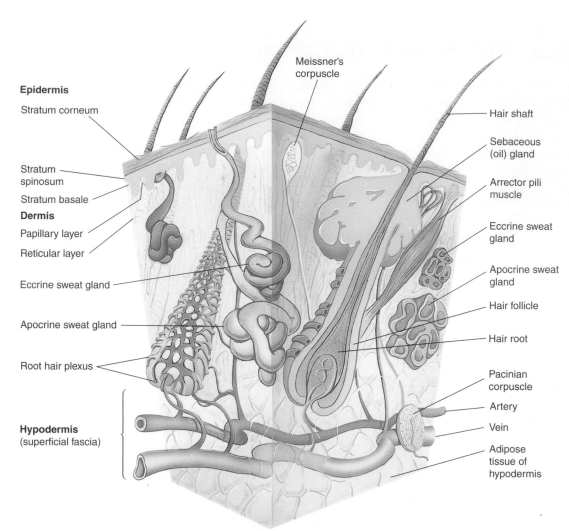

Epidermis

Stratum corneum

Stratum spinosum

Stratum basale

Dermis

Papillary layer

Reticular layer

Eccrine sweat gland

Apocrine sweat gland

Root hair plexus

Hypodermis (superficial fascia)

Meissner's corpuscle

Hair shaft

Sebaceous (oil) gland

Arrector pili muscle

Eccrine sweat gland

Apocrine sweat gland

Hair follicle

Hair root

Pacinian corpuscle

Artery

Vein

Adipose tissue of hypodermis

Skin and its appendages, **hair**, **sweat glands** (both **eccrine** and **apocrine**), **sebaceous glands**, and **nails**, are known as the **integument**. Skin may be **thick** or **thin**, depending on the thickness of its epidermis. Thick skin epidermis is composed of five distinct layers of **keratinocytes** (strata basale, spinosum, granulosum, lucidum, and corneum) interspersed with three additional cell types, **melanocytes**, **Merkel's cells**, and **Langerhans' cells**. Thin skin epidermis lacks strata granulosum and lucidum, although individual cells that constitute the absent layers are present.

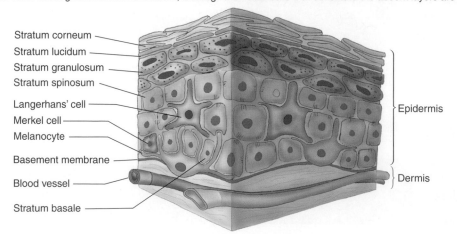

Stratum corneum

Stratum lucidum

Stratum granulosum

Stratum spinosum

Langerhans' cell

Merkel cell

Melanocyte

Basement membrane

Blood vessel

Stratum basale

Epidermis

Dermis

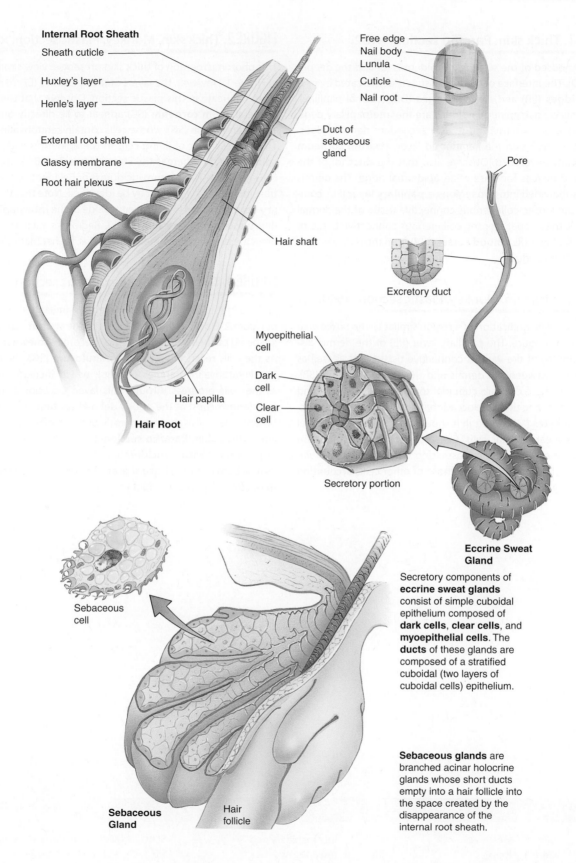

Internal Root Sheath

Sheath cuticle

Huxley's layer

Henle's layer

External root sheath

Glassy membrane

Root hair plexus

Duct of sebaceous gland

Hair shaft

Hair papilla

Hair Root

Free edge
Nail body
Lunula
Cuticle
Nail root

Pore

Excretory duct

Myoepithelial cell

Dark cell

Clear cell

Secretory portion

Eccrine Sweat Gland

Secretory components of **eccrine sweat glands** consist of simple cuboidal epithelium composed of **dark cells**, **clear cells**, and **myoepithelial cells**. The **ducts** of these glands are composed of a stratified cuboidal (two layers of cuboidal cells) epithelium.

Sebaceous cell

Sebaceous Gland

Hair follicle

Sebaceous glands are branched acinar holocrine glands whose short ducts empty into a hair follicle into the space created by the disappearance of the internal root sheath.

PLATE 11-1 · Thick Skin

FIGURE 1. Thick skin. Paraffin section. ×132.

Skin is composed of the superficial epidermis (E) and the deeper **dermis** (D). The interface of the two tissues is demarcated by **epidermal ridges** (ER) and **dermal ridges** (DR) (dermal papillae). Between successive epidermal ridges are the interpapillary pegs, which divide each dermal ridge into secondary dermal ridges. Note that in thick skin the keratinized layer, **stratum corneum** (SC), is highly developed. Observe also that the **duct** (d) of the sweat gland pierces the base of an epidermal ridge. The dermis of skin is subdivided into two regions, a **papillary layer** (PL), composed of the looser, collagenous connective tissue of the dermal ridges, and the deeper, denser, collagenous connective tissue of the **reticular layer** (RL). **Blood vessels** (BV) from the reticular layer enter the dermal ridges.

FIGURE 3. Thick skin. Monkey. Plastic section. ×540.

This is a higher magnification of a region similar to the *boxed area* in the previous figure. The papillary layer (PL) of the dermis displays **nuclei** (N) of the various connective tissue cells as well as the interface between the dermis and the **stratum basale** (SB). Observe that these cells are cuboidal to columnar in shape, and interspersed among them are occasional clear cells, probably inactive **melanocytes** (M), although it should be stressed that Merkel cells also appear as clear cells. Cells of the **stratum spinosum** (SS) are polyhedral in shape, possessing numerous intercellular bridges, which interdigitate with those of other cells, accounting for their spiny appearance.

FIGURE 2. Thick skin. Monkey. Plastic section. ×132.

This photomicrograph of thick skin presents a view similar to that in Figure 1. However, the layers of the epidermis (E) are much easier to delineate in this plastic section. Observe that the squames of the **stratum corneum** (SC) appear to lie directly on the **stratum granulosum** (SG), whose cells contain keratohyalin granules. The thickest layer of lining cells in the epidermis is the **stratum spinosum** (SS), whereas the **stratum basale** (SB) is only a single cell layer thick. The stratum lucidum is not evident, although a few transitional cells (*arrows*) may be identified. Note that the **secondary dermal ridges** (SDR), on either side of the **interpapillary peg** (IP), present **capillary loops** (CL). Regions similar to the *boxed areas* are presented in Figures 3 and 4 at higher magnification.

FIGURE 4. Thick skin. Monkey. Plastic section. ×540.

This is a higher magnification of a region similar to the *boxed area* of Figure 2. Observe that as the cells of the stratum spinosum (SS) are being pushed surfaceward, they become somewhat flattened. As the cells reach the **stratum granulosum** (SG), they accumulate keratohyalin granules (*arrows*), which increase in number as the cells progress through this layer. Occasional transitional cells (*arrowheads*) of the poorly defined stratum lucidum may be observed as well as the **squames** (S) of the **stratum corneum** (SC). *Inset.* **Thick skin. Paraffin section.** ×132. This photomicrograph displays the **stratum lucidum** (SL) to advantage. Note that this layer is between the **stratum granulosum** (SG) and **stratum corneum** (SC). Observe the **duct** (d) of a sweat gland.

KEY

BV	blood vessel	IP	interpapillary peg	SDR	secondary dermal ridges
CL	capillary loop	M	melanocytes	SG	stratum granulosum
D	dermis	N	nucleus	SB	stratum basale
d	duct	PL	papillary layer	SS	stratum spinosum
DR	dermal ridges	RL	reticular layer	S	squames
E	epidermis	SC	stratum corneum	SL	stratum lucidum
ER	epidermal ridges				

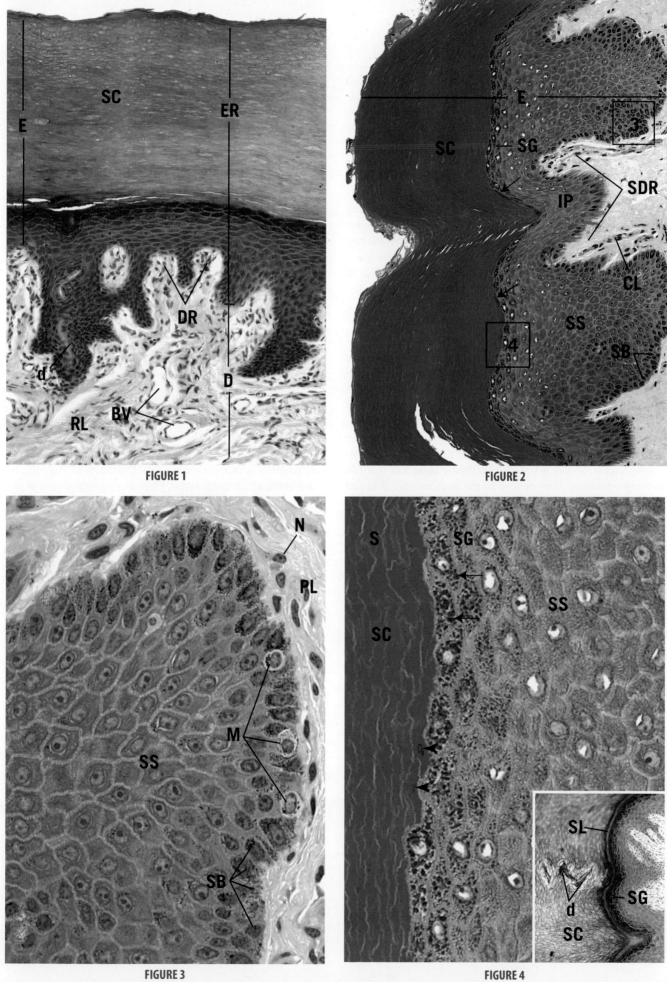

PLATE 11-1 · Thick Skin

FIGURE 1

FIGURE 2

FIGURE 3

FIGURE 4

PLATE 11-2 · Thin Skin

FIGURE 1. Thin skin. Human. Paraffin section. ×19.

Thin skin is composed of a very slender layer of epidermis (E) and the underlying **dermis** (D). Although thick skin has no hair follicles and sebaceous glands associated with it, most thin skin is richly endowed with both. Observe the **hair** (H) and the **hair follicles** (HF), whose expanded **bulb** (B) presents the connective tissue **papilla** (P). Much of the follicle is embedded beneath the skin in the superficial fascia, the fatty connective tissue layer known as the **hypodermis** (hD), which is not a part of the integument. **Sebaceous glands** (sG) secrete their sebum into short **ducts** (d), which empty into the lumen of the hair follicle. Smooth muscle bundles, **arrector pili muscle** (AP), cradle these glands, in passing from the hair follicle to the papillary layer of the dermis. **Sweat glands** (swG) are also present in the reticular layer of the dermis. A region similar to the *boxed area* is presented at a higher magnification in Figure 2.

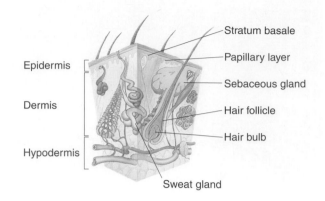

FIGURE 2. Thin skin. Human. Paraffin section. ×132.

This is a higher magnification of a region similar to the *boxed area* of the previous figure. Observe that the **epidermis** (E) is much thinner than that of thick skin and that the **stratum corneum** (SC) is significantly reduced. The epidermal ridges and **interpapillary pegs** (IP) are well represented in this photomicrograph. Note that the **papillary layer** (PL) of the dermis is composed of much finer bundles of **collagen fibers** (CF) than those of the dense irregular collagenous connective tissue of the **reticular layer** (RL). The dermis is quite vascular, as evidenced by the large number of **blood vessels** (BV) whose cross-sectional profiles are readily observed. The numerous **nuclei** (N) of the various connective tissue cells attest to the cellularity of the dermis. Note also the presence of the **arrector pili muscle** (AP), whose contraction elevates the hair and is responsible for the appearance of "goose bumps." The *boxed area* is presented at a higher magnification in the following figure.

FIGURE 3. Thin skin. Human. Paraffin section. ×270.

This photomicrograph is a higher magnification of the *boxed area* of Figure 2. Epidermis of thin skin possesses only three of four of the layers found in thick skin. The stratum basale (SB) is present as a single layer of cuboidal to columnar cells. Most of the epidermis is composed of the prickle cells of the **stratum spinosum** (SS), whereas stratum granulosum and stratum lucidum are not represented as complete layers. However, individual cells of stratum granulosum (*arrow*) and stratum lucidum are scattered at the interface of the stratum spinosum and **stratum corneum** (SC). The papillary layer of the **dermis** (D) is richly vascularized by **capillary loops** (CL), which penetrate the **secondary dermal ridges** (sDR). Observe that the **collagen fiber** (CF) bundles of the dermis become coarser as the distance from the epidermis increases.

KEY

AP	arrector pili muscle	H	hair	RL	reticular layer
B	bulb	hD	hypodermis	SC	stratum corneum
BV	blood vessels	HF	hair follicles	sDR	secondary dermal ridges
CF	collagen fibers	IP	interpapillary peg	sG	sebaceous glands
CL	capillary loops	N	nuclei	SB	stratum basale
D	dermis	P	papilla	SS	stratum spinosum
d	ducts	PL	papillary layer	swG	sweat glands
E	epidermis				

PLATE 11-2 • Thin Skin

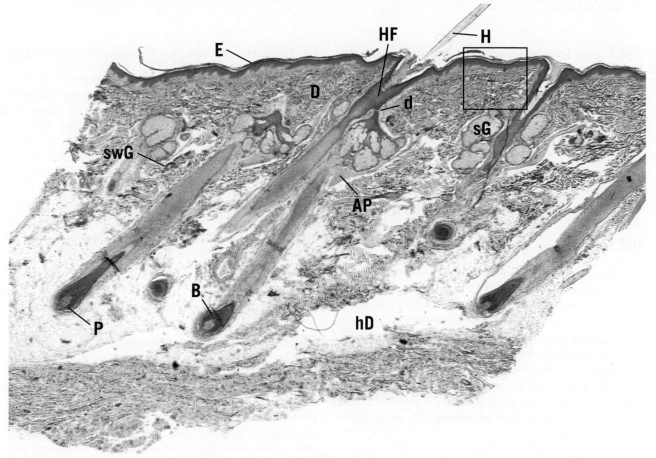

FIGURE 1

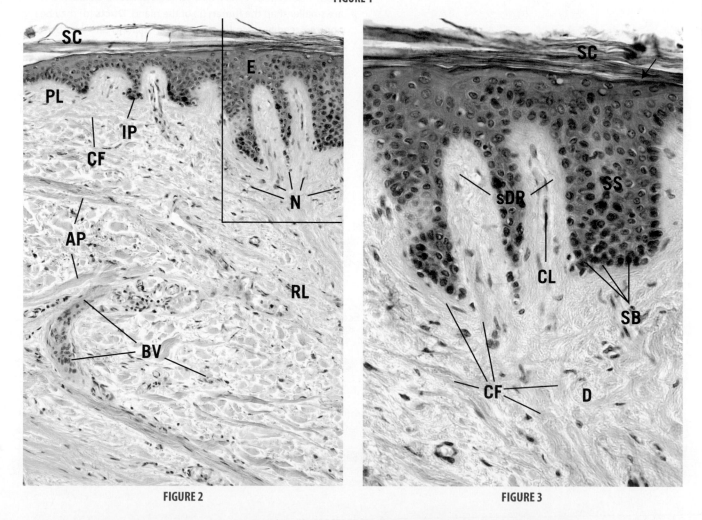

FIGURE 2

FIGURE 3

PLATE 11-3 · Hair Follicles and Associated Structures, Sweat Glands

FIGURE 1. Hair follicle. l.s. Human. Paraffin section. ×132.

The terminal expansion of the hair follicle, known as the bulb, is composed of a connective tissue, papilla (P), enveloped by epithelially derived cells of the **hair root** (HR). The mitotic activity responsible for the growth of hair occurs in the matrix, from which several concentric sheaths of epithelial cells emerge to be surrounded by a **connective tissue sheath** (CTS). Color of hair is due to the intracellular pigment that accounts for the dark appearance of some cells (*arrow*).

FIGURE 3. Sebaceous gland. Human. Paraffin section. ×132.

Sebaceous glands (sG) are branched, acinar holocrine glands, which produce an oily sebum. The secretion of these glands is delivered into the lumen of a **hair follicle** (HF), with which sebaceous glands are associated. **Basal cells** (BC), located at the periphery of the gland, undergo mitotic activity to replenish the dead cells, which, in holocrine glands, become the secretory product. Note that as these cells accumulate sebum in their cytoplasm, they degenerate, as evidenced by the gradual pyknosis of their **nuclei** (N). Observe the **arrector pili muscle** (AP), which cradles the sebaceous glands.

FIGURE 2. Hair follicle. x.s. Human. Paraffin section. ×132.

Many of the layers comprising the growing hair follicle may be observed in these cross sections. The entire structure is surrounded by a connective tissue sheath (CTS), which is separated from the epithelially derived components by a specialized basement membrane, the **inner glassy membrane** (BM). The clear polyhedral cells compose the **external root sheath** (ERS), which surrounds the **internal root sheath** (IRS), whose cells become keratinized. At the neck of the hair follicle, where the ducts of the sebaceous glands enter, the internal root sheath disintegrates, providing a lumen into which sebum and apocrine sweat are discharged. The **cuticle** (Cu) and **cortex** (Co) constitute the highly keratinized components of the hair, whereas the medulla is not visible at this magnification. Note the presence of **arrector pili muscle** (AP).

FIGURE 4. Sweat gland. Monkey. Plastic section. ×132.

The simple, coiled, tubular eccrine gland is divided into two compartments: a secretory portion (s) and a **duct** (d). The secretory portion of the gland consists of a simple cuboidal epithelium, composed of dark and clear secretory cells (which cannot be distinguished from each other unless special procedures are utilized). Intercellular canaliculi are noted between clear cells, which are smaller than the **lumen** (L) of the gland. **Ducts** (d) may be recognized readily since they are darker staining and composed of stratified cuboidal epithelium. *Insets a and b.* **Duct and secretory unit. Monkey. Plastic section.** ×540. The duct is readily evident, since its **lumen** (L) is surrounded by two layers of cuboidal cells. **Secretory cells** (s) of the eccrine sweat gland are surrounded by darker-staining **myoepithelial cells** (My). Hair root, eccrine sweat gland, and sebaceous gland.

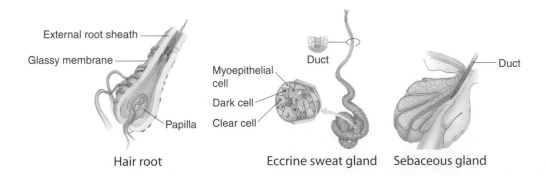

Hair root   Eccrine sweat gland   Sebaceous gland

KEY

AP	arrector pili muscle	**d**	ducts	**L**	lumen
BC	basal cells	**ERS**	external root sheath	**My**	myoepithelial cells
BM	inner glassy membrane	**HF**	hair follicle	**N**	nucleus
Co	cortex	**HR**	hair root	**P**	papilla
CTS	connective tissue sheath	**IRS**	internal root sheath	**s**	secretory
Cu	cuticle			**sG**	sebaceous glands

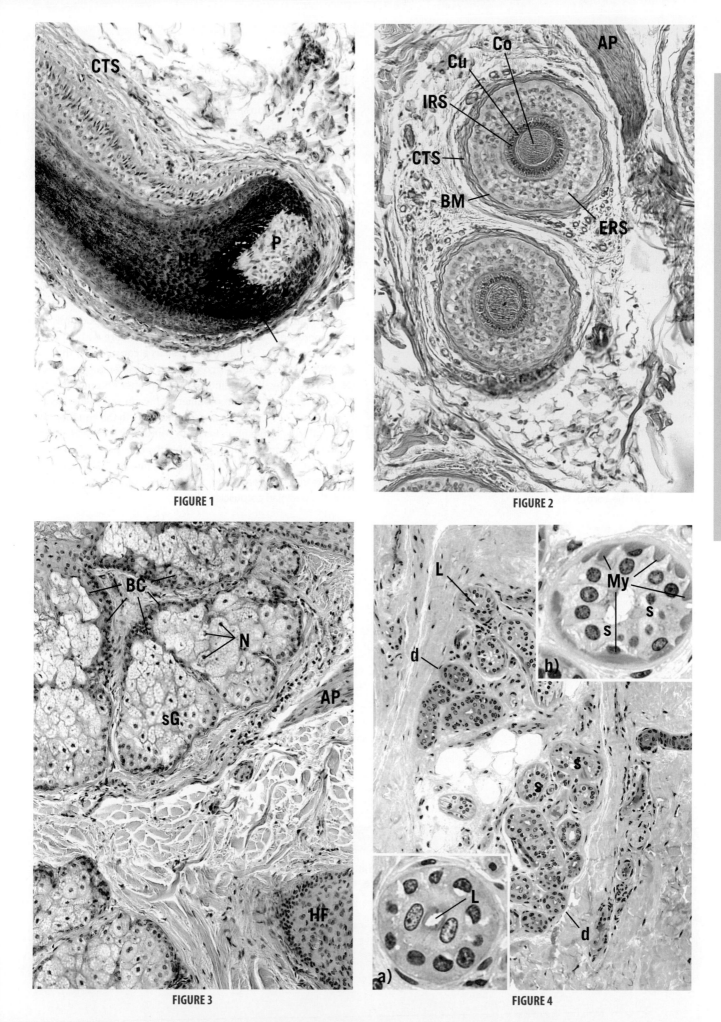

PLATE 11-3 · Hair Follicles and Associated Structures, Sweat Glands

FIGURE 1

FIGURE 2

FIGURE 3

FIGURE 4

PLATE 11-4 · Nail, Pacinian and Meissner's Corpuscles

FIGURE 1. Fingernail. l.s. Paraffin section. ×14.

The nail is a highly keratinized structure that is located on the dorsal surface of the **distal phalanx** (Ph) of each finger and toe. The horny **nail plate** (NP) extends deep into the dermis, forming the **nail root** (NR). The epidermis of the distal phalanx forms a continuous fold, resulting in the **eponychium** (Ep) or cuticle, the **nail bed** (NB) underlying the nail plate, and the **hyponychium** (Hy). The epithelium (*arrow*) surrounding the nail root is responsible for the continuous elongation of the nail. The **dermis** (D) between the nail bed and the **bone** (Bo) of the distal phalanx is tightly secured to the **fibrous periosteum** (FP). Note that this is a developing finger, as evidenced by the presence of **hyaline cartilage** (HC) and endochondral osteogenesis (*arrowheads*).

FIGURE 3. Meissner's corpuscle. Paraffin section. ×540.

Meissner's corpuscles are oval, encapsulated mechanoreceptors lying in dermal ridges just deep to the stratum basale (SB). They are especially prominent in the genital areas, lips, fingertips, and soles of the feet. A connective tissue **capsule** (Ca) envelops the corpuscle. The **nuclei** (N) within the corpuscle belong to flattened (probably modified) Schwann cells, which are arranged horizontally in this structure. The afferent **nerve fiber** (NF) pierces the base of Meissner's corpuscle, branches, and follows a tortuous course within the corpuscle.

FIGURE 2. Fingernail. x.s. Paraffin section. ×14.

The **nail plate** (NP) in cross section presents a convex appearance. On either side, it is bordered by a **nail wall** (NW), and the groove it occupies is referred to as the lateral **nail groove** (NG). The **nail bed** (NB) is analogous to four layers of the epidermis, whereas the nail plate represents the stratum corneum. The **dermis** (D), deep to the nail bed, is firmly attached to the **fibrous periosteum** (FP) of the **bone** (Bo) of the terminal phalanx. Observe that the fingertip is covered by thick skin whose **stratum corneum** (SC) is extremely well developed. The small, darkly staining structures in the dermis are **sweat glands** (swG).

FIGURE 4. Pacinian corpuscle. Paraffin section. ×132.

Pacinian corpuscles, located in the dermis and hypodermis, are mechanoreceptors. They are composed of a **core** with an **inner** (IC) and an **outer** (OC) region, as well as a **capsule** (Ca) that surrounds the core. The inner core invests the afferent **nerve fiber** (NF), which loses its myelin sheath soon after entering the corpuscle. The core cells are modified Schwann cells, whereas the components of the capsule are continuous with the endoneurium of the afferent nerve fiber. Pacinian corpuscles are readily recognizable in section since they resemble the cut surface of an onion. Observe the presence of an **arrector pili muscle** (AP) and profiles of **ducts** (d) of a sweat gland in the vicinity of, but not associated with, the pacinian corpuscle.

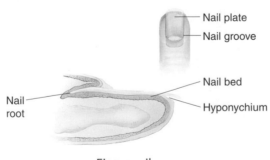

Fingernail

KEY

AP	arrector pili	**Hy**	hyponychium	**NW**	nail wall
Ca	capsule	**IC**	inner core	**OC**	outer core
Bo	bone	**N**	nuclei	**Ph**	distal phalanx
D	dermis	**NB**	nail bed	**SC**	stratum corneum
d	duct	**NF**	nerve fiber	**SB**	stratum basale
Ep	eponychium	**NG**	nail groove	**swG**	sweat glands
FP	fibrous periosteum	**NP**	nail plate		
HC	hyaline cartilage	**NR**	nail root		

PLATE 11-4 • Nail, Pacinian and Meissner's Corpuscles

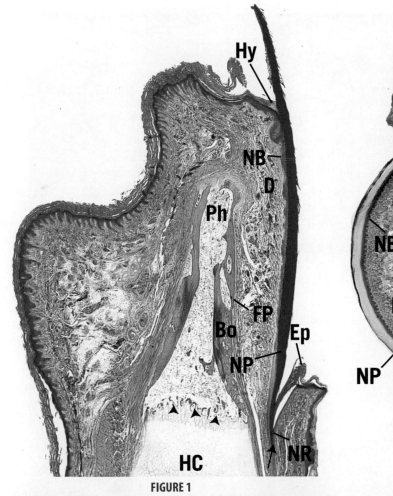

FIGURE 1

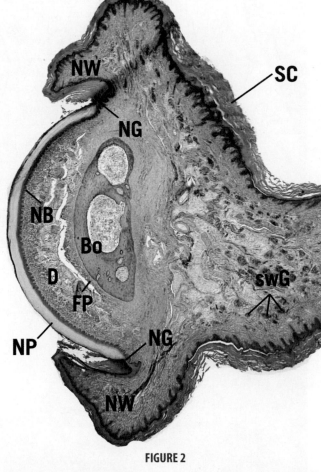

FIGURE 2

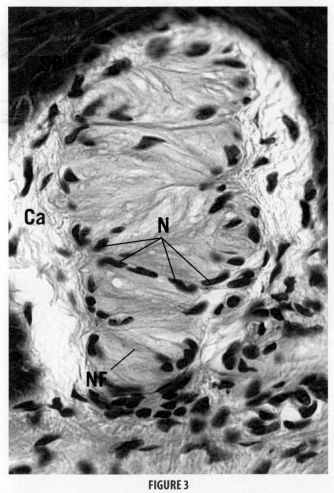

FIGURE 3

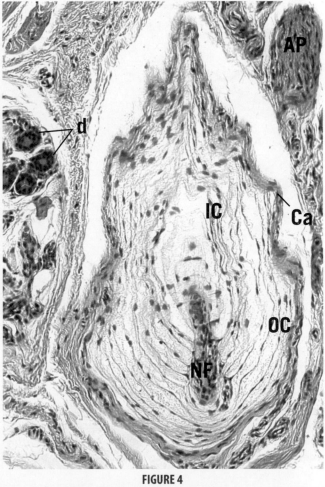

FIGURE 4

PLATE 11-5 · Sweat Gland, Electron Microscopy

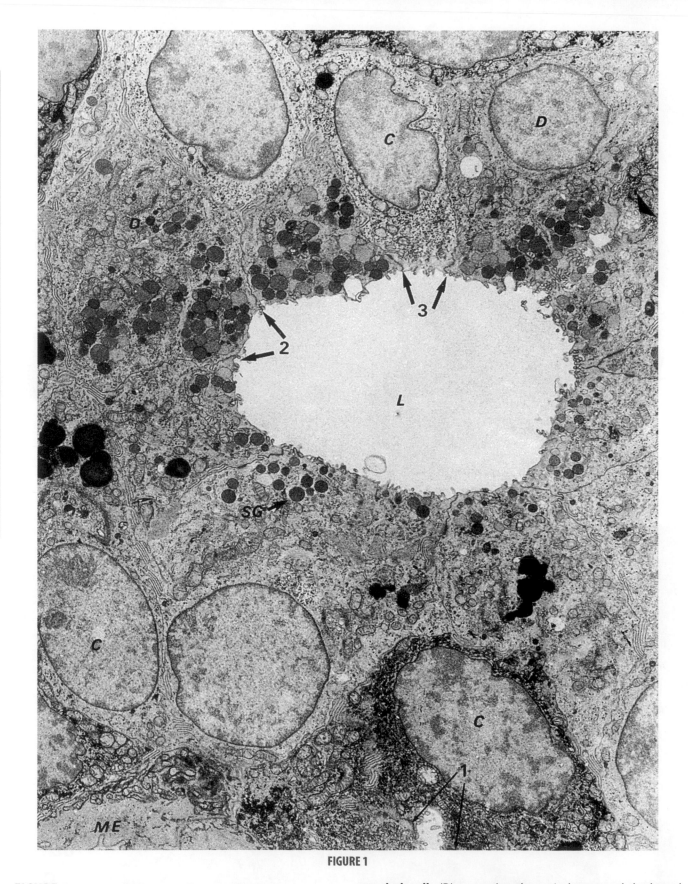

FIGURE 1

FIGURE 1. Sweat gland. x.s. Human. Electron microscopy. ×5,040.

Tight junctions (*arrows*) occur at three locations in the secretory coil of human sweat glands: (1) between **clear cells** (C) separating the lumen of the intercellular canaliculus (*arrowhead*) and the basolateral intercellular space, (2) between two **dark cells** (D) separating the main lumen and the lateral intercellular space, and (3) between a clear cell and a dark cell, separating the main lumen (L) and intercellular space. Note the presence of **secretory granules** (SG) and **myoepithelial cell** (ME). (From Briggman JV, Bank HL, Bigelow JB, et al. Structure of the tight junctions of the human eccrine sweat gland. Am J Anat 1981;162:357–368.)

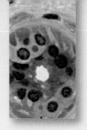

Chapter Summary

I. SKIN

A. Epidermis

The **epidermis** constitutes the superficial, epithelially derived region of skin. It is composed of four cell types: **keratinocytes, melanocytes, Langerhans cells,** and **Merkel cells.** The keratinocytes are arranged in five layers, and the remaining three cell types are interspersed among them. The five layers of the epidermis are

1. Stratum Basale

A single layer of cuboidal to columnar cells that stand on the **basement membrane.** This is a region of cell division. It also contains **melanocytes** and **Merkel cells.**

2. Stratum Spinosum

Composed of many layers of polyhedral **prickle cells** bearing **intercellular bridges.** Mitotic activity is also present. It also contains **Langerhans cells** and processes of **melanocytes.**

3. Stratum Granulosum

Cells that are somewhat flattened and contain **keratohyalin granules.** It is absent as a distinct layer in thin skin.

4. Stratum Lucidum

A thin, translucent layer that is also absent in thin skin.

5. Stratum Corneum

Composed of **squames** packed with **keratin.** Superficial squames are desquamated.

B. Dermis

The **dermis** is a **dense, irregular, collagenous connective tissue** subdivided into two layers: papillary and reticular.

1. Papillary Layer

The **dermal ridges** (dermal papillae) and **secondary dermal ridges** interdigitate with the **epidermal ridges** (and **interpapillary pegs**) of the epidermis. **Collagen fibers** are slender in comparison with those of deeper layers of the dermis. Dermal ridges house **capillary loops** and **Meissner's corpuscles.**

2. Reticular Layer

The **reticular layer** of skin is composed of coarse bundles of collagen fibers. It supports a **vascular plexus** and interdigitates with the underlying **hypodermis.** Frequently, it houses **hair follicles, sebaceous glands,** and **sweat glands. Krause's end bulbs** and **pacinian corpuscles** may also be present.

II. APPENDAGES

A. Hair

Hair is an **epidermal** downgrowth embedded into dermis or hypodermis. It has a free **shaft** surrounded by several layers of cylindrical sheaths of cells. The terminal end of the hair follicle is expanded as the **hair bulb,** composed of connective tissue **papilla** and the **hair root.** The concentric layers of the follicle are

1. Connective Tissue Sheath

2. Glassy Membrane

A modified basement membrane.

3. External Root Sheath

Composed of a few layers of polyhedral cells and a single layer of columnar cells.

4. Internal Root Sheath

Composed of three layers: **Henle's layer, Huxley's layer,** and the **cuticle.** The internal root sheath stops at the neck of the follicle, where sebaceous gland ducts open into the hair follicle, forming a **lumen** into which the sebum is delivered.

5. Cuticle of the Hair

Composed of highly keratinized cells that overlap each other.

6. Cortex

The bulk of the hair, composed of highly keratinized cells.

7. Medulla

A thin core of the hair whose cells contain soft keratin.

B. Sebaceous Glands

Sebaceous glands are in the forms of **saccules** associated with hair follicles. They are **branched alveolar holocrine glands** that produce an oily **sebum.** Secretions are delivered into the neck of the hair follicle via short, wide **ducts. Basal cells** are regenerative cells of sebaceous glands, located at the periphery of the **saccule.**

C. Arrector Pili Muscle

Arrector pili muscles are bundles of smooth muscle cells extending from the **hair follicle** to the **papillary layer** of the dermis. They cradle the **sebaceous gland**. Contractions of these muscle fibers elevate the hair, forming "goose bumps," release heat, and assist in the delivery of sebum from the gland into its duct.

D. Sweat Glands

1. Sweat Glands

Simple, coiled, tubular glands whose **secretory portion** is composed of a simple cuboidal epithelium. **Dark cells** and **light cells** are present with **intercellular canaliculi** between cells. **Myoepithelial cells** surround the secretory portion.

2. Ducts

Composed of a stratified cuboidal (two-cell-thick) epithelium. Cells of the duct are darker and smaller than those of the secretory portions. Ducts pierce the base of the epidermal ridges to deliver sweat to the outside.

E. Nail

The horny **nail plate** sits on the **nail bed**. It is bordered laterally by the **nail wall**, the base of which forms the **lateral nail groove**. The **eponychium** (cuticle) is above the nail plate. The **hyponychium** is located below the free end of the nail plate. The posterior aspect of the nail plate is the **nail root**, which lies above the **matrix**, the area responsible for the growth of the nail.

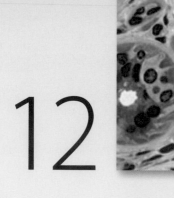

12 RESPIRATORY SYSTEM

The respiratory system functions in exchanging carbon dioxide for oxygen, which is then distributed to all of the tissues of the body. To accomplish this function, air must be brought to that portion of the respiratory system where exchange of gases can occur. The respiratory system, therefore, has two portions:

- **conducting portion**
- **respiratory portion**.

Some of the larger conduits of the conducting portion are extrapulmonary, whereas its smaller components are intrapulmonary. The respiratory portions, however, are completely intrapulmonary. The luminal diameters of the various conduits can be modified by the presence of smooth muscle cells along their length (Table 12-1).

CONDUCTING PORTION OF THE RESPIRATORY SYSTEM

The extrapulmonary region of the conducting portion consists of the nasal cavities, pharynx, larynx, trachea, and bronchi. The intrapulmonary region entails the intrapulmonary bronchi, bronchioles, and terminal bronchioles (see Graphic 12-1).

Extrapulmonary Region

The mucosa of the extrapulmonary region of the conducting portion modifies the inspired air by humidifying, cleansing, and adjusting its temperature. This **mucosa** is composed of

- **pseudostratified ciliated columnar epithelium** (respiratory epithelium) with numerous **goblet cells** and an
- underlying **connective tissue sheath** that is well endowed with **seromucous glands**.

Modulation of the temperature of the inspired air is accomplished mostly in the **nasal cavity** by the rich vascularity of the connective tissue just deep to its respiratory epithelium.

Nasal Cavity and Olfaction

In certain areas, the mucosa of the nasal cavity is modified to function in **olfaction** and is referred to as the **olfactory mucosa**. The glands in the lamina propria of this region, known as **Bowman's glands**, produce a thin mucous secretion that dissolves odoriferous substances, and the **olfactory cells** of the pseudostratified columnar olfactory epithelium perceive these sensory stimuli. Olfactory cells are

- **bipolar neurons** whose receptor ends are modified, nonmotile **cilia** that arise from a swelling, the **olfactory vesicle**, and extend into the overlying mucus. The axon

of each olfactory cell arises from the basal end of the cell and passes through the cribriform plate at the roof of the nasal cavity to enter the floor of the cranial cavity to synapse with **mitral cells** of the **olfactory bulb**. Each olfactory cell lives approximately for 4 months.

- **Odorant binding proteins** (integral membrane proteins that are odorant receptors) lying within the plasma membrane of the cilia are sensitive to molecules of specific odor groups, where each of these molecules is known as an **odorant**.
  - When an odorant binds to its corresponding odorant receptor, one of two possibilities occurs.
    - The receptor itself may be a **gated ion channel**, and, upon binding the odorant, the ion channel opens or
    - the bound receptor activates **adenylate cyclase**, causing the formation of cAMP, which, in turn, facilitates the opening of ion channels.
  - The opening of the ion channel results in ion flow into the cell with subsequent **depolarization** of the plasmalemma, and the olfactory cell becomes **excited**.
  - The action potentials generated by the depolarizations of the olfactory cells are transmitted, via synaptic contacts, to the mitral cells of the olfactory bulbs.
  - The axons of the mitral cells form the olfactory tract, which transmits signals to the amygdala of the brainstem.
  - The odorant must satisfy at least three requirements: it must be **volatile**, **water soluble**, and **lipid soluble,** so that it can:
    - enter the nasal cavity (volatility),
    - penetrate the mucus (water solubility), and
    - have access to the phospholipid membrane (lipid solubility).
- In addition to the olfactory cells, two other cell types compose the olfactory epithelium, namely, sustentacular cells (supporting cells) and basal cells.
  - **Sustentacular cells** do not possess any sensory function, but they manufacture a yellowish-brown pigment that is responsible for the coloration of the olfactory mucosa; additionally, they insulate and support the olfactory cells.
  - **Basal cells** are small, dark cells that lie on the basement membrane and probably are regenerative in function forming sustentacular, olfactory, as well as more basal cells.

Axons of the **olfactory cells** are collected into small nerve bundles that pass through the cribriform plate of the ethmoid bone as the **first cranial nerve**, the **olfactory nerve**. Thus, it should be noted that the cell bodies of the olfactory nerve (cranial nerve I) are located in a rather vulnerable place, in the surface epithelium lining the nasal cavity.

TABLE 12-1 • Summary Table of Respiratory System

Division	Region	Skeleton	Glands	Epithelium	Cilia	Goblet Cells	Special Features
Nasal cavity	Vestibule	Hyaline cartilage	Sebaceous and sweat glands	Stratified squamous keratinized	No	No	Vibrissae
	Respiratory	Bone and hyaline cartilage	Seromucous	Pseudostratified columnar	Yes	Yes	Large venous plexus
	Olfactory	Nasal conchae (bone)	Bowman's glands	Pseudostratified ciliated columnar	Yes	No	Basal cells, sustentacular cells, olfactory cells, nerve fibers
Pharynx	Nasal	Muscle	Seromucous glands	Pseudostratified ciliated columnar	Yes	Yes	Pharyngeal tonsil, eustachian tube
	Oral	Muscle	Seromucous glands	Stratified squamous nonkeratinized	No	No	Palatine tonsils
Larynx		Hyaline and elastic cartilage	Mucous and seromucous glands	Stratified squamous nonkeratinized and pseudostratified ciliated columnar	Yes	Yes	Vocal cords, epiglottis, some taste buds
Trachea and extrapulmonary (primary bronchi)		C-rings of hyaline cartilage	Mucous and seromucous glands	Pseudostratified ciliated columnar	Yes	Yes	Trachealis muscle, elastic lamina
Intrapulmonary conducting	Secondary bronchi	Plates of hyaline cartilage	Seromucous glands	Pseudostratified ciliated columnar	Yes	Yes	Two helical-oriented ribbons of smooth muscle
	Bronchioles	Smooth muscle	None	Simple columnar to simple cuboidal	Yes	Only in larger bronchioles	Clara cells
	Terminal bronchile	Smooth muscle	None	Simple cuboidal	Some	None	<0.5 mm in diameter, Clara cells
Respiratory	Respiratory bronchiole	Some smooth muscle	None	Simple cuboidal and simple squamous	Some	None	Outpocketings of alveoli
	Alveolar duct	None	None	Simple squamous	None	None	Outpocketings of alveoli; type I pneumocytes, type II pneumocytes, dust cells
	Alveolus	None	None	Simple squamous	None	None	Type I pneumocytes, type II pneumocytes, dust cells

Larynx and Trachea

The conducting portion of the respiratory system is supported by a skeleton composed of bone and/or cartilage that assists in the maintenance of a patent lumen, whose diameters are controlled by smooth muscle cells located in their walls.

- The **larynx**, a region of the conducting portion, is designed for phonation and to prevent food, liquids, and other foreign objects from gaining access to its lumen.
  - It is composed of three paired and three unpaired cartilages, numerous extrinsic and intrinsic muscles, and several ligaments.
  - The actions of these muscles on the cartilages and ligaments modulate the tension and positioning of the vocal folds, thus permitting variations in the pitch of the sound being produced.
  - The lumen of the **larynx** is subdivided into three compartments: **vestibule**, **ventricle**, and **infraglottic cavity**.
- The **trachea,** continuous with the lumen of the infraglottic cavity, is supported by 15 to 20 **C-rings**, horseshoe-shaped segments of **hyaline cartilage**. The trachea has three layers, the mucosa, submucosa, and adventitia. It is the adventitia that houses the C-rings, whose open ends face posteriorly and are connected by a smooth muscle slip, the **trachealis muscle**. Contraction of this muscle reduces the lumen of the trachea, thus increasing the velocity of air flow.
  - The tracheal lumen is lined by a pseudostratified ciliated columnar epithelium, known as respiratory epithelium. This epithelium is composed of various cell types, namely, goblet cells, ciliated cells, basal cells, brush cells, serous cells, and hormone-producing diffuse neuroendocrine system (DNES) cells.
    - **Goblet cells** constitute about 30% of the epithelial cells. Goblet cells are unicellular glands that produce **mucinogen**, a mucous substance that is released onto the wet epithelial surface where it becomes hydrated to form **mucin**. Once particular substances located in the tracheal lumen are intermixed with mucin, that viscous material becomes known as **mucus**.
    - **Ciliated cells** also compose about 30% of the cell population. They are tall, ciliated cells whose cilia sweep the mucus toward the larynx.
    - **Basal cells** also constitute approximately 30% of the epithelial cell population. They are regenerative cells that function in replacing the epithelial lining of the trachea.
    - **Brush cells** form only 3% of the cell population of the respiratory epithelium. They possess small mucinogen-containing granules in their cytoplasm and long microvilli that reach into lumen of the trachea. Brush cells may have neurosensory functions or they may be defunct goblet cells that released their mucinogen.
    - **Serous cells** are tall, columnar cells whose cytoplasm houses small vesicles containing a serous secretion whose function is not understood. Serous cells form 3% of the epithelial cell population.
    - **DNES cells** constitute 3% to 4% of the epithelial cell population, and they form polypeptide hormones that they store in small granules localized in their basal cytoplams. When released, these hormones may act locally (paracrine hormones) or at a distance (hormones) to regulate respiratory functions. Nerve fibers often contact many of these DNES cells, to form structures, known as **pulmonary neuroepithelial bodies**, that by monitoring local hypoxic conditions can alert the brain's respiratory center to increase respiration.
  - The trachea subdivides into the two primary bronchi that lead to the right and the left lungs.

Intrapulmonary Region

The intrapulmonary region is composed of **intrapulmonary bronchi** (secondary bronchi), whose walls are supported by irregular plates of hyaline cartilage.

- Each intrapulmonary bronchus gives rise to several **bronchioles**, tubes of decreasing diameter that do not possess a cartilaginous supporting skeleton.
  - The epithelial lining of the larger bronchioles is ciliated with a few goblet cells, but those of smaller bronchioles are simple columnar, with goblet cells being replaced by **Clara cells**. Moreover, the thickness of their walls also decreases, as does the luminal diameter.
  - The last region of the conduction portion is composed of **terminal bronchioles,** whose mucosa is further decreased in thickness and complexity. The patency of those airways whose walls do not possess a cartilaginous support is maintained by elastic fibers that radiate from their periphery and intermingle with elastic fibers emanating from nearby structures.

RESPIRATORY PORTION OF THE RESPIRATORY SYSTEM

The respiratory portion of the respiratory system begins with branches of the terminal bronchiole known as **respiratory bronchioles** (see Graphic 12-2).

- Respiratory bronchioles are very similar to terminal bronchioles except that they possess outpocketings

TABLE 12-2 • Components of the Blood-Air Barrier		
Endothelial Component	**Epithelial and Pneumocyte Component**	**Pneumocyte Component**
Attenuated endothelial cell	Combined basal laminae	Attenuated pneumocyte I Surfactant and fluid coating of the alveolus

known as **alveoli**, structures whose thin walls permit gaseous exchange.

- Respiratory bronchioles lead to **alveolar ducts**, each of which ends in an expanded region known as an **alveolar sac**, with each sac being composed of a number of alveoli. The epithelium of alveolar sacs and alveoli is composed of two types of cells:
  - highly attenuated **type I pneumocytes**, which form much of the lining of the alveolus and alveolar sac, and
  - **type II pneumocytes**, are cells that
    - manufacture **surfactant**, a phospholipid that reduces surface tension of the alveolar surface
    - enter the cell cycle to form more type I and type II pneumocytes.

Associated with the respiratory portion of the lungs is an extremely rich capillary network, supplied by the pulmonary arteries and drained by the pulmonary veins.

- The **capillaries** invest each alveolus, and their highly attenuated nonfenestrated, continuous endothelial cells closely approximate the type I pneumocytes.
- In many areas, the basal laminae of the type I pneumocytes and endothelial cells fuse into a single basal lamina, providing for a minimal **blood-air barrier**, thus facilitating the exchange of gases (see Table 12-2).

Since the lung contains about 300 million alveoli with a total surface area of approximately 75 m², these small spaces that crowd against each other are separated from one another by walls of various thicknesses known as **interalveolar septa**.

- The thinnest of these interalveolar septa often presents communicating **alveolar pores**, whereby air may pass between alveoli.
- A somewhat thicker septum may possess intervening connective tissue elements that may be as slender as a capillary with its attendant basal lamina, or it may have collagen and elastic fibers as well as smooth muscle fibers and connective tissue cells.
- Macrophages known as **dust cells** are often noted in interalveolar septa.
  - Dust cells are derived from **monocytes** and enter the lungs via the bloodstream.
  - Here, they mature and become extremely efficient scavengers. It is believed that dust cells are the most numerous of all cell types present in the lungs, even

though they are eliminated from the lungs at a rate of 50 million per day.

- Although it is not known whether they actively migrate to the bronchioles or reach it via fluid flow, it is known that they are transported from there within the mucus layer, via ciliary action of the respiratory epithelium, into the pharynx.
- Once they reach the pharynx, they are either expectorated or swallowed.

MECHANISM OF GASEOUS EXCHANGE (See Graphic 12-2)

The partial pressures of O_2 and CO_2 are responsible for the uptake or release of these gases by red blood cells (RBC) within the bloodstream. Since cells convert O_2 to CO_2 during their metabolism, the partial pressure of CO_2 is high in tissues, and every minute approximately 200 mL of this gas enters the bloodstream and is carried in the following manner:

- 20 mL dissolves in its molecular form in the plasma
- 40 mL forms a bond with the globin moiety of hemoglobin
- 140 mL is taken up by the RBC; within the RBC cytosol
  - where **carbonic anhydrase** catalyzes the formation of H_2CO_3 from H_2O and CO_2
  - H_2CO_3 dissociates to form H^+ and HCO_3^-.
    - HCO_3^- diffuses out of the erythrocyte cytosol into the plasma; in exchange
    - Cl^- enters the erythrocyte cytosol from the plasma, a process known as the **chloride shift**.

The converse is true in the alveoli of the lungs, where O_2 is taken up by RBC and CO_2 is released in the following manner:

- HCO_3^- **ions** enter the RBC cytosol from the plasma, and in order to maintain electrical neutrality,
  - Cl^- **ions** leave the RBC cytosol; therefore,
  - another **chloride shift** occurs but in a reverse direction
- HCO_3^- **ions** bind with H^+ **ions** to form H_2CO_3
- O_2 enters the RBC cytosol and binds to the **heme moiety** of hemoglobin

○ H_2CO_3 forms, with the assistance of the enzyme carbonic anhydrase, H_2O and CO_2

○ The CO_2 leaves the erythrocyte, enters the blood stream, and from there enters the alveolar air spaces and is exhaled.

MECHANISM OF RESPIRATION

The process of **inspiration** requires energy, in that it depends on the contraction of the **diaphragm** and elevation of the **ribs**, increasing the size of the **thoracic cavity**.

• The **visceral pleura** adheres to the lungs and is separated from the **parietal pleura** by the pleural cavity, that cavity is also enlarged, reducing the pressure within it.

• Pressure in the enlarged **pleural cavities** is less than the atmospheric pressure in the lungs, air enters the lungs (whose **elastic fibers** become stretched), and the volume of the pleural cavity is reduced.

Unlike inspiration, the process of **expiration** does not require energy, since it is dependent on **relaxation** of the muscles responsible for inspiration.

• As the muscles relax, the volume of the thoracic cage decreases, increasing the pressure inside the lung, which exceeds atmospheric pressure

• The stretched **elastic fibers** of the expanded lungs return to their **resting length**.

• These two forces drive the air out of the lungs.

CLINICAL CONSIDERATIONS

Hyaline Membrane Disease

Hyaline membrane disease is frequently observed in premature infants who lack adequate amounts of pulmonary surfactant. This disease is characterized by **labored breathing**, since a high alveolar surface tension, caused by inadequate levels of surfactant, makes it difficult to expand the alveoli. The administration of glucocorticoids prior to birth can induce synthesis of surfactant, thus circumventing the appearance of the disease.

Cystic Fibrosis

Although cystic fibrosis is viewed as a disease of the lungs, it is really a hereditary condition that alters the secretions of a number of glands, such as the liver, pancreas, salivary glands, sweat glands, and glands of the reproductive system. In the case of the lungs, liver, pancreas, and the intestines, the mucous secretions become abnormally thickened and block the lumina of these organs. In the respiratory system, the walls of the bronchioles thicken with the progression of the disease, areas of the lung become constricted, the thick secretions in the airways become infected, the lungs cease to function, and death ensues. In the most common type of cystic fibrosis, individuals possess two copies of the defective gene that code for altered ion channels, known as **cystic fibrosis transmembrane conductance regulator** (**CFTR**). In normal cells, the CFTR is embedded in the cell membrane and allows Cl^- ions to leave the cell, which decreases the salt concentration inside the cell, causing water molecules to also leave the cell. The water molecules then dilute the mucus that builds up outside the cell. The mucus can then be cleared from the extracellular space. In mutated cells the defective CFTR is either destroyed by the cell's proteasome system or is embedded in the cell membrane but remains shut so that Cl^- ions cannot leave the cell. Consequently, water does not leave the cell and the mucus becomes abnormally thick and viscous and cannot be cleared from the extracellular space. In the case of the small respiratory and terminal bronchioles as well as the larger elements of the conducting system of the respiratory system become clogged with mucus and the individual is unable to respire, succumbs to infections, and dies. Prior to the availability of antibiotics, most children with cystic fibrosis died in the first few years of life. However, with current treatment the median survival rate is 37 years of age.

Emphysema

Emphysema is a disease that results from **destruction of alveolar walls** with the consequent formation of large cyst-like sacs, reducing the surface available for gas exchange. Emphysema is marked by **decreased elasticity** of the lungs, which are unable to recoil adequately during expiration. It is associated with exposure to **cigarette smoke** and other substances that inhibit α_1-antitrypsin, a protein that normally protects the lungs from the action of elastase produced by alveolar macrophages. **Panacinar emphysema** is a form of emphysema characterized by a uniform damage to the respiratory bronchiole, alveolar ducts, alveolar sacs, and alveoli. The alveolar septa are almost completely destroyed and the lung tissue takes on a lacy appearance frequently referred to as "cotton candy lung."

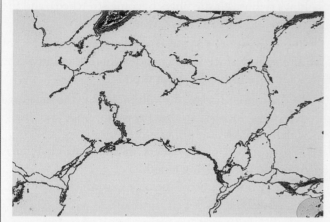

This figure is from the lung of a patient who had panacinar emphysema. Note the large air spaces and the absence of alveolar septa and the limited number of alveolar walls. (Reprinted with permission from Rubin R, Strayer D, et al., eds. Rubin's Pathology. Clinicopathologic Foundations of Medicine, 5th ed. Baltimore: Lippincott Williams & Wilkins, 2008. p. 515.)

Bronchial Asthma

Bronchial asthma is a condition in which the bronchi become partially and reversibly obstructed by airway spasm (**bronchoconstriction**), mast cell–induced inflammatory response to allergens and/or other stimuli that would not affect a normal lung, and the formation of excess mucus. Some of the most characteristic alterations are the hypertrophy of the bronchial smooth muscle coat as well as the increase in the submucosal mucous glands. Moreover, the epithelium loses its pseudostratified ciliated characteristic and assumes a squamous metaplastic appearance with an increase in basal cell and goblet cell numbers. The basal lamina is also increased in thickness, and the submucosa is edematous and infiltrated by eosinophils and other leukocytes. Asthma attacks vary with the individual; in some it is hardly noticed, whereas in others shortness of breath is very evident and wheezing accompanies breathing out. Most individuals who suffer from asthmatic conditions use nebulizers containing bronchodilators, such as albuterol, to relieve the attack.

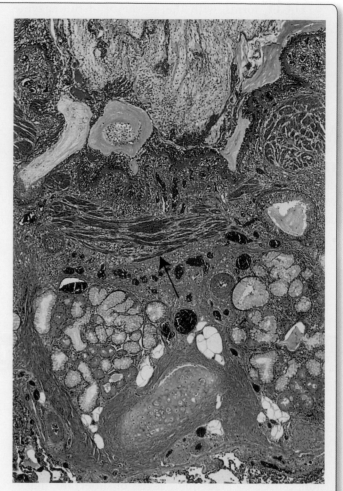

This figure is from the lung of a patient who died of asthma. Note that the lumen of the bronchus is obstructed by a mucous plug. The arrow indicates smooth muscle hyperplasia characteristic in advanced cases of asthma. (Reprinted with permission from Rubin R, Strayer D, et al., eds. Rubin's Pathology. Clinicopathologic Foundations of Medicine, 5th ed. Baltimore: Lippincott Williams & Wilkins, 2008. p. 518.)

Pneumonia

Pneumonia is a possibly lethal infection of the alveoli and the connective tissue elements of the lungs. In the United States, of the 2 million people who contract pneumonia annually, approximately 40 to 70,000 succumb to this disease. The infection is more dangerous to patients who are immunocompromised and/or suffering from chronic diseases. In third world countries, pneumonia and diarrhea-induced dehydration are the two most significant causes of death. There are numerous types of pneumonia depending on the causative agents, namely, bacterial, viral, or fungal, and the organism is either inhaled into the lungs or enters the lungs via the circulatory system. The principal diagnostic features of pneumonia are productive coughs, fever, chills, shallow breathing, hearing rasping sounds amplified by stethoscopes, and the presence of white foci in the lung as observed on chest x-rays.

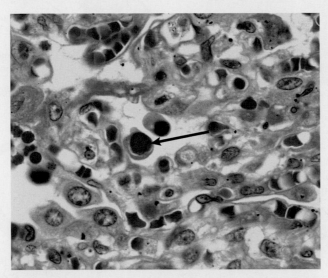

This figure is from the lung of a patient with adenovirus pneumonia. Note that the lumen of the alveolus houses cells with basophilic nuclear inclusions. These cells are referred to as "smudge cells" (*arrow*) and are characterized by a thin rim of cytoplasm surrounding the nucleus housing the basophilic inclusion. (Reprinted with permission from Rubin R, Strayer D, et al., eds. Rubin's Pathology. Clinicopathologic Foundations of Medicine, 5th ed. Baltimore: Lippincott Williams & Wilkins, 2008. p. 502.)

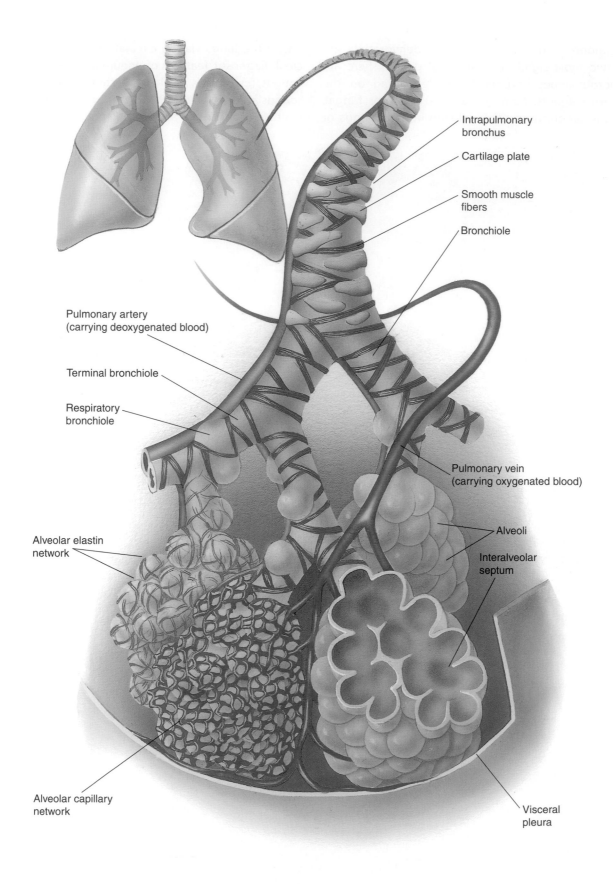

Intrapulmonary bronchus

Cartilage plate

Smooth muscle fibers

Bronchiole

Pulmonary artery (carrying deoxygenated blood)

Terminal bronchiole

Respiratory bronchiole

Pulmonary vein (carrying oxygenated blood)

Alveoli

Interalveolar septum

Alveolar elastin network

Alveolar capillary network

Visceral pleura

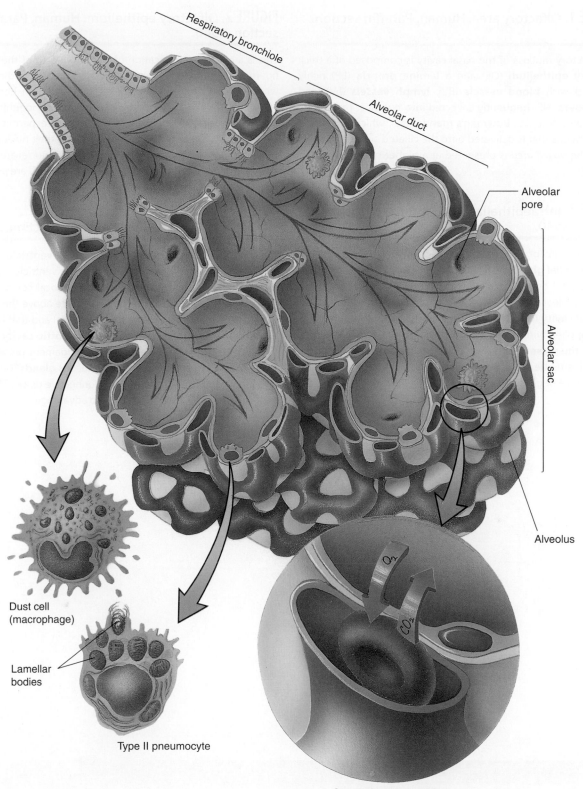

Respiratory bronchiole

Alveolar duct

Alveolar pore

Alveolar sac

Alveolus

Dust cell
(macrophage)

Lamellar
bodies

Type II pneumocyte

O_2

CO_2

Gas exchange occurring
at the alveolar-capillary
barrier

PLATE 12-1 • Olfactory Mucosa, Larynx

FIGURE 1. Olfactory area. Human. Paraffin section. ×270.

The olfactory mucosa of the nasal cavity is composed of a thick **olfactory epithelium** (OE) and a **lamina propria** (LP) richly endowed with **blood vessels** (BV), **lymph vessels** (LV), and **nerve fibers** (NF) frequently collected into bundles. The lamina propria also contains **Bowman's glands** (BG), which produce a watery mucus that is delivered onto the ciliated surface by short ducts. The *boxed area* is presented at a higher magnification in Figure 2.

FIGURE 3. Intraepithelial gland. Human. Paraffin section. ×540.

The epithelium of the nasal cavity occasionally displays small, **intraepithelial glands** (IG). Note that these structures are clearly demarcated from the surrounding epithelium. The secretory product is released into the space (*asterisk*) that is continuous with the **nasal cavity** (NC). The subepithelial **connective tissue** (CT) is richly supplied with **blood vessels** (BV) and **lymph vessels** (LV). Observe the **plasma cells** (PC), characteristic of the subepithelial connective tissue of the respiratory system, which also displays the presence of **glands** (GI).

FIGURE 2. Olfactory epithelium. Human. Paraffin section. ×540.

This is a higher magnification of the *boxed area* of the previous figure. The epithelium (OE) is pseudostratified ciliated columnar, whose **cilia** (C) are particularly evident. Although hematoxylin and eosin–stained tissue does not permit clear identification of the various cell types, the positions of the nuclei permit tentative identification. **Basal cells** (BC) are short, and their nuclei are near the basement membrane. **Olfactory cell** (OC) nuclei are centrally located, whereas nuclei of **sustentacular cells** (SC) are positioned near the apex of the cell.

FIGURE 4. Larynx. l.s. Human. Paraffin section. ×14.

The right half of the larynx, at the level of the **ventricle** (V), is presented in this survey photomicrograph. The ventricle is bounded superiorly by the **ventricular folds** (false vocal cords) (VF) and inferiorly by the **vocal folds** (VoF). The space above the ventricular fold is the beginning of the **vestibule** (Ve) and that below the vocal fold is the beginning of the **infraglottic cavity** (IC). The **vocalis muscle** (VM) regulates the vocal ligament present in the vocal fold. Acini of mucous and seromucous **glands** (GI) are scattered throughout the subepithelial connective tissue. The **laryngeal cartilages** (LC) are also shown to advantage.

KEY

BC	basal cells	LC	laryngeal cartilages	PC	plasma cells
BG	Bowman's glands	LP	lamina propria	SC	sustentacular cells
BV	blood vessels	LV	lymph vessels	V	ventricle
C	cilia	NC	nasal cavity	Ve	vestibule
CT	connective tissue	NF	nerve fibers	VF	ventricular folds
GI	glands	OC	olfactory cells	VM	vocalis muscle
IC	infraglottic cavity	OE	olfactory epithelium	VoF	vocal folds
IG	intraepithelial glands				

PLATE 12-1 · Olfactory Mucosa, Larynx p.

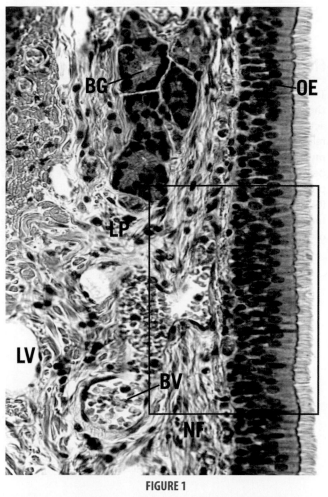

FIGURE 1

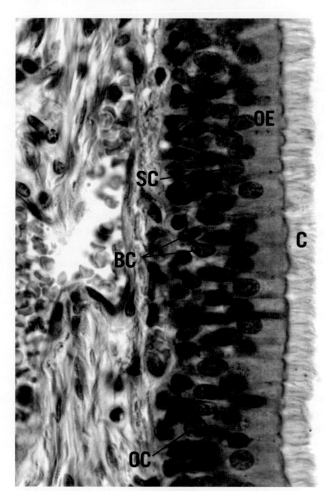

FIGURE 2

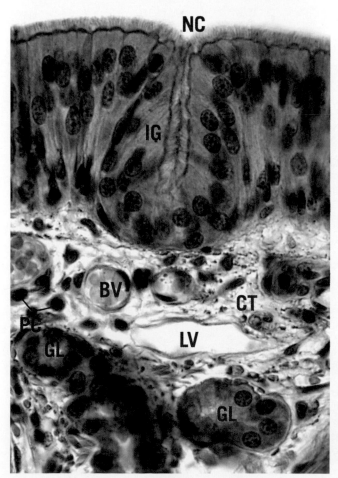

FIGURE 3

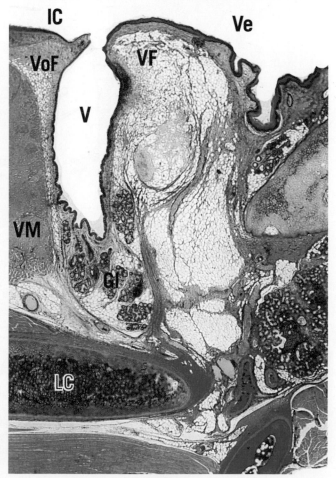

FIGURE 4

PLATE 12-2 · Trachea

FIGURE 1. Trachea. l.s. Monkey. Paraffin section. ×20.

This survey photomicrograph presents a longitudinal section of the **trachea** (Tr) and **esophagus** (Es). Observe that the **lumen** (LT) of the trachea is patent, due to the presence of discontinuous cartilaginous **C-rings** (CR) in its wall. The C-rings of the trachea are thicker anteriorly than posteriorly and are separated from each other by thick, fibrous connective tissue (*arrows*) that is continuous with the perichondrium of the C-rings. The adventitia of the trachea is adhered to the esophagus via a loose type of **connective tissue** (CT), which frequently contains adipose tissue. Note that the **lumen** (LE) of the esophagus is normally collapsed. A region similar to the *boxed area* is presented at a higher magnification in Figure 3.

FIGURE 3. Trachea. l.s. Monkey. Paraffin section. ×200.

This photomicrograph is a higher magnification of a region similar to the *boxed area* of Figure 1. The pseudostratified, ciliated columnar **epithelium** (E) lies on a basement membrane that separates it from the underlying lamina propria. The outer extent of the lamina propria is demarcated by an elastic lamina (*arrows*), deep to which is the **submucosa** (SM), containing a rich **vascular supply** (BV). The **C-ring** (CR), with its attendant **perichondrium** (Pc), constitutes the most substantive layer of the tracheal wall. The adventitia of the trachea, which some consider to include the C-ring, is composed of a loose type of connective tissue, housing some **adipose cells** (AC), **nerves** (N), and **blood vessels** (BV). Collagen fiber bundles of the adventitia secure the trachea to the surrounding structures.

FIGURE 2. Trachea. l.s. Monkey. Plastic section. ×270.

The trachea is lined by a pseudostratified ciliated columnar **epithelium** (E), which houses numerous **goblet cells** (GC) that actively secrete a mucous substance. The **lamina propria** (LP) is relatively thin, whereas the **submucosa** (SM) is thick and contains **mucous** and **seromucous glands** (GI), whose secretory product is delivered to the epithelial surface via ducts that pierce the lamina propria. The **perichondrium** (Pc) of the hyaline cartilage **C-rings** (CR) merges with the submucosal connective tissue. Note a longitudinal section of a **blood vessel** (BV), indicative of the presence of a rich vascular supply.

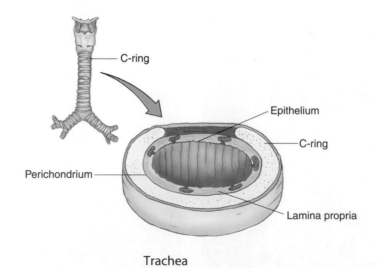

Trachea

KEY					
AC	adipose cells	**Es**	esophagus	**LT**	lumen—trachea
BV	blood vessels	**GC**	goblet cells	**N**	nerves
CR	C-rings	**GI**	mucous/seromucous glands	**Pc**	perichondrium
CT	connective tissue	**LE**	lumen—esophagus	**SM**	submucosa
E	epithelium	**LP**	lamina propria	**Tr**	trachea

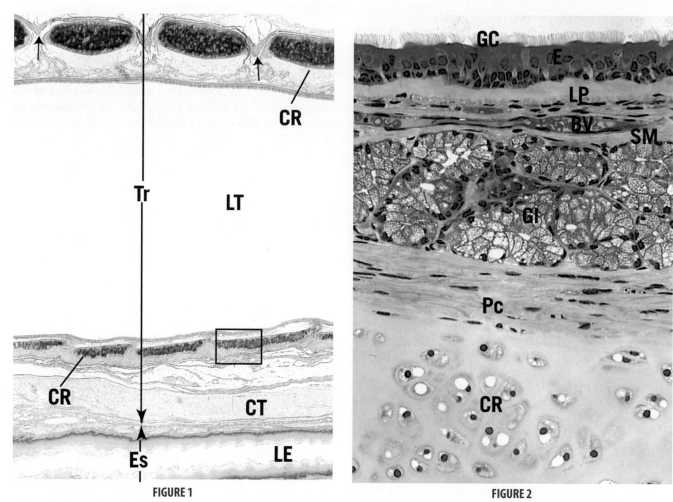

GC
E
LP
BV
SM
Gl
Pc
CR

FIGURE 2

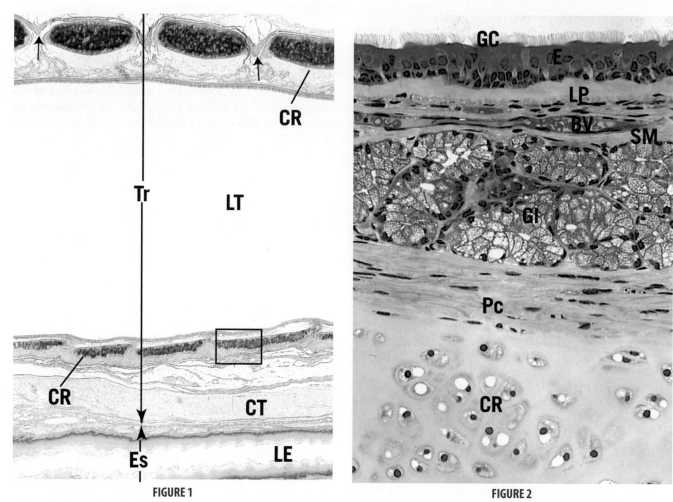

CR
Tr
LT
CR
CT
LE
Es

FIGURE 1

PLATE 12-2 · Trachea

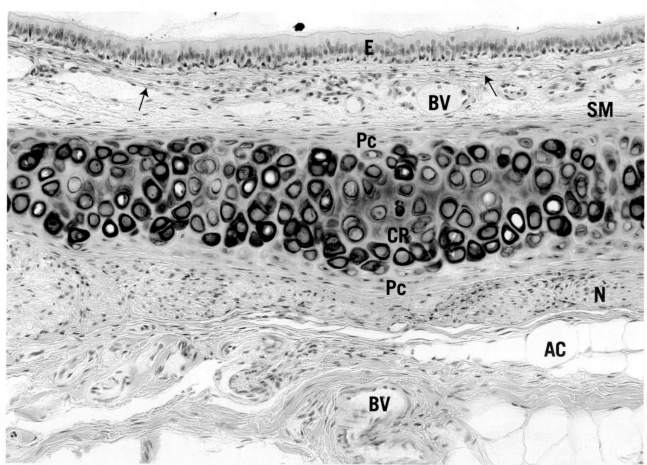

E
BV
SM
Pc
CR
Pc
N
AC
BV

FIGURE 3

PLATE 12-3 · Respiratory Epithelium and Cilia, Electron Microscopy

FIGURE 1. Tracheal epithelium. Hamster. Electron microscopy. ×7,782.

The tracheal epithelium of the hamster presents mucus-producing **goblet cells** (GC) as well as **ciliated columnar cells** (CC), whose cilia (*arrows*) project into the lumen. Note that both cell types are well endowed with **Golgi apparatus** (GA), whereas goblet cells are particularly rich in **rough endoplasmic reticulum** (rER). (Courtesy of Dr. E. McDowell.) *Inset.* **Bronchus. Human. Electron microscopy.** ×7,782. The apical region of a ciliated epithelial cell presents both **cilia** (C) and microvilli (*arrow*). (Courtesy of Dr. E. McDowell.)

KEY					
C	cilia	GA	Golgi apparatus	rER	rough endoplasmic
CC	ciliated columnar cell	GC	goblet cell		reticulum

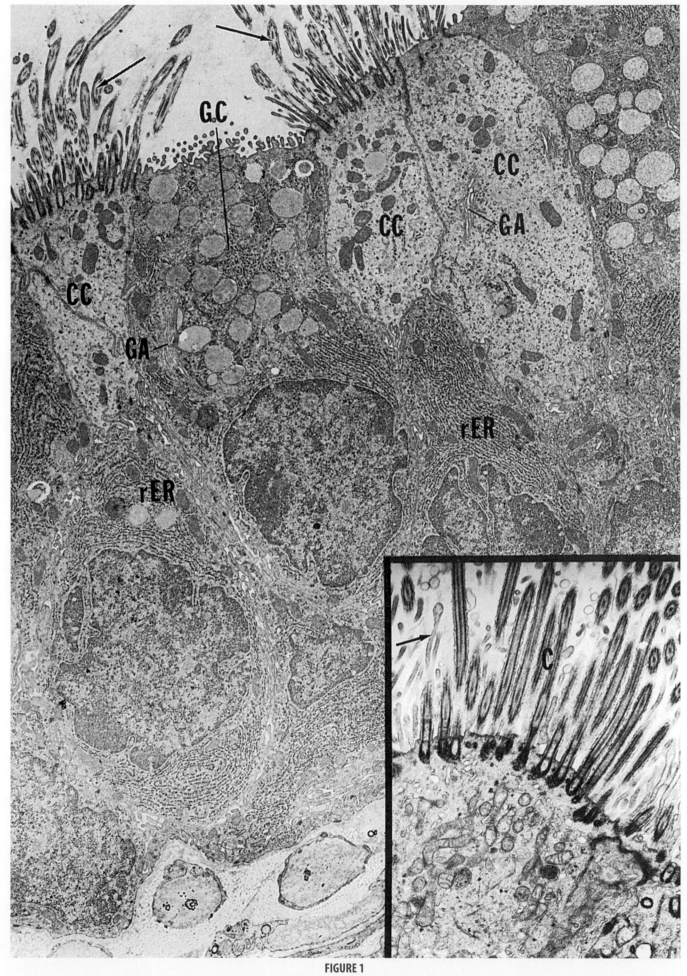

PLATE 2-3 • Respiratory Epithelium and Cilia, Electron Microscopy

FIGURE 1

PLATE 12-4 · Bronchi, Bronchioles

FIGURE 1. Lung. Paraffin section. ×14.

This survey photomicrograph presents a section of a lung that permits the observation of the various conduits that conduct air and blood to and from the lung. The intrapulmonary bronchus (IB) is recognizable by its thick wall, containing plates of **hyaline cartilage** (HC) and **smooth muscle** (Sm). Longitudinal sections of a **bronchiole** (B), **terminal bronchiole** (TB), and **respiratory bronchiole** (RB) are also evident. Smaller bronchioles (*asterisks*) may also be recognized, but their identification cannot be ascertained. *Arrows* point to structures that are probably alveolar ducts leading into alveolar sacs. Several **blood vessels** (BV), branches of the pulmonary circulatory system, may be noted. Observe that **lymphatic nodules** (LN) are also present along the bronchial tree.

FIGURE 3. Bronchiole. x.s. Paraffin section. ×270.

Bronchioles maintain their patent **lumen** (L) without the requirement of a cartilaginous support, since they are attached to surrounding lung tissue by elastic fibers radiating from their circumference. The lumina of bronchioles are lined by simple columnar to simple cuboidal **epithelium** (E), interspersed with **Clara cells** (CC), depending on the diameter of the bronchiole. The **lamina propria** (LP) is thin and is surrounded by **smooth muscle** (Sm), which encircles the lumen. Bronchioles have no glands in their walls and are surrounded by **lung tissue** (LT).

FIGURE 2. Intrapulmonary bronchus. x.s. Paraffin section. ×132.

Intrapulmonary bronchi are relatively large conduits for air, whose **lumina** (L) are lined by a typical respiratory **epithelium** (E). The **smooth muscle** (Sm) is found beneath the mucous membrane, and it encircles the entire lumen. Note that gaps (*arrows*) appear in the muscle layer, indicating that two ribbons of smooth muscle wind around the lumen in a helical arrangement. Plates of **hyaline cartilage** (HC) act as the skeletal support, maintaining the patency of the bronchus. The entire structure is surrounded by **lung tissue** (LT).

FIGURE 4. Terminal bronchioles. x.s. Paraffin section. ×132.

The smallest conducting bronchioles are referred to as **terminal bronchioles** (TB). These have very small diameters, and their lumina are lined with a simple cuboidal **epithelium** (E) interspersed with **Clara cells** (CC). The connective tissue is much reduced, and the smooth muscle layers are incomplete and difficult to recognize at this magnification. Terminal bronchioles give rise to **respiratory bronchioles** (RB), whose walls resemble those of the terminal bronchioles except that the presence of alveoli permits the exchange of gases to occur. Observe the **alveolar duct** (not labeled) in the lower right-hand corner.

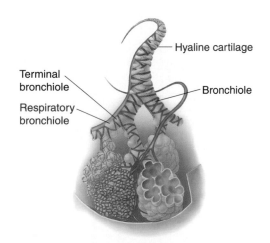

Hyaline cartilage

Terminal bronchiole

Respiratory bronchiole

Bronchiole

Bronchial system and lung

KEY

B	bronchiole	IB	intrapulmonary bronchus	RB	respiratory bronchiole
BV	blood vessels	L	lumen	Sm	smooth muscle
CC	Clara cells	LN	lymphatic nodule	TB	terminal bronchiole
E	epithelium	LP	lamina propria		
HC	hyaline cartilage	LT	lung tissue		

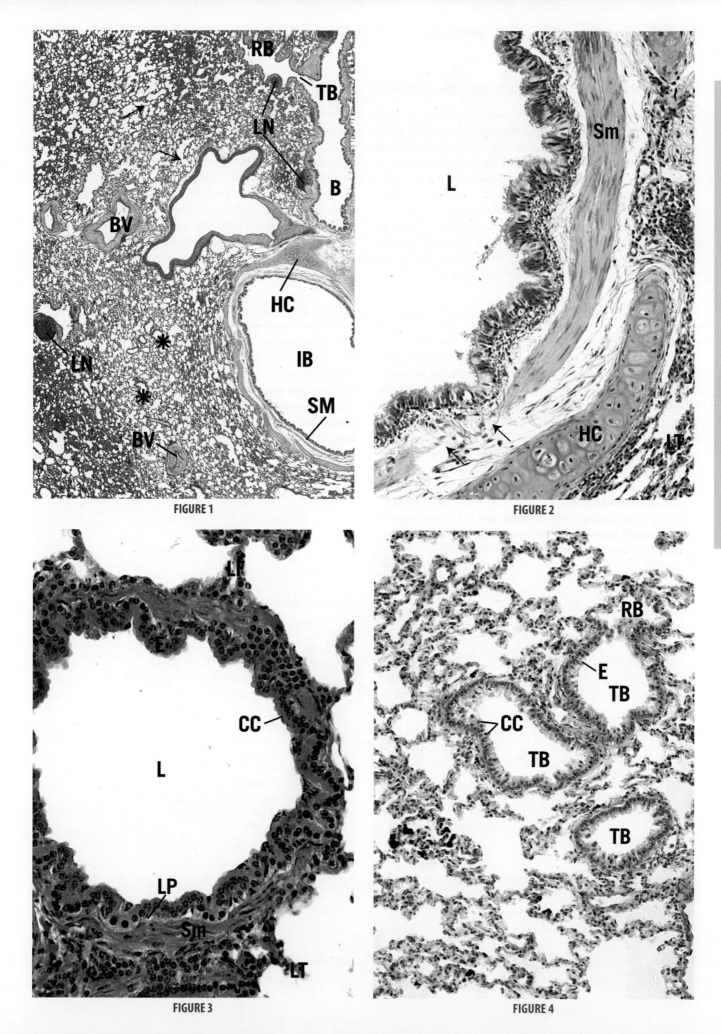

PLATE 12-4 · Bronchi, Bronchioles

FIGURE 1

FIGURE 2

FIGURE 3

FIGURE 4

PLATE 12-5 · Lung Tissue

FIGURE 1. Respiratory bronchiole. Paraffin section. ×270.

The respiratory bronchiole whose lumen (L) occupies the lower half of this photomicrograph presents an apparently thick wall with small outpocketings of **alveoli** (A). It is in these alveoli that gaseous exchanges first occur. The wall of the respiratory bronchiole is composed of a simple cuboidal epithelium consisting of some ciliated cells and **Clara cells** (CC). The remainder of the wall presents an incomplete layer of smooth muscle cells surrounded by fibroelastic connective tissue. Careful examination of this photomicrograph reveals that the wall of the respiratory bronchiole is folded upon itself, thus giving a misleading appearance of thick walls.

FIGURE 2. Alveolar duct. l.s. Human. Paraffin section. ×132.

Alveolar ducts (AD), unlike respiratory bronchioles, do not possess a wall of their own. These structures are lined by a simple squamous **epithelium** (E), composed of highly attenuated cells. Alveolar ducts present numerous outpocketings of **alveoli** (A), and they end in **alveolar sacs** (AS), consisting of groups of alveoli clustered around a common air space. Individual alveoli possess small smooth muscle cells that, acting like a purse string, control the opening into the alveolus. These appear as small knobs (*arrow*). A region similar to the *boxed area* is presented at a higher magnification in Figure 3.

FIGURE 3. Interalveolar septum. Monkey. Plastic section. ×540.

This photomicrograph is a higher magnification of a region similar to the *boxed area* of Figure 2. Two alveoli (A) are presented, recognizable as empty spaces separated from each other by an **interalveolar septum** (IS). The septum is composed of a **capillary** (Ca), the nucleus (*asterisk*) of whose endothelial lining bulges into the lumen containing **red blood cells** (RBC). The interalveolar septum as well as the entire alveolus is lined by **type I pneumocytes** (P1), which are highly attenuated squamous epithelial cells, interspersed with **type II pneumocytes** (P2). Thicker interalveolar septa house **blood vessels** (BV) and connective tissue elements including macrophages known as **dust cells** (DC). Note the presence of **smooth muscle cells** (Sm) and connective tissue elements that appear as knobs at the entrance into the alveolus.

FIGURE 4. Lung. Dust cells. Paraffin section. ×270.

The highly vascular nature of the lung is evident in this photomicrograph, since the blood vessels (BV) and the **capillaries** (Ca) of the interalveolar septa are filled with red blood cells. The dark blotches that appear to be scattered throughout the lung tissue represent **dust cells** (DC), macrophages that have phagocytosed particulate matter. *Inset*. **Lung. Dust cell. Monkey. Plastic section.** ×540. The **nucleus** (N) of a **dust cell** (DC) is surrounded by phagosomes containing particulate matter that was probably phagocytosed from an alveolus of the lung.

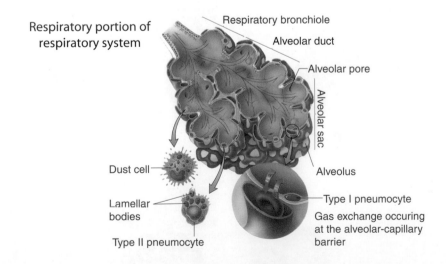

Respiratory portion of respiratory system

Respiratory bronchiole

Alveolar duct

Alveolar pore

Alveolar sac

Dust cell

Lamellar bodies

Type II pneumocyte

Alveolus

Type I pneumocyte

Gas exchange occuring at the alveolar-capillary barrier

KEY

A	alveolus	**CC**	Clara cell	**N**	nucleus
AD	alveolar duct	**DC**	dust cell	**P1**	type I pneumocytes
AS	alveolar sac	**E**	epithelium	**P2**	type II pneumocytes
BV	blood vessel	**IS**	interalveolar septum	**RBC**	red blood cells
Ca	capillary	**L**	lumen	**Sm**	smooth muscle

PLATE 12-5 • Lung Tissue

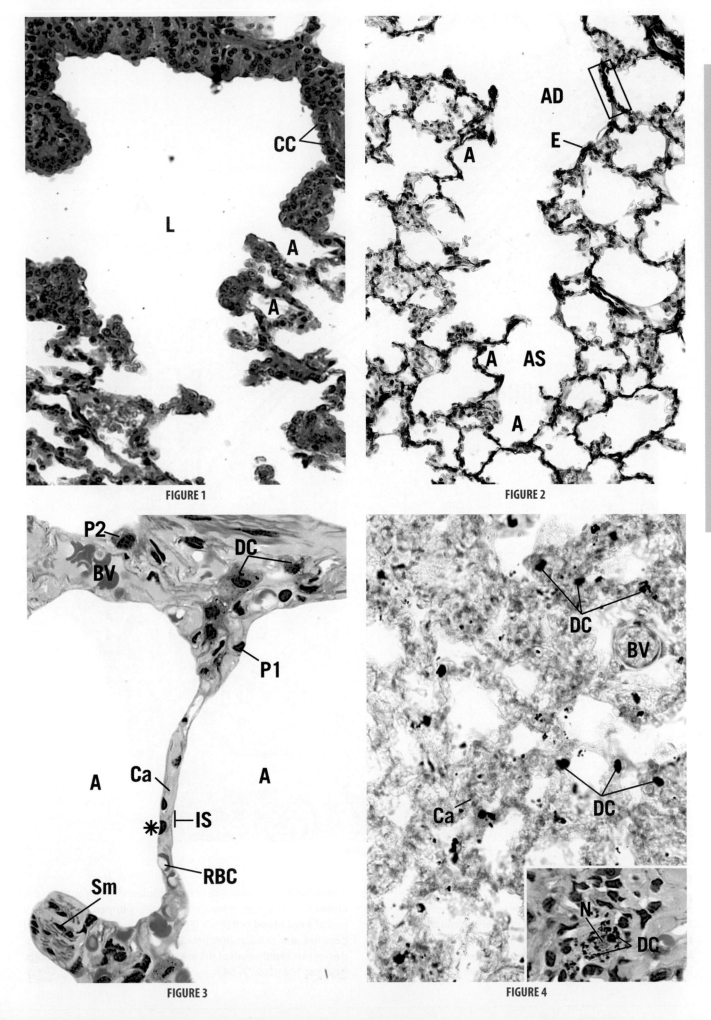

FIGURE 1

FIGURE 2

FIGURE 3

FIGURE 4

PLATE 12-6 · Blood-Air Barrier, Electron Microscopy

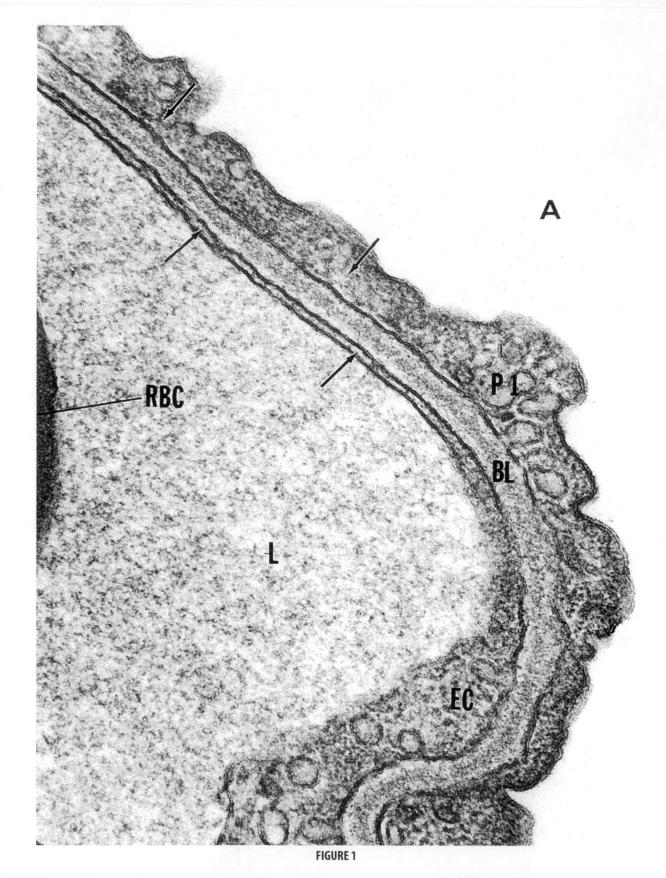

FIGURE 1

FIGURE 1. Blood-air barrier. Dog. Electron microscopy. ×85,500.

The blood-air barrier is composed of highly attenuated **endothelial cells** (EC), **type I pneumocytes** (P1), and an intervening **basal lamina** (BL). Note that the cytoplasm (*arrows*) of both cell types is greatly reduced, as evidenced by the close proximity of the plasmalemma on either side of the cytoplasm. The air space of the **alveolus** (A) is empty, whereas the capillary **lumen** (L) presents a part of a **red blood cell** (RBC). (From DeFouw D. Vesicle numerical densities and cellular attenuation: comparisons between endothelium and epithelium of the alveolar septa in normal dog lungs. Anat Rec 1984;209:77–84.)

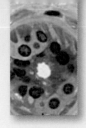

Chapter Summary

I. CONDUCTING PORTION

A. Nasal Cavity

1. Respiratory Region

The **respiratory region** is lined by **respiratory (pseudostratified ciliated columnar) epithelium**. The subepithelial connective tissue is richly vascularized and possesses seromucous glands.

2. Olfactory Region

The epithelium of the **olfactory region** is thick, **pseudostratified ciliated columnar epithelium** composed of three cell types: **basal cell**, **sustentacular cells**, and **olfactory cells**. The lamina propria is richly vascularized and possesses **Bowman's glands**, which produce a watery mucus.

B. Larynx

The **larynx** is lined by a **respiratory epithelium** except for certain regions that are lined by **stratified squamous nonkeratinized epithelium**. From superior to inferior, the **lumen** of the larynx presents three regions: the **vestibule**, **the ventricle**, and the **infraglottic cavity**. The **ventricular** and **vocal folds** are the superior and inferior boundaries of the ventricle, respectively. Cartilages, extrinsic and intrinsic muscles, as well as mucous and seromucous glands are present in the larynx.

C. Trachea

1. Mucosa

The **mucosa** of the trachea is composed of a **respiratory epithelium** with numerous **goblet cells**, a **lamina propria**, and a well-defined **elastic lamina**.

2. Submucosa

The **submucosa** houses **mucous** and **seromucous glands**.

3. Adventitia

The **adventitia** is the thickest portion of the tracheal wall. It houses the **C-rings** of **hyaline cartilage** (or thick connective tissue between the rings). Posteriorly, the **trachealis muscle** (smooth muscle) fills in the gap between the free ends of the cartilage.

D. Extrapulmonary Bronchi

Extrapulmonary bronchi resemble the trachea in histologic structure.

E. Intrapulmonary Bronchi

These and subsequent passageways are completely surrounded by lung tissue.

1. Mucosa

Intrapulmonary bronchi are lined by **respiratory epithelium** with **goblet cells**. The subepithelial connective tissue is no longer bordered by an elastic lamina.

2. Muscle

Two ribbons of **smooth muscle** are wound helically around the mucosa.

3. Cartilage

The C-rings are replaced by irregularly shaped **hyaline cartilage plates** that encircle the smooth muscle layer. **Dense collagenous connective tissue** connects the perichondria of the cartilage plates.

4. Glands

Seromucous glands occupy the connective tissue between the cartilage plates and smooth muscle. **Lymphatic nodules** and branches of the pulmonary arteries are also present.

F. Bronchioles

Bronchioles are lined by **ciliated simple columnar** to **simple cuboidal epithelium** interspersed with nonciliated **Clara cells**. **Goblet cells** are found only in larger bronchioles. The **lamina propria** possesses no glands and is surrounded by **smooth muscle**. The walls of bronchioles are not supported by cartilage. The largest bronchioles are about 1 mm in diameter.

G. Terminal Bronchioles

Terminal bronchioles are usually less than 0.5 mm in diameter. The lumen is lined by **simple cuboidal epithelium** (some ciliated) interspersed with **Clara cells**. The connective tissue and smooth muscle of the wall of the terminal bronchioles are greatly reduced.

II. RESPIRATORY PORTION

A. Respiratory Bronchiole

Respiratory bronchioles resemble terminal bronchioles, but they possess outpocketings of **alveoli** in their walls. This is the first region where exchange of gases occurs.

B. Alveolar Ducts

Alveolar ducts possess no walls of their own. They are long, straight tubes lined by **simple squamous epithelium** and display numerous outpocketings of **alveoli**. Alveolar ducts end in alveolar sacs.

C. Alveolar Sacs

Alveolar sacs are composed of groups of **alveoli** clustered around a common air space.

D. Alveolus

An **alveolus** is a small air space partially surrounded by highly attenuated epithelium. Two types of cells are present in the lining: **type I pneumocytes** (lining cells) and **type II pneumocytes** (produce surfactant). The opening of the alveolus is controlled by **elastic fibers**. Alveoli are separated from each other by richly vascularized walls known as **interalveolar septa**, some of which present **alveolar pores** (communicating spaces between alveoli). **Dust cells** (macrophages), **fibroblasts**, and other **connective tissue elements** may be noted in interalveolar septa. The **blood-air barrier** is a part of the interalveolar septum, the thinnest of which is composed of surfactant, **continuous endothelial cells**, **type I pneumocyte**, and their intervening **fused basal laminae**.

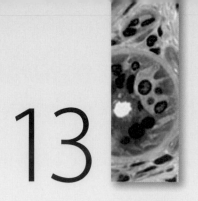

13 DIGESTIVE SYSTEM I

PROPERTY OF LIBRARY
SOUTH UNIVERSITY CLEVELAND CAMPUS
WARRENSVILLE HEIGHTS, OH 44128

CHAPTER OUTLINE

The digestive system functions in the ingestion, digestion, and absorption of food as well as in the elimination of its unusable portions. To accomplish these functions, the digestive system is organized into three major components:

- the oral cavity, where food is reduced in size, is moistened, begins to be digested, and is introduced as small spherical portions, each known as a **bolus**, into the alimentary canal;
- a muscular alimentary canal, along whose lumen the ingested foods are converted, both physically and chemically, into absorbable substances; and
- an extramural glandular portion, which provides fluids, enzymes, and emulsifying agents necessary so that the alimentary canal can perform its various functions.

ORAL CAVITY AND ORAL MUCOSA

The **oral cavity** may be subdivided into two smaller cavities: the externally positioned vestibule and the internally placed oral cavity proper.

- The **vestibule** is the space bounded by the lips and cheeks anteriorly and laterally, whereas its internal boundary is formed by the dental arches. The ducts of the parotid glands deliver their secretory products into the vestibule (see Graphics 13-1 and 13-2).
- The **oral cavity proper** is bounded by the teeth externally, the floor of the mouth inferiorly, and the hard and soft palates superiorly.
  - At its posterior extent, the oral cavity proper is separated from the oral pharynx by an imaginary plane drawn between the palatoglossal folds just anterior to the palatine tonsils.

Both the oral cavity proper and the vestibule are lined by **stratified squamous epithelium**, which, in regions that are subject to abrasive forces, is modified into **stratified squamous keratinized** (or **parakeratinized**) **epithelium** (see Table 13-1).

Oral Mucosa

The epithelium and underlining connective tissue constitute the **oral mucosa**. If the epithelium is keratinized (or parakeratinized), the mucosa is said to be masticatory mucosa, and if the epithelium is not keratinized, the mucosa is referred to as lining mucosa.

- Most of the oral cavity possesses **lining mucosa**, with the exception of the gingiva, hard palate, and the dorsal surface of the tongue, which are covered by **masticatory mucosa**.

- The oral cavity has areas of **specialized mucosa**, located mostly on the dorsal surface of the tongue, though present also on the soft palate and pharynx, where barrel-shaped intraepithelial structures known as **taste buds** function in taste perception.

SALIVARY GLANDS, PALATE, AND TONSILS

The three pairs of major salivary glands—parotid, sublingual, and submandibular—deliver their secretions into the oral cavity. The hard palate assists the tongue in the preparation of the bolus, and the soft palate, a moveable structure, seals the communication between the oral and nasal pharynges, thus preventing passage of food and fluids from the former into the latter.

- The connective tissue underlying the epithelium of the oral cavity is richly endowed with **minor salivary glands** that, secreting **saliva** in a continuous fashion, contribute to the maintenance of a moist environment.
  - Saliva functions also in assisting in the process of deglutition by acting as a lubricant for dry foods and for holding the bolus together in a semisolid mass.
  - Moreover, enzymes present in saliva initiate digestion of carbohydrates, whereas secretory antibodies protect the body against antigenic substances.

The entrance to the pharynx is guarded against bacterial invasion by the **tonsillar ring**, composed of the **lingual**, **pharyngeal**, and **palatine tonsils**.

TONGUE, TEETH, AND ODONTOGENESIS

The contents of the oral cavity are the **tongue**, a muscular structure that functions in the preparation of the bolus, tasting of the food, and beginning of deglutition (swallowing), and **teeth**, utilized in biting and mastication of food.

Tongue

The **tongue** is a mucosa-invested moveable muscular structure that has two regions, the root (base) and the body (see Graphic 13-2).

- The **root** anchors the tongue into the hyoid bone, the posterior aspect of the oral cavity and the pharynx.

TABLE 13-1 • Summary of the Oral Mucosa

Summary of the Oral Mucosa			
Mucosal Region	Type of Epithelium	Height of Connective Tissue Papillae	Special Comments
Lip			
Skin aspect	Stratified squamous keratinized	Medium	Hair, sebaceous glands, and sweat glands
Vermilion zone	Stratified squamous keratinized	High	Few sebaceous glands? The vermilion zone must be moistened by tongue
Vestibular aspect	Lining mucosa	Medium	Mucous (mixed?) salivary glands
Cheek			
Skin aspect	Stratified squamous keratinized	Medium	Hair, sebaceous glands, and sweat glands
Vestibular aspect	Lining mucosa	Medium	Mucous (mixed?) salivary glands; Fordyce's granules
Gingiva			
Free and attached	Masticatory mucosa	High	Tightly bound to periosteum
Sulcular	Lining mucosa	Low	
Junctional epithelium	Lining mucosa	None	Attached to tooth surface by hemidesmosomes
Col	Lining mucosa (junctional epithelium?)	Low to none	
Alveolar Mucosa			
	Lining mucosa	Low	Some minor salivary glands
Hard Palate			
Anterior lateral	Masticatory mucosa	High	Fat globules
Posterior lateral	Masticatory mucosa	High	Mucous salivary glands
Raphe	Masticatory mucosa	High	Tightly bound to periosteum
Soft Palate			
	Lining mucosa	Low	Elastic lamina; mucous salivary glands
Uvula	Lining mucosa	Low	Mucous salivary glands
Floor of Mouth			
	Lining mucosa	Low	Mucous salivary glands
Tongue			
Dorsal surface	Specialized mucosa		Taste buds; lingual papillae, serous, mucous, and mixed salivary glands; lingual tonsils
Ventral surface	Lining mucosa	Low	Plica fimbriata

(Reprinted with permission from Leslie P. Gartner Essentials of Oral Histology and Embryology, 3rd ed. P. 118, Jen House Publishing Company, Baltimore, MD 1999.)

- The body is freely moving in the oral cavity and its dorsal surface (facing the palate) is divided into an anterior two-thirds and a posterior one-third by a shallow, posteriorly directed V-shaped groove, the **sulcus terminalis**, whose apex is a shallow depression, the **foramen cecum**. The dorsum of the posterior one-third of the tongue has crypts that burrow into the submucosal lymphoid tissue, the **lingual tonsil**.
  - During embryogenesis, the **thyroglossal duct**, which will form the thyroid gland, originates from the foramen cecum.

The dorsum of the tongue is covered by **masticatory mucosa** sporting **lingual papillae**, and the ventral surface is covered by **lining mucosa**. The core of the tongue is composed of two groups of skeletal muscle, the **intrinsic group** and the **extrinsic group**, interspersed with connective tissue and three pairs of minor salivary glands, **posterior mucous glands**, **glands of von Ebner** (purely serous glands), and **Blandin-Nuhn glands** (mixed glands).

Lingual Papillae

The four types of **lingual papillae** are outgrowths of the mucosa of the dorsal surface:

- **Filiform papillae** are the most numerous, and they are conical in shape, have no taste buds, and their stratified squamous epithelium is **highly keratinized**.
- **Fungiform papillae** are mushroom-shaped and possess a few **taste buds** on their free surface. The epithelium of fungiform papillae is stratified squamous nonkeratinized.
- **Foliate papillae** are located on the posterolateral aspects of the anterior two-thirds of the tongue. They present as shallow furrows that possess taste buds for the first 2 years of life after which the taste buds degenerate. Glands of von Ebner release their secretion into the furrows.
- The twelve or so **circumvallate papillae**, located just anterior to the sulcus terminalis, possess numerous **taste buds** and are surrounded by a deep, moat-like furrow. Glands of von Ebner release their serous secretion into the bottom of the moat-like depression.

Taste Buds

Each taste bud is barrel-shaped, is completely intraepithelial, and is composed of 60 to 80 spindle-shaped neuroepithelial cells that are of four types:

- **basal cells (type IV)**, which act as regenerative cells;
- **dark cells (type I cells)**, which probably arise directly from basal cells and mature into
- **light cells (type II)**; and
- **intermediate cells (type III cells)**, which will undergo apoptosis and die.

The complete life cycle of these cells is about 10 days to 2 weeks, and they are continuously replaced by basal cell derivatives. The cells are compacted together and form an opening known as a **taste pore** at the epithelial surface (see Graphic 13-2).

- Basally, cell types I, II, and III form **synaptic contacts** with nerve fibers;
- apically, they possess long microvilli known as **taste hairs**, which pass through the taste pore and are exposed to the moist environment of the oral cavity.
  - The taste hairs have two types of **taste receptors (TR1** and **TR2)** that bind dissolved chemicals from the food, known as **tastants**, resulting in the activation of G proteins and/or direct opening of ion channels.
  - The end result is that the neuroepithelial cells become activated and release neurotransmitter substances at their synaptic junctions with the nerve fibers.
  - The central nervous system then registers the signal and interprets the taste that was sensed by the taste bud.
  - Each taste bud recognizes one or more of the five taste sensations: sour, sweet, salty, umami (savory), or bitter.

Teeth

Humans have two sets of dentition, there are 20 **deciduous teeth** in the mouth of a child, and as they are exfoliated, they are replaced by the **permanent dentition**, composed of 20 **succedaneous teeth** and an additional 12 **accessional teeth** for a total of 32 permanent teeth. At approximately 6 to 13 years of age, the dentition is mixed in that both deciduous and permanent teeth are present in the mouth at the same time. The increase in the number of teeth is probably a function of the greater space availability in the adult mouth. Each tooth is composed of a **crown** and a **root** and the **cervix**, where the crown and root contact each other. Three calcified substances, **enamel**, **dentin**, and **cementum** form the substance of each tooth. Dentin is located both in the crown (coronal dentin) and in the root (radicular dentin) and surrounds the **pulp**, a very vascularized and highly ordered connective tissue. Enamel covers coronal dentin, cementum covers radicular dentin, and the two meet at the cervix.

- **Enamel** is the hardest tissue in the body; it is
  - 96% inorganic matrix composed of **calcium hydroxyapatite crystals** and
  - 4% organic matrix consisting mostly of the protein **enamelin**

○ Manufactured by cells known as **ameloblasts**, which are not present after the tooth erupts into the oral cavity; therefore, enamel is acellular posteruption and cannot repair itself.

- **Dentin** is the second hardest tissue in the body, it is
  ○ 65% to 70% inorganic matrix composed of **calcium hydroxyapatite crystals** and
  ○ 30% to 35% **type I collagen fibers**
  ○ elaborated by cells known as **odontoblasts** that remain in their position in the pulp and continue to form dentin throughout the tooth's life

- **Cementum** is
  ○ 45% to 50% inorganic matrix composed of **calcium hydroxyapatite crystals**
  ○ 50% to 55% type I collagen fibers, glycosaminoglycans, and proteoglycans
  ○ Formed by cementoblasts that continue to manufacture cementum throughout the life of the tooth because the addition of cementum compensates for the erosion of enamel, thus maintaining the length of the tooth for proper occlusion.

- **Pulp** is a gelatinous, highly vascularized connective tissue that fills the **pulp cavity**, known as the **pulp chamber** in the crown of the tooth and **root canal** in the root of the tooth.
  ○ The peripheral layer of the pulp is composed of **odontoblasts**.
  ○ Deep to the odontoblasts is an acellular layer (the **cell-free zone**) and deep to that is a layer of fibroblasts and mesenchymal cells (the **cell-rich zone**)
  ○ **core of the pulp** has normal connective tissue cells and also houses blood vessels, lymph vessels, and nerve fibers.
    ▪ The nerve fibers are of two types: **autonomic** that serve blood vessels and **sensory fibers** that conduct pain information from the pulp.

The root of each tooth is suspended in its bony housing, the **alveolus**, by a dense collagenous connective tissue ligament, the **periodontal ligament**. The cervix of each tooth is surrounded by gingiva whose epithelium forms a collar, the **junctional epithelium**, whose attachment to the cervical enamel creates occluding junctions, thus isolating the connective tissue of the gingiva from the oral cavity.

Odontogenesis (See Graphic 13-2)

Odontogenesis, tooth formation, begins at 6 1/2 weeks of development as a horseshoe-shaped epithelial band, known as the **dental lamina**, arises from the oral epithelium of both the maxillary and the mandibular processes. Ten epithelial swellings, known as **tooth buds**, form on the lingual aspect of each dental lamina and press into the surrounding ectomesenchyme. It should be noted that cells of the ectomesenchyme are **neural crest** derivatives.

- Each tooth bud develops at a different rate to form a three-dimensional, three-layered epithelial structure, the **cap stage** of tooth development, composed of the **enamel organ** whose indentation is filled with ectomesenchymal cells, known as the **dental papilla**. The enamel organ and dental papilla together form the **tooth germ**.
  ○ The enamel organ's three layers are the **outer enamel epithelium** and **inner enamel epithelium** that form a rim, the **cervical loop**, at their junction, and the intervening space between the two epithelial layers are filled with cells known as **stellate reticulum.**
  ○ The concavity of the inner enamel epithelial layer is filled with ectomesenchymal cells, the dental papilla, which is responsible for the formation of **dentin** and the **pulp**.
  ○ Ectomesenchymal cells surrounding the tooth germ condense to form a connective tissue capsule, the **dental sac**, around the developing tooth germ. The dental sac is responsible for the formation of cementum, the periodontal ligament, and the bony alveolus.
  ○ A new epithelial growth develops from the dental lamina just lingually directed from the cap, known as the **succedaneous lamina**. This lamina grows deep into the ectomesenchyme; its distal terminus will form a tooth bud that will give rise to the permanent replacement of the forming deciduous tooth.
  ○ A group of cells derived from the stellate reticulum form a cluster against the inner enamel epithelium known as the **enamel knot**. These cells will either undergo apoptosis during the cap stage or they will survive into the next stage of tooth development.
  ○ The inner enamel epithelial cells will differentiate into ameloblasts and will form the **enamel** of the tooth.

- As the cap enlarges and forms a fourth layer of cells, the stratum intermedium, located between the stellate reticulum and the inner enamel epithelium, the tooth germ is in the **bell stage** of odontogenesis.
  ○ If the enamel knot survives into the bell stage, the enamel organ rearranges itself to form a **premolar** or a **molar tooth**. If the enamel knot undergoes apoptosis during the cap stage, the developing tooth will be an **incisor or a canine tooth**.
  ○ During the late bell stage, the peripheral-most cells of the dental papilla begin to differentiate into **odontoblasts** to start forming **dentin**.

- ○ In response to the formation of the odontoblasts, the cells of the inner enamel epithelium differentiate into **ameloblasts** to start forming **enamel**.
- Once the tooth germ forms dentin as well as enamel, odontogenesis has progressed into a new stage known as **apposition**.
  - ○ The appositional stage of tooth development is responsible for the formation of the crown of the tooth.
- After the enamel of the crown is completely formed, odontogenesis enters its new phase, namely, **root formation**.
  - ○ This process occurs simultaneously with **eruption**, in that as the root(s) of the tooth increase(s) in length the tooth moves toward the oral cavity and will erupt through the connective tissue and eventually the oral epithelium.
  - ○ Once the tooth reaches the oral cavity, it will continue to erupt at a rapid pace until it contacts its opposing tooth in the opposite arch.
  - ○ It is important to understand that the root does not push the tooth into its position in the oral cavity, instead, modified fibroblasts, **myofibroblasts**, of the forming periodontal ligament pull on the collagen fibers attached to the cementum of the root and "drag" the forming tooth into its proper position.

Molecular Mechanisms of Odontogenesis

Odontogenesis is induced by the ectodermally derived cells of the dental lamina that express **lymphoid enhancer factor-1** (Lef-1), a transcription factor.

- Lef-1 induces the epithelial cells to synthesize and release **bone morphogenic protein-4** (BMP-4), **sonic hedgehog** (Shh), and **fibroblast growth factor-8** (FGF-8).
- These signaling molecules act on the underlying ectomesenchymal cells to differentiate into odontogenic tissues. These neural crest–derived cells begin to express **activin βA**, **BMP-4**, the adhesive glycoprotein **tenascin,** and the membrane-bounded proteoglycan **syndecan**.
- Moreover, they also express several transcription factors, namely, **Egr-1** (early growth response-1), **Msx-1** (homeobox-containing genes), and **Msx-2**.
- This activation of the ectomesenchyme elicits their role in the induction of the tooth morphology, so that it is the ectomesenchyme that will determine, for instance, whether the developing tooth will become a molar or an incisor.
- Signaling molecules from the ectomesenchyme induce the formation of the **enamel knot**, which synthesizes and releases its own signaling molecules, namely, FGF-4, BMP-2, BMP-4, BMP-7, and Shh.
- These signaling molecules promote the differentiation of the inner enamel epithelial cells into **ameloblasts** and those of the peripheral-most layer of the dental papilla into **odontoblasts**.
- As mentioned above, continued maintenance of the enamel knot is responsible for the remodeling of the inner enamel epithelium, resulting in the morphodifferentiation of the enamel organ into a template that is the prototype of a molar tooth, whereas if the enamel knot undergoes apoptosis, morphodifferentiation is constrained and an incisor is formed.

CLINICAL CONSIDERATIONS

Herpetic Stomatitis

Herpetic stomatitis, a relatively common disease caused by the herpes simplex virus type I, is distinguished by painful **fever blisters** appearing on or in the vicinity of the lips. This is a recurring disease since the virus, in its dormant phase, inhabits the trigeminal ganglion. It travels along the axon to cause the appearance of the blisters. During the active stage, the patient is highly contagious, since the virus is shed via the seeping clear exudate.

Caries

Caries, or cavities, are formed by the action of acid-secreting bacteria that adhere to very small defects or irregularities of the enamel surface. The acids formed by the bacteria decalcify the enamel, providing larger defects that can house a much larger number of the proliferating bacteria with the formation of more acid and decalcification of more of the enamel. The carious lesion is pain-free until it reaches the underlying dentin. Since the most sensitive region of dentin is at the dentinoenamel junction, the tooth is sensitive to heat, cold, mechanical contact, and sweets. Continued bacterial activity, without the intervention of a dental health professional, could cause eventual loss of the tooth and perhaps even more serious sequelae.

Hemorrhage of the Pulp

Darkening of a tooth may be due to hemorrhage of the pulp. Although frequently the pulp is damaged severely enough that it can no longer be saved, a dental professional should be consulted because tooth discoloration does not necessarily require root canal therapy.

Necrotizing Ulcerative Gingivitis

Necrotizing ulcerative gingivitis is an acute ulcerative condition of the gingiva with accompanying necrosis, halitosis, erythematous appearance, and moderate to severe pain. Fever and regional lymphadenopathy may also be evident. This is usually a disease of the young adult who is experiencing stress and is not particularly attentive to dental hygiene. Frequently, *Treponema vincentii* and fusiform bacillus are present in large numbers, and they are also believed to be causative agents of the condition.

Spindle Cell Carcinoma

Spindle cell carcinoma is a modified type of squamous cell carcinoma where the histologic appearance of the malignant epithelial cells is spindle-shaped, resembling fibroblasts. It is highly aggressive, resulting in a survival rate of only 40% after 2 years. Spindle cell carcinoma is more commonly present in males 60 years of age or older, and in the oral region, this tumor is usually restricted to the gingiva, tongue, and lower lip. The most common causative agents of spindle cell carcinoma are alcoholism, tobacco use, and poor oral hygiene. Diagnostic features include painful inflammation, ulcers that do not heal readily, and growths that may be as large as 10 cm in diameter.

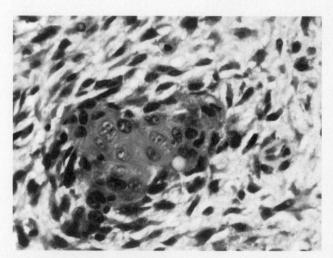

This light microscopic image from a patient with spindle cell carcinoma displays both epithelioid- and spindle-shaped malignant cells. (Reprinted with permission from Mills SE, Carter, D, et al., eds. Sternberg's Diagnostic Surgical Pathology, 5th ed., Philadelphia: Lippincott Williams & Wilkins, 2010. p. 794.)

Odontomas

Odontomas are hamartomatous anomalies (developmental malformations) that appear to be malignant, but fortunately, they are benign. These are the most frequent tumor-like structures of the maxillary and mandibular arches, and they arise from remnants of embryonic odontogenic tissues, forming tooth-like structures that are frequently calcified and display a haphazard arrangement. They are usually asymptomatic and are discovered on radiographs taken during routine dental examinations. Complex odontomas do not pose a significant health risk.

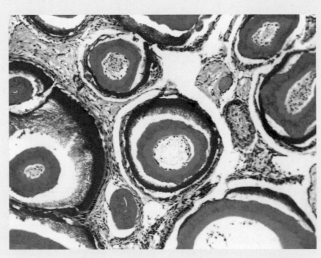

This light microscopic image from a patient with complex odontoma displays the presence of dentin, enamel, and pulp-like tissues scattered in a haphazard manner. (Reprinted with permission from Mills SE, Carter D, et al., eds. Sternberg's Diagnostic Surgical Pathology, 5th ed., Philadelphia: Lippincott Williams & Wilkins, 2010, p. 807.)

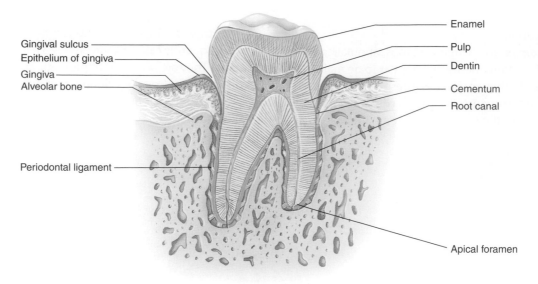

Tooth

The tooth, composed of a crown and root, is suspended in its bony socket, the alveolus, by a dense, collagenous connective tissue, the **periodontal ligament**. The crown of the tooth consists of two calcified tissues, **dentin** and **enamel**, whereas the root is composed of dentin and **cementum**. The pulp chamber of the crown and the root canal of the root are continuous with one another. They are occupied by a gelatinous connective tissue, the **pulp**, which houses blood and lymph vessels, nerve fibers, connective tissue elements, as well as **odontoblasts**, the cells responsible for the maintenance and repair of dentin. Vessels and nerves serving the pulp enter the root canal via the **apical foramen**, a small opening at the apex of the root.

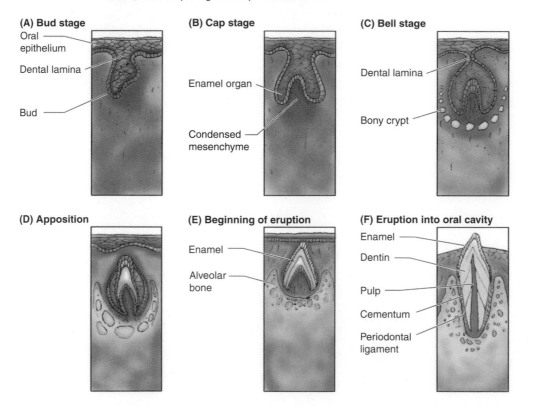

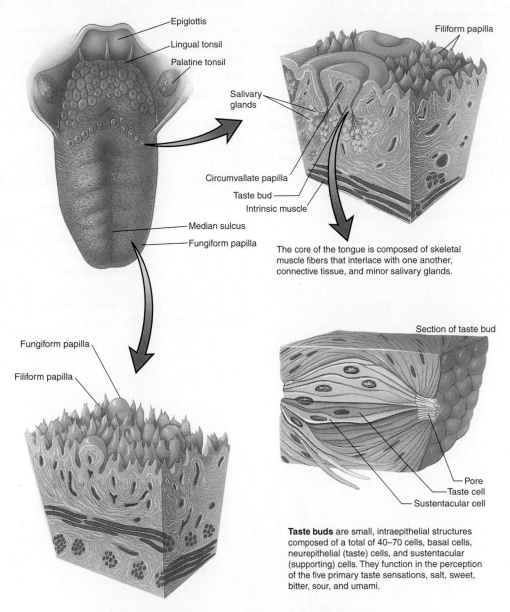

The core of the tongue is composed of skeletal muscle fibers that interlace with one another, connective tissue, and minor salivary glands.

Taste buds are small, intraepithelial structures composed of a total of 40–70 cells, basal cells, neurepithelial (taste) cells, and sustentacular (supporting) cells. They function in the perception of the five primary taste sensations, salt, sweet, bitter, sour, and umami.

The dorsal surface of the tongue is subdivided into an anterior two-thirds, populated by the four types of lingual papillae, and a posterior one-third housing the lingual tonsils. The two regions are separated from one another by a "V-shaped" depression, the sulcus terminalis. **Filiform papillae** are short, conical, and highly keratinized. **Fungiform papillae** are mushroom-shaped, and the dorsal aspect of their epithelia houses three to five taste buds. **Circumvallate papillae**, the largest of the lingual papillae, are six to twelve in number. Each circumvallate papilla is depressed into the surface of the tongue and is surrounded by a moat-like trough. The lateral aspect of the papilla as well as the lining of the trough houses numerous taste buds. **Foliate papillae** are located on the lateral aspect of the tongue.

PLATE 13-1 • Lip

FIGURE 1. Lip. Human. Paraffin section. ×14.

The human lip presents three surfaces and a core (C). The external surface is covered by skin, composed of epidermis (E) and **dermis** (D). Associated hair follicles (*arrow*) and glands are evident. The **vermillion** (**red**) **zone** (VZ) is only found in humans. The high dermal papillae (*arrowheads*) carry blood vessels close to the surface, accounting for the pinkish coloration of this region. The internal aspect is lined by a wet, stratified, squamous, nonkeratinized **epithelium** (Ep), and the underlying connective tissue houses minor salivary glands. The core of the lip is composed of skeletal muscle interspersed with fibroelastic connective tissue.

FIGURE 3. Lip. Human. External aspect. Paraffin section. ×132.

The external aspect of the lip is covered by thin skin. Neither the epidermis (E) nor the **dermis** (D) presents any unusual features. Numerous **hair follicles** (HF) populate this aspect of the lip, and **sebaceous glands** (Sg) as well as sweat glands are noted in abundance.

FIGURE 2. Lip. Human. Internal aspect. Paraffin section. ×270.

The internal aspect of the lip is lined by a mucous membrane that is continuously kept moist by saliva secreted by the three major and numerous minor salivary glands. The thick epithelium (Ep) is a stratified squamous nonkeratinized type, which presents deep **rete ridges** (RR) that interdigitate with the **connective tissue papillae** (CP). The connective tissue is fibroelastic in nature, displaying a rich **vascular supply** (BV).

FIGURE 4. Lip. Human. Vermilion zone. Paraffin section. ×132.

The vermilion zone of the lip is covered by a modified skin composed of stratified squamous keratinized epithelium (Ep) that forms extensive interdigitations with the underlying **dermis** (D). Neither hair follicles nor sweat glands populate this area (though occasional sebaceous glands may be present). Note the cross-sectional profiles of **skeletal muscle fibers** (SM) and the rich **vascular supply** (BV) of the lip.

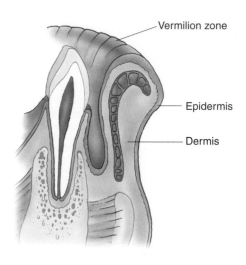

Vermilion zone

Epidermis

Dermis

Lip

KEY

BV	vascular supply	E	epidermis	Sg	sebaceous glands
C	core	Ep	epithelium	SM	skeletal muscle
CP	connective tissue papillae	HF	hair follicles	VZ	vermilion (red) zone
D	dermis	RR	rete ridges		

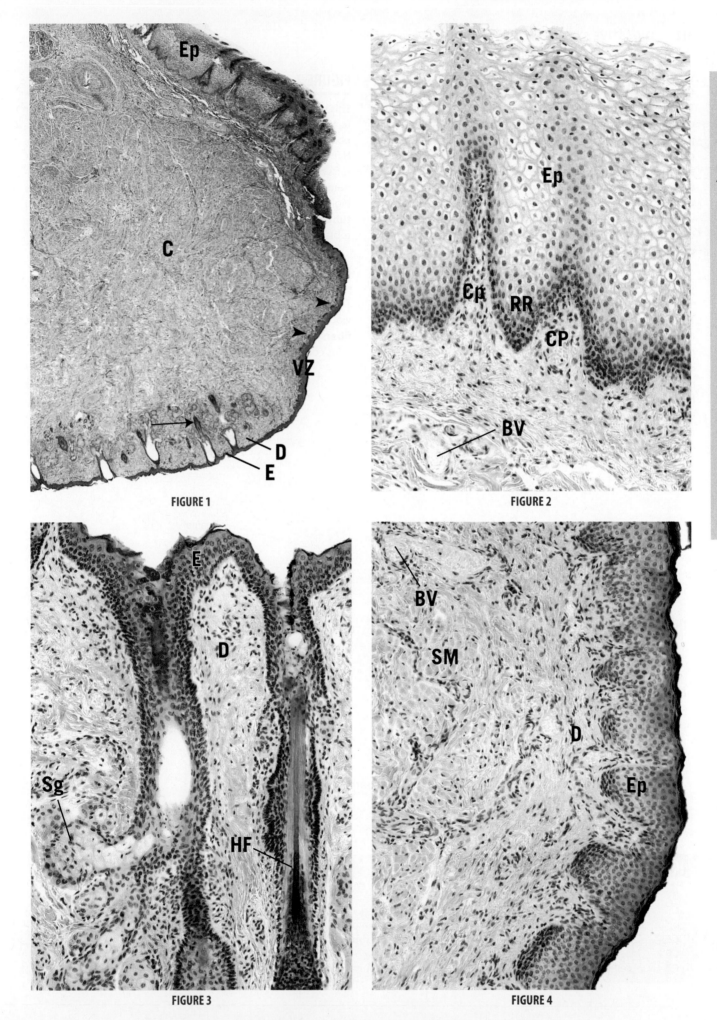

PLATE 13-1 · Lip

FIGURE 1

FIGURE 2

FIGURE 3

FIGURE 4

PLATE 13-2 · Tooth and Pulp

FIGURE 1. Tooth. Human. Ground section. ×14.

The tooth consists of a crown, neck, and root, composed of calcified tissue surrounding a chamber housing a soft, gelatinous pulp. In ground section, only the hard tissues remain. The crown is composed of **enamel** (e) and **dentin** (d), whose interface is known as the **dentinoenamel junction** (DEJ). At the neck of the tooth, enamel meets **cementum** (c), forming the **cementoenamel junction** (CEJ). The **pulp chamber** (PC) is reduced in size as the individual ages. The gap in the enamel (*arrows*) is due to the presence of a carious lesion (cavity). A region similar to the *boxed area* is presented at a higher magnification in Figure 2.

FIGURE 3. Pulp. Human. Paraffin section. ×132.

The pulp is surrounded by dentin (d) from which it is separated by a noncalcified **dentin matrix** (DM). The pulp is said to possess four regions: the **odontoblastic layer** (OL), the **cell-free zone** (CZ), the **cell-rich zone** (CR), and the **core** (C). The core of the pulp is composed of **fibroblasts** (F), delicate collagen fibers, numerous **nerve bundles** (NB), and **blood vessels** (BV). Branches of these neurovascular structures reach the periphery of the pulp, where they supply the cell-rich zone and the odontoblasts with capillaries and fine nerve fibers.

FIGURE 2. Tooth. Human. Ground section. ×132.

This photomicrograph is a higher magnification of a region similar to the *boxed area* of the previous figure. The enamel (e) is composed of enamel rods (*arrows*), each surrounded by a rod sheath. Hypomineralized regions of enamel present the appearance of tufts of grass, **enamel tufts** (ET), which extend from the **dentinoenamel junction** (DEJ) partway into the enamel. **Dentin** (d), not as highly calcified as enamel, presents long, narrow canals, **dentinal tubules** (DT), which in the living tooth house processes of odontoblasts, cells responsible for the formation of dentin.

FIGURE 4. Pulp. Human. Paraffin section. ×270.

This is a higher magnification of the lower right corner of the previous figure. Note the presence of blood vessels (BV) and **nerve fibers** (NF), as well as the numerous **fibroblasts** (F) of this gelatinous connective tissue.

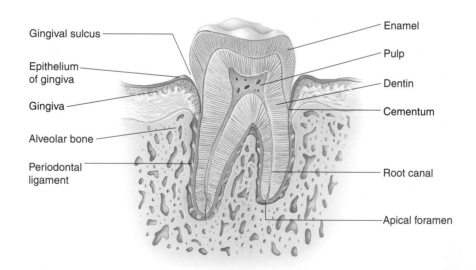

Gingival sulcus

Epithelium of gingiva

Gingiva

Alveolar bone

Periodontal ligament

Enamel

Pulp

Dentin

Cementum

Root canal

Apical foramen

Tooth

KEY

BV	blood vessel	**d**	dentin	**F**	fibroblasts
C	core	**DEJ**	dentinoenamel junction	**NB**	nerve bundles
c	cementum	**DM**	dentin matrix	**OL**	odontoblastic layer
CEJ	cementoenamel junction	**DT**	dentinal tubule	**PC**	pulp chamber
CR	cell-rich zone	**e**	enamel		
CZ	cell-free zone	**ET**	enamel tufts		

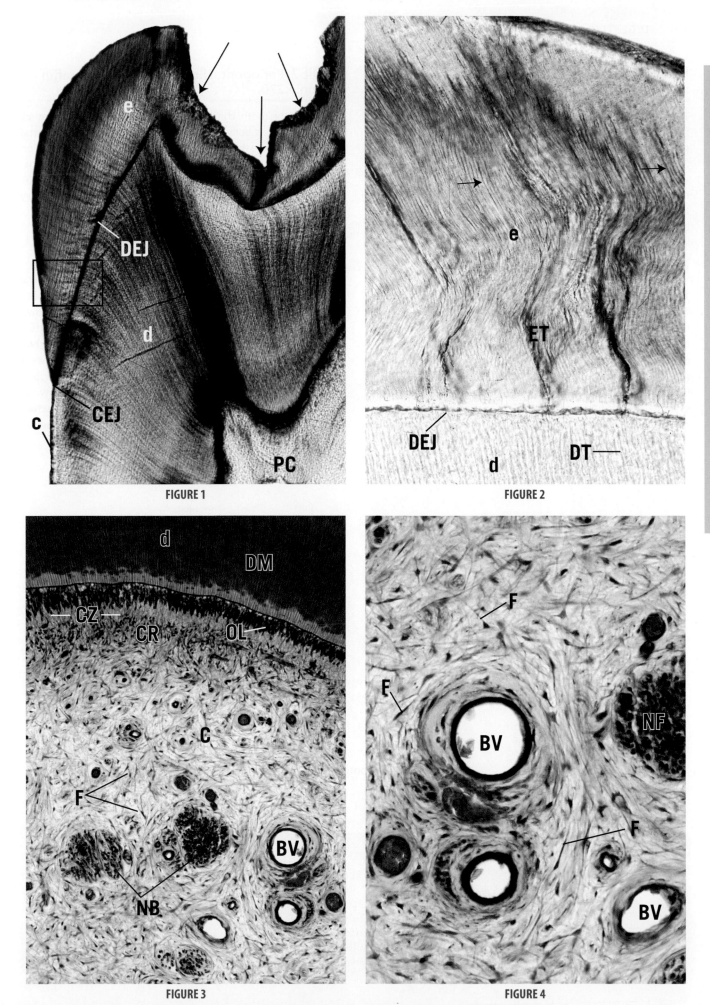

PLATE 13-2 · Tooth and Pulp

FIGURE 1

FIGURE 2

FIGURE 3

FIGURE 4

PLATE 13-3 • Periodontal Ligament and Gingiva

FIGURE 1. Periodontal ligament. Human. Paraffin section. ×132.

The root of the tooth, composed of dentin (d) and **cementum** (c), is suspended in its **alveolus** (A) by a collagenous tissue, the **periodontal ligament** (PL). The strong bands of **collagen fibers** (CF) are embedded in the bone via **Sharpey's fibers** (SF). **Blood vessels** (BV) from the bone enter and supply the periodontal ligament. The dentinocemental junction (*arrows*) is clearly evident. Near the apex of the root, the cementum becomes thicker and houses cementocytes.

FIGURE 3. Gingiva. Human. Paraffin section. ×14.

This is a decalcified longitudinal section of an incisor tooth; thus, all of the calcium hydroxyapatite crystals have been extracted from the tooth and from its bony **alveolus** (A). Since enamel is composed almost completely of calcium hydroxyapatite crystals, only the space where enamel used to be, the **enamel space** (ES), is represented in this photomicrograph. The **crest** (cr) of the alveolus is evident, as are the **periodontal ligament** (PL) and the **gingiva** (G). The **gingival margin** (GM), **free gingiva** (FG), **attached gingiva** (AG), **sulcular epithelium** (SE), **junctional epithelium** (JE), and **alveolar mucosa** (AM) are also identified.

FIGURE 2. Periodontal ligament. Human. Paraffin section. ×270.

The root of the tooth, composed of dentin (d) and **cementum** (c), is suspended in its bony **alveolus** (A) by fibers of the **periodontal ligament** (PL). Note that this photomicrograph is taken in the region of the **crest** (cr) of the alveolus, above which the periodontal ligament is continuous with the connective tissue of the **gingiva** (G). Note that both the gingiva and the periodontal ligament are highly vascular, as evident from the abundance of **blood vessels** (BV).

FIGURE 4. Gingiva. Human. Paraffin section. ×132.

This photomicrograph is a higher magnification of the gingival margin region of the previous figure. Note that the enamel space (ES) is located between the **dentin** (d) of the incisor tooth's crown and the **junctional epithelium** (JE). The **sulcular epithelium** (SE) of the **free gingiva** (FG) borders a space known as the **gingival sulcus** (GS), which would be clearly evident if the enamel were still present in this photomicrograph. Observe the well-developed interdigitations of the epithelium and connective tissue, known as the rete apparatus (*arrows*) of the **free gingiva** (FG) and **attached gingiva**, indicative of the presence of abrasive forces that act on these regions of the oral cavity.

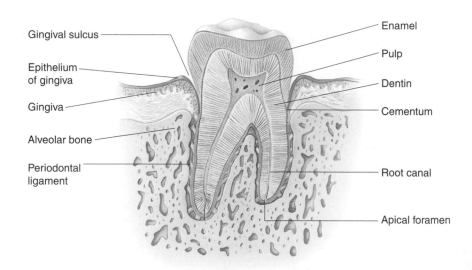

Gingival sulcus — Enamel

Epithelium of gingiva — Pulp

Gingiva — Dentin

Alveolar bone — Cementum

Periodontal ligament — Root canal

— Apical foramen

Tooth

KEY

A	alveolus	**CF**	collagen fibers	**G**	gingiva
AM	alveolar mucosa	**d**	dentin	**GM**	gingival margin
AT	attached gingiva	**DEJ**	dentinoenamel junction	**GS**	gingival sulcus
BV	blood vessel	**DT**	dentinal tubule	**JE**	junctional epithelium
c	cementum	**ES**	enamel space	**PC**	pulp chamber
cr	crest of alveolus	**ET**	enamel tufts	**PL**	periodontal ligament
CEJ	cementoenamel junction	**FG**	free gingiva	**SE**	sulcular epithelium

PLATE 13-3 · Periodontal Ligament and Gingiva

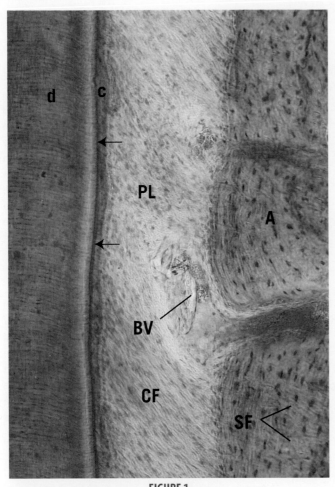

FIGURE 1

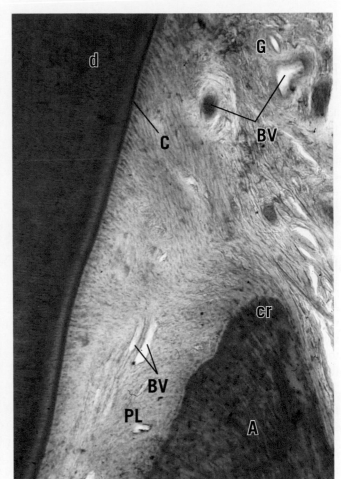

FIGURE 2

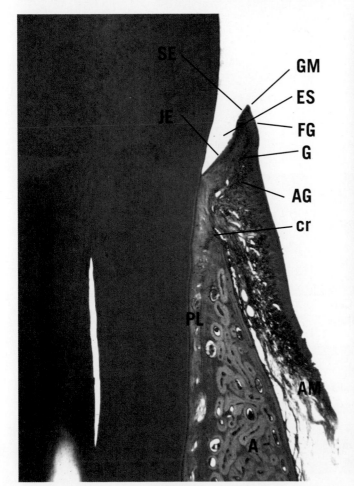

FIGURE 3

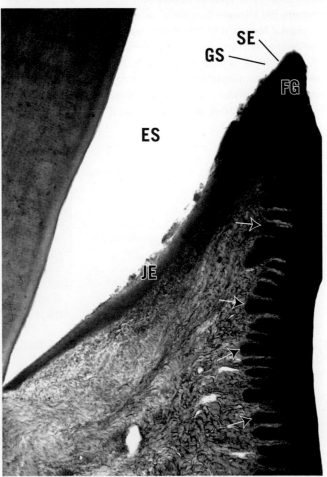

FIGURE 4

PLATE 13-4 • Tooth Development

FIGURE 1a. Tooth development. Dental lamina. Frontal section. Pig. Paraffin section. ×132.

The dental lamina (DL) is a horseshoe-shaped band of epithelial tissue that arises from the **oral epithelium** (OE) and is surrounded by **mesenchymal cells** (MC). A frontal section of the dental lamina is characterized by the club-shaped appearance in this photomicrograph. The mesenchymal cells in discrete regions at the distal aspect of the dental lamina become rounded and congregate to form the precursor of the dental papilla responsible for the formation of the pulp and dentin of the tooth.

FIGURE 1b. Tooth development. Bud stage. Frontal section. Pig. Paraffin section. ×132.

At various discrete locations along the dental lamina (DL), an epithelial thickening, the **bud** (B), makes its appearance. Each bud will provide the cells necessary for enamel formation for a single tooth. The **dental papilla** (DP) forms a crescent-shaped area at the distal aspect of the bud.

FIGURE 3. Tooth development. Bell stage. Frontal section. Pig. Paraffin section. ×132.

As the enamel organ expands in size, it resembles a bell, hence the bell stage of tooth development. This stage is characterized by four cellular layers: **outer enamel epithelium** (OEE), **stellate reticulum** (SR), **inner enamel epithelium** (IEE), and **stratum intermedium** (SI). Observe that the enamel organ is still connected to the **dental lamina** (DL). The **dental papilla** (DP) is composed of rounded mesenchymal cells, whose peripheral-most layer (*arrows*) will differentiate to form odontoblasts. Note the wide basement membrane (*arrowheads*) between the future odontoblasts and inner enamel epithelium (the future ameloblasts). Observe also the spindle-shaped cells of the **dental sac** (DS).

FIGURE 2. Tooth development. Cap stage. Frontal section. Pig. Paraffin section. ×132.

Increased mitotic activity transforms the bud into a cap-shaped structure. Observe that three epithelial layers of the enamel organ may be recognized: the outer enamel epithelium (OEE), the **inner enamel epithelium** (IEE), and the intervening **stellate reticulum** (SR). The inner enamel epithelium has begun to enclose the **dental papilla** (DP). Note that mesenchymal cells become elongated, forming the **dental sac** (DS), which will envelop the enamel organ and dental papilla. Moreover, a **bony crypt** (BC) will enclose the dental sac.

FIGURE 4. Tooth development. Apposition. Frontal section. Pig. Paraffin section. ×132.

The elaboration of dentin (d) and **enamel** (e) is indicative of apposition. Dentin is manufactured by **odontoblasts** (O), the peripheral-most cell layer of the **dental papilla** (DP). The odontoblastic processes (*arrows*) are visible in this photomicrograph as they traverse the **dentin matrix** (DM). **Ameloblasts** (A) are highly elongated, columnar cells that manufacture enamel. The long, epithelial structure located to the left is the **succedaneous lamina** (SL), which is responsible for the development of the permanent tooth.

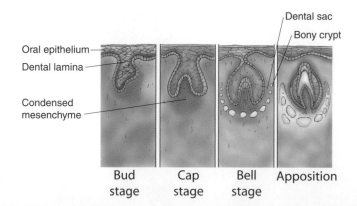

Oral epithelium
Dental lamina
Condensed mesenchyme
Dental sac
Bony crypt

Bud stage   Cap stage   Bell stage   Apposition

KEY

A	ameloblast	DP	dental papilla	OE	oral epithelium
B	bud	DS	dental sac	OEE	outer enamel epithelium
BC	bony crypt	e	enamel	SI	stratum intermedium
d	dentin	IEE	inner enamel epithelium	SL	succedaneous lamina
DL	dental lamina	MC	mesenchymal cell	SR	stellate reticulum
DM	dentin matrix	O	odontoblast		

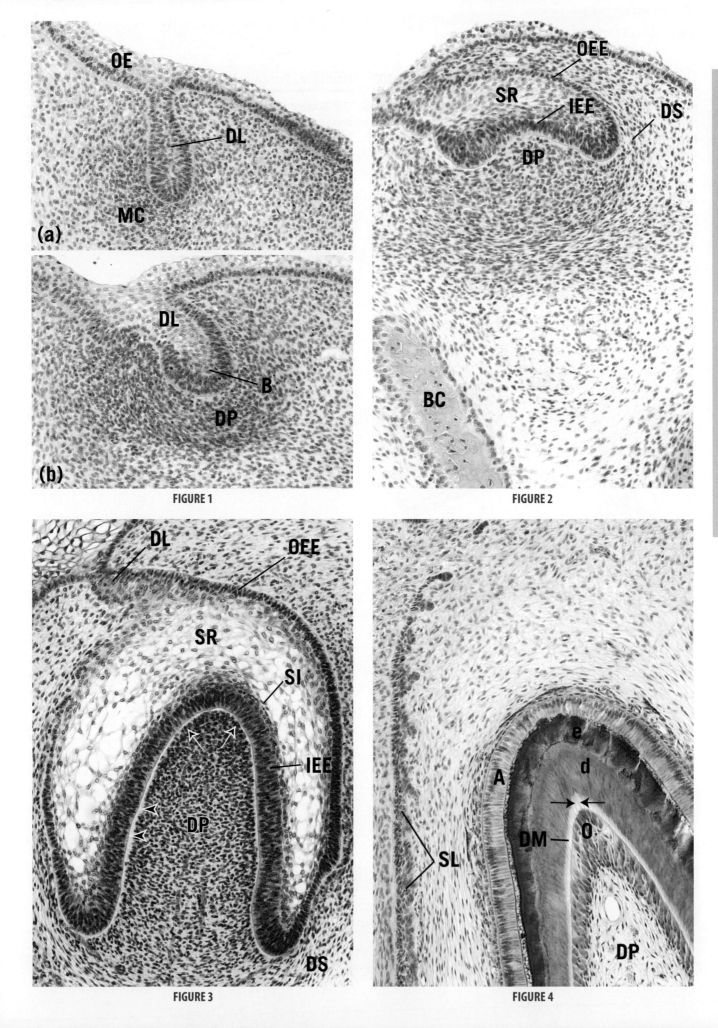

PLATE 13-4 · Tooth Development

FIGURE 1

FIGURE 2

FIGURE 3

FIGURE 4

PLATE 13-5 · Tongue

FIGURE 1. Tongue. Human. l.s. Paraffin section. ×20.

Part of the anterior two-thirds of the tongue is presented in this photomicrograph. This muscular organ bears numerous **filiform papillae** (FP) on its dorsal surface, whose stratified squamous epithelium is keratinized (*arrow*). The ventral surface of the tongue is lined by stratified squamous nonkeratinized **epithelium** (Ep). The intrinsic muscles of the tongue are arranged in four layers: **superior longitudinal** (SL), **vertical** (V), **inferior longitudinal** (IL), and horizontal (not shown here). The mucosa of the tongue tightly adheres to the perimysium of the intrinsic tongue muscles by the subepithelial **connective tissue** (CT).

FIGURE 2. Tongue. Human. l.s. Paraffin section. ×14.

The posterior aspect of the anterior two-thirds of the tongue presents circumvallate papillae (Cp). These papillae are surrounded by a deep groove (*arrow*), the base of which accepts a serous secretion via the **ducts** (Du) of the **glands of von Ebner** (GE). The **epithelium** (Ep) of the papilla houses taste buds along its lateral aspects but not on its superior surface. The core of the tongue contains **skeletal muscle** (SM) fibers of the extrinsic and intrinsic lingual muscles as well as glands and **adipose tissue** (AT). A region similar to the *boxed area* is presented at a higher magnification in Figure 3.

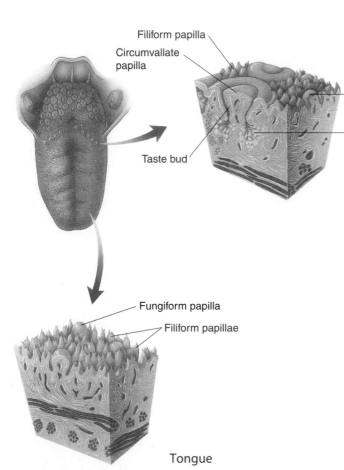

Filiform papilla
Circumvallate papilla
Taste bud
Fungiform papilla
Glands of von Ebner
Fungiform papilla
Filiform papillae
Tongue

FIGURE 3. Circumvallate papilla. Monkey. x.s. Plastic section. ×132.

This photomicrograph is a higher magnification of a region similar to the *boxed area* of the previous figure, rotated 90 degrees. Note the presence of the groove (G) separating the **circumvallate papilla** (Cp) from the wall of the groove. **Glands of von Ebner** (GE) deliver a serous secretion into this groove, whose contents are monitored by numerous intraepithelial **taste buds** (TB). Observe that taste buds are not found on the superior surface of the circumvallate papilla, only on its lateral aspect. The connective tissue core of the papilla is richly endowed by **blood vessels** (BV) and **nerves** (N).

KEY

AT	adipose tissue	**Ep**	epithelium	**N**	nerves
BV	blood vessels	**FP**	filiform papillae	**SL**	superior longitudinal muscle
Cp	circumvallate papillae	**G**	groove	**SM**	skeletal muscle
CT	connective tissue	**GE**	glands of von Ebner	**TB**	taste buds
Du	ducts	**IL**	inferior longitudinal muscle	**V**	vertical muscle

PLATE 13-5 • Tongue

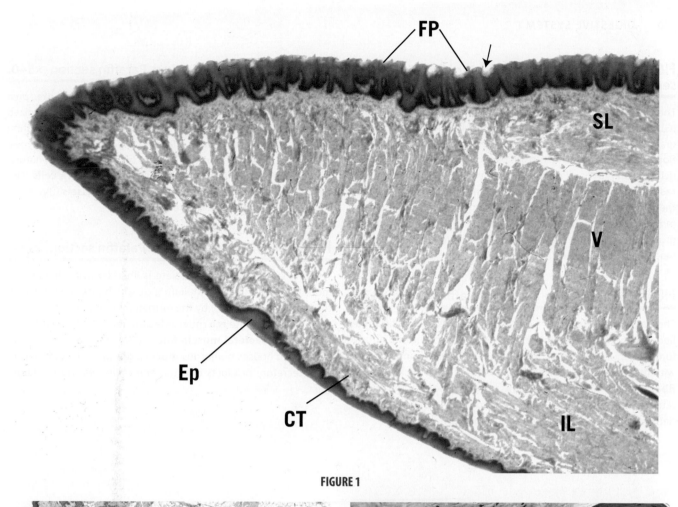

FP

↓

SL

V

Ep

CT

IL

FIGURE 1

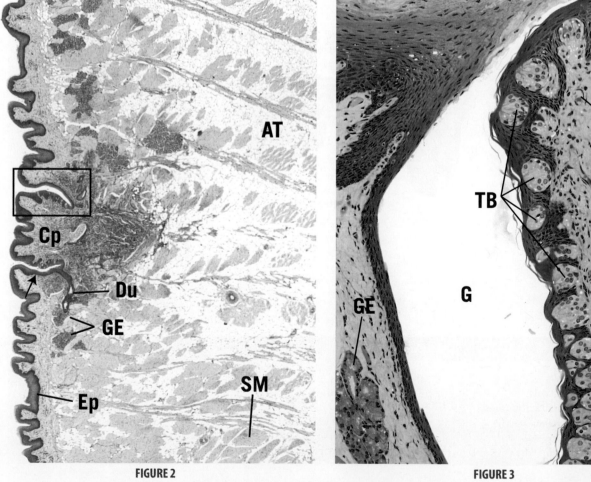

AT

Cp

Du

GE

Ep

SM

FIGURE 2

BV

TB

Cp

BV

GE

G

N

FIGURE 3

PLATE 13-6 · Tongue and Palate

FIGURE 1. Circumvallate papilla. Monkey. Paraffin section. ×132.

The base of the circumvallate papilla (Cp), the surrounding **groove** (G), and the wall of the groove are evident in this photomicrograph. The **glands of von Ebner** (GE) deliver their serous secretions via short **ducts** (Du) into the base of the groove. Observe the rich **vascular** (BV) and **nerve** (N) supply to this region. Numerous **taste buds** (TB) populate the epithelium of the lateral aspect of the circumvallate papilla. Each taste bud possesses a taste pore (*arrows*) through which taste hairs (microvilli) protrude into the groove. A region similar to the *boxed area* is presented at a higher magnification in Figure 2.

FIGURE 3. Hard palate. Human. Paraffin section. ×132.

The hard palate possesses a nasal and an oral surface. The stratified squamous parakeratinized epithelium (Ep) of the oral surface forms deep invaginations, **rete ridges** (RR), which interdigitate with the subepithelial **connective tissue** (CT). The thick **collagen fiber bundles** (CF) firmly bind the palatal mucosa to the periosteum of the underlying bone. The hard palate also houses large deposits of adipose tissue and mucous glands.

FIGURE 2. Taste bud. Monkey. Paraffin section. ×540.

This is a higher magnification of a region similar to the *boxed area* of Figure 1. Note that the stratified squamous parakeratinized epithelium (Ep) displays squames in the process of desquamation (*arrowheads*). The **taste buds** (TB) are composed of four cell types. **Basal** (lateral) **cells** (BC) are believed to be regenerative in nature, whereas **light cells** (LC), intermediate cells, and **dark cells** (DC) are gustatory. Observe the presence of **blood vessels** (BV) in the subepithelial **connective tissue** (CT).

FIGURE 4. Soft palate. Human. Paraffin section. ×132.

The oral surface of the soft palate is lined by a stratified squamous nonkeratinized epithelium (Ep), which interdigitates with the **lamina propria** (LP) by the formation of shallow **rete ridges** (RR). The soft palate is a moveable structure, as attested by the presence of **skeletal muscle fibers** (SM). The core of the soft palate also houses numerous **mucous glands** (MG) that deliver their secretory products into the oral cavity via short, straight ducts.

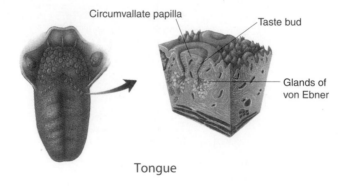

Circumvallate papilla

Taste bud

Glands of von Ebner

Tongue

KEY					
BC	basal cells	**Du**	ducts	**MG**	mucous glands
BV	blood vessels	**Ep**	epithelium	**N**	nerve
CF	collagen fiber bundles	**G**	groove	**RR**	rete ridges
Cp	circumvallate papilla	**GE**	glands of von Ebner	**SM**	skeletal muscle
CT	connective tissue	**LC**	light cells	**TB**	taste buds
DC	dark cells	**LP**	lamina propria		

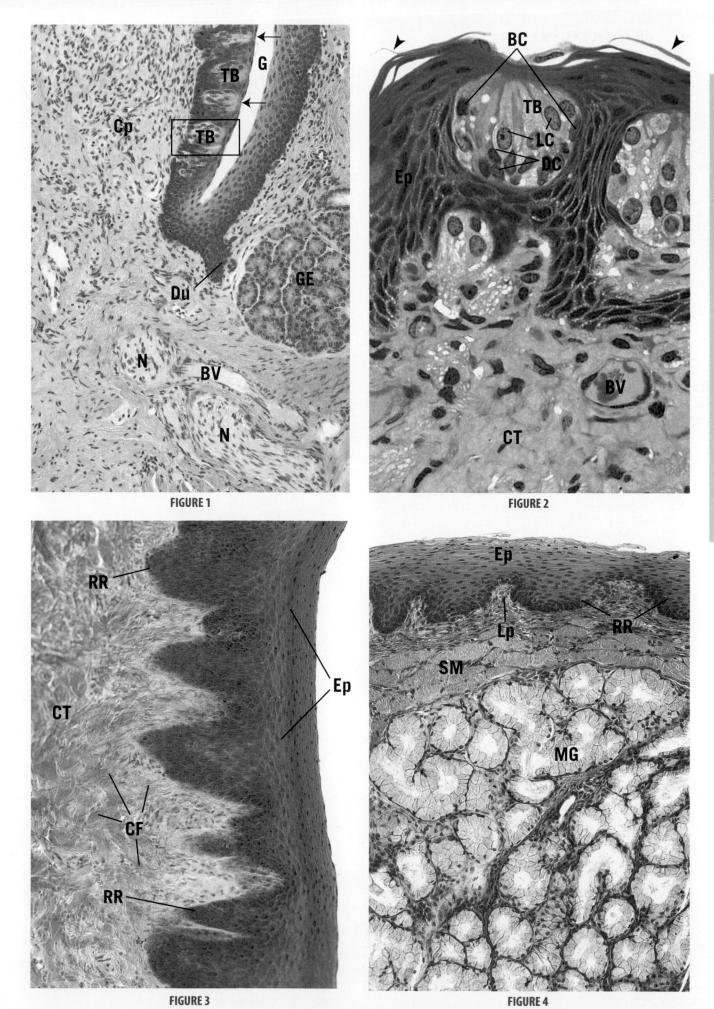

PLATE 13-6 • Tongue and Palate

FIGURE 1

FIGURE 2

FIGURE 3

FIGURE 4

PLATE 13-7 • Teeth and Nasal Aspect of the Hard Palate

FIGURE 1. Human central incisor roots. Paraffin section. ×132.

The roots of two human central incisors and their supporting tissues are noted in this composite photomicrograph. Note that the root of one incisor, Root 1, is at the top of the figure, and progressing down the page, the **hyaline layer of Hopewell-Smith** (HL) separates the **dentin** (d) of the root from the **cementum** (c). The **periodontal ligament** (PL1), with its attendant **blood vessels** (BV), of this tooth suspends tooth 1 in its alveolus. The **interdental septum** (IS), positioned between the two incisors and composed of woven bone, is formed by the fusion of the **alveolar bones proper** (ABP 1 and 2) of each root. Note the presence of **osteons** (Os) in the woven bone; the center of these osteons approximates the line of fusion between the two alveolar bones proper. The **periodontal ligament** of the other incisor (PL 2) is located between the alveolar bone proper (ABP 2) and the **cementum** of this tooth. Its **dentin** (d) and **hyaline layer of Hopewell-Smith** (HL) of root 2 are evident.

FIGURE 2. Hard palate. Human. Paraffin section. ×132.

The hard palate possesses a nasal and an oral surface. Note that the pseudostratified ciliated columnar **epithelium** (Ep) displays cilia and an **intraepithelial gland** (IeGL). Observe the presence of **glands** (Gl) and **blood vessels** (BV) in the subepithelial **connective tissue** (CT). The epithelium and the subepithelial connective tissue are collectively referred to as the **mucoperiosteum** (MP), which is firmly attached to the **bony shelf** (B) of the palate. A higher magnification of the *boxed area* is presented in Figure 3.

FIGURE 3. Hard palate. Human. Paraffin section. ×132.

This is a higher magnification of a region similar to the *boxed area* of Figure 2. Note the presence of **glands** (Gl), **blood vessels** (BV), and **lymph vessels** (LV) within the subepithelial **connective tissue** (CT). The thick **collagen fiber bundles** (CF) firmly bind the palatal mucosa to the periosteum of the underlying bone. Observe the clearly visible **cilia** (c) of the pseudostratified ciliated columnar **epithelium** (Ep) covering the nasal surface of the hard palate.

KEY

ABP	alveolar bone proper	**d**	dentin	**IeGL**	intraepithelial gland
B	bony shelf	**Ep**	epithelium	**IS**	interdental septum
BV	blood vessel	**GL**	gland	**MP**	palatal mucosa
C	cementum	**HL**	hyaline layer of	**Os**	osteon
CT	connective tissue		Hopewell-Smith	**PL**	periodontal ligament

PLATE 13-7 · Teeth and Nasal Aspect of the Hard Palate

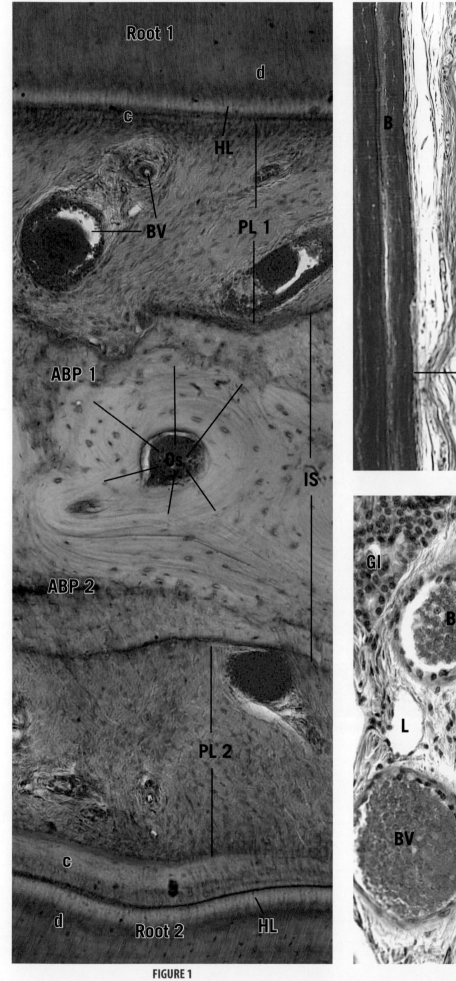

FIGURE 1

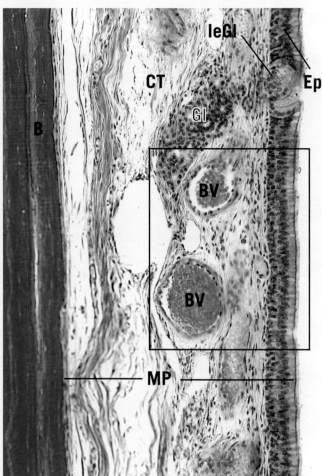

FIGURE 2

FIGURE 3

PLATE 13-8 · Teeth Scanning Electron Micrograph of Enamel

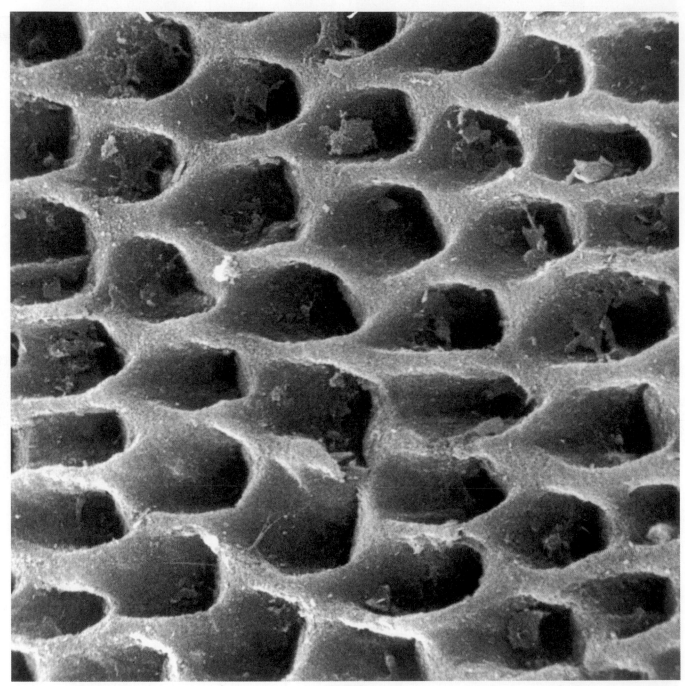

FIGURE 1

FIGURE 1. Human enamel. Scanning electron microscopy. ×3,150.

This three-dimensional view of the forming mineralized human enamel displays rod spaces (the recesses) surrounded by the interrod enamel. The rod spaces were occupied by Tomes' processes of the ameloblasts, and as the ameloblasts recede, rod spaces are filled in by the secretory mechanism, and the spaces are filled by enamel known as rod segments. The arched aspects of the rod spaces are directed occlusally. As rod segments are positioned on top of each other, they form an enamel rod whose shape resembles a keyhole. (From Fejerskov O. Human dentition and experimental animals. J Dent Res 1979;58(Special Issue B):725–734.)

PLATE 13-9 • Teeth Scanning Electron Micrograph of Dentin

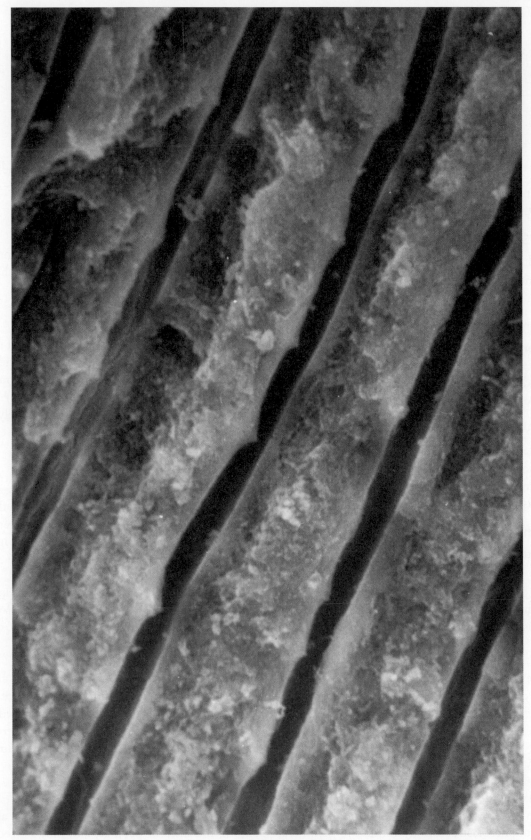

FIGURE 1

FIGURE 1. Human dentin. Scanning electron microscopy. ×3,800.

This three-dimensional view of mineralized human dentin displays a longitudinal section of dentinal tubules. In a healthy, living dentin, the tubules house the processes of odontoblasts that extend at least 1 mm into the dentinal tubule. Additionally, some of the tubules also house nerve fibers, and all of the tubules are filled completely with an extracellular fluid that originates in the pulp of the tooth. (From Thomas H. The dentin-predentin complex and its permeability: anatomical overview. J Dent Res 1985;64(Special Issue B):607–612.)

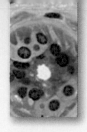

Chapter Summary

I. LIPS

The **lips** control access to the **oral cavity** from the outside environment.

A. External Surface

The external surface is covered with thin **skin** and therefore possesses **hair follicles, sebaceous glands,** and **sweat glands**.

B. Transitional Zone

The **transitional zone (vermilion zone)** is the pink area of the lip. Here the connective tissue papillae extend deep into the epidermis. Hair follicles and sweat glands are absent, whereas sebaceous glands are occasionally present.

C. Mucous Membrane

The vestibular aspect of the lip is lined by a **wet epithelium** (stratified squamous nonkeratinized) with numerous **minor mixed salivary glands** in the subepithelial connective tissue.

D. Core of the Lip

The core of the lip contains **skeletal muscle**.

II. TEETH

Teeth are composed of three calcified tissues and a loose connective tissue core, the pulp.

A. Enamel

Enamel is the hardest substance in the body. It is made by **ameloblasts,** cells no longer present in the erupted tooth. Enamel is present only in the crown.

B. Dentin

Dentin is a calcified, collagen-based material that constitutes the bulk of the **crown** and **root**; it surrounds the pulp. Dentin is made by **odontoblasts,** whose long processes remain in channels, the **dentinal tubules,** traversing dentin. The odontoblast cell body forms the peripheral extent of the pulp.

C. Cementum

Cementum is located on the **root** of the tooth, surrounding **dentin**. Cementum is a collagen-based, calcified material manufactured by **cementoblasts,** which may become entrapped and then are referred to as **cementocytes**.

Fibers of the **periodontal ligament** are embedded in cementum and bone, thus suspending the tooth in its **bony socket,** the **alveolus**.

D. Pulp

The **pulp** is a gelatinous type of mesenchymal-appearing connective tissue that occupies the **pulp chamber**. It is richly supplied by **nerves** and **blood vessels**.

III. GINGIVA

The **gingiva** (gum) is that region of the oral mucosa that is closely applied to the **neck of the tooth** and is attached to the **alveolar bone**. It is covered by a **stratified squamous partially keratinized (parakeratotic) epithelium**. The underlying connective tissue is densely populated with thick bundles of collagen fibers.

IV. TONGUE

The **tongue** is a **muscular organ** whose oral region is freely moving; its root is attached to the floor of the pharynx. **Skeletal muscle** forms the core of the tongue, among which groups of serous and seromucous glands are interspersed.

A. Oral Region (Anterior Two-Thirds)

The mucosa of the dorsal surface of the anterior two-thirds of the tongue is modified to form four types of lingual papillae.

1. Filiform Papillae

Filiform papillae are long and slender and are the most numerous. They form a roughened surface (especially in animals such as cats) and are distributed in parallel rows along the entire surface. They are covered by a **parakeratinized stratified squamous epithelium** (but bear no taste buds) over a **connective tissue core**.

2. Fungiform Papillae

Fungiform papillae are mushroom-shaped, are scattered among the filiform papillae, and may be recognized by their appearance as red dots. They contain **taste buds** along their dorsal aspect.

3. Foliate Papillae

Foliate papillae appear as longitudinal furrows along the side of the tongue near the posterior aspect of the anterior two-thirds. Their **taste buds** degenerate at an early age in humans. Serous **glands of von Ebner** are associated with these papillae.

4. Circumvallate Papillae

Circumvallate papillae are very large and form a V-shaped row at the border of the oral and pharyngeal portions of the tongue. Circumvallate papillae are each surrounded by a moat or groove, the walls of which contain **taste buds** in their **stratified squamous nonkeratinized epithelium**. Serous **glands of von Ebner** open into the base of the furrow. The connective tissue core of the circumvallate papilla possesses a rich nerve and vascular supply.

B. Pharyngeal Region (Posterior One-Third)

The **mucosa** of the posterior one-third of the tongue presents numerous **lymphatic nodules** that constitute the **lingual tonsils**.

V. PALATE

The **palate**, composed of hard and soft regions, separates the **oral** and **nasal cavities** from each other. Therefore, the palate possesses a **nasal** and an **oral aspect**. The **oral** aspect is covered by **stratified squamous epithelium** (**partially keratinized** on the hard palate), whereas the **nasal** aspect is covered by a **respiratory epithelium**. The **subepithelial connective tissue** presents dense collagen fibers interspersed with **adipose tissue** and **mucous glands**. The **core** of the hard palate houses a **bony shelf**, whereas that of the soft palate is composed of **skeletal muscle**.

VI. TOOTH DEVELOPMENT

Tooth development (odontogenesis) may be divided into several stages (see Graphic 13-1). These are named according to the morphology and/or the functional state of the developing tooth. **Dental lamina formation** is followed by **bud**, **cap**, and **bell stages**. Dentin formation initiates the **apposition stage**, followed by **root formation** and **eruption**. These stages occur in both **primary** (deciduous teeth) and **secondary** (permanent teeth) **dentition**.

14 DIGESTIVE SYSTEM II

CHAPTER OUTLINE

The **digestive tract (alimentary canal)** is an approximately 9-m-long, hollow, tubular structure that extends from the oral cavity to the anus whose wall is modified along its length to perform the various facets of digestion.

- The oral cavity receives food and, via mastication and bolus formation, delivers it into the oral pharynx, from where it enters the esophagus and eventually the stomach.
- The gastric contents are reduced to an **acidic chyme**, which is transferred in small aliquots into the small intestine, where most digestion and absorption occur.
- The liquefied food residue passes into the large intestine, where the digestion is completed and water is resorbed.
- The solidified feces are then passed to the rectum for elimination through the anus.

A common architectural plan is evident for the digestive tract from the esophagus to the anus, in that four distinct concentric layers may be recognized to constitute the wall of this long, tubular structure.

LAYERS OF THE WALL OF THE DIGESTIVE TRACT

The layers of the **digestive tract** are the mucosa, submucosa, muscularis externa, and the serosa/adventitia. These layers are described from the lumen outward, and they form the general plan of the **digestive tract**. The cellular composition and the general plan are modified along the digestive tract as one proceeds from the esophagus to the anus (see Table 14-1, which depicts these alterations).

- The innermost layer directly surrounding the lumen is known as the **mucosa**, which is composed of three concentric layers:
  - a wet epithelial lining with secretory and absorptive functions;
  - a connective tissue lamina propria containing glands and components of the circulatory system;
  - and a muscularis mucosae, usually consisting of two thin, smooth muscle layers, responsible for the mobility of the mucosa.
- The **submucosa** is a coarser connective tissue component that physically supports the mucosa and provides neural, vascular, and lymphatic supply to the mucosa. Moreover, in some regions of the digestive tract, the submucosa houses glands.
- The **muscularis externa** usually consists of an **inner circular** and an **outer longitudinal smooth muscle layer**, which is modified in certain regions of the digestive tract.

- Although these layers are described as circularly or longitudinally arranged, they are actually wrapped around the digestive tract in tight and loose helices, respectively.
- Vascular and neural plexuses (**Auerbach's** and **Meissner's**) reside between the muscle layers.
- The muscularis externa functions in churning and propelling the luminal contents along the digestive tract via peristaltic action.
- Thus, as the circular muscles reduce the diameter of the lumen, preventing the movement of the luminal contents in a proximal direction (toward the mouth), the longitudinal muscles contract in such a fashion as to push the luminal contents in a distal direction (toward the anus).
- The outermost layer of the digestive tract is either a **serosa** or an **adventitia**.
  - The intraperitoneal regions of the digestive tract, that is, those that are suspended by peritoneum, possess a **serosa**. This structure consists of connective tissue covered by a **mesothelium** (simple squamous epithelium), which reduces frictional forces during digestive movements.
  - Other regions of the digestive tract are firmly attached to surrounding structures by connective tissue fibers. These regions possess an **adventitia**.

REGIONS OF THE DIGESTIVE TRACT

Esophagus

The **esophagus** is a short, muscular tube whose lumen is usually collapsed unless a bolus of food is traversing its length for delivery from the pharynx into the stomach.

- The **mucosa** of the esophagus is composed of a **stratified squamous nonkeratinized epithelium**; the lamina propria, a loose type of connective tissue, housing mucus-producing esophageal **cardiac glands;** and a **muscularis mucosae** composed only of longitudinally oriented smooth muscle fibers.
- The submucosa of this organ is composed of dense, irregular collagenous connective tissue interspersed with elastic fibers. This is one of the two regions of the digestive tract (the other is the duodenum) that houses glands in its submucosa. These glands are the mucus-producing **esophageal glands proper**.
- The **muscularis externa** of the esophagus is composed of **inner circular** and **outer longitudinal** layers. Those in the proximal (upper) one-third are **skeletal**; those in the middle one-third are **skeletal** and **smooth**, whereas those in the distal (lower) one-third are **smooth muscle**.

TABLE 14-1 • Selected Histological Features of the Alimentary Canal

Region	Epithelium	Lamina Propria	Layers of Muscularis Mucosae*	Submucosa	Layers of Muscularis Externa[†]
Esophagus	Stratified squamous	Esophageal cardiac glands	Longitudinal	Collagenous CT, esophageal glands proper	Inner circular, outer longitudinal
Stomach	Simple columnar, no goblet cells	Gastric glands	Inner circular, outer longitudinal, sometimes outermost circular	Collagenous CT, no glands	Inner oblique, middle circular, outer longitudinal
Small intestine	Simple columnar with goblet cells	Villi, crypts of Lieberkühn, Peyer patches in ileum (extend into submucosa), lymphoid nodules	Inner circular, outer longitudinal	Fibroelastic CT, Brunner glands in duodenum	Inner circular, outer longitudinal
Large intestine, cecum, colon	Simple columnar with goblet cells	Crypts of Lieberkühn (lack Paneth cells), lymphoid nodules	Inner circular, outer longitudinal	Fibroelastic CT, no glands	Inner circular, outer longitudinal (modified to form teniae coli)
Rectum	Simple columnar with goblet cells	Crypts of Lieberkühn (fewer but deeper than in colon) lymphoid nodules	Inner circular, outer longitudinal	Fibroelastic CT, no glands	Two layers: inner circular, outer longitudinal
Anal canal	Simple columnar cuboidal (proximal), stratified squamous nonkeratinized (distal to anal valves), stratified squamous keratinized (anus)	Sebaceous glands, circumanal glands, lymphoid nodules, rectal columns or Morgagni (involve entire mucosa), hair follicles (anus)	Inner circular, outer longitudinal	Fibroelastic CT with large veins, no glands	Inner circular (forms internal anal sphincter), outer longitudinal
Appendix	Simple columnar with goblet cells	Crypts of Lieberkühn (shallow), lymphoid nodules (large, numerous and may extend into the submucosa)	Inner circular, outer longitudinal	Fibroelastic CT, confluent lymphoid nodules, no glands, fat tissue (sometimes)	Inner circular, outer longitudinal

*The muscularis mucosae is composed entirely of smooth muscle throughout the alimentary canal.

[†]The muscularis externa is composed entirely of smooth muscle in all regions except the esophagus. The upper third of the esophageal muscularis externa is all skeletal muscle; the middle third is a mixture of skeletal and smooth muscle; and the lower third is all smooth muscle.

CT, connective tissue.

TABLE 14-2 • Principal Secretions of the Epithelial Cells of the Stomach

Gastric Glands of the Stomach	Approximate Life Span of the Cells	Secretions
Surface lining cells	3–5 days	Visible mucus
Mucous neck cells	6 days	Soluble mucus
Parietal cells	200 days	Hydrochloric acid, gastric intrinsic factor
Chief cells	60–90 days	Pepsin, rennin, lipase precursors
Diffuse neuroendocrine system cells	60–90 days	Gastrin, somatostatin, secretin, cholecystokinin
Regenerative cells	Function to replace epithelial lining of stomach and cells of glands	

Stomach

The **stomach** functions in acidifying and converting the semisolid **bolus** into the viscous fluid, **chyme**, which undergoes initial digestion and is delivered into the **duodenum** in small quantities.

The gastric mucosa is lined by a simple columnar epithelium whose **surface lining cells** (not goblet cells) produce a mucous substance that coats and protects the stomach lining from the low pH environment and from autodigestion.

The lamina propria of the stomach houses **gastric glands**; depending on the region of the stomach, these are cardiac, fundic, or pyloric (see Graphic 14-1).

- The **mucosa** of the empty stomach is thrown into longitudinal folds, known as **rugae**. The luminal surface, lined by a simple columnar epithelium (**surface lining cells**), displays **foveolae (gastric pits)**, whose base is perforated by several gastric glands of the lamina propria. All **gastric glands** are composed of **parietal cells (oxyntic cells)**, **mucous neck cells**, **surface lining cells**, **diffuse neuroendocrine system (DNES,** formerly known as **APUD) cells**, and **regenerative cells**. Fundic glands, in addition, also house **chief (zymogenic) cells**.
  - Parietal cells live for approximately 200 days before being replaced by stem cells.
    - They secrete hydrochloric acid (HCl) into their **intracellular canaliculi**. These cells alter their morphology during HCl secretion, in that they increase their number of **microvilli** that project into the intracellular canaliculi. It is believed that these microvilli are stored as the **tubulovesicular system**, flanking the intracellular canaliculi when the cell is not secreting HCl. The production of HCl is dependent on gastrin, histamine H_2, and acetylcholine M_3 binding to their respective receptors on the parietal cell basal membrane.
    - Parietal cells also secrete **gastric intrinsic factor**, a glycoprotein that binds to and forms a complex

with vitamin B_{12} in the gastric lumen. When this complex reaches the ileum, it binds to specific receptors on the surface absorptive cells, and the vitamin becomes absorbed (see Table 14-2).
  - **Mucous neck cells** live for approximately 6 days. They are located in the neck of gastric glands, and they manufacture *soluble mucus* that becomes part of and lubricates chyme.
  - **Surface lining cells** live for about 3 to 5 days and manufacture *visible mucus* that adheres to the lining of the stomach, protecting it from autodigestion.
  - The various types of **DNES** cells live for about 60 to 90 days. They produce hormones such as **gastrin**, **somatostatin**, **secretin**, and **cholecystokinin**. Table 14-3 presents other hormones produced by the entire digestive tract.
  - **Regenerative cells**, located mainly in the neck and isthmus, replace the epithelial lining of the stomach and the cells of the glands.
  - **Chief cells**, located in the base of the fundic glands, live for about 60 to 90 days. They produce precursors of enzymes (**pepsin, rennin**, and **lipase**).

Small Intestine

The **small intestine** is composed of the **duodenum, jejunum,** and **ileum**. The mucosa of all three regions displays **villi** (singular: **villus**), extensions of the lamina propria, covered by a simple columnar type of epithelium. The epithelium is composed of goblet, surface absorptive, and DNES cells.

- **Goblet cells** produce **mucinogen** that becomes hydrated to form **mucin**, which, when mixed with the luminal contents of the stomach, becomes known as **mucus**.
- **DNES cells** release various hormones (e.g., **secretin, motilin, neurotensin, cholecystokinin, gastric inhibitory peptide,** and **gastrin**) (see Table 14-3 for hormones produced by the digestive tract).

TABLE 14-3 • Hormones Produced by Cells of the Digestive Tract

Hormone	Location	Action
Cholecystokinin	Small intestine	Contraction of gallbladder; release of pancreatic enzymes
Gastric inhibitory peptide	Small intestine	Inhibits hydrochloric acid (HCl) secretion
Gastrin	Stomach	Stimulates secretion of HCl and gastric enzymes
Ghrelin	Stomach	Maintains constant intraluminal pressure in the stomach; induces hunger; modulates smooth muscle tension in muscularis externa
Glycentin	Stomach; large intestine	Stimulates hepatocytic glycogenolysis
Glucagon	Stomach; duodenum	Stimulates hepatocytic glycogenolysis
Motilin	Small intestine	Increases intestinal peristalsis
Neurotensin	Small intestine	Decreases intestinal peristalsis; stimulates blood flow to the ileum
Secretin	Small intestine	Stimulates bicarbonate secretion by the pancreas
Serotonin	Stomach; small intestine; large intestine	Increases intestinal peristalsis
Somatostatin	Stomach; duodenum	Inhibits diffuse neuroendocrine system cells in the vicinity of the release
Substance P	Stomach; small intestine; large intestine	Increases intestinal peristalsis
Human epidermal growth factor (urogastrone)	Duodenal (Brunner's) glands	Inhibits HCl secretion; increases epithelial cell mitosis
Vasoactive intestinal peptide	Stomach; small intestine; large intestine	Increases intestinal peristalsis; stimulates secretion of ions and water by the digestive tract

- The tall, columnar **surface absorptive cells** possess dense accumulations of microvilli, forming the **striated border**. Their tips have a thick coat of **glycocalyx**, rich in **disaccharidases** and **dipeptidases**. These cells function in absorption of sugars, amino acids, fatty acids, monoglycerides, electrolytes, water, and many other substances. These epithelial cells also participate in the immune defense of the body by manufacturing **secretory protein**, which binds to the **J protein** component of the antibody and protects **immunoglobulin A (IgA)** as it traverses the epithelial cell and enters the intestinal lumen. Long-chained lipids, in the form of **chylomicrons**, are delivered to the **lacteals**, blindly ending lymphatic channels of the villus.

Simple tubular glands of the mucosa, **the crypts of Lieberkühn**, open into the intervillar spaces. These crypts are composed of simple columnar cells (similar to surface absorptive cells), goblet (and oligomucous) cells, DNES, and regenerative cells, as well as **Paneth's cells**. The last are located in the base of the crypts and house large secretory granules believed to contain **lysozyme, defensin and TNF-α**.

- The lamina propria of the ileum houses large accumulations of lymphatic nodules, **Peyer's patches**. The surface epithelium interposed between Peyer's patches and the lumen of the ileum instead of being composed of simple columnar cells is formed by **microfold cells (M cells)** (see below).

The submucosa of the duodenum contains numerous glands, **duodenal (Brunner's) glands**, that produce an alkaline, mucin-containing fluid that protects the intestinal lining. They also manufacture **human epidermal growth factor** (also known as **urogastrone**), a polypeptide that inhibits HCl production and enhances epithelial cell division.

Large Intestine

The **large intestine** is subdivided into the **cecum**, the **colon** (**ascending**, **transverse**, **descending**, and **sigmoid**), the **rectum**, the **anal canal**, and the **appendix** (see Graphic 14-2). The large intestine possesses no villi but does house **crypts of Lieberkühn** in its lamina propria.

- The epithelial lining of the lumen and of the crypts is composed of **goblet** (and **oligomucous**) **cells**, **surface absorptive cells**, **regenerative cells**, and occasional **DNES cells**. There are no Paneth's cells in the large intestine, with the possible exception of the appendix.

The large intestine functions in the absorption of the remaining amino acids, lipids, and carbohydrates, as well as fluids, electrolytes, and certain vitamins, and it also is responsible for the compaction of feces.

GUT-ASSOCIATED LYMPHOID TISSUE

The lumen of the digestive tract is rich in antigenic substances, bacteria, and toxins; in fact, it has been estimated that the intestinal tract houses several trillion microbes with a total weight of approximately 2 kg. Since only a thin, simple columnar epithelium separates the richly vascularized connective tissue from this threatening milieu, the lamina propria of the intestines is well endowed with lymphoid elements. These include

- scattered cells (B cells, T cells, plasma cells, mast cells, macrophages, etc.),
- individual lymphatic nodules, and,
- in the ileum, **Peyer's patches**, clusters of lymphatic nodules.

Regions where lymphatic nodules come in contact with the epithelial lining of the intestines display flattened cells that form the interface between the lumen and the lymphatic nodule. These are **M cells (microfold cells)**, which phagocytose antigens and transport them (*without* breaking them down into epitopes), via clathrin-coated vesicles, to the basal aspect of the cell. The antigens are released into the lamina propria for uptake by antigen-presenting cells and dendritic cells.

It is interesting to note that the lamina propria of the colon has no lymph vessels, thus, generally, cancers of the colon metastasize at a much slower rate than do other cancers of the digestive tract.

DIGESTION AND ABSORPTION

Carbohydrates

- **Amylases**, present in the saliva and in the pancreatic secretion, hydrolyze carbohydrates to disaccharides.
- **Oligo-** and **disaccharidases**, present in the glycocalyx of surface absorptive cells, break down oligo- and disaccharides into monosaccharides (glucose and galactose) that enter the surface absorptive cell, requiring active transport using sugar-glucose transporter-1. The cells then release the glucose and galactose into the lamina propria, where these sugars enter the circulatory system for transport to the liver.

Proteins

- **Proteins**, denatured by HCl in the lumen of the stomach, are hydrolyzed (by the enzyme **pepsin**) into **polypeptides**.
- These are further broken down into **tri-** and **dipeptides** by proteases of the pancreatic secretions.
- **Tri-** and **dipeptidases** of the glycocalyx hydrolyze dipeptides into individual amino acids, which enter the surface absorptive cells, involving active transport, and are transferred into the lamina propria, where they enter the capillary network to be transported to the liver.

Lipids

- **Pancreatic lipase** breaks lipids down into **fatty acids**, **monoglycerides**, and **glycerol** within the lumen of the duodenum and proximal jejunum.
- Bile salts, delivered from the gallbladder, emulsify the fatty acids and monoglycerides, forming **micelles**, which, along with glycerol, diffuse into the surface absorptive cells.
- Within these cells, they enter the **smooth endoplasmic reticulum**, are reesterified to **triglycerides**, and are covered by a coat of protein within the Golgi apparatus, forming lipoprotein droplets known as **chylomicrons**.
- Chylomicrons exit these cells at their basolateral membranes and enter the **lacteals** of the villi, contributing to the formation of **chyle**.
- Chyle enters the lymph vascular system, makes its way to the thoracic duct, and then into the venous system at the junction of the left internal jugular vein and left brachiocephalic vein.
- Fatty acids that are shorter than 12 carbon chains in length pass through the surface absorptive cells without being reesterified and gain entrance to the blood capillaries of the villi.

Water and Ions

Water and ions are absorbed through the surface absorptive cells of the small and the large intestines.

CLINICAL CONSIDERATIONS

Crohn's Disease

Crohn's disease is a subcategory of **inflammatory bowel disease**, a condition of unknown etiology. It usually involves the small intestine or the colon but may affect any region of the digestive tract, from the esophagus to the anus, as well as extra-alimentary canal structures such as the skin, the kidney, and the larynx. It is characterized by patchy ulcers and deep fistulas in the intestinal wall. Clinical manifestations include abdominal pain, diarrhea, and fever, and these recur after various periods of ever shortening remission.

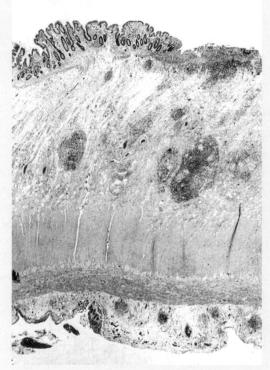

This figure is from the colon of a patient with Crohn's disease displaying ulceration of the mucosa, a hypertrophied submucosa with clusters of lymphoid elements, as well as smaller aggregates of lymphoid elements in the subserosal connective tissue adjacent to the muscularis externa. (Reprinted with permission from Rubin R, Strayer D, et al., eds. Rubin's Pathology. Clinicopathologic Foundations of Medicine, 5th ed. Baltimore: Lippincott Williams & Wilkins, 2008, p. 595.)

Mallory-Weiss Syndrome

Approximately 4% to 6% of the bleeding from the upper gastrointestinal tract is attributable to **Mallory-Weiss syndrome**. This is a laceration of the lower esophagus or the cardiac/fundic region of the stomach as a result of

powerful vomiting or sometimes strenuous hiccuping. Frequently, the bleeding is self-limiting, but occasionally, it requires surgical intervention.

Peptic Ulcers

Peptic ulcers are areas of the stomach, but mostly of the duodenum, that are denuded of the epithelial lining due to the action of the acid chyme. Most commonly, the underlying reasons are *Helicobacter pylori* infections and the use of aspirin, corticosteroids, and nonsteroidal antiinflammatory drugs. The bacteria, *H. pylori*, are able to live in the mucous substance lining the gastric epithelium probably by forming a protective envelope of bicarbonate buffer around themselves that neutralizes the acidic milieu. It is now believed that strains of this bacterium that possess *cagA* gene are the causative agents of peptic ulcers. Interestingly, people who smoke and/or drink alcoholic beverages develop peptic ulcers more frequently than do nonsmokers and nondrinkers. The symptoms involve mild to sharp pain in the midline of the lower thoracic and upper abdominal regions.

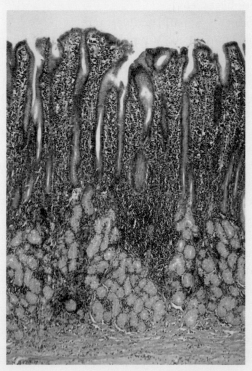

A. This figure is from a patient with an active *H. pylori* infection that resulted in chronic gastritis, a condition that may progress to peptic ulcer disease. Observe that the lamina propria has a heavy infiltrate of lymphocytes and plasma cells.

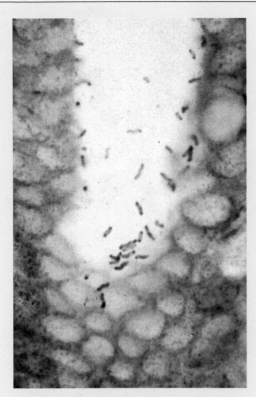

B. A higher magnification of the surface lining cells stained with silver display the presence of *H. pylori* as small, curved rods. (Reprinted with permission from Rubin R, Strayer D, et al., eds. Rubin's Pathology. Clinicopathologic Foundations of Medicine, 5th ed. Baltimore, MD: Lippincott, Williams & Wilkins, 2008, p. 563.)

Zollinger-Ellison Syndrome

Zollinger-Ellison syndrome is a cancerous lesion of gastrin-producing cells in the stomach, duodenum, or the pancreas, resulting in the overproduction of HCl by parietal cells of the stomach and the formation of numerous recurrent peptic ulcers. A high blood level of gastrin, especially after intravenous administration of secretin, usually is a strong indicator of this syndrome.

Antibiotic-Associated Colitis

Antibiotics such as ampicillin, cephalosporin, and clindamycin often cause an imbalance in the intestinal bacterial flora, permitting the vigorous proliferation of *Clostridium difficile*, resulting in infection by this organism. The two major toxins (Toxin A and Toxin B) produced by *C. difficile* frequently cause inflammation of the sigmoid colon. Depending on the severity of the infection, the patient will suffer from abdominal cramps, loose stool, bloody diarrhea, fever, and, in extreme cases, dehydration and perforation of the bowel.

Hiatal Hernia

Hiatal hernia is a condition in which a region of the stomach herniates through the **esophageal hiatus** of the diaphragm. It may be of two types, sliding and paraesophageal hiatal hernia. In the former condition, the cardioesophageal junction and the cardiac region of the stomach slides in and out of the thorax, whereas in the latter case the cardioesophageal junction remains in its normal place, below the diaphragm, but a part (or occasionally all) of the stomach pushes into the thorax and is positioned next to the esophagus. Usually, hiatal hernia is asymptomatic, although acid reflux disease is common in patients afflicted with this condition.

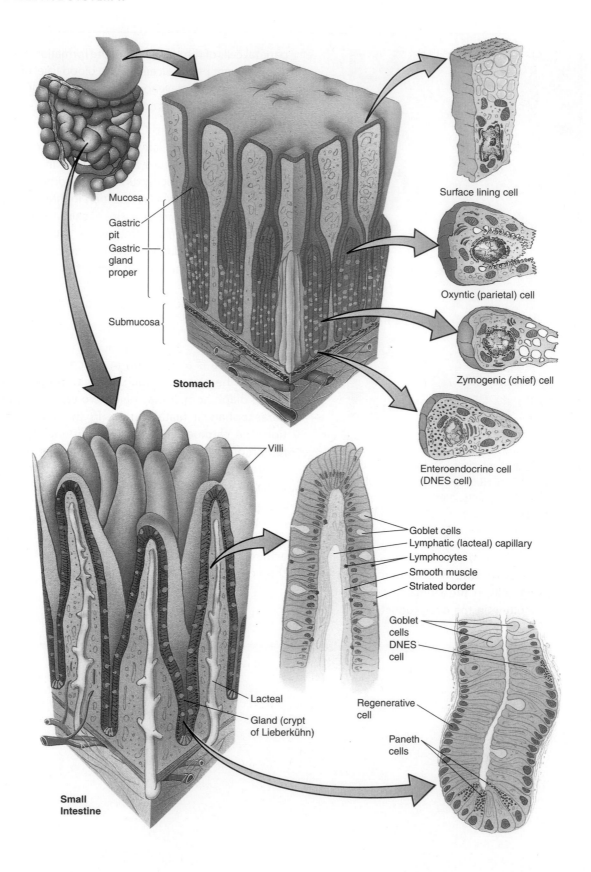

Mucosa

Gastric pit

Gastric gland proper

Submucosa

Stomach

Surface lining cell

Oxyntic (parietal) cell

Zymogenic (chief) cell

Enteroendocrine cell (DNES cell)

Villi

Goblet cells
Lymphatic (lacteal) capillary
Lymphocytes
Smooth muscle
Striated border

Goblet cells

DNES cell

Regenerative cell

Paneth cells

Lacteal

Gland (crypt of Lieberkühn)

Small Intestine

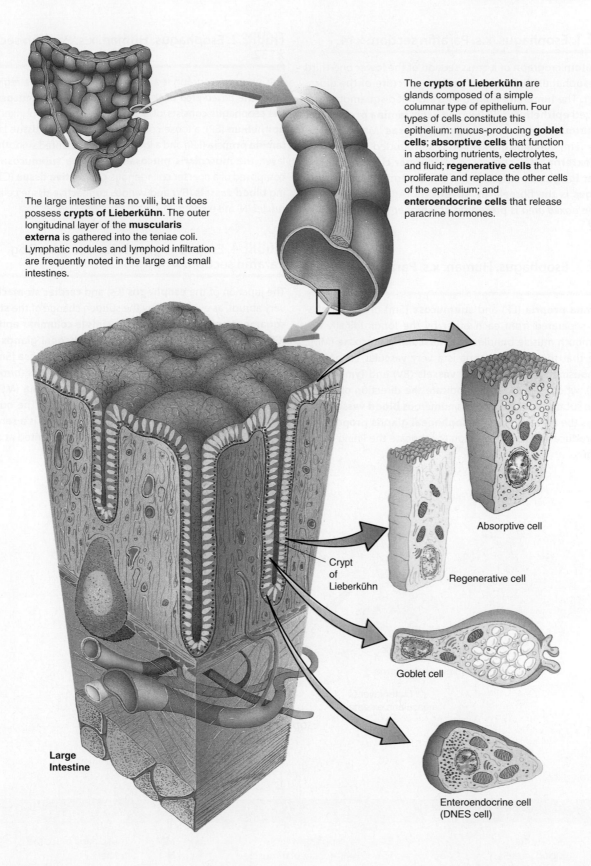

The **crypts of Lieberkühn** are glands composed of a simple columnar type of epithelium. Four types of cells constitute this epithelium: mucus-producing **goblet cells**; **absorptive cells** that function in absorbing nutrients, electrolytes, and fluid; **regenerative cells** that proliferate and replace the other cells of the epithelium; and **enteroendocrine cells** that release paracrine hormones.

The large intestine has no villi, but it does possess **crypts of Lieberkühn**. The outer longitudinal layer of the **muscularis externa** is gathered into the teniae coli. Lymphatic nodules and lymphoid infiltration are frequently noted in the large and small intestines.

Crypt of Lieberkühn

Absorptive cell

Regenerative cell

Goblet cell

Enteroendocrine cell (DNES cell)

Large Intestine

PLATE 14-1 · Esophagus

FIGURE 1. Esophagus. x.s. Paraffin section. ×14.

This photomicrograph of a cross section of the lower one-third of the esophagus displays the general structure of the digestive tract. The **lumen** (L) is lined by a stratified squamous nonkeratinized **epithelium** (EP) lying on a thin **lamina propria** (LP) that is surrounded by the **muscularis mucosae** (MM). The **submucosa** (Sm) contains glands and is surrounded by the **muscularis externa** (ME), composed of an **inner circular** (IC) and an **outer longitudinal** (OL) layer. The outermost tunic of the esophagus is the fibroelastic **adventitia** (Ad). A region similar to the *boxed area* is presented at a higher magnification in Figure 2.

FIGURE 3. Esophagus. Human. x.s. Paraffin section. ×132.

The **lamina propria** (LP) and **submucosa** (Sm) of the esophagus are separated from each other by the longitudinally oriented smooth muscle bundles, the **muscularis mucosae** (MM). Observe that the lamina propria is a very vascular connective tissue, housing numerous **blood vessels** (BV) and **lymph vessels** (LV), whose valves (*arrow*) indicate the direction of lymph flow. The submucosa also displays numerous **blood vessels** (BV) as well as the presence of the **esophageal glands proper** (EG), which produce a mucous secretion to lubricate the lining of the esophagus.

FIGURE 2. Esophagus. Human. x.s. Paraffin section. ×132.

This photomicrograph is a higher magnification of a region similar to the *boxed area* of the previous figure. The **mucosa** (M) of the esophagus consists of a stratified squamous nonkeratinized **epithelium** (EP); a loose collagenous connective tissue layer, the **lamina propria** (LP); and a longitudinally oriented smooth muscle layer, the **muscularis mucosae** (MM). The **submucosa** (Sm) is composed of a coarser collagenous **connective tissue** (CT), housing **blood vessels** (BV) and various connective tissue cells whose **nuclei** (N) are evident.

FIGURE 4. Esophagogastric junction. l.s. Dog. Paraffin section. ×14.

The junction of the **esophagus** (Es) and **cardiac stomach** (CS) is very abrupt, as evidenced by the sudden change of the **stratified squamous epithelium** (SE) to the **simple columnar epithelium** (CE) of the stomach. Note that the **esophageal glands proper** (EG) continue for a short distance into the **submucosa** (Sm) of the stomach. Observe also the presence of gastric pits (*arrows*) and the increased thickness of the **muscularis externa** (ME) of the stomach compared with that of the esophagus. The outermost tunic of the esophagus inferior to the diaphragm is a **serosa** (Se) rather than an adventitia. The *boxed area* is presented at a higher magnification in Figure 1 of the next plate.

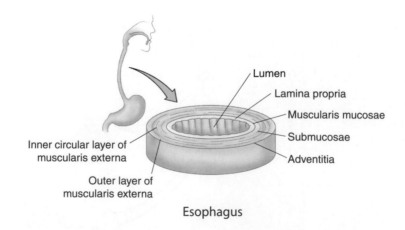

Lumen
Lamina propria
Muscularis mucosae
Submucosae
Adventitia
Inner circular layer of muscularis externa
Outer layer of muscularis externa

Esophagus

KEY					
Ad	adventitia	**Es**	esophagus	**MM**	muscularis mucosae
BV	blood vessels	**IC**	inner circular muscle	**N**	nucleus
CE	simple columnar epithelium	**L**	lumen	**OL**	outer longitudinal muscle
CS	cardiac stomach	**LP**	lamina propria	**SE**	stratified squamous epithelium
CT	connective tissue	**LV**	lymph vessels	**Se**	serosa
EG	esophageal glands proper	**M**	mucosa	**Sm**	submucosa
EP	epithelium	**ME**	muscularis externa		

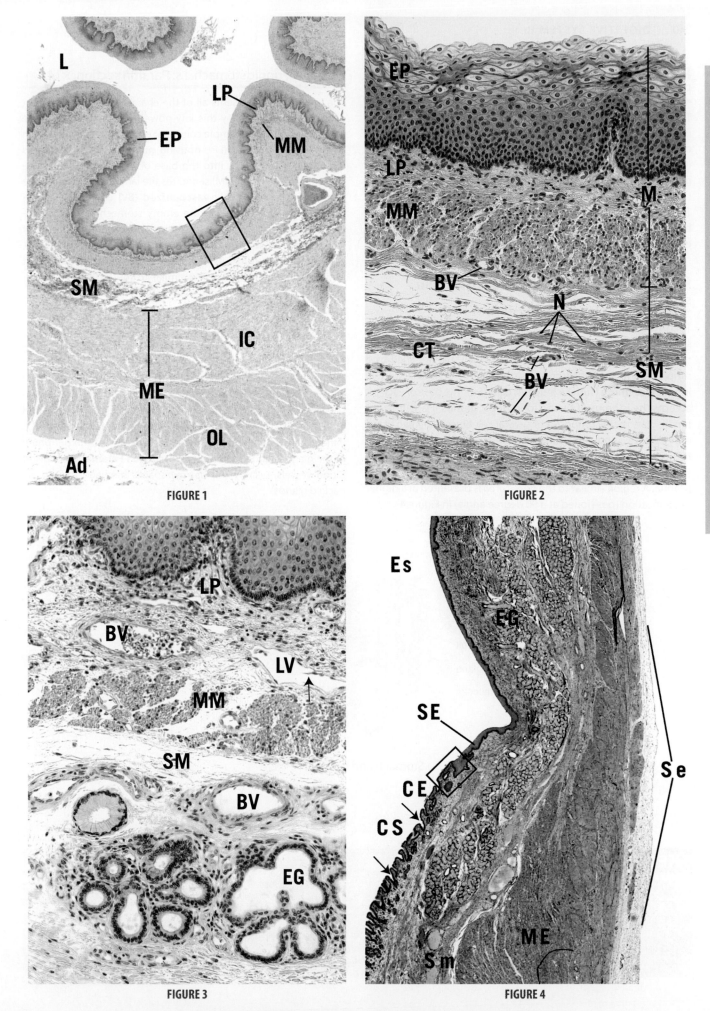

PLATE 14-1 · Esophagus

FIGURE 1

FIGURE 2

FIGURE 3

FIGURE 4

PLATE 14-2 · Stomach

FIGURE 1. Esophagogastric junction. l.s. Dog. Paraffin section. ×132.

This photomicrograph is a higher magnification of the *boxed region* of Figure 4, Plate 14-1. The **stratified squamous epithelium** (SE) of the esophagus is replaced by the **simple columnar epithelium** (CE) of the stomach in a very abrupt fashion (*arrow*). The **lamina propria** (LP) displays **gastric pits** (GP), lined by the typical mucus-secreting **surface lining cells** (SC), characteristic of the stomach. The structure labeled with an *asterisk* is not a lymphatic nodule but is a more or less tangential section through the esophageal epithelium. Note the presence of the **muscularis mucosae** (MM).

FIGURE 3. Fundic stomach. x.s. Dog. Paraffin section. ×132.

This photomicrograph presents a higher magnification of a region similar to the *boxed area* of Figure 2. The mucosa of the fundic stomach displays numerous **gastric pits** (GP) that are lined by a simple columnar epithelium, consisting mostly of mucus-producing **surface lining** (surface mucous) **cells** (SC). The base of each pit accepts the isthmus of two to four **fundic glands** (FG). Although fundic glands are composed of several cell types, only two, **parietal cells** (PC) and **chief cells** (CC), are readily distinguishable in this preparation. The **lamina propria** (LP) is richly **vascularized** (BV). Note the **muscularis mucosae** (MM) beneath the lamina propria. A region similar to the *boxed area* is presented at a higher magnification (positioned at a 90 degree angle) in Figure 4.

FIGURE 2. Fundic stomach. l.s. Paraffin section. ×14.

The fundic region presents all of the characteristics of the stomach, as demonstrated by this low-power photomicrograph. The **lumen** (L) is lined by a simple columnar epithelium, deep to which is the **lamina propria** (LP), housing numerous **gastric glands** (GG). Each gland opens into the base of a **gastric pit** (GP). The **muscularis mucosae** (MM) separates the lamina propria from the **submucosa** (Sm), a richly **vascularized** (BV) connective tissue, thrown into folds (rugae) in the empty stomach. The **muscularis externa** (ME) is composed of three poorly defined layers of smooth muscle: **innermost oblique** (IO), **middle circular** (MC), and **outer longitudinal** (OL). Serosa (*arrow*) forms the outermost tunic of the stomach. A region similar to the *boxed area* is presented at a higher magnification in Figure 3.

FIGURE 4. Fundic glands. x.s. Paraffin section. ×540.

This photomicrograph presents a higher magnification (positioned at a 90 degree angle) of a region similar to the *boxed area* of Figure 3. The **lumina** (L) of several glands can be recognized. Note that **chief cells** (CC) are granular in appearance and are much smaller than the round, plate-like **parietal cells** (PC). Parietal cells, as their name implies, are located at the periphery of the gland. Slender **connective tissue (CT) elements**, housing blood vessels, occupy the narrow spaces between the closely packed glands.

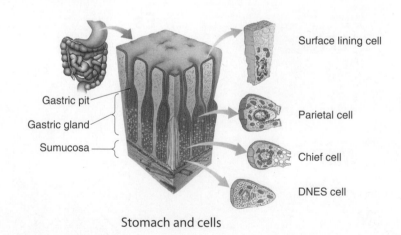

Surface lining cell

Gastric pit

Gastric gland

Sumucosa

Parietal cell

Chief cell

DNES cell

Stomach and cells

KEY

BV	blood vessels	GP	gastric pits	MM	muscularis mucosae
CC	chief cells	IO	innermost oblique muscle	OL	outer longitudinal muscle
CE	columnar epithelium	L	lumen	PC	parietal cells
CT	connective tissue	LP	lamina propria	SC	surface lining cells
FG	fundic glands	ME	muscularis externa	SE	squamous epithelium
GG	gastric glands	MC	middle circular muscle	Sm	submucosa

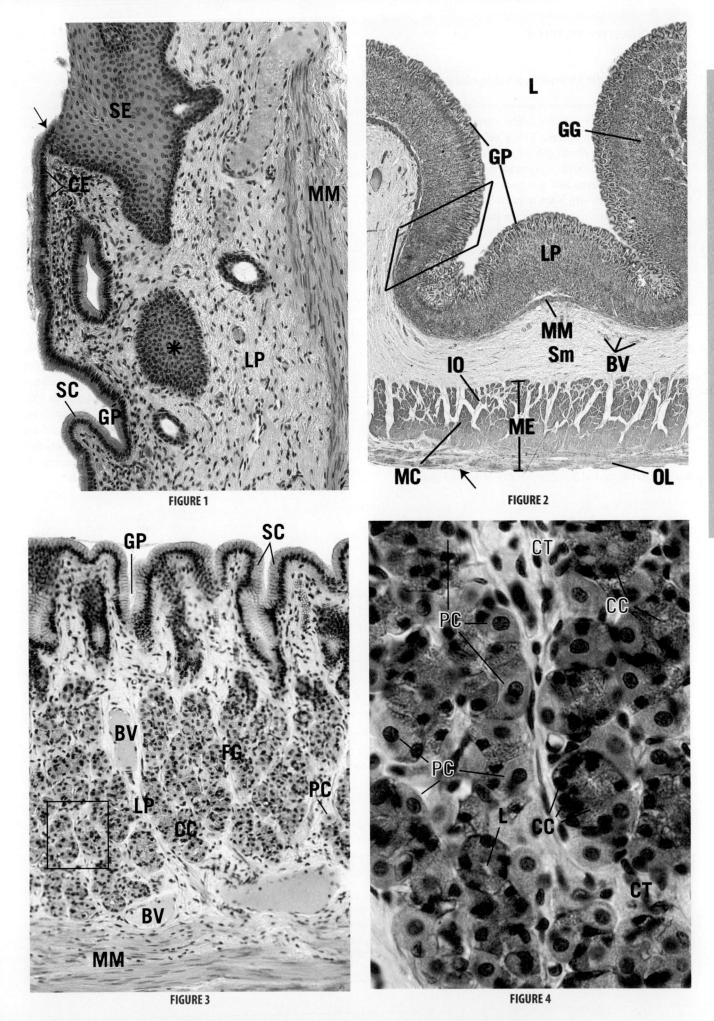

PLATE 14-2 • Stomach

FIGURE 1

FIGURE 2

FIGURE 3

FIGURE 4

PLATE 14-3 · Stomach

FIGURE 1. Fundic stomach. x.s. Monkey. Plastic section. ×270.

The **gastric pits** (GP) of the fundic stomach are lined mostly by mucus-producing **surface lining cells** (SC). Each gastric pit receives two to four fundic glands, simple tubular structures that are subdivided into three regions: isthmus, neck, and base. The isthmus opens directly into the gastric pit and is composed of **immature cells** (Ic), which are responsible for the renewal of the lining of the gastric mucosa, **surface lining cells** (SC), and **parietal cells** (PC). The neck and base of these glands are presented in Figure 2.

FIGURE 3. Pyloric gland. Stomach. x.s. Monkey. Plastic section. ×132.

The mucosa of the pyloric region of the stomach presents **gastric pits** (GP) that are deeper than those of the cardiac or fundic regions. The deep aspects of these pits are coiled (*arrows*). As in the other regions of the stomach, the **epithelium** (Ep) is simple columnar, consisting mainly of **surface lining cells** (SC). Note that the **lamina propria** (LP) is loosely packed with **pyloric glands** (PGs) and that considerable **connective tissue** (CT) is present. The pyloric glands are composed mainly of **mucous cells** (mc). Observe the two muscle layers of the **muscularis mucosae** (MM). A region similar to the *boxed area* is presented in Figure 4.

FIGURE 2. Fundic gland. Stomach. x.s. Monkey. Plastic section. ×270.

The **neck** (n) and **base** (b) of the fundic gland both contain the large, plate-shaped **parietal cells** (PC). The neck also possesses a few immature cells as well as **mucous neck cells** (Mn), which manufacture a mucous substance. The base of the fundic glands contains numerous acid-manufacturing **parietal cells** (PC) and **chief cells** (CC), which produce digestive enzymes. Note that the lamina propria is tightly packed with glands and that the intervening **connective tissue** (CT) is flimsy. The bases of these glands extend to the **muscularis mucosae** (MM).

FIGURE 4. Pyloric gland. Stomach. x.s. Human. Paraffin section. ×270.

This is a photomicrograph of a region similar to the *boxed area* of Figure 3. The simple columnar **epithelium** (Ep) of the **gastric pit** is composed mostly of surface lining cells. These pits are not only much deeper than those of the fundic or cardiac regions but are also somewhat coiled (*arrow*), as are the **pyloric glands** (PG), which empty into the base of the pits. These glands are populated by **mucus-secreting cells** (mc) similar to mucous neck cells, whose **nuclei** (N) are flattened against the basal cell membrane. Note that the glands are not closely packed and that the **lamina propria** (LP) is very cellular and possesses a rich **vascular supply** (BV).

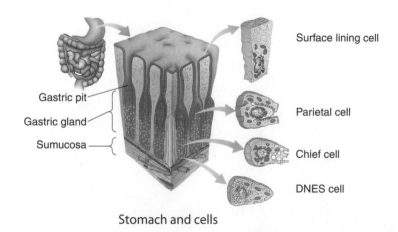

Gastric pit
Gastric gland
Sumucosa

Surface lining cell
Parietal cell
Chief cell
DNES cell

Stomach and cells

KEY

B	base	**IC**	immature cells	**N**	neck
BV	blood vessels	**LP**	lamina propria	**PC**	parietal cells
CC	chief cells	**Mc**	mucous cells	**PG**	pyloric glands
CT	connective tissue	**MM**	muscularis mucosae	**SC**	surface lining cells
EP	epithelium	**Mn**	mucous neck cell		
GP	gastric pits	**N**	nucleus		

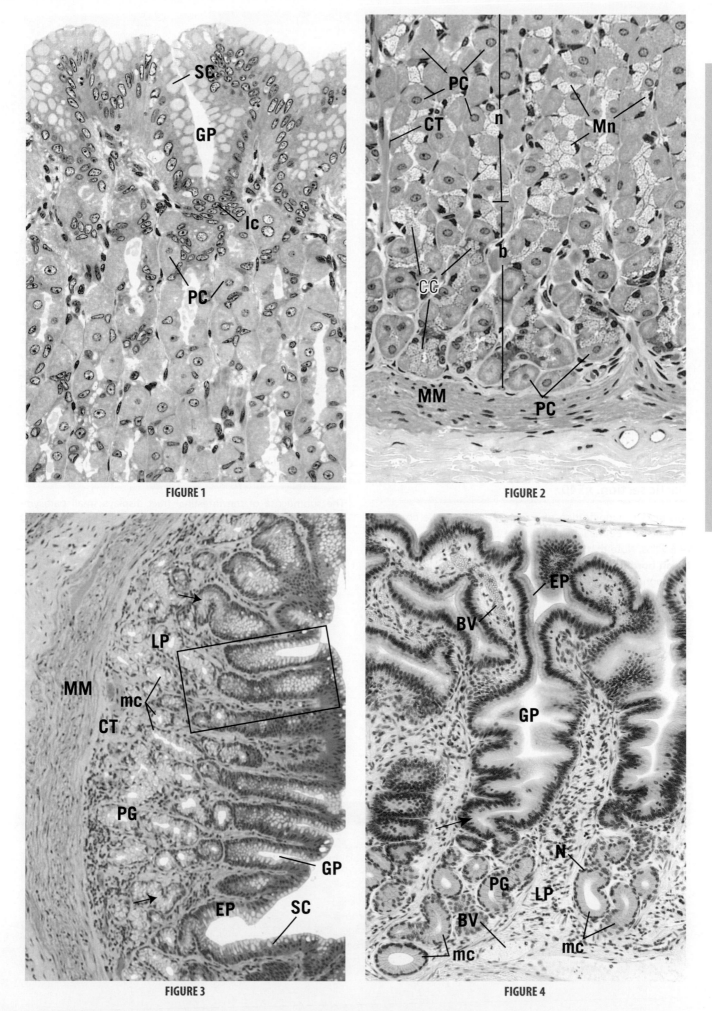

PLATE 14-3 · Stomach

FIGURE 1

FIGURE 2

FIGURE 3

FIGURE 4

PLATE 14-4 · Duodenum

FIGURE 1a. Duodenum. l.s. Monkey. Plastic section. Montage. ×132.

The lamina propria of the duodenum possesses finger-like evaginations known as **villi** (V), which project into the **lumen** (L). The villi are covered by **surface absorptive cells** (SA), a simple columnar type of epithelium with a brush border. Interspersed among these surface absorptive cells are **goblet cells** (GC) as well as occasional APUD cells. The **connective tissue** (CT) core (lamina propria) of the villus is composed of lymphoid and other cellular elements whose nuclei stain very intensely. Blood vessels also abound in the lamina propria, as do large, blindly ending lymphatic channels known as **lacteals** (I), recognizable by their large size and lack of red blood cells. Frequently, these lacteals are collapsed. The deeper aspect of the lamina propria houses glands, the **crypts of Lieberkühn** (CL). These simple tubular glands deliver their secretions into the intervillar spaces. The bases of these crypts reach the **muscularis mucosae** (MM), composed of inner circular and outer longitudinal layers of smooth muscle. Deep to this muscle layer is the submucosa, which, in the duodenum, is occupied by compound tubular **glands of Brunner** (GB). These glands deliver their mucous secretion via **ducts** (D), which pierce the muscularis mucosae, into the crypts of Lieberkühn. A region similar to the *boxed area* is presented at a higher magnification in Figure 1b.

FIGURE 1b. Epithelium and core of villus. Monkey. Plastic section. ×540.

This higher magnification of a region similar to the *boxed area* presents the epithelium and part of the connective tissue core of a villus. Note that the **surface absorptive cells** (SA) display a **brush border** (BB), terminal bars (*arrow*), and **goblet cells** (GC). Although APUD cells are also present, they constitute only a small percentage of the cell population. The **lamina propria** (LP) core of the villus is highly cellular, housing **lymphoid cells** (LC), **smooth muscle cells** (SM), mast cells, **macrophages** (Ma), and fibroblasts, among others.

FIGURE 2. Duodenum. l.s. Monkey. Plastic section. ×132.

This photomicrograph is a continuation of the montage presented in Figure 1a (compare *asterisks*). Note that the **submucosa** (Sm), occupied by **glands of Brunner** (GB), is a **vascular** structure (BV) and also houses Meissner's submucosal plexus. The submucosa extends to the **muscularis externa** (ME), composed of an **inner circular** (IC) and **outer longitudinal** (OL) smooth muscle layer. Note the presence of **Auerbach's myenteric plexus** (AP) between these two muscle layers. The duodenum, in part, is covered by a **serosa** (Se), whose mesothelium provides this organ with a smooth, moist surface.

FIGURE 3a. Duodenum. x.s. Monkey. Plastic section. ×540.

The base of the crypt of Lieberkühn displays the several types of cells that compose this gland. **Paneth's cells** (Pc) are readily recognizable due to the large granules in their apical cytoplasm. **DNES cells** (APD) are clear cells with fine granules usually located basally. **Goblet cells** (GC), **columnar cells** (Cc), and **stem cells** (Sc) constitute the remaining cell population.

FIGURE 3b. Duodenum. x.s. Monkey. Plastic section. ×540.

The submucosa of the intestinal tract displays small parasympathetic ganglia, Meissner's submucosal plexus. Note the large **postganglionic cell bodies** (PB) surrounded by elements of **connective tissue** (CT).

KEY

AP	Auerbach's plexus	GC	goblet cell	OL	outer longitudinal muscle
APD	DNES cell	IC	inner circular muscle	PB	postganglionic cell body
BB	brush border	I	lacteal	Pc	Paneth's cell
BV	blood vessels	L	lumen	SA	surface absorptive cell
Cc	columnar cell	LC	lymphoid cell	Sc	stem cell
CL	crypts of Lieberkühn	LP	lamina propria	Se	serosa
CT	connective tissue	Ma	macrophage	Sm	submucosa
D	duct	ME	muscularis externa	SM	smooth muscle cell
GB	glands of Brunner	MM	muscularis mucosae	V	villi

PLATE 14-4 • Duodenum

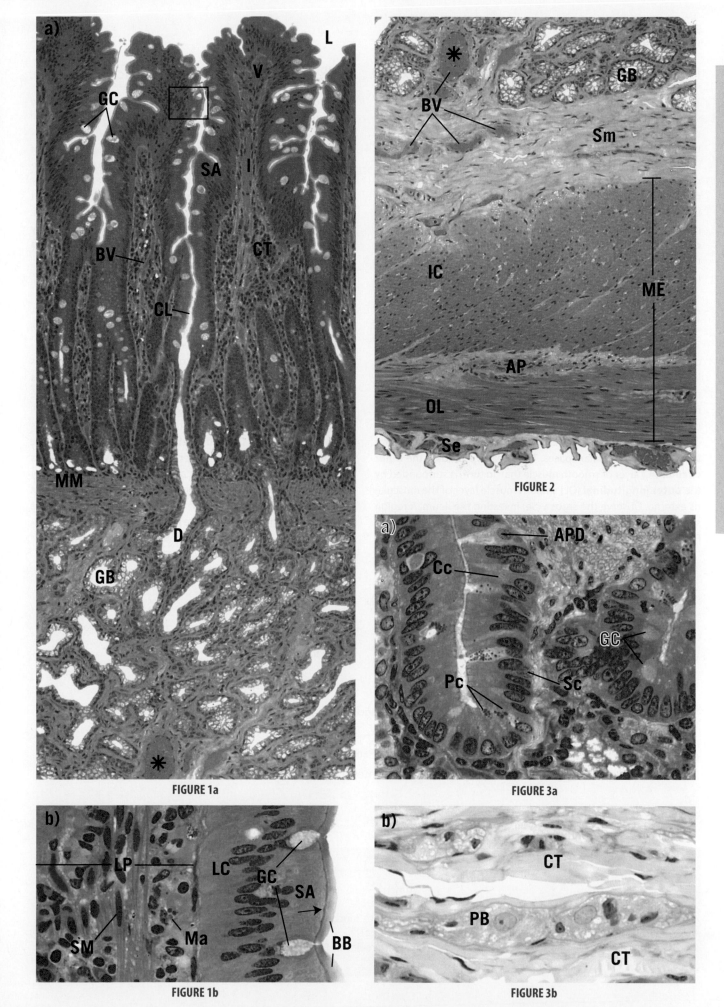

FIGURE 1a

FIGURE 2

FIGURE 3a

FIGURE 1b

FIGURE 3b

PLATE 14-5 · Jejunum, Ileum

FIGURE 1. Jejunum. x.s. Monkey. Plastic section. ×132.

The **mucosa** (M) and **submucosa** (Sm) of the jejunum are presented in this photomicrograph. The **villi** (V) of this region possess more **goblet cells** (GC) than those of the duodenum. Observe that the **crypts of Lieberkühn** (CL) open into the intervillar spaces (*arrow*) and that the lamina propria displays numerous dense nuclei, evidence of lymphatic infiltration. The flimsy **muscularis mucosae** (MM) separates the lamina propria from the submucosa. Large **blood vessels** (BV) occupy the submucosa, which is composed of a loose type of collagenous connective tissue. The **inner circular** (IC) layer of the muscularis externa is evident at the bottom of the photomicrograph. The *boxed region* is presented at a higher magnification in Figure 2.

FIGURE 3. Ileum. l.s. Human. Paraffin section. ×14.

The entire wall of the ileum is presented, displaying spiral folds of the submucosa that partially encircle the lumen. These folds, known as **plicae circulares** (Pci), increase the surface area of the small intestines. Note that the lamina propria is clearly delineated from the **submucosa** (Sm) by the muscularis mucosae. The lamina propria forms numerous **villi** (V) that protrude into the **lumen** (L); glands known as **crypts of Lieberkühn** (CL) deliver their secretions into the intervillar spaces. The submucosa abuts the **inner circular** (IC) layer of smooth muscle that, in turn, is surrounded by the **outer longitudinal** (OL) smooth muscle layer of the muscularis externa. Observe the **serosa** (Se) investing the ileum. A region similar to the *boxed area* is presented at a higher magnification in Figure 4.

FIGURE 2. Jejunum. x.s. Monkey. Plastic section. ×540.

This photomicrograph is a higher magnification of the *boxed area* of Figure 1. The crypts of Lieberkühn are composed of several cell types, some of which are evident in this figure. **Goblet cells** (GC) that manufacture mucus may be noted in various degrees of mucus production. Narrow **stem cells** (Sc) undergo mitotic activity (*arrowhead*), and newly formed cells reconstitute the cell population of the crypt and villus. **Paneth's cells** (PC) are located at the base of crypts and may be recognized by their large granules. **DNES cells** (APD) appear as clear cells, with fine granules usually basally located. The lamina propria displays numerous **plasma cells** (PlC).

FIGURE 4. Ileum. x.s. Monkey. Plastic section. ×132.

This is a higher magnification of a region similar to the *boxed area* of Figure 3. Note that the **villi** (V) are covered by a simple columnar epithelium, whose cellular constituents include numerous **goblet cells** (GC). The core of the villus displays **blood vessels** (BV) as well as a large lymphatic vessel known as a **lacteal** (I). The **crypts of Lieberkühn** (CL) open into the intervillar spaces (*arrow*). The group of lymphatic nodules of the ileum are known as **Peyer's patches** (PP). *Inset a*. **Crypt of Lieberkühn. l.s. Monkey. Plastic section.** ×540. The crypts of Lieberkühn also possess **DNES cells** (APD), recognizable by their clear appearance and usually basally oriented fine granules. *Inset b*. **Crypt of Lieberkühn. l.s. Monkey. Plastic section.** ×540. The base of the crypt of Lieberkühn displays cells with large granules. These are **Paneth's cells** (PC), which produce the bacteriocidal agent lysozyme and other substances.

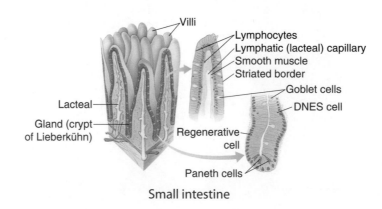

Small intestine

KEY

APD	DNES cell	**L**	lumen	**PP**	Peyer's patch
BV	blood vessels	**M**	mucosa	**OL**	outer longitudinal muscle
CL	crypts of Lieberkühn	**MM**	muscularis mucosae	**Sc**	stem cell
GC	goblet cell	**PC**	Paneth's cell	**Se**	serosa
IC	inner circular muscle	**PCi**	plicae circulares	**Sm**	submucosa
I	lacteal	**PIC**	plasma cell	**V**	villi

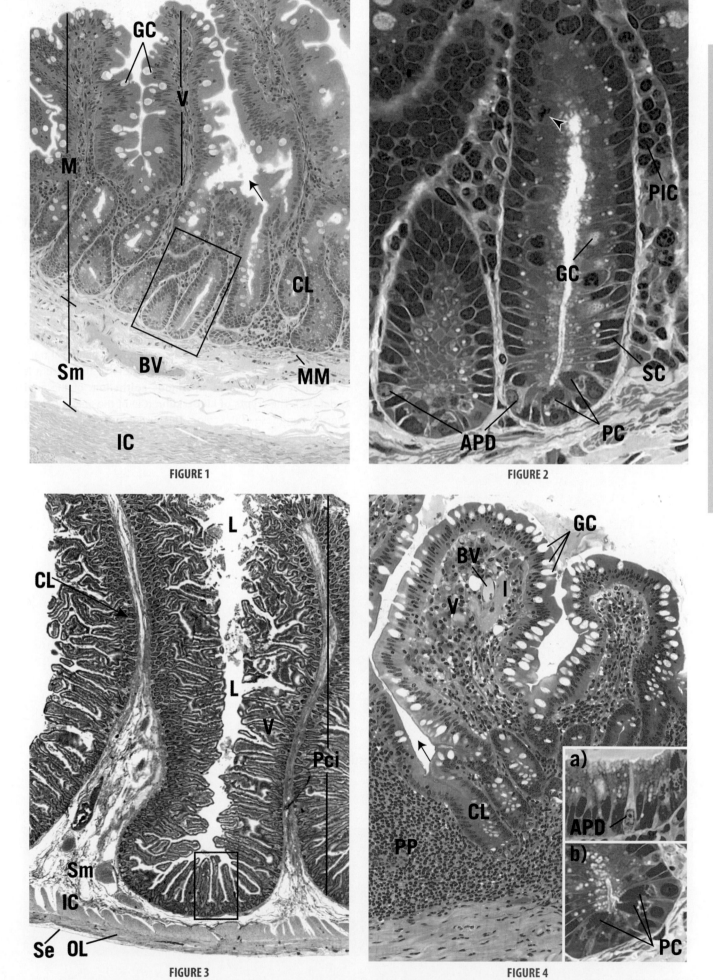

PLATE 14-5 • Jejunum, Ileum

FIGURE 1

FIGURE 2

FIGURE 3

FIGURE 4

PLATE 14-6 · Colon, Appendix

FIGURE 1. Colon. l.s. Monkey. Plastic section. ×132.

This photomicrograph depicts the mucosa and part of the submucosa of the colon. Note the absence of surface modifications such as pits and villi, which indicate that this section is not of the stomach or small intestines. The **epithelium** (Ep) lining the **lumen** (L) is simple columnar with numerous **goblet cells** (GC). The straight tubular glands are **crypts of Lieberkühn** (CL), which extend down to the **muscularis mucosae** (MM). The **inner circular** (IC) and **outer longitudinal** (OL) layers of smooth muscle comprising this region of the mucosa are evident. The **submucosa** (Sm) is very **vascular** (BV) and houses numerous **fat cells** (FC). The *boxed area* is presented at a higher magnification in Figure 2.

FIGURE 2. Colon. l.s. Monkey. Plastic section. ×540.

This photomicrograph is a higher magnification of the *boxed area* of Figure 1. The cell population of the **crypts of Lieberkühn** (CL) is composed of numerous **goblet cells** (GC), which deliver their mucus into the **lumen** (L) of the crypt. **Surface epithelial cells** (SEC) as well as undifferentiated stem cells are also present. The latter undergo mitosis (*arrow*) to repopulate the epithelial lining. **DNES cells** (APD) constitute a small percentage of the cell population. Note that Paneth's cells are not present in the colon. The **lamina propria** (LP) is very cellular, housing many **lymphoid cells** (LC). The **inner circular** (IC) and **outer longitudinal** (OL) smooth muscle layers of the **muscularis mucosae** (MM) are evident.

FIGURE 3. Appendix. x.s. Paraffin section. ×132.

The cross section of the appendix displays a **lumen** (L) that frequently contains debris (*arrow*). The lumen is lined by a simple columnar **epithelium** (Ep), consisting of many **goblet cells** (GC). **Crypts of Lieberkühn** (CL) are relatively shallow in comparison with those of the colon. The **lamina propria** (LP) is highly infiltrated with **lymphoid cells** (LC), derived from **lymphatic nodules** (LN) of the **submucosa** (Sm) and lamina propria. The **muscularis mucosae** (MM) delineates the border between the lamina propria and the submucosa.

FIGURE 4. Anorectal junction. l.s. Human. Paraffin section. ×132.

The anorectal junction presents a superficial similarity to the esophagogastric junction because of the abrupt epithelial transition. The **simple columnar epithelium** (CE) of the rectum is replaced by the **stratified squamous epithelium** of the **anal canal** (AC). The **crypts of Lieberkühn** (CL) of the anal canal are shorter than those of the colon. The **lamina propria** (LP) is infiltrated by **lymphoid cells** (LC).

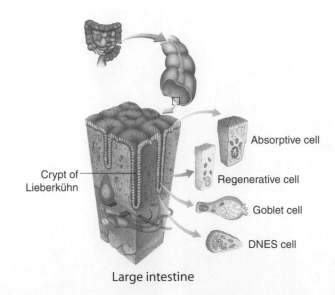

Crypt of Lieberkühn

Absorptive cell
Regenerative cell
Goblet cell
DNES cell

Large intestine

KEY					
AC	anal canal	**FC**	fat cell	**LP**	lamina propria
APD	DNES cell	**GC**	goblet cell	**MM**	muscularis mucosae
BV	blood vessels	**IC**	inner circular muscle	**OL**	outer longitudinal muscle
CE	simple columnar epithelium	**L**	lumen	**SE**	stratified squamous epithelium
CL	crypts of Lieberkühn	**LC**	lymphoid cell	**SEC**	surface epithelial cell
EP	epithelium	**LN**	lymphatic nodule	**Sm**	submucosa

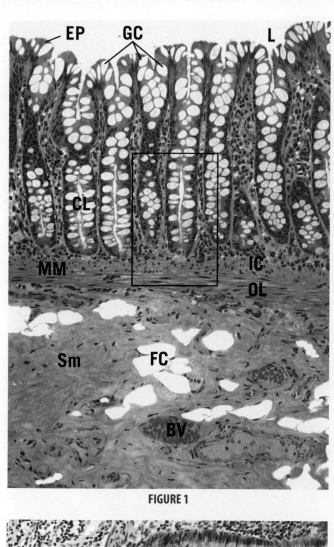

FIGURE 1

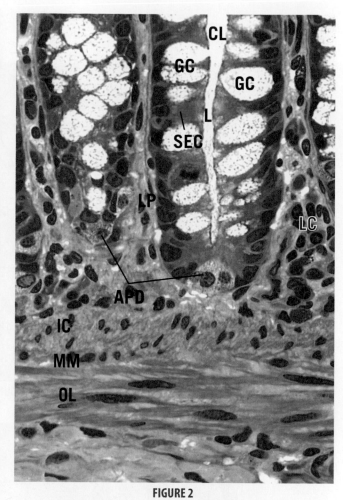

FIGURE 2

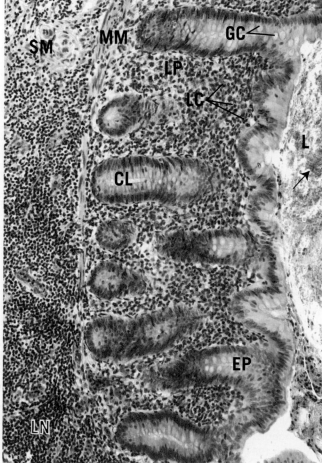

FIGURE 3

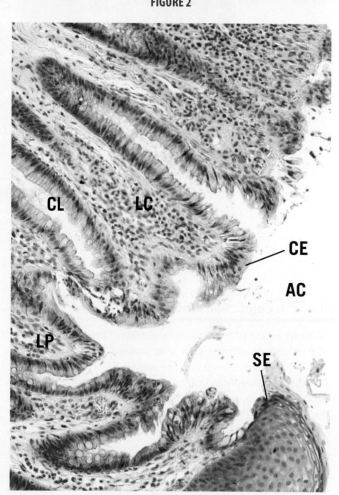

FIGURE 4

PLATE 14-6 · Colon, Appendix

PLATE 14-7 • Colon, Electron Microscopy

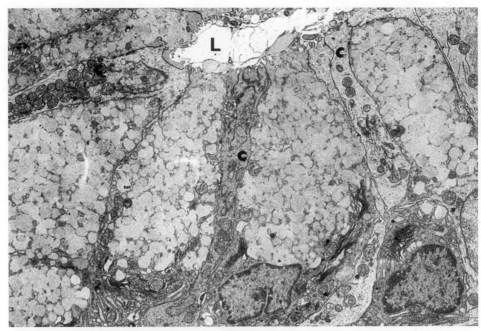

FIGURE 1

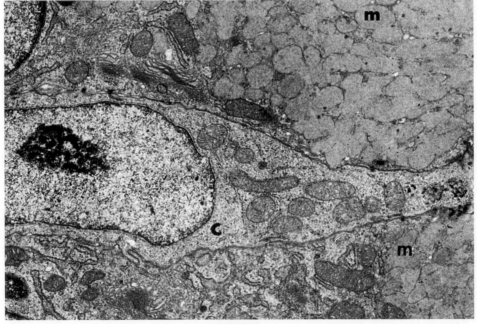

FIGURE 2

FIGURE 1. Colon. Rat. Electron microscopy. ×3,780.

The deep aspect of the crypt of Lieberkühn presents **columnar cells** (c) and deep crypt cells that produce a mucous type of secretion that is delivered into the **lumen** (L) of the crypt. (From Altmann GG. Morphological observations on mucus-secreting nongoblet cells in the deep crypts of the rat ascending colon. Am J Anat 1983;167:95–117.)

FIGURE 2. Colon. Rat. Electron microscopy. ×12,600.

At a higher magnification of the deep aspect of the crypt of Lieberkühn, the deep crypt cells present somewhat electron-dense **vacuoles** (m). Note that many of these vacuoles coalesce, forming amorphous vacuolar profiles. The slender **columnar cell** (C) displays no vacuoles but does possess numerous mitochondria and occasional profiles of rough endoplasmic reticulum. Observe the large, oval nucleus and clearly evident nucleolus. (From Altmann GG. Morphological observations on mucus-secreting nongoblet cells in the deep crypts of the rat ascending colon. Am J Anat 1983;167:95–117.)

PLATE 14-8 • Colon, Scanning Electron Microscopy

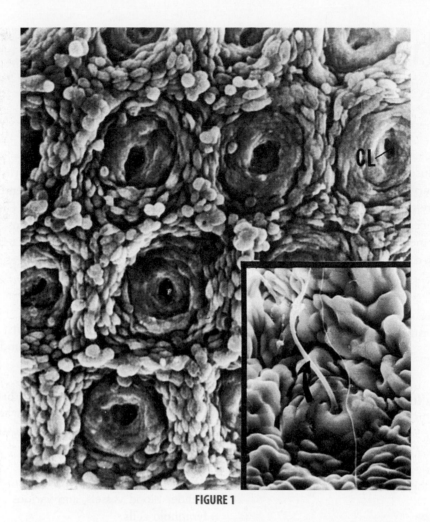

FIGURE 1

FIGURE 1. Colon. Monkey. Scanning electron microscopy. ×614.

This scanning electron micrograph displays the openings of the **crypts of Lieberkühn** (CL) as well as the cells lining the mucosal surface. (From Specian RD, Neutra MR. The surface topography of the colonic crypt in rabbit and monkey. Am J Anat 1981;160:461–472.) *Inset.* **Colon. Rabbit. Scanning electron microscopy.** ×778. The openings of the crypts of Lieberkühn are not as regularly arranged in the rabbit as in the monkey. Observe the mucus arising from the crypt opening (*arrow*). (From Specian RD, Neutra MR. The surface topography of the colonic crypt in rabbit and monkey. Am J Anat 1981;160:461–472.)

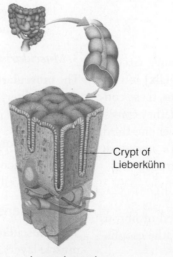

Crypt of Lieberkühn

Large intestine

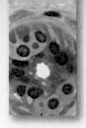

Chapter Summary

I. ESOPHAGUS

The **esophagus** is a muscular tube that delivers the **bolus** of food from the **pharynx** to the **stomach**. The esophagus, as well as the remainder of the digestive tract, is composed of four concentric layers: **mucosa**, **submucosa**, **muscularis externa**, and **adventitia**. The **lumen** of the esophagus is normally collapsed.

A. Mucosa

The **mucosa** has three regions: **epithelium**, **lamina propria**, and **muscularis mucosae**. It is thrown into longitudinal folds.

1. Epithelium

The **epithelium** is **stratified squamous nonkeratinized**.

2. Lamina Propria

The **lamina propria** is a loose connective tissue that contains mucus-producing **esophageal cardiac glands** in some regions of the esophagus.

3. Muscularis Mucosae

The **muscularis mucosae** is composed of a single layer of **longitudinally** oriented **smooth muscle**.

B. Submucosa

The **submucosa**, composed of fibroelastic connective tissue, is thrown into longitudinal folds. The **esophageal glands proper** of this layer produce a mucous secretion. **Meissner's submucosal plexus** houses postganglionic parasympathetic nerve cells.

C. Muscularis Externa

The **muscularis externa** is composed of **inner circular** (tight helix) and **outer longitudinal** (loose helix) **muscle layers**. In the upper one-third of the esophagus, these consist of **skeletal muscle**; in the middle one-third, they consist of **skeletal** and **smooth muscle**; and in the lower one-third, they consist of **smooth muscle**. **Auerbach's myenteric plexus** is located between the two layers of muscle.

D. Adventitia

The **adventitia** of the esophagus is composed of fibrous connective tissue. Inferior to the diaphragm, the esophagus is covered by a **serosa**.

II. STOMACH

The **stomach** is a sac-like structure that receives food from the **esophagus** and delivers its contents, known as chyme, into the **duodenum**. The stomach has three histologically recognizable regions: **cardiac**, **fundic**, and **pyloric**. The **mucosa** and **submucosa** of the empty stomach are thrown into folds, known as **rugae**, that disappear in the distended stomach.

A. Mucosa

The **mucosa** presents **gastric pits**, the bases of which accept the openings of **gastric glands**.

1. Epithelium

The **simple columnar epithelium** has no goblet cells. The cells composing this epithelium are known as **surface lining cells** and extend into the gastric pits.

2. Lamina Propria

The **lamina propria** houses numerous **gastric glands**, slender blood vessels, and various connective tissue and **lymphoid cells**.

a. *Cells of Gastric Glands*
   Gastric glands are composed of the following cell types: **parietal (oxyntic) cells**, **chief (zymogenic) cells**, **mucous neck cells**, **DNES (enteroendocrine) cells**, and **stem cells**. Glands of the **cardiac region** have no **chief** and only a few **parietal cells**. Glands of the **pyloric region** are short and possess no chief cells and only a few parietal cells. Most of the cells are mucus-secreting cells resembling **mucous neck cells**. Glands of the **fundic region** possess all five cell types.

3. Muscularis Mucosae

The **muscularis mucosae** is composed of an **inner circular** and an **outer longitudinal smooth muscle** layer. A third layer may be present in certain regions.

B. Submucosa

The **submucosa** contains no glands. It houses a vascular plexus as well as **Meissner's submucosal plexus**.

C. Muscularis Externa

The **muscularis externa** is composed of three smooth muscle layers: the **inner oblique**, the **middle circular**, and the **outer longitudinal**. The middle circular forms the **pyloric sphincter. Auerbach's myenteric plexus** is located between the circular and longitudinal layers.

D. Serosa

The stomach is covered by a connective tissue coat enveloped in visceral peritoneum, the **serosa**.

III. SMALL INTESTINE

The **small intestine** is composed of three regions: **duodenum**, **jejunum**, and **ileum**. The **mucosa** of the small intestine presents folds, known as **villi**, that change their morphology and decrease in height from the duodenum to the ileum. The submucosa displays spiral folds, **plicae circulares** (valves of Kerckring).

A. Mucosa

The **mucosa** presents **villi**, evaginations of the epithelially covered **lamina propria**.

1. Epithelium

The **simple columnar epithelium** consists of **goblet, surface absorptive**, and **DNES cells**. The number of goblet cells increases from the duodenum to the ileum.

2. Lamina Propria

The **lamina propria**, composed of **loose connective tissue**, houses glands, known as the **crypts of Lieberkühn**, that extend to the muscularis mucosae. The cells composing these glands are **goblet cells, columnar cells**, and, especially at the base, **Paneth's cells, DNES cells**, and **stem cells**. An occasional **caveolated cell** may also be noted. A central **lacteal**, a blindly ending lymphatic vessel, **smooth muscle cells, blood vessels**, solitary **lymphatic nodules**, and **lymphoid cells** are also present. **Lymphatic nodules**, with **M cell** epithelial caps, are especially abundant as **Peyer's patches** in the ileum.

3. Muscularis Mucosae

The **muscularis mucosae** consists of an **inner circular** and an **outer longitudinal** layer of **smooth muscle**.

B. Submucosa

The **submucosa** is not unusual except in the **duodenum**, where it contains **Brunner's glands**.

C. Muscularis Externa

The **muscularis externa** is composed of the usual **inner circular** and **outer longitudinal** layers of **smooth muscle**, with **Auerbach's myenteric plexus** intervening.

D. Serosa

The duodenum is covered by **serosa** and **adventitia**, whereas the jejunum and ileum are covered by a serosa.

IV. LARGE INTESTINE

The **large intestine** is composed of the **appendix**, the **cecum**, the **colon** (**ascending, transverse**, and **descending**), the **rectum**, and the **anal canal**. The appendix and anal canal are described separately, although the remainder of the large intestine presents identical histologic features.

A. Colon

1. Mucosa

The **mucosa** presents no specialized folds. It is thicker than that of the small intestine.

a. Epithelium
The **simple columnar epithelium** has goblet cells and columnar cells.

b. Lamina Propria
The **crypts of Lieberkühn** of the **lamina propria** are longer than those of the small intestine. They are composed of numerous **goblet cells**, a few **DNES cells**, and **stem cells. Lymphatic nodules** are frequently present.

c. Muscularis Mucosae
The **muscularis mucosae** consists of **inner circular** and **outer longitudinal smooth muscle** layers.

2. Submucosa

The **submucosa** resembles that of the jejunum or ileum.

3. Muscularis Externa

The **muscularis externa** is composed of **inner circular** and **outer longitudinal smooth muscle** layers. The outer longitudinal muscle layer is modified into **teniae coli**, three flat ribbons of longitudinally arranged smooth muscles. These are responsible for the formation of **haustra coli** (sacculations). **Auerbach's plexus** occupies its position between the two layers.

4. Serosa

The colon possesses both **serosa** and **adventitia**. The serosa presents small, fat-filled pouches, the **appendices epiploicae**.

B. Appendix

The **lumen** of the **appendix** is usually stellate-shaped, and it may be obliterated. The **simple columnar epithelium** covers a **lamina propria** rich in **lymphatic nodules** and some **crypts of Lieberkühn**. The **muscularis mucosae**, **submucosa**, and **muscularis externa** conform to the general plan of the digestive tract. It is covered by a **serosa**.

C. Anal Canal

The **anal canal** presents longitudinal folds, **anal columns**, which become joined at the orifice of the anus to form **anal valves**, and intervening **anal sinuses**. The epithelium changes from the **simple columnar** of the rectum to **simple cuboidal** at the **anal valves**, to **stratified squamous** distal to the anal valves, and to **epidermis** at the orifice of the anus. **Circumanal glands, hair follicles**, and **sebaceous glands** are present here. The **submucosa** is rich in vascular supply. The **muscularis externa** forms the internal anal sphincter muscle. An **adventitia** connects the anus to the surrounding structures.

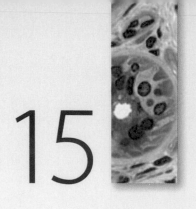

15 DIGESTIVE SYSTEM III

The major **glands of the digestive system** are located outside the wall of the digestive tract but are connected to its lumen via ducts. These glands include the major salivary glands, pancreas, and liver.

MAJOR SALIVARY GLANDS

The major salivary glands are the **parotid, submandibular,** and **sublingual glands**. These produce about 1 L of saliva per day, approximately 95% of the daily salivary secretion, which they deliver into the oral cavity.

- The three pairs of salivary glands possess a secretory component that is responsible for the formation of **primary saliva (isotonic saliva)**, which is modified by the initial portion of the **duct** system (**striated ducts**) to form the **secondary saliva (hypotonic saliva)**.
- Saliva is a **hypotonic** solution whose functions include lubrication and cleansing of the oral cavity (and reducing bacterial flora by the **lysozyme, lactoferrin, peroxidases**, histidine-rich proteins, and **immunoglobulin A [IgA]** that it contains), initial digestion of carbohydrates by **salivary amylase**, and assisting in the process of **taste** (by dissolving food substances).
  - ○ Saliva also acts as a buffer due to its contents of bicarbonates produced by cells of the striated duct.
- The parotid gland produces **serous secretions**, whereas the submandibular and sublingual glands manufacture **mixed secretions** (a combination of serous and mucous saliva).

PANCREAS

The **pancreas** is a mixed gland, in that it has exocrine and endocrine functions (see Graphic 15-1). Every day, the **exocrine pancreas** produces approximately 1 L of an alkaline fluid rich in digestive enzymes and proenzymes, which is delivered to the duodenum via the pancreatic duct.

- **Enzymes** are manufactured by the acinar cells (see Table 15-1 which lists these enzymes and their function), whereas the **alkaline fluid** is released by centroacinar cells and cells of the intercalated ducts.
  - ○ The pancreas, unlike the salivary glands, does not possess striated ducts.
- The release of the enzymes and alkaline fluid is intermittent and is controlled by the hormones **cholecystokinin** and **secretin**, respectively, as well as acetylcholine released by nerve cells of the enteric nervous system. The two types of secretions may be delivered independent of each other.

- ○ These hormones are produced by the **DNES cells** of the epithelial lining of the alimentary tract mucosa.

The **endocrine** pancreas is composed of scattered spherical aggregates of richly vascularized cords of endocrine cells, known as **islets of Langerhans**. Five cell types are present in these structures (see Table 15-2 Hormones produced by cells of the Islets of Langerhans):

- α cells, producing **glucagon,**
- β cells, manufacturing **insulin,**
- δ cells, manufacturing **somatostatin,**
- **PP cells,** secreting **pancreatic polypeptide,** and
- **G cells,** producing **gastrin.**

LIVER

The **liver** is the largest gland of the body. It performs a myriad of functions, many of which are *not* glandular in nature (see Graphic 15-2). It is believed that the parenchymal cells of the liver, known as **hepatocytes,** have a lifespan of about 5 months and they are capable of performing each of the approximately 100 different functions of the liver.

- Since each hepatocyte is bordered by a vascular **sinusoid**, liver cells can absorb toxic materials and byproducts of digestion, which they detoxify and store for future use.
- **Hepatic sinusoids** receive oxygen-rich blood from branches of the **hepatic artery** and nutrient-laden blood from branches of the **portal vein**.
- The **sinusoidal lining cells** possess
  - ○ large **fenestrae** that lack diaphragms and they display
  - ○ discontinuities between adjoining cells that, although large, are too small for the passage of blood cells or platelets.
- Monocyte-derived macrophages, known as **Kupffer cells**, participate in the formation of the sinusoidal endothelial lining.
  - ○ **Kupffer cells** participate in removing defunct red blood cells and other undesirable particulate matter from the bloodstream.

Fat-storing (Ito) cells are located in the space of Disse, the narrow space between the sinusoidal lining cells and the hepatocytes. Ito cells are believed to function in the accumulation and storage of **vitamin A**, but in the case of alcoholic cirrhosis, these cells also manufacture type I collagen, responsible for fibrosis of the liver.

Hepatocytes are arranged in radiating **plates of liver cells** that are arranged in such a fashion that they form hexagonal lobules (2 mm long and 0.7 mm in diameter). These structures are referred to as **classical lobules** (see Graphic 15-2).

TABLE 15-1 • Enzymes Produced by the Acinar Cells of the Pancreas*

Enzymes	Function
Trypsinogen[†]	As trypsin: converts proenzymes into active enzymes, cleaves dietary proteins present in the chyme
Chymotrypsinogen	As chymotrypsin: cleaves dietary proteins present in the chyme
Carboxypeptidase	Cleaves peptide bonds at the carboxyl terminus of a protein
Aminopeptidase	Cleaves peptide bonds at the amino terminus of a protein
Amylase	Cleaves carbohydrates
Lipase	Digests lipids liberating free fatty acids
DNase (**deoxyribonuclease**)	Hydrolyses phosphodiester links of the deoxyphosphate backbone of DNA
RNase (**ribonuclease**)	Hydrolyses phosphodiester links of the phosphate backbone of RNA
Elastase	Digests elastic fibers

*Some of these are proenzymes that are activated in the lumen of the duodenum by trypsin
†Trypsinogen and chymotrypsinogen are activated by enterokinases present on the microvilli of the surface absorptive cells forming trypsin and chymotrypsin, respectively.

TABLE 15-2 • Hormones Produced by the Cells of the Islets of Langerhans

Cells (and % of Total)	Hormone	Molecular Weight (Da)	Function
β cell (70%)	Insulin	6,000	Decreases blood glucose level by inducing the uptake, storage, and glycolysis of glucose; stimulates formation of glycerol; hinders lipid digestion by adipocytes
α cell (20%)	Glucagon	3,500	Decreases blood glucose level, induces glycogenolysis and gluconeogenesis
δ_1 cell (~5%)	Somatostatin	1,640	Inhibits hormone release from other cells of the Islet of Langerhans, inhibits enzyme release by acinar cells of the pancreas, reduces smooth muscle activity of the digestive tract and gallbladder
Δ_2 cell (~2%)	VIP (vasoactive intestinal peptide)	3,800	Stimulates glycogenolysis; reduces smooth muscle activity of the digestive tract; modulates H_2O and ion movements in intestinal epithelial cells
PP cell (~1%)	Pancreatic polypeptide	4,200	Inhibits secretory activity of the exocrine pancreas
G cell (~1%)	Gastrin	2,000	Induces HCl manufacture by parietal cells of the stomach

- Where three **classical lobules** meet, their slender connective tissue elements merge to form **portal areas** that house branches of the hepatic artery, portal vein, bile duct, and lymph vessel.
- The center of each classical lobule houses a single **central vein,** which receives blood from the numerous hepatic sinusoids, thus forming the beginning of the blood drainage system.
- Central veins lead to **sublobular veins** that merge with other sublobular veins forming larger veins that eventually drain into the **right** and **left hepatic veins** that deliver their blood into the **inferior vena cava.**

In addition to the classical lobule, two other conceptual lobulations have been suggested for the liver, **portal lobule**, a triangular structure whose three apices are three neighboring central veins (see Graphic 15-2), and **liver acinus (of Rappaport)**, a diamond-shaped structure whose long axis connects two adjacent central veins and short axis connects two portal areas (see Graphic 15-2).

- **Portal lobules** were suggested since in a classical lobule blood flows toward the center of the lobule and bile flows to the periphery of the lobule. Whereas in the portal lobule concept the bile flows to the center of the lobule.
- **Liver acinus** was suggested to describe blood flow and oxygen supply of the hepatic lobule because it reflects pathological changes in the liver during hypoxia and toxin-induced alterations.
  - Each acinus is subdivided into three more or less equal zones,
    - the zone in the vicinity of the central vein (zone 3) receives the least amount of oxygen,
    - the zone in the vicinity of the short axis, between the two portal areas (zone 1), receives the most oxygen, and
    - zone 2, the region between zones 1 and 3, receives an intermediate amount of oxygen.

Exocrine Function of the Liver

- The liver forms about 1 L of **bile** per day, which is its **exocrine secretion.**
  - **Bile** is delivered into a system of conduits: **bile canaliculi, cholangioles, canals of Hering, interlobular bile ducts,** and **right** and **left hepatic ducts,** which then directs the bile into the **common hepatic duct** and from there, via the **cystic duct** into the **gallbladder,** a storage organ associated with the liver.
  - The release of concentrated bile into the duodenum via the cystic and common bile ducts is regulated by hormones of the DNES cells in the alimentary tract.

- Bile is a green, somewhat viscous fluid composed of water, ions, cholesterol, phospholipids, bilirubin glucuronide, and bile acids.
  - One of these components, **bilirubin glucuronide**, is a water-soluble conjugate of nonsoluble **bilirubin**, a toxic breakdown product of **hemoglobin**.
  - It is in the **smooth endoplasmic reticulum (sER)** of the hepatocytes that detoxification of bilirubin occurs.

Endocrine and Other Functions of the Liver

- the synthesis and release of numerous **plasma proteins** and components, such as fibrinogen, urea, albumin, prothrombin, and lipoproteins;
- manufacture of proteins that regulate the transfer and metabolism of **iron**;
- **storage** of glycogen and lipids for release during intervals between eating;
- synthesis of glucose;
- synthesis of the five classes of **lipoproteins** (see Table 15-3)
- **gluconeogenesis** from noncarbohydrate sources (amino acids and lipids); and
- **transport** of IgA into the bile and, subsequently, into the lumen of the small intestine.
- **Detoxification** of various drugs, toxins, metabolic by-products, and chemicals occurs either by the **microsomal mixed-function oxidase system** of the sER or by **peroxidases** of peroxisomes.

GALLBLADDER

The **gallbladder** is a small, pear-shaped organ that receives bile from the liver.

- It not only stores but also concentrates bile and, in response to the **cholecystokinin** released by the DNES cells of the alimentary tract, forces the bile into the lumen of the duodenum via the cystic and common bile ducts.
- The gallbladder can store as much as 50 mL of bile.
  - The **bile** emulsifies fats, facilitating the action of the enzyme **pancreatic lipase.**
- The lamina propria, lined by a simple columnar epithelium, is thrown into highly convoluted folds in the empty gallbladder. These folds disappear on distention.
  - Occasionally, tubuloalveolar mucous glands are present.

TABLE 15-3 • The Classes of Lipoproteins

Lipoprotein Class	Density (g/mL)	Characteristics and Function
Chylomicrons	<0.95	Manufactured in the small intestine and released into the lacteals of the lamina propria as relatively large globules (as large as 500 μm in diameter). Composed of ~2% protein, ~90% triglycerides, ~2% cholesterol, and ~6% phospholipids. The protein moiety enables the chylomicron to be miscible with the aqueous plasma.
VLDL	0.95–1.006	Manufactured in the liver and to a much lesser extent in the small intestine and is modified in the bloodstream by the acquisition of additional proteins. These are much smaller (~60 nm in diameter) than chylomicrons. The blood-circulating enzyme lipoprotein lipase cleaves triglycerides from VLDL.
IDL	1.006–1.019	Is formed in the bloodstream as lipoprotein lipase continues to remove triglycerides from VLDL. It is rich in apolipoprotein E and is about 30 nm in diameter.
LDL	1.019–1.063	Is formed in the bloodstream as IDL loses its apolipoprotein E. LDL is ~20 nm in diameter. They have a relatively high cholesterol content, and they are considered to be the principal causative agents of plaque buildup in blood vessels with ensuing cardiovascular disease which may result in death. LDL appears to block the quorum sensing in *Staphylococcus aureus* permitting excessive proliferation of the bacteria.
HDL	1.063–1.210	Is manufactured in the liver is about 12 nm in diameter and consists of as much as 50% protein, 40% triglyceride, and 15% cholesterol. They transport cholesterol to the liver and to glands synthesizing steroid hormones. HDLs can remove cholesterol from vascular plaques; therefore, high HDL concentration in the blood decreases the possibility of cardiovascular disease.

VLDL, very-low-density lipoprotein; IDL, intermediate-density lipoprotein; LDL, low-density lipoprotein; HDL, high-density lipoprotein.

CLINICAL CONSIDERATIONS

Gastrinoma

Gastrinoma is a disease in which the **G cells** of the pancreas undergo **excess proliferation** (frequently cancerous), resulting in an **overproduction of the hormone gastrin**. This hormone is responsible for binding to parietal cells of the stomach, causing them to oversecrete hydrochloric acid with a resultant formation of peptic ulcers in the stomach and the duodenum.

Chronic Pancreatitis

Chronic pancreatitis, chronic inflammation of the pancreas, is caused by a plethora of factors, genetic as well as environmental, most frequently excessive alcohol consumption and, to a lesser extent, obstruction of the pancreatic duct. The pathologic features include injury to the acinar cells of the exocrine pancreas due to the release of a variety of inflammatory pharmaceutical agents by the connective tissue cells. The chronic inflammation induces type I and type III collagen formation with the resultant fibrosis of the organ.

Kaposi's Sarcoma of the Liver

Kaposi's sarcoma of the liver is almost solely present in patients with immunodeficient diseases and has been observed in as many as a quarter of

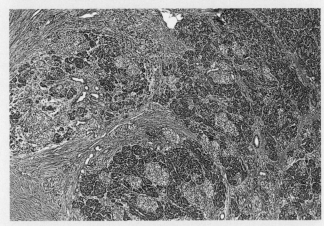

This photomicrograph is of a patient suffering from chronic pancreatitis. Observe that the connective tissue elements are highly exaggerated, the acini are greatly reduced in number, and the Islets of Langerhans are very close to each other because of the reduction in acinar population. (Reprinted with permission from Mills SE, Carter D, et al., eds. Sternberg's Diagnostic Surgical Pathology, 5th ed., Philadelphia: Lippincott Williams & Wilkins, 2010, p. 1438.)

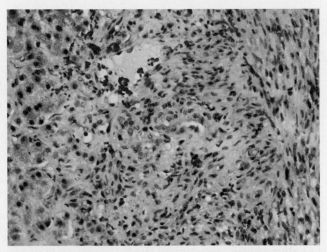

This photomicrograph is of a patient suffering from Kaposi's sarcoma of the liver. Observe the presence of relatively normal hepatocytes in the upper left, whereas much of the right-hand side displays the presence of spindle-shaped cells, typical of Kaposi's sarcoma cells. An additional typical feature of this disease is the presence of extravasated erythrocytes. (Reprinted with permission from Mills SE, Carter D, et al., eds. Sternberg's Diagnostic Surgical Pathology, 5th ed., Philadelphia: Lippincott Williams & Wilkins, 2010, p. 1584.)

the patient population who succumbed to AIDS. Additionally, a Kaposi's sarcoma–associated herpesvirus has also been determined to be a causative factor in this disease. The autopsied livers presented with numerous darkened nodules of a soft consistency most of which occupied expanded connective tissue of the intrahepatic biliary tract.

Type I Diabetes

Type I (**insulin-dependent**) diabetes is characterized by **polyphagia** (insatiable hunger), **polydipsia** (unquenchable thirst), and **polyuria** (excessive urination). It usually has a sudden onset before 20 years of age, is distinguished by damage to and destruction of beta cells, and results from a **low level of plasma insulin**.

Type II Diabetes Mellitus

Type II (**non–insulin-dependent**) diabetes mellitus commonly occurs in overweight individuals over 40 years of age. It does not result from low levels of plasma insulin and is **insulin resistant**, which is a major factor in its pathogenesis. The resistance to insulin is due to decreased binding of insulin to its plasmalemma receptors and to defects in postreceptor insulin action. Type II diabetes is usually controlled by diet.

Hepatitis

Hepatitis is inflammation of the liver, and although it could have various causes such as abuse of alcohol and certain drugs, its most common cause is one of the five types of hepatitis viruses, denoted by the first five letters of the alphabet, A through E. **Hepatitis A** is usually spread by poor hygiene (fecal-oral route and contaminated water) as well as by sexual contact. Usually, there are no symptoms; the patient recovers and does not become a carrier. **Hepatitis B**, a more serious condition than hepatitis A, is usually transmitted by body fluids and, in case of drug addicts, by the sharing of needles. Patients can become carriers of the virus, and in 10% of the patients, the condition may become chronic, leading to cirrhosis and cancer of the liver. In the past, **hepatitis C** was transmitted by blood transfusions, but screening has almost completely eradicated that route and now it is transmitted mostly by shared needles among drug addicts. About three-quarters of people who have the hepatitis C virus will reach the chronic stage, and of these, 20% to 25% will develop cirrhosis and then liver cancer. **Hepatitis D** is also transmitted by the sharing of needles and is always accompanied by hepatitis B. The double infection is a more severe condition. **Hepatitis E** is spread by the fecal-oral route and is responsible for epidemics but mostly in underdeveloped countries. Neither chronic nor carrier states are present with this form of the hepatitis virus. Universal vaccination is recommended to protect the population from hepatitis B, and this has the added benefit of protection against hepatitis D; it is recommended that travelers to underdeveloped countries where hepatitis A is prevalent be vaccinated against hepatitis A. There are no vaccines currently available against hepatitis C or E.

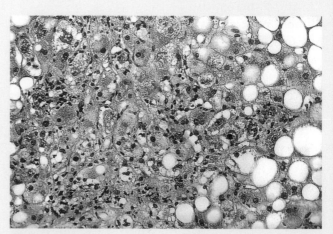

This photomicrograph is of a patient suffering from acute alcohol-induced hepatitis. Observe that the specimen presents some of the earliest histopathological signs of alcohol-induced hepatitis, namely, macrovascular fatty changes, Mallory hyaline, and the infiltration by neutrophils. (Reprinted with permission from Mills SE, Carter D, et al., eds. Sternberg's Diagnostic Surgical Pathology, 5th ed., Philadelphia: Lippincott Williams & Wilkins, 2010. p. 1513.)

Jaundice (Icterus)

Jaundice (icterus) is characterized by excess bilirubin in the blood and deposition of **bile pigment** in the skin and sclera of the eyes, resulting in a yellowish appearance. It may be hereditary or due to pathologic conditions such as excess destruction of red blood cells (**hemolytic jaundice**), liver dysfunction, and obstruction of the biliary passages (**obstructive jaundice**).

Gallstones (Biliary Calculi)

Gallstones (biliary calculi) are concretions, usually of fused crystals of **cholesterol** that form in gallbladder or bile duct. They may accumulate to such an extent that the cystic duct is blocked, thus preventing emptying of the gallbladder, and they may require surgical removal if less invasive methods fail to dissolve or pulverize them. If the obstruction occurs in an abrupt manner due to the gallstones, the gallbladder can rapidly become inflamed, a condition known as **chronic cholecystitis**.

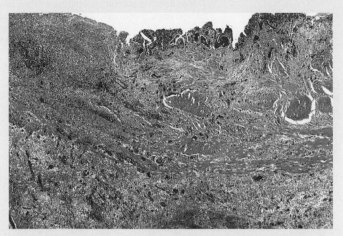

This photomicrograph is from a gallbladder whose cystic duct was obstructed by the presence of gallstones resulting in acute cholecystitis. Observe that much of the luminal surface of the mucosa lacks an epithelial lining and that the lamina propria is edematous. Moreover, the adventitia is thicker than normal. (Reprinted with permission from Mills SE, Carter D, et al., eds. Sternberg's Diagnostic Surgical Pathology, 5th ed., Philadelphia: Lippincott Williams & Wilkins, 2010. p. 1606.)

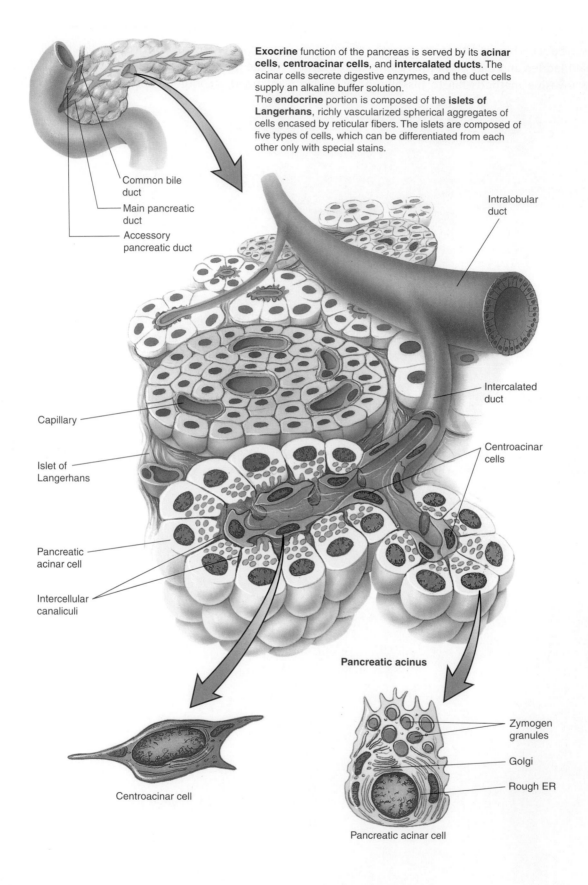

Exocrine function of the pancreas is served by its acinar cells, centroacinar cells, and intercalated ducts. The acinar cells secrete digestive enzymes, and the duct cells supply an alkaline buffer solution.

The endocrine portion is composed of the islets of Langerhans, richly vascularized spherical aggregates of cells encased by reticular fibers. The islets are composed of five types of cells, which can be differentiated from each other only with special stains.

Common bile duct

Main pancreatic duct

Accessory pancreatic duct

Intralobular duct

Intercalated duct

Centroacinar cells

Capillary

Islet of Langerhans

Pancreatic acinar cell

Intercellular canaliculi

Pancreatic acinus

Centroacinar cell

Zymogen granules

Golgi

Rough ER

Pancreatic acinar cell

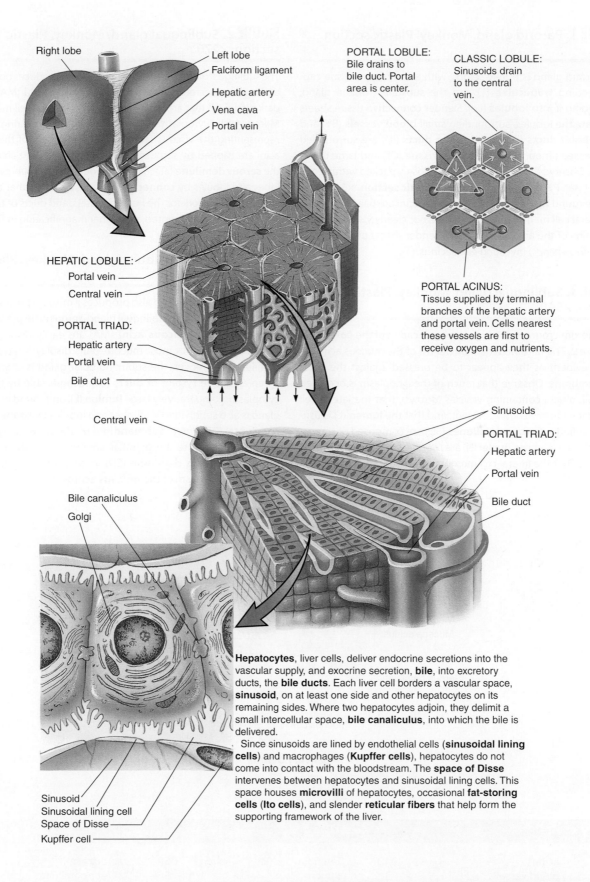

Right lobe

Left lobe
Falciform ligament
Hepatic artery
Vena cava
Portal vein

PORTAL LOBULE:
Bile drains to
bile duct. Portal
area is center.

CLASSIC LOBULE:
Sinusoids drain
to the central
vein.

HEPATIC LOBULE:
Portal vein
Central vein

PORTAL TRIAD:
Hepatic artery
Portal vein
Bile duct

PORTAL ACINUS:
Tissue supplied by terminal
branches of the hepatic artery
and portal vein. Cells nearest
these vessels are first to
receive oxygen and nutrients.

Central vein

Sinusoids

PORTAL TRIAD:
Hepatic artery
Portal vein
Bile duct

Bile canaliculus
Golgi

Sinusoid
Sinusoidal lining cell
Space of Disse
Kupffer cell

Hepatocytes, liver cells, deliver endocrine secretions into the
vascular supply, and exocrine secretion, **bile**, into excretory
ducts, the **bile ducts**. Each liver cell borders a vascular space,
sinusoid, on at least one side and other hepatocytes on its
remaining sides. Where two hepatocytes adjoin, they delimit a
small intercellular space, **bile canaliculus**, into which the bile is
delivered.
   Since sinusoids are lined by endothelial cells (**sinusoidal lining
cells**) and macrophages (**Kupffer cells**), hepatocytes do not
come into contact with the bloodstream. The **space of Disse**
intervenes between hepatocytes and sinusoidal lining cells. This
space houses **microvilli** of hepatocytes, occasional **fat-storing
cells (Ito cells)**, and slender **reticular fibers** that help form the
supporting framework of the liver.

PLATE 15-1 · Salivary Glands

FIGURE 1. Parotid gland. Monkey. Plastic section. ×132.

The parotid gland is purely serous, with a connective tissue capsule sending **trabeculae** (T) into the substance of the gland, subdividing it into **lobules** (Lo). Slender connective tissue sheets penetrate the lobules, surrounding small **blood vessels** (BV) and **intralobular ducts** (iD). **Interlobular ducts** (ID) are surrounded by increased amounts of **connective tissue** (CT) and large blood vessels. Observe that the **acini** (Ac) are closely packed within each lobule. *Inset.* **Parotid gland. Monkey. Plastic section.** ×540. Note that the round **nuclei** (N) of these serous acini are basally located. The lateral cell membranes (*arrows*) are not clearly visible, nor are the lumina of the acini. Observe the slender sheets of connective tissue (*arrowheads*) investing each acinus.

FIGURE 3. Sublingual gland. Monkey. Plastic section. ×540.

This photomicrograph is a higher magnification of the *boxed area* of Figure 2. The flattened, dark **nuclei** (N) of the mucous acini are clearly evident as they appear to be pressed against the basal cell membrane. Observe that much of the cytoplasm is occupied by small, mucin-containing vesicles (*arrows*), that the lateral cell membrane (*arrowheads*) is evident, and that the **lumen** (L) is usually identifiable. **Serous demilunes** (SD) are composed of serous-producing cells whose **nuclei** (N) are round to oval in morphology. Note also that the lateral cell membranes are not distinguishable in serous cells.

FIGURE 2. Sublingual gland. Monkey. Plastic section. ×270.

The sublingual gland is a mixed gland in that it produces both serous and mucous secretory products. The **mucous acini** (MA) possess dark **nuclei** (N) that are flattened against the basal cell membrane. Moreover, the cytoplasm is filled with a frothy-appearing material, representing the viscous secretory product. Many of the mucous acini are capped by serous cells, forming a crescent-shaped cap, the **serous demilune** (SD). The sublingual gland is subdivided into lobes and lobules by **connective tissue septa** (CT) that act as the supporting network for the nerves, vessels, and ducts of the gland. The *boxed area* is presented at a higher magnification in Figure 3.

FIGURE 4. Submandibular gland. Monkey. Plastic section. ×132.

The submandibular gland also produces a mixed type of secretion; however, unlike in the sublingual gland, serous acini predominate. **Serous** (SA) and **mucous acini** (MA) are easily distinguishable from each other, but most mucous units display a cap of serous demilunes. Moreover, the submandibular gland is characterized by an extensive system of **ducts** (D), recognizable by their pale cytoplasm, comparatively large **lumina** (L), and round nuclei. This gland is also subdivided into lobes and lobules by **connective tissue septa** (CT). *Inset.* **Submandibular gland. Monkey. Plastic section.** ×540. Note the granular appearance of the cells comprising the **serous demilune** (SD) in contrast with the "frothy" appearing cytoplasm of the **mucous acinus** (MA).

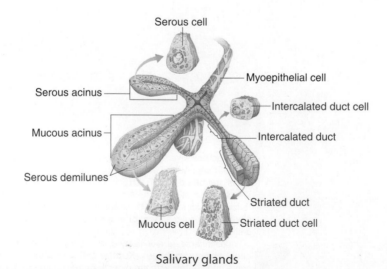

Salivary glands

KEY					
Ac	acinus	**ID**	interlobular duct	**SA**	serous acini
BV	blood vessel	**L**	lumen	**SD**	serous demilune
CT	connective tissue	**Lo**	lobule	**T**	trabeculae
D	duct	**MA**	mucous acini		
iD	intralobular duct	**N**	nucleus		

PLATE 15-1 • Salivary Glands

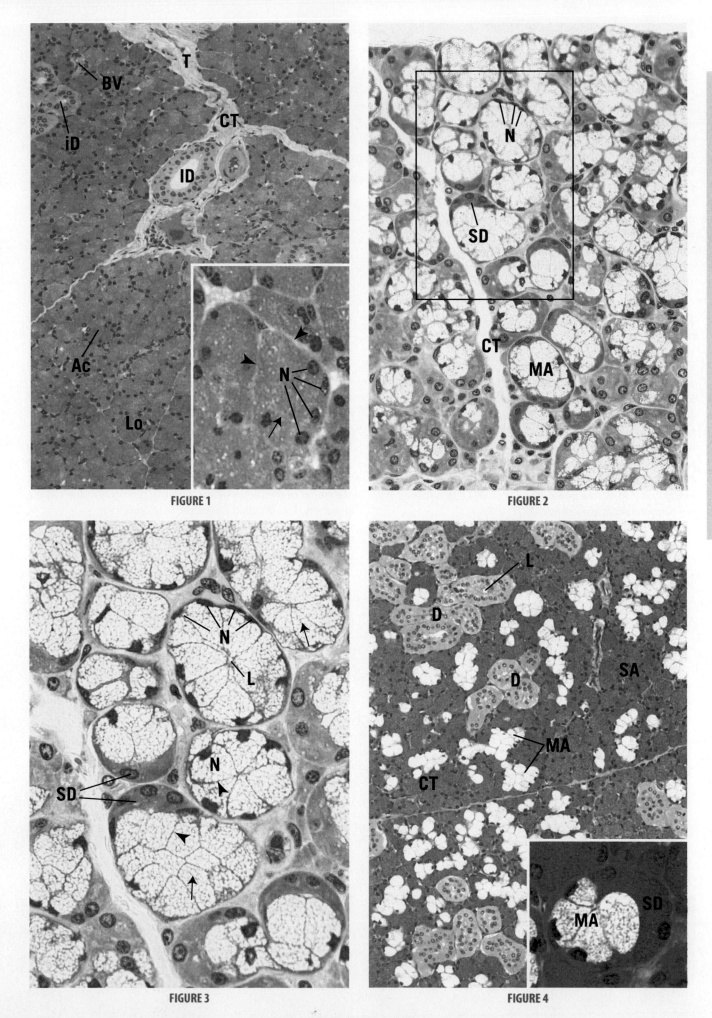

FIGURE 1

FIGURE 2

FIGURE 3

FIGURE 4

PLATE 15-2 · Pancreas

FIGURE 1. Pancreas. Human. Paraffin section. ×132.

The pancreas is a complex gland since it has both exocrine and endocrine components. The exocrine portion comprises the bulk of the organ as a compound tubuloalveolar gland, secreting a serous fluid. The gland is subdivided into lobules by **connective tissue septa** (CT). Each **acinus** (Ac) is composed of several pyramid-shaped cells, possessing round nuclei. Cells located in the center of the acinus, **centroacinar cells** (CA), form the smallest ducts of the gland. The endocrine portion of the pancreas is composed of small, spherical clumps of cells, **islets of Langerhans** (IL), which are richly endowed by capillaries. These islets of Langerhans are haphazardly scattered among the serous acini of the pancreas. The *boxed area* is presented at a higher magnification in Figure 2.

FIGURE 3. Pancreas. Monkey. Plastic section. ×540.

With the use of plastic sections, the morphology of the pancreatic acinus is well defined. Observe that in fortuitous sections the acinus resembles a pie, with the individual cells clearly delineated (*arrows*). The **nucleus** (N) of each trapezoid-shaped cell is round and the basal cytoplasm (*arrowhead*) is relatively homogeneous, whereas the apical cytoplasm is packed with **zymogen granules** (ZG). **Centroacinar cells** (CA) may be recognized both by their locations as well as by the pale appearance of their nuclei. *Inset.* **Pancreas. Monkey. Plastic section.** ×540. Observe the **centroacinar cell** (CA), whose pale nucleus is readily differentiated from the surrounding acinar cell nuclei.

FIGURE 2. Pancreas. Human. Paraffin section. ×270.

This photomicrograph is a higher magnification of the *boxed area* of Figure 1. Note that the **connective tissue septa** (CT), while fairly extensive in certain regions, are quite slender in the interlobular areas. The trapezoidal morphologies of individual cells of the serous acini are clearly evident in fortuitous sections (*arrow*). Observe also the **centroacinar cells** (CA), located in the center of acini, which represent the smallest units of the pancreatic duct system.

FIGURE 4. Islets of Langerhans. Monkey. Plastic section. ×270.

The **islets of Langerhans** (IL), the endocrine portion of the pancreas, are a more or less spherical configuration of cells randomly scattered throughout the exocrine portion of the gland. As such, each islet is surrounded by serous **acini** (Ac). The islets receive their rich **blood supply** (BV) from the **connective tissue elements** (CT) of the exocrine pancreas. *Inset.* **Islets of Langerhans. Monkey. Plastic section.** ×540. Observe the rich vascularity of the islets of Langerhans, as evidenced by the presence of **erythrocyte** (RBC)-engorged blood vessels. Although each islet is composed of A, B, C, and D cells, they can only be distinguished from each other by the use of special stains. However, it should be noted that, in the human, B cells are the most populous and are usually located in the center of the islet, whereas A cells are generally found at the periphery. This situation is reversed in the monkey.

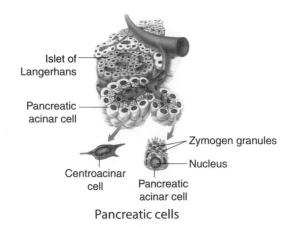

Pancreatic cells

KEY

Ac	acinus	**CT**	connective tissue septa	**RBC**	erythrocyte
BV	blood vessel	**IL**	islets of Langerhans	**ZG**	zymogen granule
CA	centroacinar cell	**N**	nucleus		

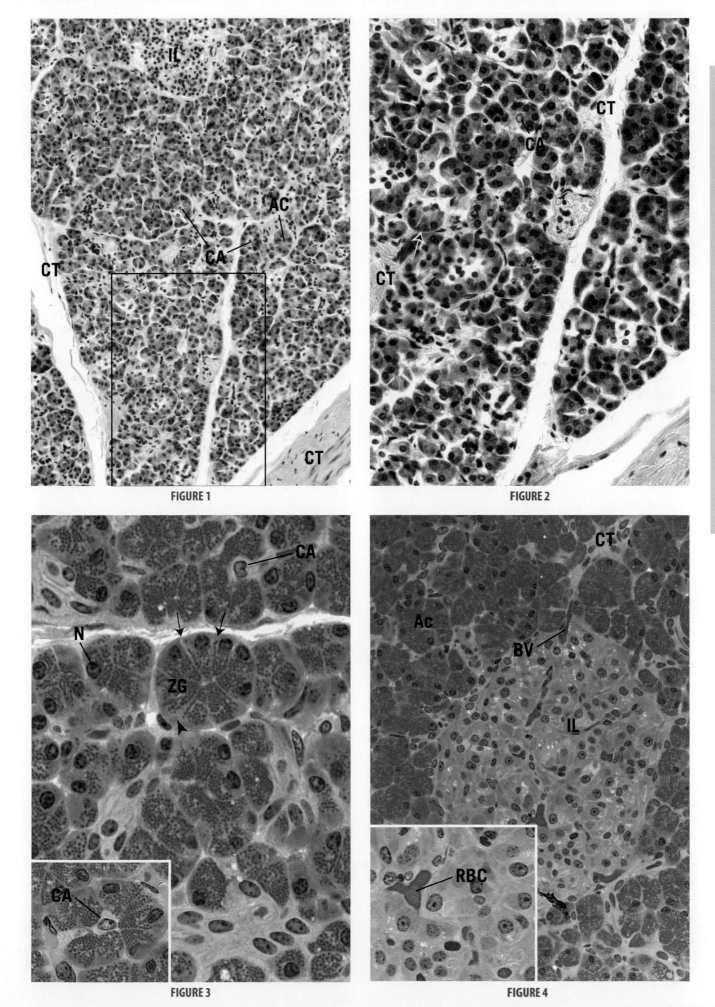

PLATE 15-2 • Pancreas

FIGURE 1

FIGURE 2

FIGURE 3

FIGURE 4

PLATE 15-3 · Liver

FIGURE 1. Liver. Pig. Paraffin section. ×14.

Note that the liver is invested by a connective tissue capsule, **Glisson's capsule** (GC), from which, in the pig, **septa** (S) extend to subdivide the gland into more or less hexagon-shaped classical **lobules** (Lo). Blood vessels, lymph vessels, and bile ducts travel within the connective tissue septa to reach the apices of the classic lobules, which are known as the **portal areas** (PA). Bile reaches the portal areas from within the lobules, whereas blood enters the substance of the lobules from the portal areas. Within each lobule, the blood flows through tortuous channels, the liver sinusoids, to enter the **central vein** (CV) in the middle of the classical lobule.

FIGURE 3. Liver. Monkey. Plastic section. ×132.

The **central vein** (CV) of the liver lobule (a terminal radix of the hepatic vein) collects blood from the **sinusoids** (Si) and delivers it to sublobular veins. The **plates of liver cells** (PL) and hepatic sinusoids appear to radiate, as spokes of a wheel, from the central vein. The *boxed area* is presented at a higher magnification in Figure 4.

FIGURE 2. Liver. Dog. Paraffin section. ×132.

The portal area of the liver houses terminal branches of the **hepatic artery** (HA) and **portal vein** (PV). Note that the vein is much larger than the artery, and its wall is very thin in comparison to the size of its lumen. Branches of **lymph vessels** (LV) and **bile ducts** (BD) are also present in the portal area. Bile ducts may be recognized by their cuboidal-to-columnar epithelium. Observe that unlike in the pig, connective tissue septa do not demarcate the boundaries of classic liver lobules, although the various structures of the portal area are invested by connective tissue elements. **Plates of liver cells** (PL) and **sinusoids** (Si) extend from the portal areas.

FIGURE 4. Liver. Monkey. Plastic section. ×270.

This photomicrograph is a higher magnification of the *boxed area* of the previous figure. Note that the lumen of the **central vein** (CV) is lined by a simple squamous **epithelium** (Ep), which is continuous with the endothelial lining of the hepatic **sinusoids** (Si), tortuous vascular channels that freely communicate with each other. Observe also that the **liver plates** (LP) are composed of **hepatocytes** (H), one to two cell layers thick, and that each plate is bordered by sinusoids.

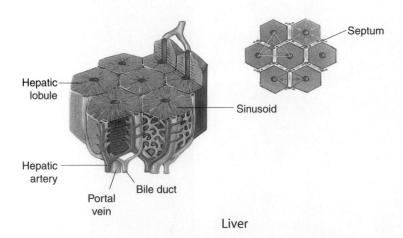

Hepatic lobule

Septum

Sinusoid

Hepatic artery

Bile duct

Portal vein

Liver

KEY

BD	bile duct	**HA**	hepatic artery	**PL**	plates of liver cells
CV	central vein	**Lo**	lobule	**PV**	portal vein
Ep	epithelium	**LP**	liver plates	**S**	septa
GC	Glisson's capsule	**LV**	lymph vessel	**Si**	sinusoid
H	hepatocyte	**PA**	portal area		

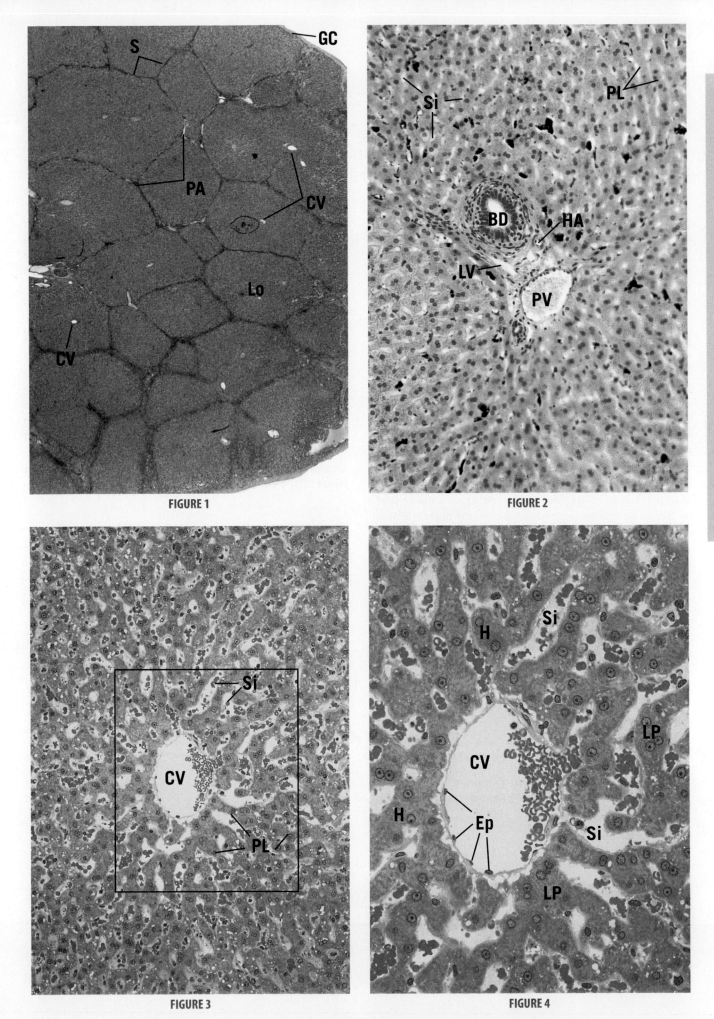

PLATE 15-3 · Liver

FIGURE 1

FIGURE 2

FIGURE 3

FIGURE 4

PLATE 15-4 · Liver, Gallbladder

FIGURE 1. Liver. Monkey. Plastic section. ×540.

This photomicrograph is a high magnification of **liver plates** (LP). Observe that individual **hepatocytes** (H) are polygonal in shape. Each hepatocyte possesses one or two nuclei, although occasionally some have three nuclei. Plates of hepatocytes enclose hepatic **sinusoids** (Si) that are lined by **sinusoidal lining cells** (SC); therefore, hepatocytes do not come into direct contact with the bloodstream. The space between the sinusoidal lining cells and the hepatocytes, the space of Disse, is at the limit of resolution of the light microscope. *Inset.* **Liver. Human. Paraffin section.** ×540. The hepatocyte cell membranes are clearly evident in this photomicrograph. Note that in fortuitous sections, small intercellular spaces (*arrows*) are recognizable. These are bile canaliculi through which bile flows to the periphery of the lobule.

FIGURE 3. Gallbladder. Human. Paraffin section. ×132.

The gallbladder is a pear-shaped, hollow organ that functions in storing and concentrating bile. Its histologic structure is relatively simple, but its appearance may be deceiving. The mucosa of an empty gallbladder, as in this photomicrograph, is thrown into numerous folds (*arrows*), providing it with a glandular morphology. However, close observation of the **epithelium** (Ep) demonstrates that all of the simple columnar cells of the mucous membrane are identical. A loose **connective tissue** (CT), sometimes referred to as a lamina propria, lies deep to the epithelium. Observe that a muscularis mucosae is lacking, and the **smooth muscle** (SM) surrounding the connective tissue is the muscularis externa. The outermost coat of the gallbladder is a serosa or adventitia. A region similar to the *boxed area* is presented in Figure 4.

FIGURE 2. Liver. Paraffin section. ×540.

A system of macrophages known as **Kupffer cells** (KC) are found interspersed among the endothelial lining cells of liver **sinusoids** (Si). These macrophages are larger than the epithelial cells and may be recognized by the presence of phagocytosed material within them. Kupffer cells may be demonstrated by injecting an animal intravenously with india ink, as is the case in this specimen. Observe that some cells appear as large, black smudges since they are filled with phagocytosed ink (*asterisk*), whereas other cells possess only small quantities of the phagocytosed material (*arrowheads*). Note also that much of the sinusoidal lining is devoid of ink, indicating that the endothelial cells are probably not phagocytic.

FIGURE 4. Gallbladder. Human. Paraffin section. ×540.

This photomicrograph is a higher magnification of a region similar to the *boxed area* of Figure 3. Note that the **epithelium** (Ep) is composed of identical-appearing tall columnar cells, whose **nuclei** (N) are basally oriented. The lateral cell membranes are evident in certain regions (*arrows*), whereas the apical brush border is usually not visible in hematoxylin and eosin–stained specimens. Observe that a relatively thick **basal membrane** (BM) separates the epithelium from the underlying loose **connective tissue** (CT).

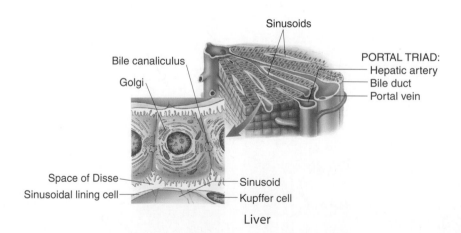

Liver

KEY

BM	basal membrane	KC	Kupffer cell	Si	sinusoid
CT	connective tissue	LP	liver plate	SM	smooth muscle
Ep	epithelium	N	nucleus		
H	hepatocyte	SC	sinusoidal lining cell		

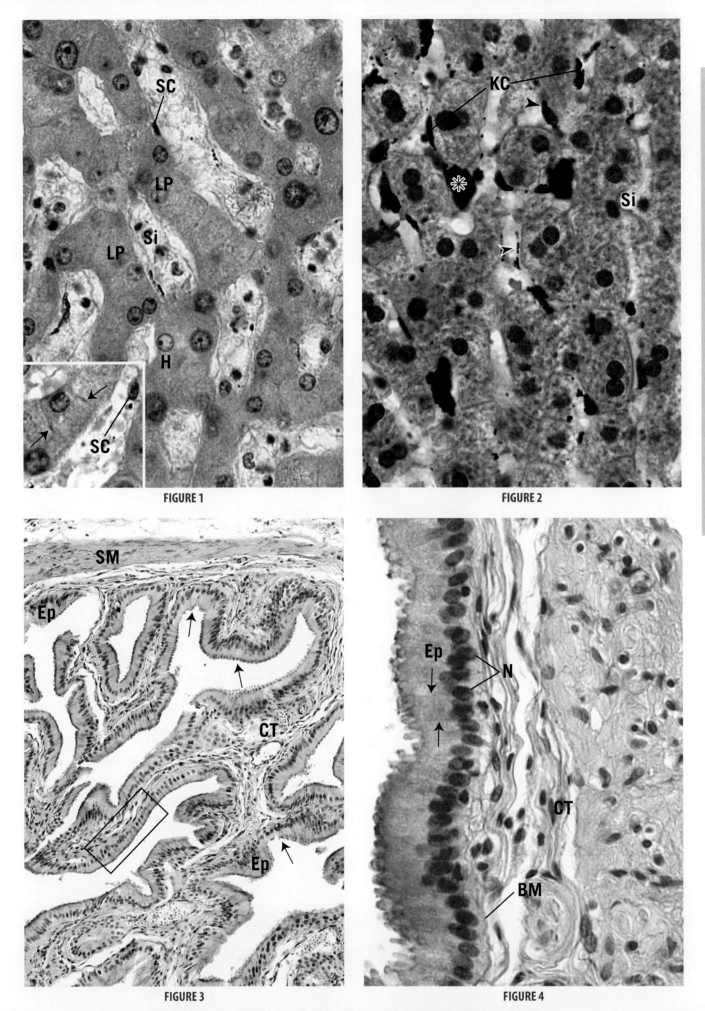

PLATE 15-4 • Liver, Gallbladder

FIGURE 1

FIGURE 2

FIGURE 3

FIGURE 4

PLATE 15-5 • Salivary Gland, Electron Microscopy

FIGURE 1. Sublingual gland. Human. Electron microscopy. ×4,050.

The human sublingual gland is composed mostly of mucous acini capped by serous demilunes. The **mucous cells** (mc) display numerous **filamentous bodies** (f) and secretory granules, which appear to be empty (*asterisks*). The **serous cells** (dc) may be recognized by their paler cytoplasm and the presence of secretory granules (*arrows*) housing electron-dense materials. Note also the presence of **myoepithelial cells** (myo), whose processes (*arrowheads*) encircle the acinus. (Courtesy of Dr. A. Riva.)

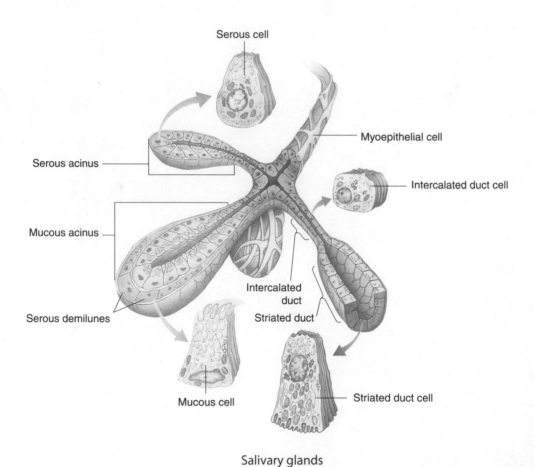

Salivary glands

KEY			
dc	serous cells	**mc**	mucous cells
f	filamentous bodies	**myo**	myoepithelial cells

PLATE 15-5 • Salivary Gland, Electron Microscopy

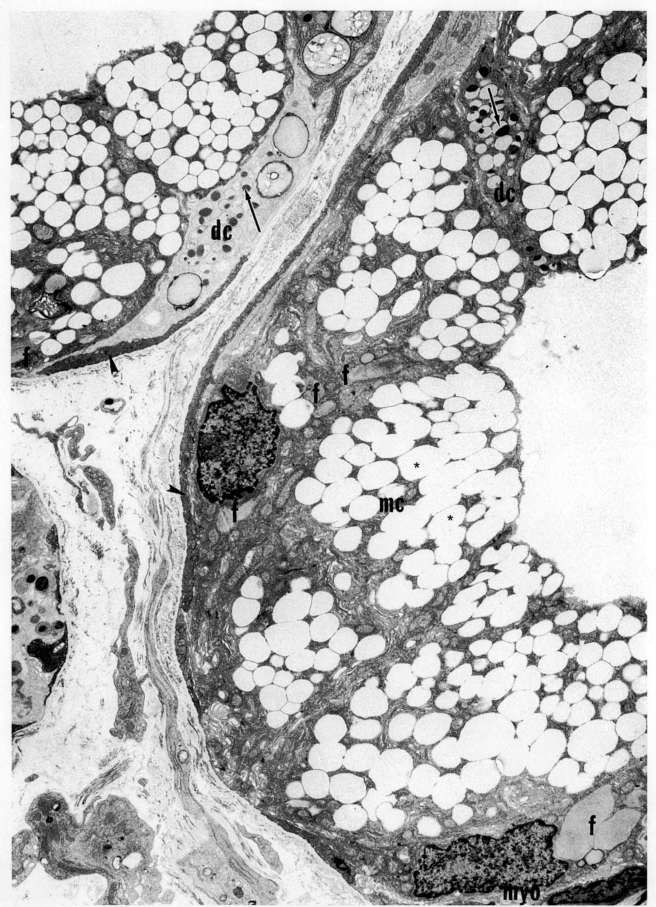

FIGURE 1

PLATE 15-6 • Liver, Electron Microscopy

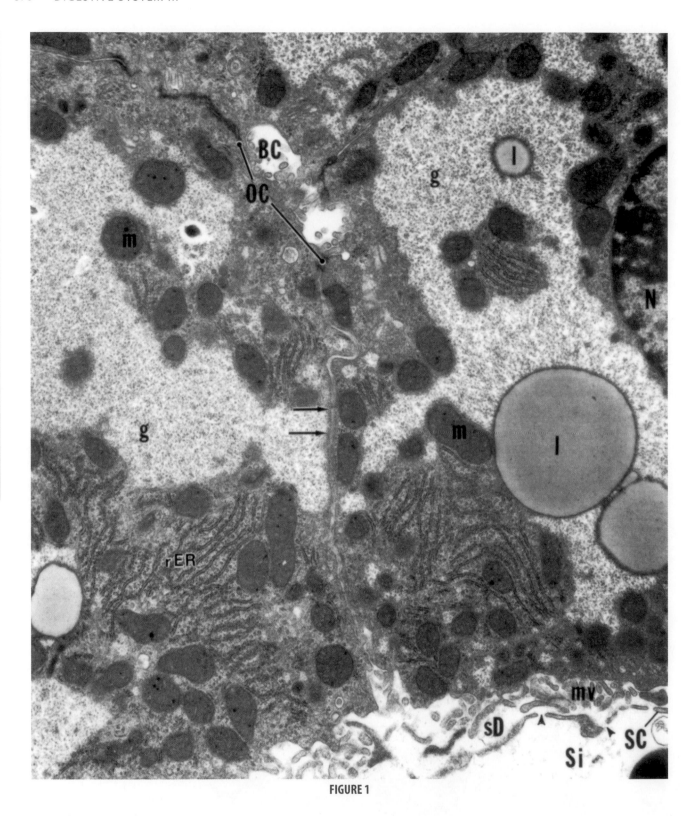

FIGURE 1

FIGURE 1. Liver. Mouse. Electron microscopy. ×11,255.

The hepatocytes of this electron micrograph display two of their surfaces, one bordering a **sinusoid** (Si) and the other where two parenchymal cells contact each other (*arrows*). The sinusoidal surface displays **microvilli** (mv) that extend into the **space of Disse** (sD). They almost contact **sinusoidal lining cells** (SC) that present numerous fenestrae (*arrowheads*). The parenchymal contacts are characterized by the presence of **bile canaliculi** (BC), intercellular spaces that are isolated by the formation of **occluding junctions** (OC). The cytoplasm of hepatocytes houses the normal cellular complements, such as numerous **mitochondria** (m), elements of **rough endoplasmic reticulum** (rER), Golgi apparatus, smooth endoplasmic reticulum, lysosomes, and inclusions such as **glycogen** (g) and **lipid droplets** (l). The **nucleus** (N) of one of the hepatocytes is evident.

PLATE 15-7 • Islet of Langerhans, Electron Microscopy

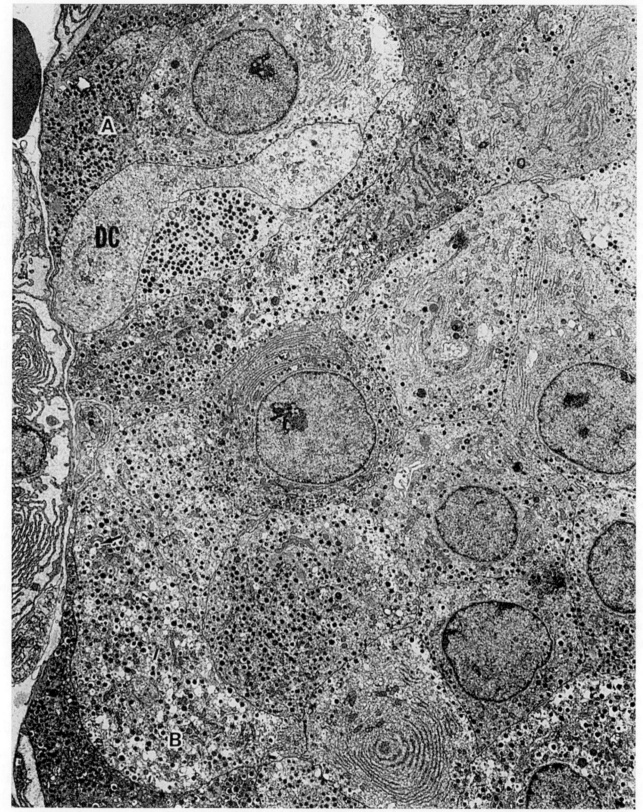

FIGURE 1

FIGURE 1. Islet of Langerhans. Rabbit. Electron microscopy. ×3,578.

The islets of Langerhans house four types of parenchymal cells, namely, A, B, C, and D cells. **B cells** (B) are the most numerous and may be recognized by the presence of secretory granules whose electron-dense core is surrounded by a clear zone (*arrows*).

A cells (A), the second most numerous secretory cell, also house many secretory granules; however, these lack an electron-lucent periphery. **D cells** (DC) are the least numerous and are characterized by secretory granules that are much less electron-dense than those of the other two cell types. (From Sato T, Herman L. Stereological analysis of normal rabbit pancreatic islets. Am J Anat 1981;161:71–84.)

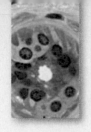

Chapter Summary

I. MAJOR SALIVARY GLANDS

Three **major salivary glands** are associated with the oral cavity. These are the **parotid, submandibular,** and **sublingual glands.**

A. Parotid Gland

The **parotid gland** is a purely serous **compound tubuloalveolar gland** whose **capsule** sends **septa** (frequently containing adipose cells) into the substance of the gland, dividing it into **lobes** and **lobules. Serous acini,** surrounded by **myoepithelial cells,** deliver their secretions into **intercalated ducts.**

B. Submandibular Gland

This compound **tubuloalveolar gland** is mostly **serous,** although it contains enough **mucous units,** capped by **serous demilunes,** to manufacture a mixed secretion. **Acini** are surrounded by **myoepithelial (basket) cells.** The **capsule** sends **septa** into the substance of the gland, subdividing it into **lobes** and **lobules.** The **duct** system is extensive.

C. Sublingual Gland

The **sublingual gland** is a **compound tubuloalveolar gland** whose capsule is not very definite. The gland produces a **mixed** secretion, possessing mostly **mucous acini** capped by **serous demilunes** and surrounded by **myoepithelial (basket) cells.** The **intralobular duct** system is not very extensive.

II. PANCREAS

The **exocrine pancreas** is a **compound tubuloalveolar serous gland** whose connective tissue **capsule** sends **septa** to divide the parenchyma into lobules. **Acini** present **centroacinar cells,** the beginning of the ducts that empty into **intercalated ducts,** which lead to **intralobular,** then **interlobular ducts.** The **main duct** receives secretory products from the interlobular ducts. The **endocrine pancreas** with its **islets of Langerhans** (composed of **A, B, G,** and **D cells**) are scattered among the serous acini.

III. LIVER

A. Capsule

Glisson's capsule invests the liver and sends **septa** into the substance of the liver at the **porta hepatis** to subdivide the parenchyma into lobules.

B. Lobules

1. Classical Lobule

Classical lobules are hexagonal with **portal areas (triads)** at the periphery and a **central vein** in the center. **Trabeculae (plates)** of liver cells anastomose. **Sinusoids** are lined by **sinusoidal lining cells** and **Kupffer cells** (macrophages). Within the **space of Disse, fat-accumulating cells** may be noted. **Portal areas** housing **bile ducts, lymph vessels,** and branches of the **hepatic artery** and the **portal vein** are surrounded by **terminal plates** composed of **hepatocytes.** Bile passes peripherally within **bile canaliculi,** intercellular spaces between liver cells, to enter **bile ductules,** then **canals of Hering** (and **cholangioles**), to be delivered to **bile ducts** at the portal areas.

2. Portal Lobule

The apices of triangular cross sections of **portal lobules** are **central veins.** Thus, **portal areas** form the centers of these lobules. The portal lobule is based on bile flow.

3. Acinus of Rappaport (Liver Acinus)

The **acinus of Rappaport** in section is a diamond-shaped area of the liver whose long axis is the straight line between neighboring **central veins** and whose short axis is the intersecting line between neighboring portal areas. The liver acinus is based on **blood flow.**

IV. GALLBLADDER

The **gallbladder** is connected to the liver via its **cystic duct,** which joins the **common hepatic duct.**

A. Epithelium

The gallbladder is lined by a **simple columnar epithelium.**

B. Lamina Propria

The **lamina propria** is thrown into intricate folds that disappear in the distended gallbladder. **Rokitansky-Aschoff sinuses** (epithelial diverticula) may be present.

C. Muscularis Externa

The **muscularis externa** is composed of an obliquely oriented **smooth muscle** layer.

D. Serosa

Adventitia attaches the gallbladder to the capsule of the liver, whereas **serosa** covers the remaining surface.

16 URINARY SYSTEM

The urinary system, composed of the kidneys, ureters, urinary bladder, and urethra, functions in the formation of urine, regulation of blood pressure and fluid volume of the body, acid-base balance, and formation and release of certain hormones.

The functional unit of the kidney is the **uriniferous tubule** (see Graphic 16-1), consisting of the **nephron** and the **collecting tubule**, each of which is derived from a different embryologic primordium.

KIDNEY

The **kidneys** possess a convex and a concave border, the latter of which is known as the **hilum**. It is here that arteries enter and the ureter, veins, and lypmh vessels leave the kidney. Each kidney has a capsule that has two layers, the outer fibrous layer and an inner, more cellular layer.

- Outer fibrous layer is composed of type I and type III collagen and occasional fibroblasts
- The inner layer consists of types I and III collagen and myofibroblasts

Each kidney is divided into a **cortex** and a **medulla**.

- The **cortex** is subdivided into the cortical labyrinth and the medullary rays (see Table 16-1),
  - The **cortical labyrinth** is composed of the renal corpuscles and the convoluted tubular portions of the nephron
  - Each **medullary ray** is an extension of the renal medulla into the cortex, where it forms the core of a kidney **lobule**.
    - Each of the 500 or so medullary rays are composed of pars recta of proximal and distal convoluted tubules as well as of collecting ducts
- the **medulla** is composed of 10 to 18 **renal pyramids**, each of which is said to constitute a **lobe** of the kidney.
  - The apex of each pyramid is perforated by 15 to 20 **papillary ducts** (of Bellini) at the **area cribrosa**.
  - The region of the medulla between neighboring renal pyramids is occupied by cortical-like material known as **renal columns** (of Bertin).

The vascular supply of the kidney must be appreciated to understand the histophysiology of the kidney. Each kidney is supplied by a renal artery, a direct branch of the abdominal aorta. This vessel subdivides into several major branches as it enters the hilum of the kidney, each of which subsequently divides to give rise to two or more interlobar arteries.

- **Interlobar arteries** pass between neighboring pyramids toward the cortex and, at the corticomedullary junction, give rise to
- **arcuate arteries** that follow the base of the pyramid.

- Small, **interlobular arteries** derived from arcuate arteries enter the cortical labyrinth, equidistant from neighboring medullary rays, to reach the **renal capsule**. Along the extent of the interlobular arteries, smaller vessels, known as
- **afferent glomerular arterioles**, arise, become enveloped by **Bowman's capsule**, and form a capillary plexus known as the **glomerulus**.
  - Collectively, Bowman's capsule and the glomerulus are referred to as the **renal corpuscle** (see Graphic 16-2).
- **Efferent glomerular arterioles** drain the glomerulus, passing into the cortex.
  - In the cortex, they form the **peritubular capillary network**
  - In the medulla, they form the **arteriae spuriae**, a part of the vasa recta.
- The interstitium of the cortical labyrinth and the capsule of the kidney are drained by **interlobular veins**, most of which enter the **arcuate veins**, tributaries of the **interlobar veins**.
- Blood from the interlobar veins enters the **renal vein**, which delivers its blood to the inferior vena cava.

Uriniferous Tubule

The functional unit of the kidney is the **uriniferous tubule** (see Table 16-1), consisting of the **nephron** and the **collecting tubule**, each of which is derived from a different embryologic primordium.

Nephron

There are three types of nephrons, classified by the location of their renal corpuscles in the kidney cortex:

- **juxtamedullary nephrons**, possessing long, thin limbs of Henle's loop,
- **cortical (subcapsular) nephrons** located just beneath the capsule, and
- **midcortical (intermediate) nephrons**, whose renal corpuscles are located in the midcortical region.

It is the long, thin limbs of Henle's loop that assist in the establishment of a concentration gradient in the renal medulla, permitting the formation of hypertonic urine.

Bowman's Capsule

- The nephron begins at **Bowman's capsule**, a distended, blindly ending, invaginated region of the tubule.
  - The modified cells of the inner, **visceral layer** are known as **podocytes**. Some of their
    - **primary (major)** processes but mainly their secondary processes and terminal **pedicels** wrap around the glomerular capillaries.

TABLE 16-1 • Location of the Various Regions of the Uriniferous Tubule

Location	Region of the Uriniferous Tubule
Cortical labyrinth	Renal corpuscle Proximal convoluted tubule Distal convoluted tubule Connecting tubule/arched collecting tubule
Medullary ray	Pars recta of proximal tubule Pars recta of distal tubule Collecting tubules (cortical collecting tubules)
Medulla	Pars recta of proximal tubules Pars recta of distal tubules Descending and ascending thin limbs of Henle's loop Henle's loop Medullary collecting tubules Papillary ducts

- The spaces between adjoining pedicels, known as **filtration slits**, are bridged by thin **slit diaphragms** that extend from one pedicel to the next.
- Pedicels are richly endowed with actin filaments permitting slight movement of the pedicels to adjust the size of the filtration slits.
  - **Glomerular capillaries** are fenestrated with large pores (60 to 90 nm in diameter) lacking diaphragms (see Graphic 16-2). The endothelial cell membranes possess aquaporin-1 channels designed for the rapid passage of water through them.
  - A thick **glomerular basal lamina** (see Table 16-2), manufactured by the podocytes and the endothelial cells of the capillary, is interposed between them.
  - Interstitial tissue composed of **intraglomerular mesangial cells** (see Table 16-3) and **extraglomerular**

mesangial cells and the extracellular matrix they manufacture is also associated with the glomerulus.
  - Intraglomerular mesangial cells share the basal lamina of the glomerular capillaries.
- The ultrafiltrate from the capillaries enters **Bowman's (urinary) space** by passing through the **filtration barrier** and is drained from there by the neck of the proximal tubule (see below).

Proximal Tubule

The **proximal tubule** has two regions, the convoluted portion (proximal convoluted tubule) and the straight portion (pars recta). The simple cuboidal epithelium of the proximal tubule adjoins the simple squamous epithelium of the parietal layer of Bowman's capsule.

- The simple cuboidal cells of the **proximal convoluted tubule** possess an extensive **brush border** (microvilli) on their luminal surface.
  - Their lateral and basal plasma membranes are considerably convoluted, and the lateral membranes form numerous interdigitations with membranes of adjoining cells.
  - The exaggerated folding of the basal plasmalemma presents a region rich in mitochondria and provides a striated appearance when viewed with the light microscope.
- The straight portion, or **pars recta**, of the proximal tubules is also referred to as the **descending thick limb of Henle's loop**. It is histologically similar to the convoluted portion; however, its brush border becomes shorter at its distal terminus, where it joins the descending thin limb of Henle's loop.

Henle's Loop

Henle's loop is composed of a simple squamous epithelium and has three regions: descending thin limb, Henle's loop, ascending thin limb.

TABLE 16-2 • Components, Location, and Function of the Glomerular Basement Membrane

Region of the Basement Membrane	Location	Components	Function
Lamina rara externa	Adjacent to the podocyte	Laminin, fibronectin, entactin, and very rich in heparan sulfate	Retards movement of negatively charged molecules
Lamina densa	Between the two laminae rarae	Type IV collagen	Filters plasma to form ultrafiltrate
Lamina rara interna	Adjacent to the capillary endothelium	Laminin, fibronectin, entactin, and very rich in heparan sulfate	Retards movement of negatively charged molecules

TABLE 16-3 • Functions of Intraglomerular Mesangial Cells
Phagocytosis of glomerular basement membrane and molecules trapped in it (69,000 Da or greater)
Physically support podocytes and their primary and secondary processes
Secretion of cytokines (e.g., PDGF, IL-1)* to facilitate repair of damaged glomerular components
Contractile elements assist in reducing the luminal diameter of glomerular capillaries to increase filtration rate
*PDGF, platelet-derived growth factor; IL-1, Interleukin 1.

- The **descending thin limb of Henle's loop** of juxtaglomerular nephrons extends to the apex of the medullary pyramid (those of midcortical and cortical nephrons are very short and will not be discussed).
- **Henle's loop** is near the apex of the medullary pyramid, and it connects the descending and ascending thin limbs in a hairpin-like loop.
- The **ascending thin limb of Henle's loop** parallels the descending thin limb as the corticalward continuation of Henle's loop.
- The descending and ascending thin limbs of Henle's loop are composed of simple squamous epithelial cells (types I through IV) whose structure varies according to their permeability to water, organelle content, and complexity of tight junctions. **Type I cells** are present only in cortical nephrons, whereas **types II, III, and IV cells** are present in juxtaglomerular nephrons.

Distal Tubule

The **distal tubule** is composed of two regions, distal convoluted tubule and pars recta of the distal tubule. Since the present discussion follows the path of the nephron and the ascending thin limb of Henle's loop ends in the pars recta of the distal tubule, the pars recta is discussed first.

- The **ascending thick limb of Henle's loop**, also known as the **pars recta of the distal tubule**, is composed of simple cuboidal cells that resemble the cells of the **distal tubule**.
  - The pars recta of the distal tubule begins much *deeper in the medulla* than the end of the pars recta of the proximal tubule.
  - The pars recta of the distal tubule ascends into the cortex to contact the afferent and efferent glomerular arterioles *of its own renal corpuscle*.
- Cells of the distal tubule that contact the afferent (and efferent) glomerular arteriole are modified, in that

they are thin, tall cuboidal cells whose nuclei are close to one another. This region is referred to as the **macula densa** of the distal tubule.
  - Cells of the macula densa communicate with modified smooth muscle cells, **juxtaglomerular (JG) cells**, of the afferent (and efferent) glomerular arterioles.
  - The macula densa and the JG cells together form the **juxtaglomerular apparatus**.
    - The **extraglomerular mesangial cells**, modified interstitial tissue cells, also known as **lacis cells**, are likewise considered to belong to the juxtaglomerular apparatus.
- The **distal convoluted tubule** is shorter than the proximal convoluted tubule; therefore, in any histological section of the renal cortex, there are fewer profiles of it surrounding the renal corpuscle. The cells of the distal convoluted tubule resemble those of the pars recta of the distal tubule, and instead of cilia, they possess short, blunt microvilli.

Collecting Tubules

Collecting tubules begin at the terminal ends of distal convoluted tubules as either **connecting tubules** or **arched collecting ducts**. Several distal convoluted tubules join each **collecting tubule**, a structure composed of a simple cuboidal epithelium whose lateral cell membranes are evident with the light microscope.

- The **cortical collecting tubules** descend from the medullary rays of the cortex to enter the renal pyramids of the medulla.
- As they enter the medulla, they are known as **medullary collecting tubules**.
- Several medullary collecting tubules merge to form the **papillary ducts (ducts of Bellini)**, which terminate at the area cribrosa.

The cuboidal cells of the collecting tubule are of two types, the lightly staining **principal cells** and the **intercalated cells** that stain darker.

- **Principal cells (light cells)** possess a single, nonmotile, apically situated cilium that probably functions as a mechanosensor that monitors fluid flow along the lumen of the tubule.
  - Principal cells possess **antidiuretic hormone (ADH)–sensitive aquaporin-2 channels** that permit the cell to be permeable to water.
  - They also have polycystin-1 and polycystin-2 in their plasmalemma. The latter of the two proteins is a calcium channel.
- **Intercalated cells (dark cells)** are fewer in number and are of two types, A and B:
  - Type A cells secrete H^+ into the tubular lumen and

○ Type B cells resorb H$^+$ and
○ secrete HCO$_3^-$

- The **papillary ducts** then deliver the urine formed by the uriniferous tubule to the intrarenal passage, namely, the **minor calyx**, to be drained into a **major calyx** and then into the **pelvis** of the **ureter**.

These excretory passages, lined by **transitional epithelium**, possess a fibroelastic subepithelial connective tissue, a smooth muscle tunic composed of **inner longitudinal** and **outer circular** layers, as well as a fibroelastic adventitia.

FORMATION OF URINE FROM ULTRAFILTRATE

Fluid, leaving the glomeruli, enters Bowman's space of the renal corpuscle, flows through the various components of the uriniferous tubule to be modified and concentrated, and leaves the papillary ducts as urine.

Formation of the Ultrafiltrate

Since the renal artery is a direct branch of the abdominal aorta, the two kidneys receive 20% of the total blood volume per minute.

- Most of this blood enters the glomeruli, where the high arterial pressure expresses approximately 10% of its fluid volume, 125 mL/min, into Bowman's spaces.
- Vascular pressure is opposed by two forces, the **colloid osmotic pressure** of the blood and the pressure exerted by the ultrafiltrate present in Bowman's space.
- The average net **filtration force**, expressing ultrafiltrate from the blood into Bowman's space, is relatively high, about 25 mm Hg.

The renal **filtration barrier**, composed of the fenestrated endothelial cells, the fused **basal laminae** of the podocyte and capillary, and the diaphragm-bridged filtration slits between pedicels, permits only the passage of water, ions, and small molecules into Bowman's space.

- The presence of the polyanionic **heparan sulfate** in the **lamina rara** of the basal lamina impedes the passage of large and negatively charged proteins through the barrier (see Table 16-2).
- Type IV collagen of the **lamina densa** acts as a molecular sieve and traps proteins larger than 69,000 Da or 7-nm diameter.

To maintain the efficiency of the filtering system, **intraglomerular mesangial cells**

- phagocytose the lamina densa, which then is renewed by the combined actions of the podocytes and endothelial cells.

- form the mesangial matrix around themselves and release prostaglandins, interleukin-1, and other cytokines.
- have contractile properties that, by constricting the glomerulus, modulate blood pressure within the glomerular network.
- form a structural support for the glomerulus.

The modified plasma that enters Bowman's space is known as the **ultrafiltrate**.

Functions of the Proximal Tubule

In a healthy individual, the **proximal tubule** resorbs approximately

- As much as eighty percent of the water, sodium, and chloride, as well as
- Hundred percent of the proteins, amino acids, and glucose from the ultrafiltrate.

The resorbed materials are eventually returned into the **peritubular capillary network** of the cortical labyrinth for distribution to the remainder of the body.

- The movement of sodium is via an active transport mechanism utilizing a **sodium-potassium-ATPase pump** in the basal plasmalemma, with chloride and water following passively.
- Since salt and water are resorbed in equimolar concentrations, the **osmolarity** of the ultrafiltrate is **not** altered in the proximal tubule but remains the same as that of blood.
- The endocytosed proteins are degraded into amino acids that are also released into the renal interstitium for distribution by the vascular system.
- The proximal tubule also secretes organic acids, bases, and other substances into the ultrafiltrate.

Functions of the Thin Limbs of Henle's Loop

- The **descending thin limb of Henle's loop** is completely permeable to water and only somewhat permeable to salts; hence, the ultrafiltrate in the lumen will attempt to equilibrate its osmolarity with the renal interstitium in its vicinity.
- The **ascending thin limb** is mostly impermeable to water but is relatively permeable to salts; thus, the movement of water is impeded but that of sodium and chloride is not.
- The ultrafiltrate will maintain the same osmolarity as the renal interstitium in its immediate surroundings as the concentration gradient decreases, approaching the cortex.

Functions of the Distal Tubule

- The **pars recta** of the distal tubule (ascending thick limb of Henle's loop) is impermeable to water but possesses a $Na^+/K^+/2Cl^-$ cotransporter on the luminal surface of the its cells that actively pumps sodium and chloride from the lumen into the cell.

- The basally located Na^+/K^+ ATPase pump transfers sodium and chloride out of the cell into the renal interstitium.
- Since water cannot enter or leave the lumen, the ultra-filtrate is **hypoosmotic** by the time it reaches the macula densa region.

Cells of the **distal convoluted tubule** possess **aldosterone receptors**. In the presence of aldosterone, the distal convoluted tubule resorbs sodium ions from and secretes hydrogen, potassium, and ammonium ions into the ultra-filtrate in its lumen, which it then delivers to the collecting duct.

Functions of the Juxtaglomerular Apparatus (see Table 16-4)

It is believed that the **macula densa cells** monitor the osmolarity and volume of the ultrafiltrate.

- If osmolarity and/or volume of the ultrafiltrate is decreased, the macula densa cells, via gap junctions,
  - instruct **juxtaglomerular cells** to release their stored proteolytic enzyme, renin, into the bloodstream and
  - instruct the smooth muscle cells of the afferent glomerular arterioles to relax thereby increasing blood flow into the glomerular capillary network
- **Renin** cleaves two amino acids from the circulating decapeptide **angiotensinogen**, changing it to **angiotensin I**, which, in turn, is cleaved by **converting enzyme** located on the luminal surfaces of capillaries (especially in the lungs), forming **angiotensin II**.
  - Angiotensin II is a powerful vasoconstrictor that
    - increases systemic vascular resistance, including that of the efferent glomerular arteriole, which increases glomerular hydrostatic pressure thus increasing glomerular filtration rate,
    - prompts the release of the mineralocorticoid aldosterone from the suprarenal cortex.
- **Aldosterone** binds to receptors on cells of the distal convoluted tubules, prompting them to resorb sodium (and chloride) from the ultrafiltrate. The addition of sodium to the extracellular compartment causes the retention of fluid with the subsequent elevation in blood pressure.

Concentration of Urine in the Nephron (Countercurrent Multiplier System)

The concentration of urine occurs only in juxtamedullary nephrons, whose long, thin limbs of Henle's loop function in the establishment of an **osmotic concentration gradient**. This gradient gradually increases from about 300 mOsm/L in the interstitium of the outer medulla to as much as 1,200 mOsm/L at the renal papilla.

Ascending Thick Limb
- The $Na^+/K^+/2Cl^-$ cotransporter of the **ascending thick limb of Henle's loop** transfers chloride and sodium ions from the lumen into the renal interstitium.
- Water is *not* permitted to leave; hence, the salt concentration of the interstitium increases.
- Since the supply of sodium and chloride inside the ascending thick limb decreases as the ultrafiltrate proceeds toward the cortex (because it is constantly being removed from the lumen), less and less sodium and chloride is available for transport; consequently, the interstitial salt concentration decreases closer to the cortex.
- The osmotic concentration gradient of the inner medulla, deep to the junction of the thin and thick ascending limbs of Henle's loop, is controlled by **urea** rather than sodium and chloride.

TABLE 16-4 • The Renin-Angiotensin-Aldosterone System

Low Ultrafiltrate Level in Pars Recta of Distal Tubule at the Macula Densa	Low Sodium Level in Pars Recta of Distal Tubule at the Macula Densa
Juxtaglomerular cells release renin, and smooth muscle cells of the afferent glomerular arterioles relax.	
Renin cleaves angiotensinogen to form angiotensin I.	
Angiotensin-converting enzyme cleaves angiotensin I to form angiotensin II.	
Angiotensin II increases systemic vascular resistance, including that of the efferent glomerular arteriole.	Angiotensin II causes release of aldosterone from the suprarenal cortex.
Glomerular filtration rate is increased.	Aldosterone prompts additional resorption of sodium and chloride from the ultrafiltrate located in the distal convoluted tubule.
Volume of ultrafiltrate is increased.	More sodium is available for the bloodstream.

Descending Thin Limb

- As the ultrafiltrate passes down the **descending thin limb of Henle's loop**, it reacts to the increasing gradient of osmotic concentration in the interstitium.
- Water leaves, and a limited amount of salts enters the lumen, **reducing the volume** and **increasing the salt concentration** of the ultrafiltrate (which becomes **hypertonic**).

Ascending Thin Limb

- In the **ascending thin limb of Henle's loop**, water is conserved, but salts are permitted to leave the ultrafiltrate, decreasing its osmolarity and contributing to the maintenance of the osmotic concentration gradient.

Concentration of Urine in the Collecting Tubule

The ultrafiltrate that enters the collecting tubule is **hypoosmotic**. As it passes down the collecting tubule, it is subject to the increasing osmotic gradient of the renal interstitium.

- If **antidiuretic hormone (ADH)** is released from the pars nervosa of the pituitary, the cells of the collecting tubules become permeable to water, which leaves the lumen of the collecting tubule, increasing the concentration of the urine.
- In the absence of ADH, the cells of the collecting tubule are impermeable to water, and the urine remains **hypotonic**.
- The collecting tubule is also responsible for permitting **urea** to diffuse into the interstitium of the **inner medulla**. The high interstitial osmolarity of this region is attributed to the urea concentration.

Role of the Vasa Recta in Urine Concentration (Countercurrent Exchange System)

The **vasa recta** assists in the maintenance of the osmotic concentration gradient of the renal medulla, since these capillary loops are completely permeable to salts and water.

- Thus, as the blood descends in the arteria recta, it becomes hyperosmotic, but as it ascends in the vena recta, its osmolarity returns to normal.
- It is also important to realize that the arteria recta carries a smaller volume than the vena recta, permitting

the removal of the fluid and salts transported into the renal interstitium by the uriniferous tubules.

EXTRARENAL EXCRETORY PASSAGES

The **extrarenal excretory passages** consist of the ureters, urinary bladder, and urethra.

- The ureters and bladder are lined by **transitional epithelia**.
- The **ureters** possess a fibroelastic lamina propria and two to three layers of smooth muscle arranged in an inner longitudinal and an outer circular fashion. The third muscle layer, the **outermost longitudinal layer**, appears in the lower one-third of the ureter.
- The **transitional epithelial lining** of the **bladder** and of the other urinary passages offers an impermeable barrier to urine.
- The plasma membrane of the surface-most cells of a transitional epithelium is thicker than the average plasma membrane and is composed of a lattice structure consisting of hexagonally arrayed elements.
- Furthermore, since cells of the transitional epithelium must line an ever larger surface as the urinary bladder distends, the plasma membrane is folded in a mosaic-like fashion.
  - Folding occurs at the **interplaque regions**, whereas the thickened **plaque regions** present **vesicular profiles**, which probably become unfolded as urine accumulates in the bladder.
- The subepithelial connective tissue of the bladder is composed, according to most, of a lamina propria and a submucosa.
- The three smooth muscle layers of the muscularis are extensively interlaced, making them indistinguishable in some areas.
- The **urethra** of the male differs from that of the female not only in its length but also in its function and epithelial lining.
  - The lamina propria of both sexes contains mucous **glands of Littré** and **intraepithelial glands**, which lubricate the lining of the urethra, facilitating the passage of urine to the outside.

The urethra is described in Chapter 17, "Female Reproductive System," and Chapter 18, "Male Reproductive System."

CLINICAL CONSIDERATIONS

Odor and Color of Urine

The odor and color of urine may provide clues to the individual's disease state. Normal urine is either colorless or has a yellow color if the urine is concentrated. Similarly, dilute urine has very little odor, whereas concentrated urine has a pungent smell. If the color of urine is reddish, the individual may have porphyria or there is fresh blood in the urine; if the color is brown, the possibility is that breakdown by-products of damaged muscle or breakdown by-products of hemoglobin are in the urine. Black discoloration could be due to the presence of melanin pigment in the urine, whereas cloudy urine could be an indication of the presence of acidic crystals or the presence of pus derived from urinary tract infection. Additionally, certain medications can discolor the urine, and the patient should be warned in advance about the color change. Changes in the odor of urine can be due to diabetes that is not being controlled (a sweet odor); fetid odor could indicate the presence of a urinary tract infection; and a musty odor of urine in a young patient may suggest phenylketonuria.

Tubular Necrosis

Tubular necrosis may result in **acute renal failure**. Cells of the renal tubules die either by being poisoned due to exposure to toxic chemicals, such as mercury or carbon tetrachloride, or die because of severe cardiovascular shock that reduces blood flow to the kidneys. The dead cells become sloughed off and occlude the lumina of their tubules. If the basal laminae remain intact, epithelial cell division may be able to repair the damage in less than 3 weeks.

Acute Glomerulonephritis

Acute glomerulonephritis is usually the result of a localized beta streptococcal infection in a region of the body other than the kidney (e.g., strep throat). Plasma cells secrete antibodies that complex with streptococcal antigens, forming an insoluble antigen-antibody complex that is filtered by the basal lamina between the podocytes and the endothelial cells of the glomerulus. As the immune complex builds up in the glomerular basal lamina, the epithelial cells and mesangial cells proliferate. Additionally, leukocytes accumulate in the glomerulus, congesting and blocking it. Moreover, pharmacologic agents released at the site of damage cause the glomerulus to become leaky, and proteins, platelets, and erythrocytes may enter the glomerular filtrate. Usually after the acute inflammation abates, the glomeruli repair themselves and the normal kidney function returns. Occasionally, however, the damage is extensive and kidney function becomes permanently impaired.

Diabetes Insipidus

Diabetes insipidus occurs because of damage to the cells of the hypothalamus that manufacture ADH (antidiuretic hormone). The low levels of ADH interfere with the ability of the collecting tubules of the kidney to concentrate urine. The excess fluid loss in the formation of copious quantities of dilute urine results in **polydipsia** (excessive thirst) and dehydration.

Diabetic Glomerulosclerosis

Diabetes mellitus causes vascular pathologies that involve blood vessels throughout the body, including those of the glomerular capillary network where synthesis of the basement membrane components increases to such an extent that it interferes with normal filtration. Additionally, hypercellularity of the mesangial cell population also interferes with the function of the normal

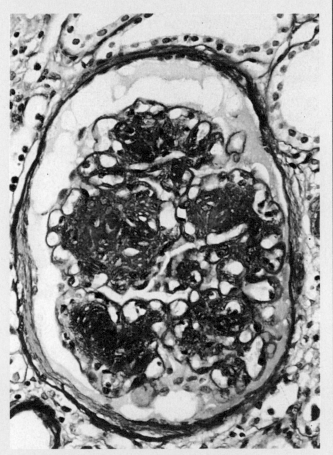

This figure is from the kidney of a patient with end-stage renal disease as a result of diabetes mellitus. Note that the glomerular capillaries are engorged with blood, the intraglomerular cell population is increased, and the glomerular basement membrane displays evidence of being thickened. (Reprinted with permission from Rubin R, Strayer D, et al., eds. Rubin's Pathology. Clinicopathologic Foundations of Medicine, 5th ed., Baltimore: Lippincott Williams & Wilkins, 2008, p. 709.)

filtration barrier and sclerosis ensues. Electron micrography demonstrates that the lamina densa of the glomerular basal membrane may increase as much as 10-fold, which becomes engorged with various plasma proteins. In the United States, approximately 35% of patients in end-stage renal disease suffer from diabetic glomerulosclerosis caused by both type I and type II diabetes mellitus.

Urate Nephropathy

Urate nephropathy is the deposition of uric acid crystals in the kidney tubules or in the renal interstitium as a result of elevated levels of uric acid in the blood. In most cases this condition is due to the patient suffering from primary gout; however, high uric acid blood levels also occur in cases of chemotherapy in cancer treatment as well as in patients who have reduced excretions of uric acid, such as in cases of lead poisoning. Although in most patients urate nephropathy is not life threatening, it may result in acute renal failure with fatal consequences.

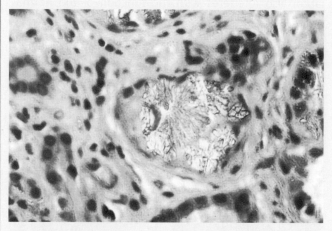

This figure is from the kidney of a patient demonstrating the deposition of uric acid crystals in the collecting tubule, indicating that the individual is suffering from urate nephropathy. (Reprinted with permission from Rubin R, Strayer D, et al., eds. Rubin's Pathology. Clinicopathologic Foundations of Medicine, 5th ed., Baltimore: Lippincott Williams & Wilkins, 2008, p. 736.)

Kidney Stones

Kidney stones usually form due to the condition known as **hyperparathyroidism**, in which the formation of excess parathyroid hormone (PTH) by the parathyroid glands results in an increased level of osteoclastic activity. The resorption of bone, as well as the increased absorption of calcium and phosphates from the gastrointestinal tract, eventuates higher than normal blood calcium levels. As the kidneys excrete higher than normal concentrations of calcium and phosphates, their presence in the urine, especially under alkaline conditions, causes their precipitation in the kidney tubules. Continued accretion of these ions onto the crystal surface causes an increase in the size of the crystals, and they become known as **kidney stones**.

Cancers of the Kidney

Cancers of the kidney are usually solid tumors, whereas cysts of the kidney are usually benign. The most common symptom of kidney cancer is **blood in the urine**, although the amount of blood may be undetectable without a microscopic examination of the urine. Usually, kidney cancers are accompanied by pain and fever, but frequently, they are discovered by abdominal palpation during routine physicals when the physician detects a lump in the region of the kidney. Since kidney cancers spread early and usually to the lung, the prognosis is poor.

Bladder Cancer

Annually, there are more than 50,000 new cases of transitional cell carcinomas of the bladder in the United States. Interestingly, almost 65% of the affected individuals are male, and about half of these patients smoke cigarettes. The most prominent symptom of bladder cancer is blood in the urine, followed by burning sensation and pain on urination, as well as an increased frequency of the urge to urinate. Although these symptoms are frequently confused with cystitis, the condition becomes suspicious once the antibiotics fail to alleviate the problem, and cytology of the urine demonstrates the presence of cancerous transitional cells. If caught early, before the carcinoma invades the deeper tissues, the survival rate is as great as 95%; however, if the tumor is a rapidly dividing one that invades the muscular layers of the bladder and reaches the lymph nodes, the 5-year survival rate drops to less than 45%.

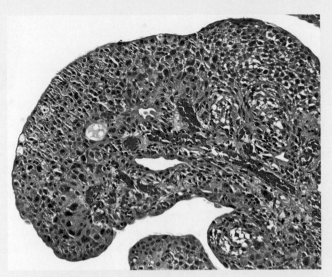

This figure is from a urinary bladder with high-grade papillary urothelial carcinoma. Note that the transitional epithelium is disorganized and the individual epithelial cells display dense, pleomorphic nuclei. (Reprinted with permission from Rubin R, Strayer D, et al., eds. Rubin's Pathology. Clinicopathologic Foundations of Medicine, 5th ed., Baltimore: Lippincott Williams & Wilkins, 2008, p. 757.)

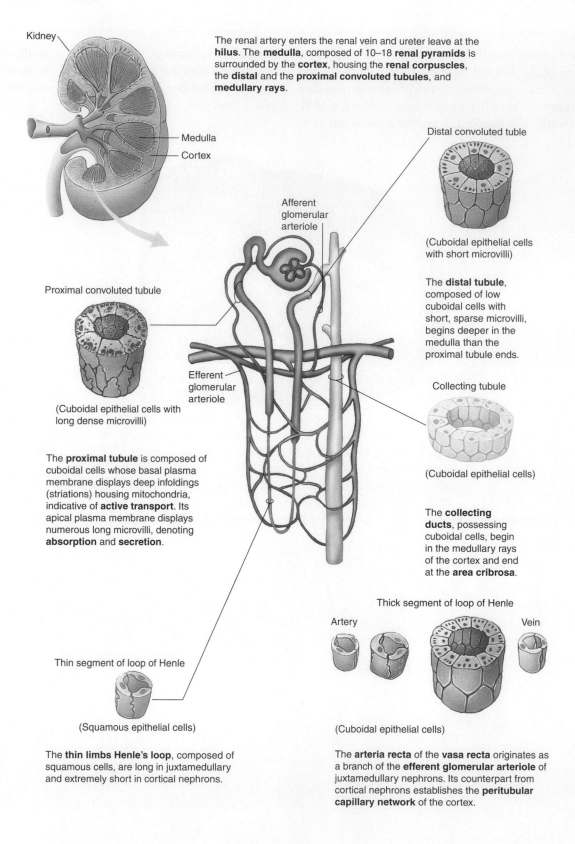

Kidney

Medulla

Cortex

The renal artery enters the renal vein and ureter leave at the **hilus**. The **medulla**, composed of 10–18 **renal pyramids** is surrounded by the **cortex**, housing the **renal corpuscles**, the **distal** and the **proximal convoluted tubules**, and **medullary rays**.

Distal convoluted tuble

(Cuboidal epithelial cells with short microvilli)

The **distal tubule**, composed of low cuboidal cells with short, sparse microvilli, begins deeper in the medulla than the proximal tubule ends.

Afferent glomerular arteriole

Proximal convoluted tubule

(Cuboidal epithelial cells with long dense microvilli)

Efferent glomerular arteriole

The **proximal tubule** is composed of cuboidal cells whose basal plasma membrane displays deep infoldings (striations) housing mitochondria, indicative of **active transport**. Its apical plasma membrane displays numerous long microvilli, denoting **absorption** and **secretion**.

Collecting tubule

(Cuboidal epithelial cells)

The **collecting ducts**, possessing cuboidal cells, begin in the medullary rays of the cortex and end at the **area cribrosa**.

Thick segment of loop of Henle

Artery   Vein

Thin segment of loop of Henle

(Squamous epithelial cells)

(Cuboidal epithelial cells)

The **thin limbs Henle's loop**, composed of squamous cells, are long in juxtamedullary and extremely short in cortical nephrons.

The **arteria recta** of the **vasa recta** originates as a branch of the **efferent glomerular arteriole** of juxtamedullary nephrons. Its counterpart from cortical nephrons establishes the **peritubular capillary network** of the cortex.

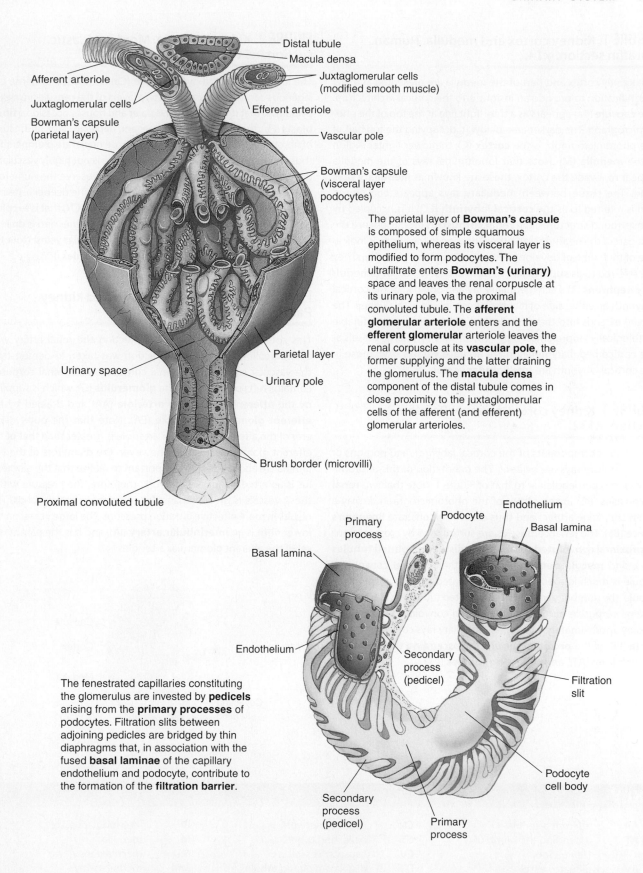

Distal tubule

Macula densa

Juxtaglomerular cells (modified smooth muscle)

Afferent arteriole

Juxtaglomerular cells

Efferent arteriole

Bowman's capsule (parietal layer)

Vascular pole

Bowman's capsule (visceral layer podocytes)

Parietal layer

Urinary space

Urinary pole

Brush border (microvilli)

Proximal convoluted tubule

The parietal layer of **Bowman's capsule** is composed of simple squamous epithelium, whereas its visceral layer is modified to form podocytes. The ultrafiltrate enters **Bowman's (urinary)** space and leaves the renal corpuscle at its urinary pole, via the proximal convoluted tubule. The **afferent glomerular arteriole** enters and the **efferent glomerular** arteriole leaves the renal corpuscle at its **vascular pole**, the former supplying and the latter draining the glomerulus. The **macula densa** component of the distal tubule comes in close proximity to the juxtaglomerular cells of the afferent (and efferent) glomerular arterioles.

Endothelium

Basal lamina

Podocyte

Primary process

Basal lamina

Endothelium

Secondary process (pedicel)

Filtration slit

Podocyte cell body

Secondary process (pedicel)

Primary process

The fenestrated capillaries constituting the glomerulus are invested by **pedicels** arising from the **primary processes** of podocytes. Filtration slits between adjoining pedicels are bridged by thin diaphragms that, in association with the fused **basal laminae** of the capillary endothelium and podocyte, contribute to the formation of the **filtration barrier**.

PLATE 16-1 · Kidney, Survey and General Morphology

FIGURE 1. Kidney cortex and medulla. Human. Paraffin section. ×14.

The kidney cortex and part of the medulla are presented at a low magnification to provide an insight into the cortical architecture. The **capsule** (Ca) appears as a thin, light line at the top of the photomicrograph. The darker area below it, occupying the top half of the photomicrograph, is the **cortex** (C); the lower lighter region is the **medulla** (M). Note that longitudinal rays of the medulla appear to invade the cortex; these are known as **medullary rays** (MR). The tissue between medullary rays appears convoluted and is referred to as the **cortical labyrinth** (CL). It is occupied by dense, round structures, the **renal corpuscles** (RC). These are the first part of the nephrons, and their location in the cortex is indicative of their time of development as well as of their function. They are referred to as **superficial** (1), **midcortical** (2), or **juxtamedullary nephrons** (3). Each medullary ray and one-half of the cortical labyrinth on either side of it constitutes a lobule of the kidney. The lobule extends into the medulla, but its borders are undefinable histologically (approximated by vertical lines). The large vessels at the corticomedullary junction are **arcuate vessels** (AV); those in the cortical labyrinth are **interlobular vessels** (IV).

FIGURE 3. Kidney cortex. Human. Paraffin section. ×132.

The various components of the cortical labyrinth and portions of two medullary rays are evident. The orientation of this photomicrograph is perpendicular to that of Figure 1. Note that two **renal corpuscles** (RC) in the center of the photomicrograph display a slight shrinkage artifact and thus clearly demonstrate **Bowman's space** (BS). The renal corpuscles are surrounded by cross sections of **proximal convoluted tubules** (PT), **distal convoluted tubules** (DT), and **macula densa** (MD). Since the proximal convoluted tubule is much longer than the convoluted portion of the distal tubule, the number of proximal convoluted tubule profiles around a renal corpuscle outnumbers the distal convoluted tubule profiles by approximately 7 to 1. The medullary rays contain the **pars recta** (PR) of the **proximal tubule,** the **ascending thick limbs of Henle's loop** (AT), and **collecting tubules** (CT).

FIGURE 2. Kidney capsule. Monkey. Plastic section. ×540.

The kidney is invested by a **capsule** (Ca) composed of dense collagenous connective tissue. The two layers of the capsule are clearly evident, in that the **outer layer** is paler and houses occasional **fibroblasts** (Fb); the **inner layer** is thinner and darker in color, and instead of fibroblasts, it has **myofibroblasts** whose nuclei are plumper than those of fibroblasts. Although this structure is not highly vascular, it does possess some **capsular vessels** (CV). Observe the numerous red blood cells in the lumina of these vessels. The deeper aspect of the capsule possesses a rich **capillary network** (CN) that is supplied by the terminal branches of the interlobular arteries and is drained by the stellate veins, tributaries of the interlobular veins. Note the cross sections of the **proximal convoluted tubules** (PT).

FIGURE 4. Colored colloidin-injected kidney. Paraffin section. ×132.

This specimen was prepared by injecting the renal artery with colored colloidin, and a thick section was taken to demonstrate the vascular supply of the renal corpuscle. Each renal corpuscle contains tufts of capillaries, the **glomerulus** (G), which is supplied by the **afferent glomerular arteriole** (AA) and drained by the **efferent glomerular arteriole** (EA). Note that the outer diameter of the afferent glomerular arteriole is greater than that of the efferent glomerular arteriole; however, the diameters of the two lumina are about equal. It is important to realize that the glomerulus is an arterial capillary network; therefore, the pressure within these vessels is greater than that of normal capillary beds. This results in more effective filtration pressure. The large vessel on the lower right is an **interlobular artery** (IA), and it is the parent vessel of the afferent glomerular arterioles.

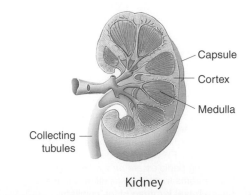

Capsule
Cortex
Medulla
Collecting tubules

Kidney

KEY

AA	afferent arteriole	CN	capillary network	IV	interlobular vessel
AT	ascending thick limb of Henle's loop	CT	collecting tubule	M	medulla
		CV	capsular vessel	MD	macula densa
AV	arcuate vessel	DT	distal convoluted tubule	MR	medullary ray
BS	Bowman's space	EA	efferent arteriole	PR	pars recta
C	cortex	Fb	fibroblast	PT	proximal convoluted tubule
Ca	capsule	G	glomerulus	RC	renal corpuscle
CL	cortical labyrinth	IA	interlobular artery		

PLATE 16-1 · Kidney, Survey and General Morphology

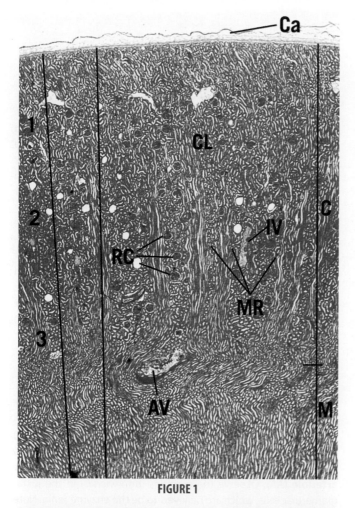

FIGURE 1

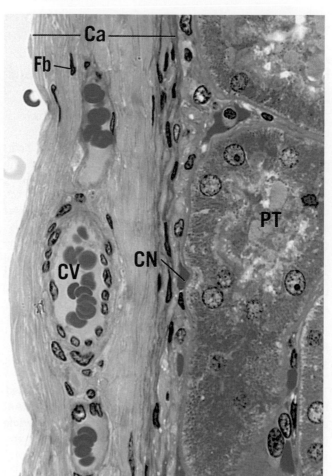

FIGURE 2

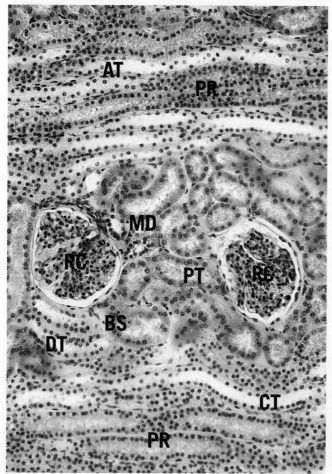

FIGURE 3

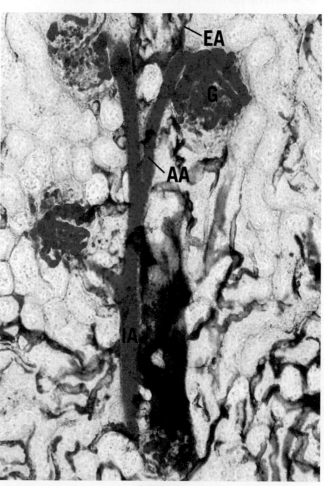

FIGURE 4

PLATE 16-2 · Renal Cortex

FIGURE 1. Kidney cortical labyrinth. Monkey. Plastic section. ×270.

The center of this photomicrograph is occupied by a renal corpuscle. The urinary pole is evident as the short neck empties into the convoluted portion of the **proximal tubule** (PT). The renal corpuscle is composed of the **glomerulus** (G), tufts of capillaries, the visceral layer of Bowman's capsule (podocytes) that is intimately associated with the glomerulus, **Bowman's space** (BS) into which the ultrafiltrate is expressed from the capillaries, and the **parietal layer** (PL) of Bowman's capsule, consisting of a simple squamous epithelium. Additionally, mesangial cells are also present in the renal corpuscle. Most of the tubular profiles surrounding the renal corpuscle are transverse sections of the darker-staining **proximal tubules** (PT), which outnumber the cross sections of the lighter-staining **distal tubules** (DT).

FIGURE 3. Kidney cortical labyrinth. Monkey. Plastic section. ×270.

The vascular pole of this renal corpuscle is very clearly represented. It is in this region that the **afferent glomerular arteriole (AA)** enters the renal corpuscle and the **efferent glomerular arteriole** (EA) leaves, draining the glomerulus. Observe that these two vessels and their capillaries are supported by **mesangial cells** (Mg). Note that although the outer diameter of the afferent glomerular arteriole is greater than that of the efferent glomerular arteriole, their luminal diameters are approximately the same. The renal corpuscle is surrounded by cross-sectional profiles of **distal** (DT) and **proximal** (PT) **tubules**. The *boxed area* is presented at a higher magnification in Figure 4. *Inset.* **Glomerulus. Kidney. Monkey. Plastic section.** ×720. The glomerulus is composed of capillaries whose **endothelial cell** (En) nuclei bulge into the lumen. The endothelial cells are separated from **podocytes** (P), modified visceral cell layer of Bowman's capsule, by a thick basal lamina (*arrows*). **Mesangial cells** (Mg) form both supporting and phagocytic elements of the renal corpuscle. Note that major processes (*asterisks*) of the podocytes are also distinguishable in this photomicrograph.

FIGURE 2. Kidney cortical labyrinth. Monkey. Plastic section. ×270.

The renal corpuscle in the center of the photomicrograph displays all of the characteristics identified in Figure 1, except that instead of the urinary pole, the **vascular pole** (VP) is presented. That is the region where the afferent and efferent glomerular arterioles enter and leave the renal corpuscle, respectively. Some of the smooth muscle cells of the afferent (and sometimes efferent) glomerular arterioles are modified in that they contain renin granules. These modified cells are known as **juxtaglomerular cells** (JC). They are closely associated with the **macula densa** (MD) region of the distal tubule. Again, note that most of the cross-sectional profiles of tubules surrounding the renal corpuscle belong to the convoluted portion of the **proximal tubules** (PT), whereas only one or two are distal tubules. Observe the rich **vascularity** (BV) of the renal cortex as well as the scant amount of connective tissue elements (*arrows*) associated with these vessels.

FIGURE 4. Juxtaglomerular apparatus. Kidney. Monkey. Plastic section. ×1,325.

The *boxed area* of Figure 3 is magnified to present the juxtaglomerular apparatus. This is composed of the **macula densa** (MD) region of the distal tubule and apparent **juxtaglomerular cells** (JC), modified smooth muscle cells of the **afferent glomerular arteriole** (AA). Observe the granules (*arrowheads*) in the juxtaglomerular cells, which are believed to be the enzyme renin. Note the nuclei (*asterisks*) of the endothelial cells lining the afferent glomerular arteriole.

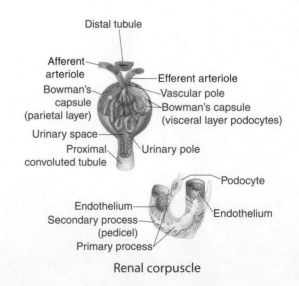

Renal corpuscle

KEY

AA	afferent arteriole	**En**	endothelial cell	**P**	podocyte
BS	Bowman's space	**G**	glomerulus	**PL**	parietal layer
BV	blood vessel	**JC**	juxtaglomerular cell	**PT**	proximal tubule
DT	distal tubule	**MD**	macula densa	**VP**	vascular pole
EA	efferent arteriole	**Mg**	mesangial cell		

PLATE 16-2 • Renal Cortex

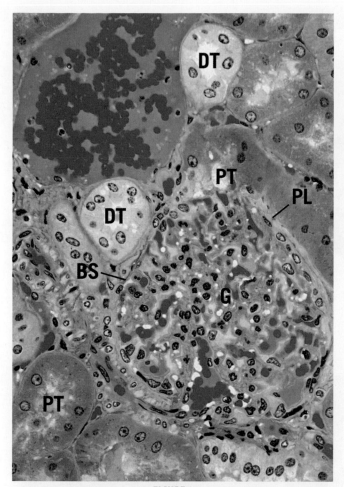

FIGURE 1

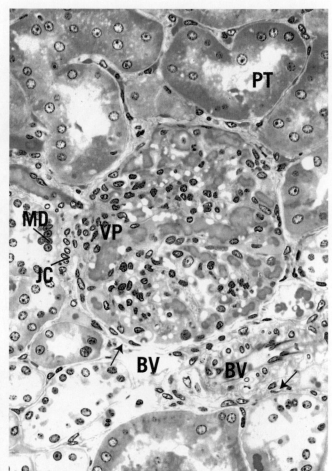

FIGURE 2

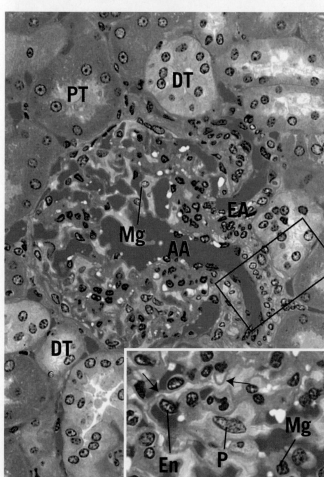
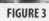

FIGURE 3

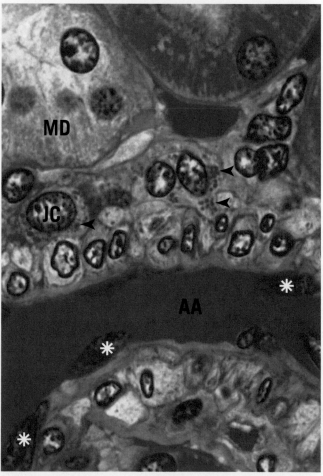

FIGURE 4

PLATE 16-3 · Glomerulus, Scanning Electron Microscopy

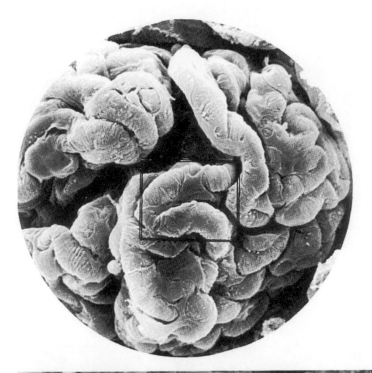

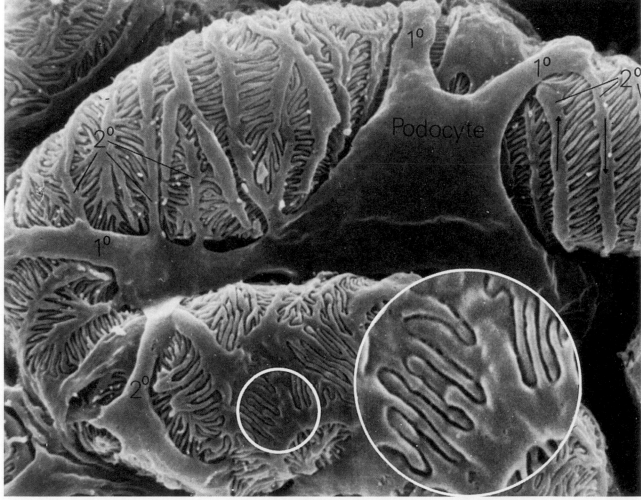

FIGURE 1

FIGURE 1. Scanning electron micrograph of a glomerulus, displaying the primary and secondary processes and pedicels of podocytes. Top, ×700; bottom, ×4,000; and *inset*, ×6,000. (From Ross MH, Reith EJ, Romrell LJ. Histology: A Text and Atlas. 2nd ed., Baltimore: Williams & Wilkins, 1989, p. 536.)

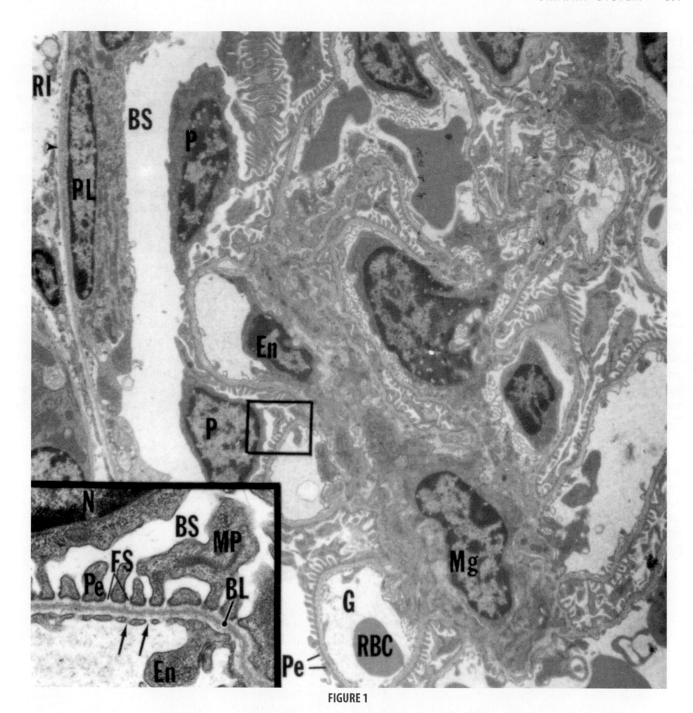

FIGURE 1

FIGURE 1. Kidney cortex. Renal corpuscle. Mouse. Electron microscopy. ×3,780.

Various components of the renal corpuscle are displayed in this electron micrograph. Note the basal lamina (*arrowhead*) separating the simple squamous cells of the **parietal layer** (PL) of Bowman's capsule from the **renal interstitium** (RI). **Bowman's space** (BS) and the **podocytes** (P) are shown to advantage, as are the **glomeruli** (G) and surrounding **pedicels** (Pe). **Mesangial cells** (Mg) occupy the space between capillary loops, and several

red blood cells (RBC) and **endothelial cells** (En) are also evident. *Inset.* **Podocyte and glomerulus. Mouse. Electron microscopy. ×6,300.** This is a higher magnification of the *boxed area*, presenting a portion of a podocyte. Observe its **nucleus** (N), **major process** (MP), and **pedicels** (Pe). Note that the pedicels lie on a **basal lamina** (BL) that is composed of a lamina rara externa, lamina densa, and lamina rara interna. Observe the fenestrations (*arrows*) in the **endothelial lining** (En) of the glomerulus. The spaces between the pedicels, known as **filtration slits** (FS), lead into **Bowman's space** (BS).

PLATE 16-5 · Renal Medulla

FIGURE 1. Renal medulla. Monkey. Plastic section. ×270.

This photomicrograph of the renal medulla demonstrates the arrangement of the various tubular and vascular structures. The formed connective tissue elements among the tubules and vessels are very sparse and constitute mainly fibroblasts, macrophages, and fibers (*asterisks*). The major tubular elements in evidence are the **collecting tubules** (CT), recognizable by the conspicuous lateral plasma membranes of their tall cuboidal (or low columnar) cells, **thick limbs of Henle's loop** (TH), and occasional **thin limbs of Henle's loop** (TL). Many vascular elements are noted; these are the vasa recta spuria, whose thicker-walled descending limbs are the **arteriolae rectae spuriae** (AR) and thinner-walled ascending limbs are the **venulae rectae spuriae** (VR).

FIGURE 3. Renal papilla. x.s. Monkey. Plastic section. ×540.

In the deeper aspect of the medulla, collecting tubules merge with each other, forming larger and larger structures. The largest of these ducts are known as **papillary ducts** (PD), or ducts of Bellini, which may be recognized by their tall, pale columnar cells and their easily discernible lateral plasma membranes (*arrows*). These ducts open at the apex of the renal papilla, in the region known as the area cribrosa. The **thin limbs of Henle's loop** (TL) are evident. These structures form the hairpin-like loops of Henle in this region, where the ascending thin limbs recur to ascend in the medulla, eventually to become thicker, forming the straight portion of the distal tubule. Note that the **arteriolae rectae spuriae** (AR) and the **venulae rectae spuriae** (VR) follow the thin limbs of Henle's loop deep into the renal papilla. Some of the connective tissue elements are marked by *asterisks*.

FIGURE 2. Renal papilla. x.s. Human. Paraffin section. ×270.

The most conspicuous tubular elements of the renal papilla are the **collecting tubules** (CT), with their cuboidal cells, whose lateral plasma membranes are evident. The numerous thin-walled structures are the **thin limbs of Henle's loop** (TL) as well as the **arteriolae rectae spuriae** (AR) and **venulae rectae spuriae** (VR) that may be identified by the presence of blood in their lumina. The formed connective tissue elements (*asterisks*) may be discerned in the interstitium among the various tubules of the kidney. An occasional thick limb of Henle's loop (TH) may also be observed.

FIGURE 4. Renal medulla. l.s. Monkey. Plastic section. ×270.

This photomicrograph is similar to Figure 1, except that it is a longitudinal rather than a transverse section of the renal medulla. The center is occupied by a **collecting tubule** (CT), as is distinguished by the tall cuboidal cells whose lateral plasma membranes are evident. The collecting tubule is flanked by **thick limbs of Henle's loop** (TH). The vasa recta are filled with blood, and the thickness of their walls identifies whether they are **arteriolae rectae spuriae** (AR) or **venulae rectae spuriae** (VR). A **thin limb of Henle's loop** (TL) is also identifiable.

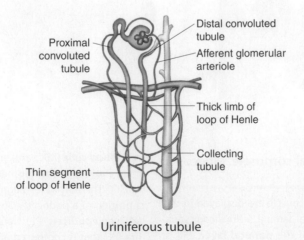

Proximal convoluted tubule

Distal convoluted tubule

Afferent glomerular arteriole

Thick limb of loop of Henle

Collecting tubule

Thin segment of loop of Henle

Uriniferous tubule

KEY

AR	arteriolae rectae spuriae	**PD**	papillary duct	**TL**	thin limb of Henle's loop
CT	collecting tubule	**TH**	thick limb of Henle's loop	**VR**	venulae rectae spuriae

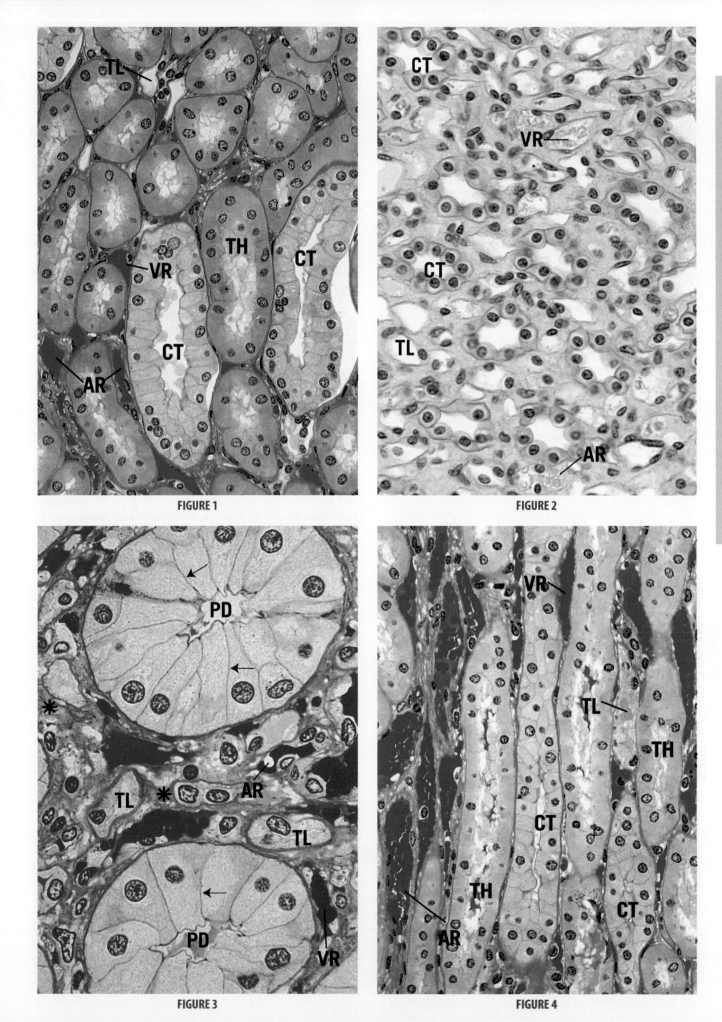

PLATE 16-5 • Renal Medulla

FIGURE 1

FIGURE 2

FIGURE 3

FIGURE 4

PLATE 16-6 · Ureter and Urinary Bladder

FIGURE 1. Ureter. x.s. Human. Paraffin section. ×14.

This low-power photomicrograph of the ureter displays its stellate-shaped **lumen** (L) and thick lining **epithelium** (E). The interface between the **subepithelial connective tissue** (SCT) and the **smooth muscle coat** (SM) is indicated by *arrows*. The muscle coat is surrounded by a fibrous **adventitia** (Ad), which houses the numerous vascular channels and nerve fibers that travel with the ureter. Thus, the wall of the ureter consists of the mucosa (epithelium and underlying connective tissue), muscularis, and adventitia.

FIGURE 3. Urinary bladder. Monkey. Plastic section. ×14.

The urinary bladder stores urine until it is ready to be voided. Since the volume of the bladder changes with the amount of urine it contains, its mucosa may or may not display folds. This particular specimen is not distended, hence the numerous folds (*arrows*). Moreover, the **transitional epithelium** (TE) of this preparation is also thick, whereas in the distended phase, the epithelium would be much thinner. Note also that the thick **muscularis** is composed of three layers of smooth muscle: **inner longitudinal** (IL), **middle circular** (MC), and **outer longitudinal** (OL). The muscle layers are surrounded either by an adventitia composed of loose connective tissue—as is the case in this photomicrograph—or by a serosa, depending on the region of the bladder being examined.

FIGURE 2. Ureter. x.s. Monkey. Plastic section. ×132.

The mucosa is highly convoluted and consists of a thick, transitional epithelium whose free surface possesses characteristic **dome-shaped cells** (D). The basal cell layer sits on a basal lamina (*arrows*), which separates the epithelium from the underlying fibrous connective tissue. The **muscularis** consists of three layers of smooth muscle: **inner longitudinal** (IL), **middle circular** (MC), and **outer longitudinal** (OL). These three layers are not always present, for the outer longitudinal layer is found only in the inferior one-third of the ureter, that is, the portion nearest the urinary bladder. The **adventitia** (Ad) is composed of fibrous connective tissue that anchors the ureter to the posterior body wall and adjacent structures.

FIGURE 4. Urinary bladder. Monkey. Plastic section. ×132.

The bladder is lined by **transitional epithelium** (TE), whose typical surface dome-shaped cells are shown to advantage. Some of these cells are binucleated. The epithelium is separated from the underlying connective tissue by a basal lamina (*arrows*). This subepithelial connective tissue is frequently said to be divided into a **lamina propria** (LP) and a **submucosa** (Sm). The vascularity of this region is demonstrated by the numerous **venules** (V) and **arterioles** (A). These vessels possess smaller tributaries and branches that supply the regions closer to the epithelium. *Inset*. **Transitional epithelium. Monkey. Plastic section.** ×540. The *boxed region* of the transitional epithelium is presented at a higher magnification to demonstrate the large, dome-shaped cells (*arrow*) at the free surface. These cells are characteristic of the empty bladder. When that structure is distended with urine, the dome-shaped cells assume a flattened morphology, and the entire epithelium becomes thinner (being reduced from five to seven to only three cell layers thick). Note that occasional cells may be binucleated.

PROPERTY OF LIBRARY
SOUTH UNIVERSITY CLEVELAND CAMPUS
WARRENSVILLE HEIGHTS, OH 44128

KEY

A	arteriole	**LP**	lamina propria	**SM**	smooth muscle coat
Ad	adventitia	**MC**	middle circular muscularis	**Sm**	submucosa
D	dome-shaped cell	**OL**	outer longitudinal muscularis	**TE**	transitional epithelium
E	epithelium			**V**	venule
IL	inner longitudinal muscularis	**SCT**	subepithelial connective tissue		
L	lumen				

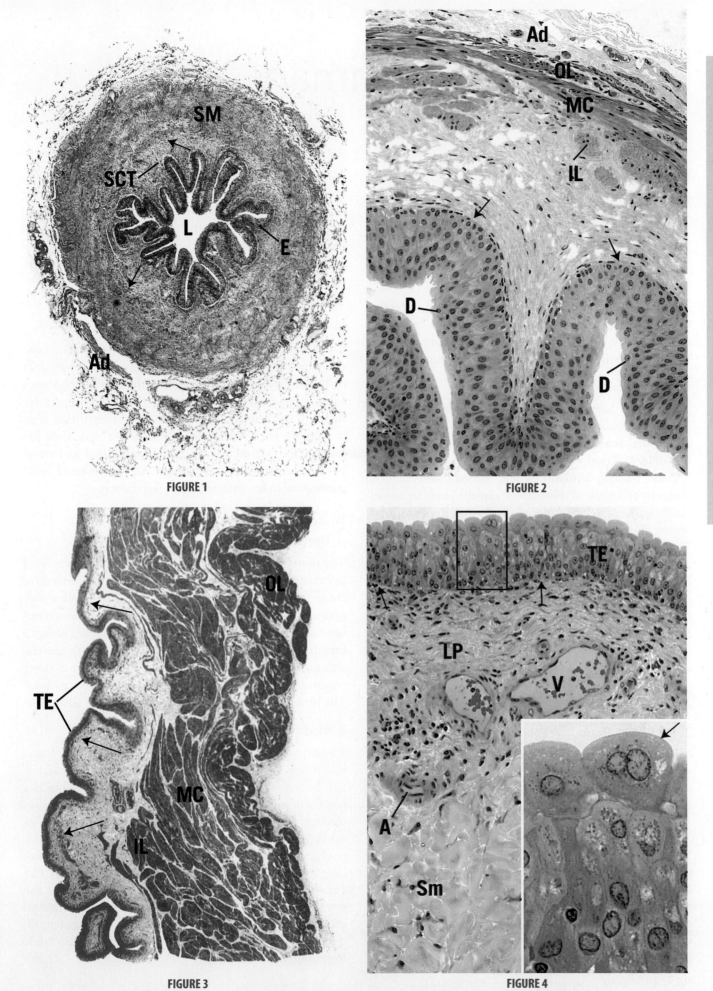

PLATE 16-6 • Ureter and Urinary Bladder

FIGURE 1

FIGURE 2

FIGURE 3

FIGURE 4

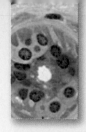

Chapter Summary

I. KIDNEY

A. Capsule

The **capsule** is composed of dense, irregular collagenous connective tissue. Occasional **fibroblasts** and blood vessels may be seen.

B. Cortex

The **cortex** consists of parts of **nephrons** and **collecting tubules** arranged in **cortical labyrinths** and **medullary rays**. Additionally, blood vessels and associated connective tissue (**renal interstitium**) are also present.

1. Cortical Labyrinth

The **cortical labyrinth** is composed of **renal corpuscles** and cross sections of **proximal convoluted tubules, distal convoluted tubules**, and the **macula densa** region of **distal tubules**. Renal corpuscles consist of **mesangial cells, parietal** (simple squamous) and **visceral** (modified to **podocytes**) **layers** of **Bowman's capsule**, and an associated capillary bed, the **glomerulus**, as well as the intervening **Bowman's space**, which receives the ultrafiltrate. The **afferent** and **efferent glomerular arterioles** supply and drain the glomerulus, respectively, at its vascular pole. **Bowman's space** is drained at the **urinary pole** into the **proximal convoluted tubule,** composed of eosinophilic simple cuboidal epithelium with a brush border. The **distal convoluted tubule** profiles are fewer in number and may be recognized by the pale cuboidal epithelial cells. The **macula densa** region of the distal tubule is associated with the **juxtaglomerular** (modified smooth muscle) **cells** of the afferent (and sometimes efferent) glomerular arterioles.

2. Medullary Rays

Medullary rays are continuations of medullary tissue extending into the cortex. They are composed mostly of **collecting tubules, pars recta of proximal tubules, ascending thick limbs of Henle's loop**, and blood vessels.

C. Medulla

The **medulla** is composed of **renal pyramids** that are bordered by **cortical columns**. The renal pyramids consist of **collecting tubules** whose simple cuboidal epithelium displays (1) clearly defined lateral cell membranes; (2) **thick descending limbs of Henle's loop**, whose cells resemble those of the proximal tubule; (3) **thin limbs of Henle's loop**, resembling capillaries but containing no blood; and (4) **ascending thick limbs of Henle's loop**, whose cells are similar to those of the distal tubule. Additionally, numerous blood vessels, the **vasa recta**, are also present, as well as slight connective tissue elements, the **renal interstitium**. The apex of the renal pyramid is the **renal papilla**, whose perforated tip is the **area cribrosa**, where the large **collecting ducts (of Bellini)** open to deliver the urine into the **minor calyx**.

D. Pelvis

The **renal pelvis**, drained by the **minor** and **major calyces**, constitutes the beginning of the main excretory duct of the kidney. The **transitional epithelium** of the minor calyx is reflected onto the renal papilla. The calyces are lined by transitional epithelium. The subepithelial connective tissue of both is loosely arranged and abuts the **muscularis**, composed of **inner longitudinal** and **outer circular** layers of **smooth muscle**. An **adventitia** of loose connective tissue surrounds the muscularis.

II. EXTRARENAL PASSAGES

A. Ureter

The **ureter** possesses a stellate-shaped lumen that is lined by **transitional epithelium**. The subepithelial connective tissue (sometimes said to be subdivided into **lamina propria** and **submucosa**) is composed of a fibroelastic connective tissue. The **muscularis** is again composed of **inner longitudinal** and **outer circular** layers of **smooth muscle**, although in its lower portion near the bladder a third, **outermost longitudinal** layer of **smooth muscle** is present. The muscularis is surrounded by a fibroelastic **adventitia**.

B. Bladder

The **urinary bladder** resembles the ureter except that it is a much larger structure and does not possess a stellate lumen, although the mucosa of the empty bladder is thrown into folds. The **lamina propria** is fibroelastic in character and may contain occasional **mucous glands** at the internal orifice of the urethra. The **muscularis** is composed of three indefinite layers of smooth muscle: **inner longitudinal, middle circular**, and **outer longitudinal**. The circular muscle coat forms the **internal sphincter** at the neck of the bladder. An **adventitia** or **serosa** surrounds the bladder. The urethra is described in Chapter 17, "Female Reproductive System," and Chapter 18, "Male Reproductive System."

17

FEMALE REPRODUCTIVE SYSTEM

The female reproductive system (see Graphic 17-1) is composed of the ovaries, genital ducts, external genitalia, and the mammary glands, although, in a strict sense, the mammary glands are not considered to be genital organs. The reproductive system functions in the propagation of the species and is under the control of a complex interplay of hormonal, neural, and, at least in the human, psychologic factors.

OVARY

Each **ovary** is a small, almond-shaped structure whose thick connective tissue capsule, the **tunica albuginea**, is covered by a **simple squamous** to **cuboidal mesothelium** known as the **germinal epithelium** (a modified mesothelium). The ovary is divisible into the **cortex**, rich in ovarian follicles and the **medulla**, a highly vascular connective tissue stroma.

- The **cortex**, located just deep to the tunica albuginea, houses the female germ cells, **oogonia**, which have undergone a series of cell divisions to form numerous **primary oocytes**.
  ○ Each primary oocyte is surrounded by a layer of epithelial cells known as **follicular cells** (whose origin is controversial), and these two structures together constitute an **ovarian follicle**.
  ○ Follicular cells secrete **meiosis-preventing substance** that prevents the continuation of meiosis and maintains the primary oocyte in the prophase of meiosis I.
  ○ Under the influence initially of local factors and later of **follicle-stimulating hormone (FSH)**, follicles enlarge, are modified, become encapsulated by the ovarian **stroma** (connective tissue), and mature.
- The **medulla** is a highly vascularized loose connective tissue stroma rich in fibroblasts and estrogen-secreting **interstitial cells**.
  ○ Additionally, occasional **hilar cells** are present in the medulla; these cells resemble interstitial cells of the testis, and they manufacture a small amount of androgens.

Ovarian Follicles

Each **ovarian follicle** passes through various maturational stages, from the primordial follicle (or non-growing follicle), through the **growing follicles** which have four stages, namely, unilaminar primary, multilaminar primary, secondary, and, finally, the Graafian (mature) follicle (see Table 17-1).
- The **primordial follicle** is composed of a **primary oocyte** surrounded by a single layer of flattened follicular cells.

- As maturation progresses, the follicular cells become cuboidal in shape, and the follicle is referred to as a **unilaminar primary follicle**.
- **Multilaminar primary follicles** display a primary oocyte surrounded by several layers of follicular cells (at this stage also referred to as **granulosa cells**).
  ○ **The zona pellucida**, manufactured by the primary oocyte is composed of three glycoproteins, ZP_1, ZP_2, and ZP_3, begins to be evident as it is interposed between the follicular cells and the primary oocyte.
  ○ Filopodia of the follicular cells adjacent to the zona pellucida and the microvilli of the primary oocyte contact and form **gap junctions** with each other in the zona pellucida.
  ○ The connective tissue stroma coalesces around the follicular cells but is separated from them by a basement membrane. This connective tissue layer is the **theca folliculi** and has two layers, a cellular **theca interna** adjacent to the basement membrane and a fibromuscular **theca externa**, surrounding the theca interna.
- With further growth of the follicle, accumulations of follicular fluid form in the extracellular spaces of the **follicular cells**. At this point, the entire structure is known as a **secondary follicle**, and it presents a well-developed **zona pellucida**,
  ○ as well as a clearly distinguishable basement membrane that is interposed between the follicular cells and the highly cellular **theca interna**
  ○ the theca interna is surrounded by a more fibrous **theca externa**.
- As maturation progresses, the **Graafian follicle** (also referred to as the **mature follicle**) **stage** is reached.
  ○ This large structure is characterized by a follicular fluid containing the central antrum, whose wall is composed of the **membrana granulosa** (follicular cells are also known as **granulosa cells**).
  ○ Jutting into the antrum is the **cumulus oophorus**, housing the primary oocyte and its attendant zona pellucida and **corona radiata**.
  ○ The membrana granulosa is separated from the theca interna by the basement membrane.
  ○ The theca externa merges imperceptibly with the surrounding ovarian stroma.
  ○ Several Graafian follicles develop during an ovulatory cycle, but (usually) only one will release its oocyte and that is known as the **dominant (Graafian) follicle**.
  ○ The dominant follicle, mostly because of the activity of **luteinizing hormone (LH)**, ruptures, thus releasing the oocyte with its attendant follicular cells.

TABLE 17-1 • Characteristics of Ovarian Follicles

Stage of Follicle	Primary Oocyte Diameter	Follicular Cells	Hormone Dependency	Theca Folliculi
Primordial	25 μm	Single layer, squamous	Local factors	Not present
Unilaminar primary	100–120 μm	Single layer, cuboidal	Local factors	Not present
Multilaminar primary	150 μm	Several layers, cuboidal	Local factors	Present
Secondary	200 μm	Several layers, cuboidal with some follicular fluid in the extracellular spaces	Follicle-stimulating hormone (FSH)	Present
Graafian	200 μm	Membrana granulosa, cumulus oophorus, corona radiata, antrum filled with liquor folliculi	FSH	Present
Dominant Graafian	200 μm	Same as in Graafian follicle	Is not FSH dependent, luteinizing hormone (for ovulation)	Present

Regulation of Follicle Maturation and Ovulation

Early development of the follicle from the primordial through the secondary follicle stage is dependent on local factors. Later development depends on **gonadotropin-releasing hormones (GnRHs)** from the hypothalamus, which activate gonadotrophs of the adenohypophysis to release **follicle-stimulating hormone (FSH)** and **luteinizing hormone (LH)**.

- **FSH** not only induces secondary follicles to mature into Graafian follicles but also causes cells of the **theca interna** to secrete **androgens**.
- Additionally, FSH prompts **granulosa cells** to develop **LH receptors**, to convert androgens to **estrogens**, and to secrete **inhibin**, **activin**, and **folliculostatin**.
  - These hormones assist in the feedback regulation of FSH release. Moreover, as estrogen reaches a threshold level, it causes a **surge of LH** release.
- The **LH** surge results not only in resumption of meiosis I in the primary oocyte and initiation of meiosis II in the (now) **secondary oocyte,** but also in **ovulation**.
  - Additionally, LH induces the development of the **corpus luteum** from the theca interna and membrana granulosa, and this can occur only when the granulosa cells respond to FSH to produce **LH receptors**.
  - Locally produced **prostaglandins** stimulate smooth muscle cells of the theca externa to undergo contraction thus assisting in ovulation.

Corpus Luteum and Corpus Albicans

Once the Graafian follicle loses its oocyte, it becomes transformed into the **corpus hemorrhagicum**. Within a couple of days, the corpus hemorrhagicum is transformed into the **corpus luteum.** The transformation into the corpus luteum involves

- the breakdown of the basement membrane between the theca interna and the granulosa cells
- collapse and folding of the former Graafian follicle upon itself
- resorption of the blood from the corpus hemorrhagicus and its replacement by fibrous connective tissue.
- transformation of the theca interna cells into theca lutein cells
- transformation of the granulosa cells into granulosa lutein cells

The transformation into the corpus luteum is due to both local factors such as IGF-I (insulin-like growth factor-I), IGF-II, as well as the following hormones LH and prolactin.

- The **corpus luteum,** a yellow glandular structure, secretes **progesterone,** a hormone that suppresses LH release by inhibiting GnRH and facilitates the thickening of the uterine **endometrium**.
- Additionally, **estrogen** (inhibitor of FSH) and **relaxin** (which causes the fibrocartilage of the pubic symphysis to become more pliable) are also released by the corpus luteum.

In case pregnancy does not occur, the corpus luteum **atrophies,** a process known as **luteolysis,** and the absence of estrogen and progesterone will once again permit the release of FSH and LH from the adenohypophysis. In this case, the corpus luteum is known as the **corpus luteum of menstruation** and will degenerate into the **corpus albicans**.

In case pregnancy does occur, the **syncytiotrophoblasts** of the forming placenta

- release **human chorionic gonadotropin (hCG)**, a hormone that maintains the placenta well into the second trimester.
- secrete **human chorionic mammotropin** (facilitates milk production and growth), **thyrotropin, corticotropin, relaxin**, and **estrogen**.
  - A few months into the pregnancy, when the placenta has been well established, the corpus luteum, known as the **corpus luteum of pregnancy**, is no longer needed, and it also undergoes luteolysis to form the fibrotic **corpus albicans**.

GENITAL DUCTS

Oviduct

Each **oviduct (fallopian tube)** is a short muscular tube leading from the vicinity of the ovary to the uterine lumen (see Graphic 17-1). The oviduct is subdivided into four regions:

- **infundibulum** (whose fimbriae approximate the ovary),
- **ampulla**,
- **isthmus**, and
- **intramural portion**, which pierces the wall of the uterus.

The mucosa of the oviduct, composed of a simple columnar epithelium and a vascular lamina propria, is extensively folded in the infundibulum and ampulla, but the folding is reduced in the isthmus and intramural portions. The simple columnar epithelium is composed of two types of cells

- **ciliated columnar**, whose cilia beat toward the uterus to transport the fertilized egg into the uterus for implantation, and
- **peg cells**, that are also columnar but have no cilia. Their apical region is expanded and houses the secretory product that these cells release, namely:
  - **factors for the capacitation** of spermatozoa and
  - **nutrient-rich medium** that nourishes the spermatozoa as well as the fertilized ovum traveling toward the uterus.

The mucosa is surrounded by a thick smooth muscle coat composed of a poorly defined inner circular and outer longitudinal layers, which, via peristaltic action, assists the cilia to propel the fertilized egg to the uterus. The muscular coat of the oviduct is covered by a serosa, whereas its intramural portion is embedded in the uterus and is surrounded by uterine connective tissue.

Uterus

The **uterus**, a pear-shaped viscus, is divisible into a **fundus, body**, and **cervix**. During pregnancy, this organ houses and supports the developing embryo and fetus.

Fundus and Body of the Uterus

The uterus is composed of a thick, muscular **myometrium** (covered by **serosa** and/or **adventitia**) and a spongy mucosal layer, the **endometrium**.

- The endometrium, composed of simple cuboidal epithelium covering the lamina propria with its secretory glands, has a superficial **functional layer** and deep **basal layer**, each with its own blood supply.
  - The **basal layer**, which remains intact during menstruation, is served by short, **straight arteries** and is occupied by the base of the **uterine glands**.
  - The **functional layer**, served by the **helicine (coiled) arteries**, undergoes hormonally modulated cyclic changes during the menstrual cycle of a postpubertal and premenarche female.

The three phases of the endometrium during the menstrual cycle are the proliferative, secretory, and menstrual phases (see Table 17-2).

- **Follicular (proliferative) phase**, during which the free surface of the endometrium is reepithelialized, and the glands, connective tissue elements, and vascular supply of the endometrium are reestablished.
  - FSH facilitates the **proliferative phase**, a thickening of the endometrium and the renewal of the connective tissue, glandular structures, and blood vessels (**helicine arteries**) subsequent to the menstrual phase.
- **Luteal (secretory) phase**, occurring within a few days after ovulation, during which the glands further enlarge and become tortuous and their lumina become filled with secretory products. Additionally, the helical arteries become more coiled, and fibroblasts of the stroma accumulate glycogen and fat.
  - LH facilitates the **secretory phase**, characterized by the further thickening of the endometrium, coiling of the endometrial glands, accumulation of glandular secretions, and further coiling and lengthening of the **helicine arteries**.
- **Menstrual phase**, during which the functional layer of the endometrium is desquamated, resulting in menstrual flow, whereas the basal layer remains more or less undisturbed.
  - Decreased levels of LH and progesterone are responsible for the **menstrual phase**, which begins with long-term, intermittent **vasoconstriction** of the helicine arteries, with subsequent necrosis of the vessel walls as well as of the endometrial tissue of the functional layer.
  - It should be understood that the basal layer is unaffected because it is being supplied by the straight arteries.
  - During relaxation (between events of vasoconstriction), the helicine arteries rupture, and the rapid

TABLE 17-2 • Phases of the Menstrual Cycle

Phases of the Cycle	Length (d)	Hormone Involved	Endometrial Characteristics
Menstrual	3–4	Reduced levels of estrogens and progesterone	Helical arteries are shut down, resulting in necrosis and sloughing of functionalis layer of the endometrium; epithelial cells in the base of the uterine glands (located in the basal layer of the endometrium) start to reepithelialize the uterine endometrium.
Proliferative (follicular)	10	Increased blood levels of follicle-stimulating hormone (FSH) and estrogens; at the end of the proliferative phase, estrogen, FSH, and luteinizing hormone (LH) blood levels peak.	The denuded surface of the endometrium becomes reepithelialized, the functionalis layer becomes thickened (~3 mm thick), and its helical arteries are reestablished and begin to become coiled; uterine glands are not as yet coiled but begin secretion.
Secretory (luteal)	14	Estrogen levels rise in the blood and progesterone blood levels peak; FSH and LH blood levels are decreased.	Helical arteries and uterine glands of the functionalis become highly coiled; the functionalis reaches its full thickness (~5 mm thick); the uterine glands are filled with their secretory products; cells of the stroma undergo decidual reaction and accumulate glycogen and lipids that provide nutrients for the blastocyst embedding itself in the endometrium.

blood flow dislodges the blood-filled necrotic functional layer, which becomes sloughed as the **hemorrhagic discharge**, so that only the basal layer of the endometrium remains as the lining of the uterus.

During pregnancy, the smooth muscle cells of the **myometrium** undergo estrogen-induced **hypertrophy** and **hyperplasia**, increasing the thickness of the muscle wall of the uterus. The smooth muscle cells increase from the 50-μm length of the nonpregnant uterus to as much as 500 μm in the gravid uterus.

- These smooth muscle cells acquire **gap junctions** that facilitate their coordinated contractile actions.
- At parturition, **oxytocin** and **prostaglandins** cause the uterine muscles to undergo rhythmic contractions that assist in expelling the fetus.
  - Subsequent to delivery, the lack of estrogen is responsible for **apoptosis** of many of the smooth muscle cells with a consequent reduction in the thickness of the myometrium.

Cervix of the Uterus

The **cervix** is the inferior aspect of the uterus and it protrudes into the vagina. The lumen (canal) of the cervix is continuous with the lumen of the uterus (superiorly) and the vaginal canal (inferiorly).

- The **wall of the cervix** is thick and is composed of a dense irregular fibroelastic connective tissue housing some smooth muscle cells and branched cervical glands.

  - The **cervical glands** produce a serous secretion that lubricates the vagina.
    - After fertilization, these glands produce a thick, viscous mucous that impedes the entry of spermatozoa and microorganisms into the uterine lumen.
- Its lumen is lined by a **simple columnar epithelium** whose cells secrete a mucous substance.
- The inferior aspect of the lumen is lined by a stratified squamous nonkeratinized epithelium, which is continuous with the vaginal epithelium.
- The thick cervical wall becomes thinner and less rigid at parturition due to the effects of the hormone **oxytocin**.

FERTILIZATION, IMPLANTATION, AND THE PLACENTA

Fertilization and Implantation

The union of the haploid sperm pronucleus with the pronucleus of the haploid ovum is known as **fertilization**, whereby a new diploid cell, the **zygote**, is formed. Fertilization usually occurs in the **ampulla** of the oviduct.

- As the zygote travels along the oviduct, it undergoes mitotic cell division, known as **cleavage**, to form a solid cluster of cells, known as the **morula**. Approximately

3 days after fertilization, the morula enters the lumen of the uterus.

- Once in the uterus, the cells of the morula rearrange themselves to form a hollow structure, the **blastocyst,** whose fluid-filled cavity also houses a small cluster of cells, the **inner cell mass (embryoblasts)** responsible for the formation of the embryo.
- Approximately 5 to 6 days after fertilization, the cells at the periphery of the blastocyst, the **trophoblasts,** proliferate and initiate the process of **implantation** into the endometrium. By the ninth day, implantation is complete.
- As the trophoblasts proliferate, they form an inner cellular layer, the **cytotrophoblast,** and an outer syncytial layer, the **syncytiotrophoblast.**
  ○ The syncytiotrophoblasts will initiate the formation of the **embryonic portion of the placenta.**
  ○ In response to the invasion of the syncytiotrophoblasts, the endometrium will initiate the formation of the **maternal portion of the placenta.**

Placenta

During pregnancy, the uterus participates in the formation of the **placenta,** a highly vascular structure that permits the exchange of various materials between the maternal and fetal circulatory systems (see Graphic 17-2). It must be stressed that the exchange occurs without the commingling of the maternal and fetal bloods and that the placenta is derived from both maternal and fetal tissues. The roles of the trophoblasts and the endometrium are as follows:

- The syncytiotrophoblasts and cytotrophoblasts form the **chorion,** the precursor of the **chorionic plate** from which the chorionic villi will arise.
- The **endometrium** in contact with the chorion becomes modified to form the **decidua** with its three regions:
  ○ **Decidua basalis,** the richly vascularized maternal portion of the placenta that induces the trophoblasts to form the chorionic villi.
  ○ **Decidua capsularis,** the tissue separating the lumen of the uterus from the embryo and will be known as the **chorion laeve,** and
  ○ **Decidua parietalis,** the endometrial tissue between the uterine lumen and the myometrium.

Initially, the **chorionic villi** are slender structures and are known as **primary villi.** Once they are invaded by mesenchymal cells and fetal capillary networks, they become more substantial and their population of cytotrophoblasts decreases because they become incorporated into the syncytiotrophoblasts; in this manner, the primary villi become known as **secondary villi.**

- As the placenta is forming, the decidua basalis develops large, blood-filled vascular channels, known as **lacunae,** and the secondary villi protrude into these "lakes" of maternal blood, supplied by maternal arterioles and drained by maternal venules.
- Secondary villi grow into these lacunae and some of the villi contact and fuse with the decidua basalis (**anchoring villi**), whereas other secondary villi (**free villi**) resemble fingers that are immersed in water.
  ○ The fetal capillary beds of the anchoring and free villi are located adjacent to the syncytiotrophoblasts and lie in close proximity of the maternal blood in the lacunae.
  ○ Oxygen and nutrients in the maternal blood diffuse through the villi to reach the fetal capillaries.
  ○ Carbon dioxide and waste products in the fetal blood also diffuse through the villi to reach the maternal blood in the lacunae.
  ○ The exchange of gases and material occurs by passing through the **placental barrier** whose components are listed in Table 17-3.

In addition to its role in the delivery of nutrients and oxygen to the fetus and exchanging it for the fetal waste products, the placenta also manufactures hormones and factors necessary for the maintenance of pregnancy and the delivery of the fetus (see Table 17-4).

VAGINA

The **vagina,** an 8- to 9-cm long muscular sheath, extending from the cervix of the uterus to the vestibule, is adapted for the reception of the penis during copulation and for the passage of the fetus from the uterus during birth. The wall of the vagina is composed of three layers: the mucosa, muscularis, and the adventitia.

- The **mucosa** consists of a stratified squamous epithelium and a loose, fibroelastic connective tissue layer, the lamina propria.

TABLE 17-3 • Components of the Placental Barrier
Endothelial cells of the fetal capillary
Basal lamina of the fetal endothelium
Connective tissue of the secondary villus
Basal lamina of the cytotrophoblasts
Cytotrophoblasts
Syncytiotrophoblasts

TABLE 17-4 • Principal Hormones and Factors Produced by the Various Components of the Placenta

Syncytiotrophoblasts	Cytotrophoblasts	Decidua Cells
Estrogens	Gonadotropin-releasing hormone	Insulin-like growth factor binding proteins
Progesterone	Corticotropin-releasing hormone	Relaxin
Chorionic gonadotrophin	Thyrotropin-releasing hormone	Prolactin
Chorionic somatotropin	Growth hormone–releasing hormone	Prostaglandins
Placental growth hormone	Inhibin	
Leptin	Activin	
	Leptin	
	Insulin-like growth factors I and II	

○ Frequently, in a virgin, the external orifice of the vagina is partially occluded by the **hymen**, a thin, somewhat vascular connective tissue membrane, covered on both sides by stratified squamous epithelium.

- The **muscularis** is composed of a mostly longitudinally disposed smooth muscle layer interspersed with some circularly arranged fibers. At its external orifice, the muscularis of the vagina possesses a sphincter, composed of circularly arrayed smooth muscle fibers.

- The **adventitia** is a dense fibroelastic connective tissue that affixes the vagina to the surrounding pelvic connective tissue.

EXTERNAL GENITALIA

The **external genitalia**, composed of **labia majora**, **labia minora**, **clitoris**, and **vestibular glands**, are also referred to as the **vulva**. These structures are richly innervated and function during sexual arousal and copulation.

MAMMARY GLANDS

The **mammary glands**, highly modified **sweat glands**, are identical in males and females until the onset of puberty, when, due to hormonal influences, the female breasts develop.

- The mammary gland is composed of numerous individual compound glands, each of which is considered a lobe.
  ○ Each lobe is drained by a **lactiferous duct** that delivers **milk**, the secretion of the mammary glands, onto the surface of the nipple.

- The pigmented region of the skin surrounding the nipple, known as the **areola**, is richly endowed by sweat, sebaceous, and areolar glands.

- During pregnancy, several hormones interact to promote the development of the secretory units of the mammary gland. Cells of the **terminal interalveolar ducts** proliferate to form secretory **alveoli**.
  ○ The hormones involved in promoting this process are **progesterone**, **estrogen**, and **human chorionic mammotropin** from the placenta and **lactogenic hormone (prolactin)** from the **acidophils** of the adenohypophysis.

- Alveoli and terminal interalveolar ducts are surrounded by **myoepithelial cells** that contract as a result of the release of **oxytocin** from the neurohypophysis (in response to suckling), forcing milk out of the breast (**milk ejection reflex**).
  ○ **Milk** is composed of water, proteins, lipids, and lactose.
    - However, milk secreted during the first few days (**colostrum**) is different, in that it is rich in vitamins, minerals, **lymphoid cells**, and proteins, especially **immunoglobulin A**, providing antibodies for the neonate for the first few months of life.

CLINICAL CONSIDERATIONS

Papanicolaou Smear

The Papanicolaou (Pap) smear is performed as part of routine gynecological examination to examine stained exfoliative cells of the lining of the cervix and vagina. Evaluation of the smeared cells permits the recognition of precancerous conditions as well as cancer of the cervix. An annual smear test is recommended since cervical cancer is relatively slow growing and the Pap smear is an extremely cost-effective procedure that has been responsible for the early detection of cervical cancer and for saving lives of affected individuals.

Gonorrhea

Gonorrhea is a sexually transmitted bacterial infection caused by the gram-negative diplococcus *Neisseria gonorrhoeae*. In the United States, over a million cases of gonorrhea occur annually. Frequently, this sexually transmitted disease is responsible for pelvic inflammatory disease (PID) and for acute salpingitis.

Pelvic Inflammatory Disease

PID an infection of the cervix, uterus, fallopian tubes, and/or ovary, is usually a sequel to microbial infection. Individuals suffering from PID exhibit tenderness and pain in the lower abdominal region, fever, unpleasant-smelling vaginal discharge, and episodes of abnormal bleeding.

Adenomyosis

Adenomyosis is a common condition in which the endometrial glands invade the myometrium and cause the uterus to enlarge, occasionally becoming two or three times its normal dimensions. In most women, adenomyosis has no symptoms, and it is only on gynecological examination that the condition is discovered. When it becomes symptomatic, the woman is usually between 35 and 50 years of age, she may experience pain during intercourse, and she notices an increase in menstrual flow as well as bleeding between periods. Although the condition is benign, if the symptoms are severe and uncontrollable, hysterectomy may be indicated.

Endometriosis

Endometriosis is distinguished by the presence of ectopic endometrial tissue dispersed to various sites along the peritoneal cavity. Occasionally, the tissues may migrate to extraperitoneal areas, including the eyes and brain. The etiology of this disease is not known. In some cases the lesions of endometriosis involve small cysts attached separately or in small clumps on the visceral or parietal peritoneum.

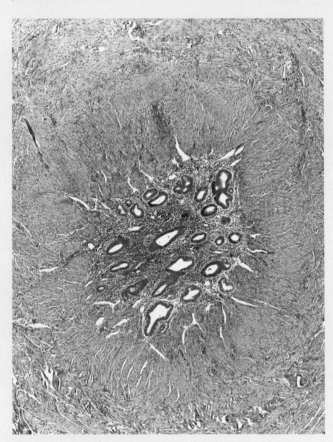

This photomicrograph is from the fallopian tube of a female patient with endometriosis. Observe that uterine glands and stroma occupy the lumen of the oviduct. (Reprinted with permission from Mills SE, Carter D, et al., eds. Sternberg's Diagnostic Surgical Pathology, 5th ed. Philadelphia: Lippincott Williams & Wilkins, 2010, p. 2377.)

Endometrial Carcinoma

Endometrial carcinoma is a malignancy of the uterine endometrium usually occurring in postmenopausal women. The most common type of endometrial cancer is adenocarcinoma. Since during the early stages the cancer cells do not invade the cervix, Pap smears are not very effective in diagnosing this disease until it has entered its later stages. The major symptom of endometrial cancer is abnormal uterine bleeding.

Hydatidiform Mole

Occasionally, an ovum does not develop normally and instead of becoming a fetus forms a mass of tissue that initially mimics pregnancy, or in some patients, after delivery, remnants of placental tissue may proliferate. Known as a hydatidiform mole, these growths increase in size much faster than would a fetus. When the physician does not hear a heartbeat, the patient's abdomen swells more than expected, and the patient complains of vomiting and severe nausea, a hydatidiform mole should be suspected. This is especially true in individuals who complain of a vaginal discharge of grape-like clusters of tissue. In most of the cases, the hydatidiform mole resorbs on its own. Only in about 20% of the cases does it become invasive, and in very rare cases does it becomes malignant (then it is known as a choriocarcinoma).

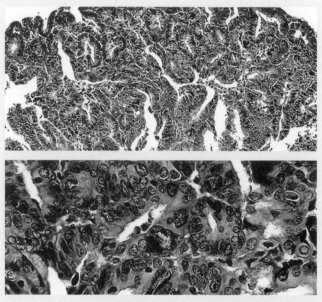

This photomicrograph is from the uterus of a female patient with Grade 1 carcinoma of the endometrium. **Top**: Observe that the uterine glands are very crowded with a scant amount of connective tissue between the glands. **Bottom**: The cells of the gland are interspersed with malignant cells displaying cytologic atypia. (Reprinted with permission from Mills SE, Carter D, et al., eds. Sternberg's Diagnostic Surgical Pathology, 5th ed. Philadelphia: Lippincott Williams & Wilkins, 2010, p. 2208.)

Paget's Disease of the Nipple

Paget's disease of the nipple usually occurs in elderly women and is associated with breast cancer of ductal origin. Initially, the disease manifests as scaly or crusty nipple frequently accompanied by a fluid discharge from the nipple. Usually, the patient has no other symptoms and frequently neglects the condition.

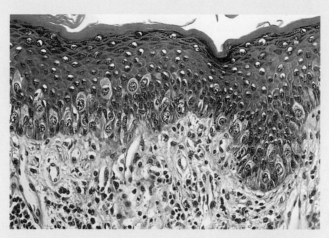

This photomicrograph is from the nipple of a female patient with Paget's disease of the nipple. Note the large Paget's cells throughout the basal aspect of the stratified squamous keratinized epithelium, with their light pink cytoplasm, vesicular-appearing nuclei, and large nucleoli. (Reprinted with permission from Mills SE, Carter D, et al., eds. Sternberg's Diagnostic Surgical Pathology, 5th ed. Philadelphia: Lippincott Williams & Wilkins, 2010, p. 293.)

GRAPHIC 17-1 • Female Reproductive System

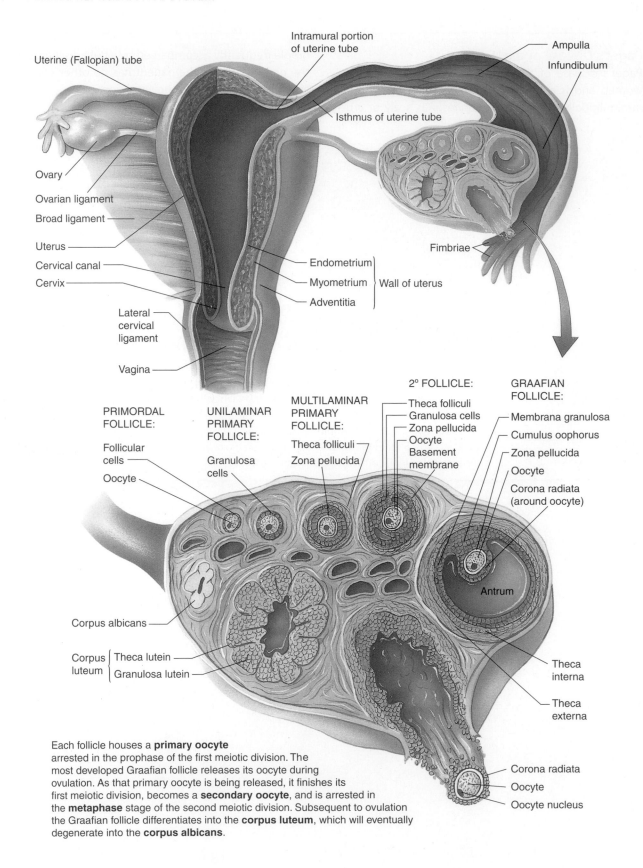

Uterine (Fallopian) tube

Intramural portion of uterine tube

Ampulla

Infundibulum

Isthmus of uterine tube

Ovary

Ovarian ligament

Broad ligament

Uterus

Cervical canal

Cervix

Endometrium

Myometrium | Wall of uterus

Adventitia

Fimbriae

Lateral cervical ligament

Vagina

PRIMORDAL FOLLICLE:

Follicular cells

Oocyte

UNILAMINAR PRIMARY FOLLICLE:

Granulosa cells

MULTILAMINAR PRIMARY FOLLICLE:

Theca folliculi

Zona pellucida

2° FOLLICLE:

Theca folliculi

Granulosa cells

Zona pellucida

Oocyte

Basement membrane

GRAAFIAN FOLLICLE:

Membrana granulosa

Cumulus oophorus

Zona pellucida

Oocyte

Corona radiata (around oocyte)

Antrum

Theca interna

Theca externa

Corpus albicans

Corpus luteum | Theca lutein

Granulosa lutein

Corona radiata

Oocyte

Oocyte nucleus

Each follicle houses a **primary oocyte** arrested in the prophase of the first meiotic division. The most developed Graafian follicle releases its oocyte during ovulation. As that primary oocyte is being released, it finishes its first meiotic division, becomes a **secondary oocyte**, and is arrested in the **metaphase** stage of the second meiotic division. Subsequent to ovulation the Graafian follicle differentiates into the **corpus luteum**, which will eventually degenerate into the **corpus albicans**.

Placental Structure

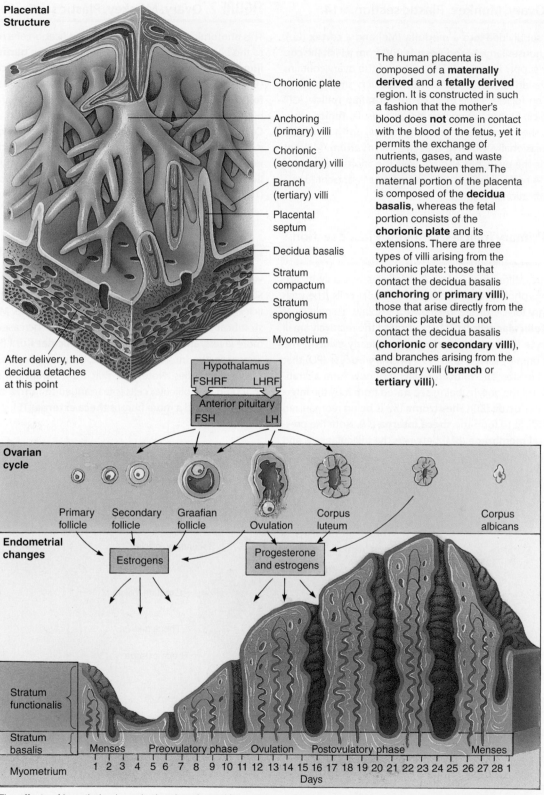

Chorionic plate

Anchoring (primary) villi

Chorionic (secondary) villi

Branch (tertiary) villi

Placental septum

Decidua basalis

Stratum compactum

Stratum spongiosum

Myometrium

After delivery, the decidua detaches at this point

The human placenta is composed of a **maternally derived** and a **fetally derived** region. It is constructed in such a fashion that the mother's blood does **not** come in contact with the blood of the fetus, yet it permits the exchange of nutrients, gases, and waste products between them. The maternal portion of the placenta is composed of the **decidua basalis**, whereas the fetal portion consists of the **chorionic plate** and its extensions. There are three types of villi arising from the chorionic plate: those that contact the decidua basalis (**anchoring** or **primary villi**), those that arise directly from the chorionic plate but do not contact the decidua basalis (**chorionic** or **secondary villi**), and branches arising from the secondary villi (**branch** or **tertiary villi**).

Hypothalamus

FSHRF   LHRF

Anterior pituitary

FSH   LH

Ovarian cycle

Primary follicle

Secondary follicle

Graafian follicle

Ovulation

Corpus luteum

Corpus albicans

Endometrial changes

Estrogens

Progesterone and estrogens

Stratum functionalis

Stratum basalis

Menses   Preovulatory phase   Ovulation   Postovulatory phase   Menses

Myometrium   1 2 3 4 5 6 7 8 9 10 11 12 13 14 15 16 17 18 19 20 21 22 23 24 25 26 27 28 1

Days

The effects of hypothalamic and adenohypophyseal hormones on the ovarian cortex and uterine endometrium.

FIGURE 1. Ovary. Monkey. Plastic section. ×14.

The ovary is subdivided into a **medulla** (Me) and a **cortex** (Co). The medulla houses large **blood vessels** (BV) from which the cortical vascular supply is derived. The cortex of the ovary contains numerous ovarian follicles, most of which are very small (*arrows*); a few maturing follicles have reached the **Graafian follicle** (GF) stage. The thick, fibrous connective tissue capsule, **tunica albuginea** (TA), is shown to advantage; the **germinal epithelium** (GE) is evident occasionally. Observe that the **mesovarium** (Mo) not only suspends the ovary but also conveys the vascular supply to the medulla. A region similar to the *boxed area* is presented at a higher magnification in Figure 2.

FIGURE 3. Primary follicles. Monkey. Plastic section. ×270.

Primary follicles differ from primordial follicles not only in size but also in morphology and number of follicular cells. The uniltaminar primary follicle of the *inset* (×270) displays a single layer of **cuboidal follicular cells** (FC) that surround the relatively small **primary oocyte** (PO), whose **nucleus** (N) is clearly evident. The multilaminar primary follicle displays a **primary oocyte** (PO) that has increased in size. The **follicular cells** (FC) now form a stratified layer around the oocyte, being separated from it by the intervening **zona pellucida** (ZP). The **stroma** (St) is being reorganized around the follicle to form the **theca interna** (TI). Note the presence of a **basal membrane** (BM) between the follicular cells and the theca interna.

FIGURE 2. Ovary. Monkey. Plastic section. ×132.

This photomicrograph is a higher magnification of a region similar to the *boxed area* of Figure 1. Observe that the **germinal epithelium** (GE) covers the collagenous capsule, the **tunica albuginea** (TA). This region of the **cortex** (Co) houses numerous **primordial follicles** (PF). Observe that the connective tissue of the ovary is highly cellular and is referred to as the **stroma** (St). *Inset.* **Ovary. Cortex. Monkey. Plastic section.** ×540. The primordial follicle is composed of a **primary oocyte** (PO), whose **nucleus** (N) and **nucleolus** (*arrow*) are evident. Observe the single layer of flat **follicular cells** (FC) surrounding the oocyte. The **tunica albuginea** (TA) and the **germinal epithelium** (GE) are also shown to advantage in this photomicrograph.

FIGURE 4. Secondary follicle. Rabbit. Paraffin section. ×132.

Secondary follicles are very similar to primary multilaminar follicles, the major difference being their larger size. Moreover, the stratification of the **follicular cells** (FC) has increased, displaying more layers, and more important, a **follicular fluid** (FF) begins to appear in the intercellular spaces, which coalesces into several Call-Exner bodies. Note also that the stroma immediately surrounding the follicular cells is rearranged to form a cellular **theca interna** (TI) and a more fibrous **theca externa** (TE).

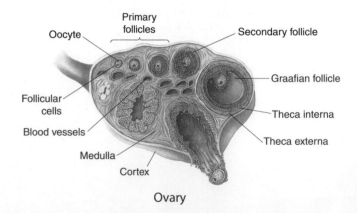

Ovary

KEY

BM	basal membrane	**GF**	Graafian follicle	**St**	stroma
BV	blood vessel	**Me**	medulla	**TA**	tunica albuginea
Co	cortex	**Mo**	mesovarium	**TE**	theca externa
FC	follicular cell	**N**	nucleus	**TI**	theca interna
FF	follicular fluid	**PF**	primordial follicle	**ZP**	zona pellucida
GE	germinal epithelium	**PO**	primary oocyte		

PLATE 17-1 · Ovary

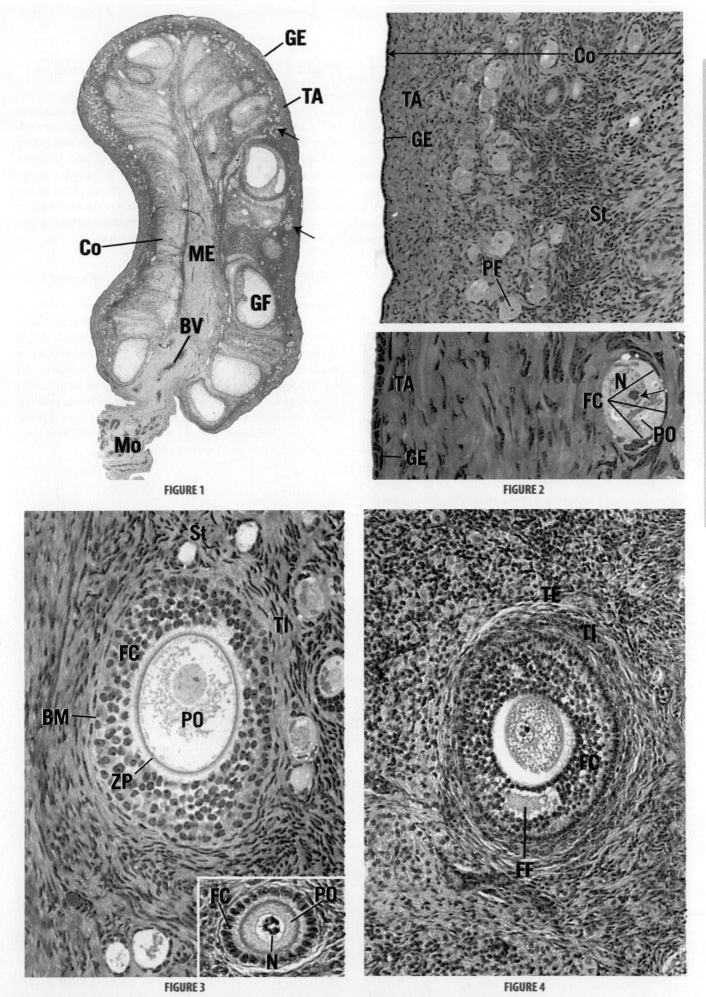

FIGURE 1

FIGURE 2

FIGURE 3

FIGURE 4

PLATE 17-2 • Ovary and Corpus Luteum

FIGURE 1. Graafian follicle. Paraffin section. ×132.

The Graafian follicle is the most mature of all ovarian follicles and is ready to release its primary oocyte in the process of ovulation. The **follicular fluid** (FL) fills a single chamber, the antrum, which is surrounded by a wall of granulosa (follicular) cells known as the **membrana granulosa** (MG). Some of the granulosa cells, which surround the **primary oocyte** (PO), jut into the antrum as the **cumulus oophorus** (CO). Observe the **basal membrane** (BM), which separates the granulosa cells from the **theca interna** (TI). The fibrous **theca externa** (TE) merges almost imperceptibly with the surrounding stroma. The *boxed area* is presented at a higher magnification in Figure 2.

FIGURE 3. Corpus luteum. Human. Paraffin section. ×14.

Subsequent to ovulation, the Graafian follicle becomes modified to form a temporary structure, the corpus hemorrhagicum, which will become the corpus luteum. The cells comprising the membrana granulosa enlarge, become vesicular in appearance, and are referred to as **granulosa lutein cells** (GL), which become folded; the spaces between the folds are occupied by connective tissue elements, blood vessels, and cells of the theca interna (*arrows*). These theca interna cells also enlarge, become glandular, and are referred to as the theca lutein cells. The remnants of the antrum are filled with fibrin and serous exudate that will be replaced by connective tissue elements. A region similar to the *boxed area* is presented at a higher magnification in Figure 4.

FIGURE 2. Graafian follicle. Cumulus oophorus. Paraffin section. ×270.

This photomicrograph is a higher magnification of the *boxed area* of Figure 1. Observe that the cumulus oophorus houses the **primary oocyte** (PO), whose **nucleus** (N) is just visible in this section. The **zona pellucida** (ZP) surrounds the oocyte, and processes (*arrows*) of the surrounding follicular cells extend into this acellular region. The single layer of follicular cells appears to radiate as a crown at the periphery of the primary oocyte and is referred to as the **corona radiata** (CR). Note the **basal membrane** (BM) as well as the **theca interna** (TI) and the **theca externa** (TE).

FIGURE 4. Corpus luteum. Human. Paraffin section. ×132.

This photomicrograph is a higher magnification of a region similar to the *boxed area* of Figure 3. The **granulosa lutein cells** (GL) of the corpus luteum are easily distinguished from the **connective tissue** (CT) elements, since the former display round **nuclei** (N), mostly in the center of large round cells (*arrowheads*). The center of the field is occupied by a fold, housing **theca lutein cells** (TL) amid numerous **connective tissue** (CT) and **vascular** (BV) elements. A region similar to the *boxed area* is presented at a higher magnification in Figure 1 of the next plate.

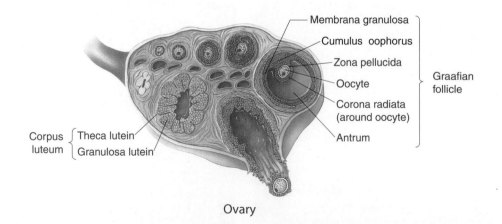

Membrana granulosa
Cumulus oophorus
Zona pellucida
Oocyte
Corona radiata (around oocyte)
Antrum
Graafian follicle

Corpus luteum { Theca lutein / Granulosa lutein

Ovary

KEY

BM	basal membrane	**FL**	follicular fluid	**TE**	theca externa
BV	vascular elements	**GL**	granulosa lutein cells	**TI**	theca interna
CO	cumulus oophorus	**MG**	membrana granulosa	**TL**	theca lutein cells
CR	corona radiata	**N**	nucleus	**ZP**	zona pellucida
CT	connective tissue	**PO**	primary oocyte		

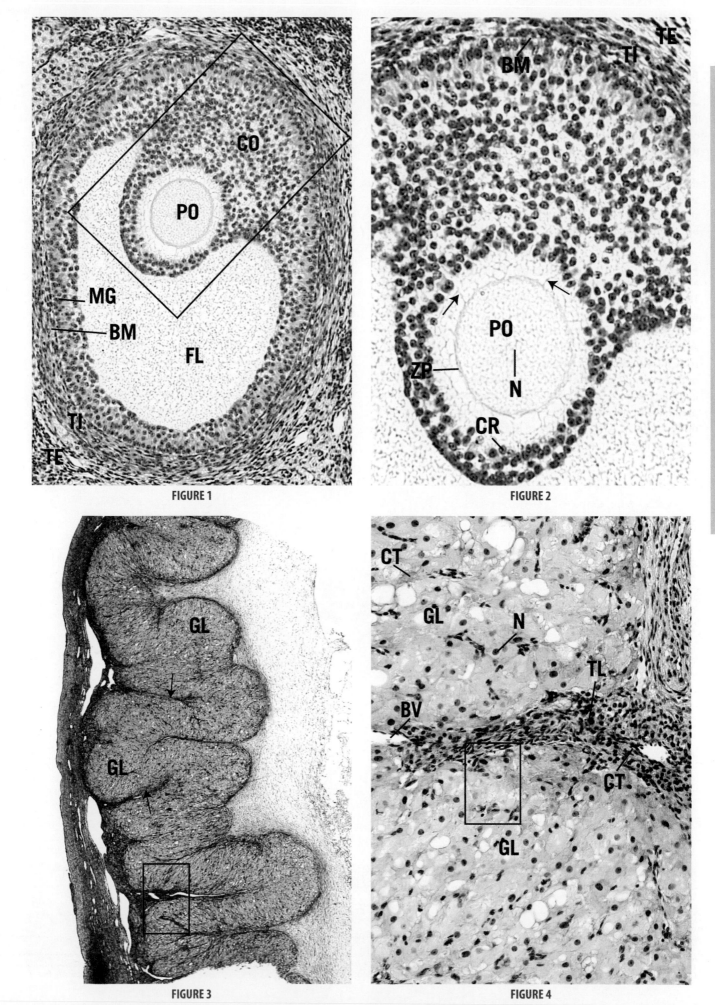

PLATE 17-2 · Ovary and Corpus Luteum

FIGURE 1

FIGURE 2

FIGURE 3

FIGURE 4

FIGURE 1. Corpus luteum. Human. Paraffin section. ×540.

This photomicrograph is similar to the *boxed area* of Figure 4 of the previous plate. Observe the large **granulosa lutein cells** (GL), whose cytoplasm appears vesicular, representing the spaces occupied by lipids in the living tissue. Note that the **nuclei** (N) of these cells are farther away from each other than the nuclei of the smaller **theca lutein cells** (TL), which also appear to be darker staining (*arrowheads*). The flattened nuclei (*arrows*) belong to various connective tissue cells.

FIGURE 3. Oviduct. x.s. Human. Paraffin section. ×14.

The oviduct, also referred to as the fallopian or uterine tube, extends from the ovary to the uterine cavity. It is suspended from the body wall by the **broad ligament** (BL), which conveys a rich **vascular supply** (BV) to the **serosa** (S) of the oviduct. The thick **muscularis** (M) is composed of ill-defined inner circular and outer longitudinal muscle layers. The **mucosa** (Mu) is thrown into longitudinal folds, which are so highly exaggerated in the infundibulum and ampulla that they subdivide the **lumen** (L) into labyrinthine spaces. A region similar to the *boxed area* is presented at a higher magnification in Figure 4.

FIGURE 2. Corpus albicans. Human. Paraffin section. ×132.

As the corpus luteum involutes, its cellular elements degenerate and undergo autolysis. The corpus luteum becomes invaded by macrophages that phagocytose the dead cells, leaving behind relatively acellular **fibrous tissue** (FT). The previously rich **vascular supply** (BV) also regressed, and the entire corpus albicans appears pale in comparison to the relatively dark staining of the surrounding ovarian **stroma** (St). The corpus albicans will regress until it becomes a small scar on the surface of the ovary.

FIGURE 4. Oviduct. x.s. Monkey. Plastic section. ×132.

This photomicrograph is a higher magnification of a region similar to the *boxed area* of Figure 3. The entire thickness of the wall of the oviduct displays its **vascular** (BV) **serosa** (S) that envelops the thick muscularis, whose **outer longitudinal** (OL) and **inner circular** (IC) layers are not very well delineated. The **mucosa** (Mu) is highly folded and is lined by a simple columnar **epithelium** (Ep). The loose connective tissue of the **lamina propria** (LP) is richly vascularized (*arrows*). The *boxed area* is presented in a higher magnification in Figure 1 in the following plate.

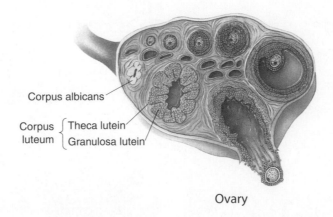

Corpus albicans

Corpus luteum { Theca lutein / Granulosa lutein

Ovary

KEY

BL	broad ligament	IC	inner circular muscle	N	nucleus
BV	vascular supply	L	lumen	OL	outer longitudinal muscle
Ep	epithelium	LP	lamina propria	S	serosa
FT	fibrous tissue	M	muscularis	ST	stroma
GL	granulosa lutein cell	Mu	mucosa	TL	theca lutein cell

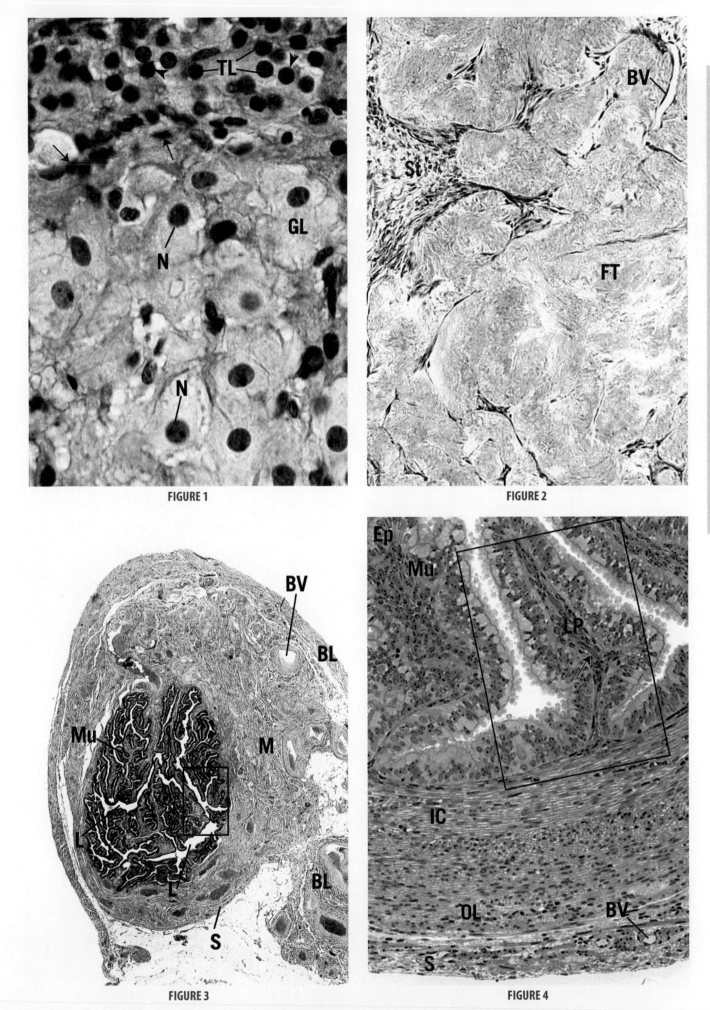

PLATE 17-3 • Ovary and Oviduct

FIGURE 1

FIGURE 2

FIGURE 3

FIGURE 4

PLATE 17-4 · Oviduct, Light and Electron Microscopy

FIGURE 1. Oviduct. x.s. Monkey. Plastic section. ×270.

This photomicrograph is a higher magnification of the *boxed area* of Figure 4 of the previous plate. Observe the **inner circular muscle** (IC) layer of the muscularis. The **lamina propria** (LP) is very narrow in this region (*arrows*) but presents longitudinal epithelially lined folds. The core of these folds is composed of a **vascular** (BV), loose but highly cellular **connective tissue** (CT). The simple columnar **epithelium** (Ep) lines the labyrinthine **lumen** (L) of the oviduct. A region similar to the *boxed area* is presented at a higher magnification in Figure 2.

FIGURE 3. Oviduct epithelium. Human. Electron microscopy. ×4,553.

The human oviduct at midcycle (day 14) presents two types of epithelial cells, the **peg cell** (PC) and the **ciliated cell** (CC). The former are secretory cells, as indicated by their extensive **Golgi apparatus** (GA) situated in the region of the cell apical to the **nucleus** (N). Observe the electron-dense secretory products (*arrows*) in the expanded, apical free ends of these cells. Note also that some ciliated cells display large accumulations of **glycogen** (Gl) at either pole of the nucleus. (From Verhage H, Bareither M, Jaffe R, Akbar M. Cyclic changes in ciliation, secretion and cell height of the oviductal epethelium in women. Am J Anat 1979;156:505–522.)

FIGURE 2. Oviduct. x.s. Monkey. Plastic section. ×540.

This photomicrograph is a higher magnification of a region similar to the *boxed area* of Figure 1. The **lamina propria** (LP) is a highly cellular, loose connective tissue that is richly **vascularized.** The **basal membrane** (BM) separating the connective tissue from the epithelial lining is clearly evident. Note that the epithelium is composed of two different cell types, a thinner **peg cell** (PC), which bears no cilia but whose apical extent bulges above the ciliated cells. These bulges (*arrowheads*) contain nutritive materials that nourish gametes. The second cell type of the oviduct epithelium is a **ciliated cell** (CL), whose cilia move in unison with those of neighboring cells, propelling the nutrient material toward the uterine lumen.

KEY

BV	vascular elements	Ep	epithelium	L	lumen
BM	basal membrane	GA	Golgi apparatus	LP	lamina propria
CC	ciliated cell	GL	glycogen	N	nucleus
CT	connective tissue	IC	inner circular muscle	PC	peg cell

PLATE 17-4 • Oviduct, Light and Electron Microscopy

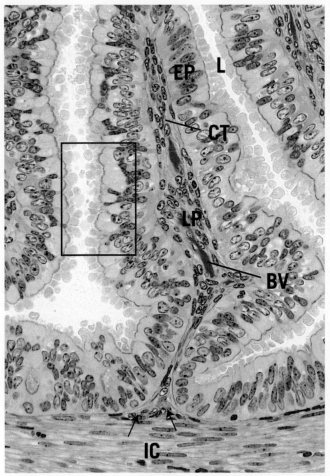

FIGURE 1

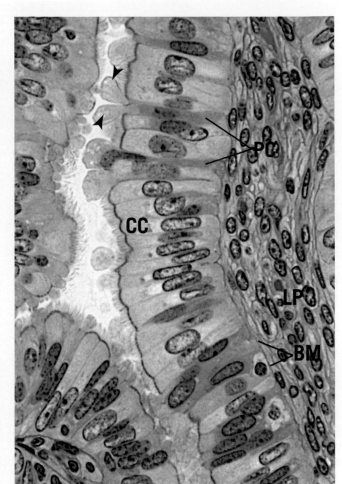

FIGURE 2

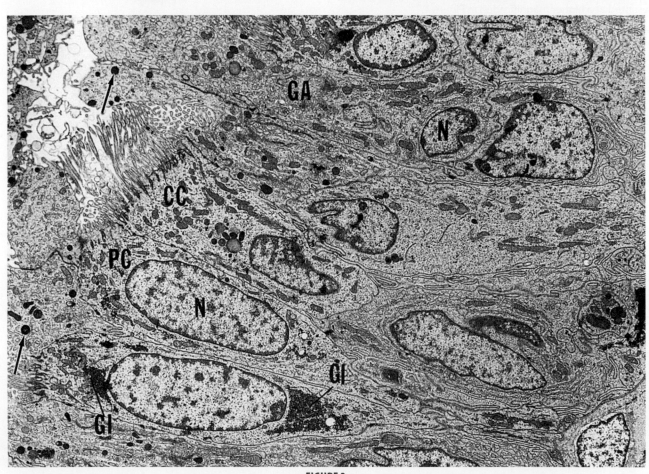

FIGURE 3

FIGURE 1. Uterus. Follicular phase. Human. Paraffin section. ×14.

The uterus is a thick-walled organ whose wall consists of three layers. The external serosa (or in certain regions, adventitia) is unremarkable and is not presented in this photomicrograph. The thick **myometrium** (My) is composed of smooth muscle, subdivided into three poorly delineated layers: **outer longitudinal** (OL), **middle circular** (MC), and **inner longitudinal** (IL). The **endometrium** (En) is subdivided into a **basal layer** (B) and a **functional layer** (F). The functional layer varies in thickness and constitution and passes through a sequence of phases during the menstrual cycle. Note that the functional layer is in the process of being built up and that the forming **glands** (GL) are straight. The deeper aspects of some of these glands display branching (*arrow*). The *boxed area* is presented at a higher magnification in Figure 2.

FIGURE 3. Uterus. Luteal phase. Human. Paraffin section. ×14.

The **myometrium** (My) of the uterus remains constant during the various endometrial phases. Observe its three layers, noting especially that the middle circular layer of smooth muscle is richly vascularized and is therefore frequently referred to as the **stratum vasculare** (SV). The **endometrium** (En) is richly endowed with **glands** (GL) that become highly tortuous in anticipation of the blastocyst that will be nourished by secretions of these glands subsequent to implantation. A region similar to the *boxed area* is presented at a higher magnification in Figure 4.

FIGURE 2. Uterus. Follicular phase. Human. Paraffin section. ×132.

This photomicrograph is a higher magnification of the *boxed area* of Figure 1. Note that the **functional layer** (F) of the endometrium is lined by a simple columnar **epithelium** (Ep) that is displaying mitotic activity (*arrows*). The forming **glands** (GL) also consist of a simple columnar **epithelium** (Ep) whose cells are actively dividing. The **stroma** (St) is highly cellular, as evidenced by the numerous connective tissue cell nuclei visible in this field. Note also the rich **vascular supply** (BV) of the endometrial stroma.

FIGURE 4. Uterus. Early luteal phase. Human. Paraffin section. ×132.

This photomicrograph is a higher magnification of a region similar to the *boxed area* of Figure 3. The functional layer of the endometrium is covered by a simple columnar **epithelium** (Ep), separating the endometrial **stroma** (St) from the uterine **lumen** (L). Note that the **glands** (GL), also composed of simple columnar epithelium, are more abundant than those in the follicular phase (Figure 2, above). Observe also that these glands appear more tortuous and are dilated and their lumina contain a slight amount of secretory product (*arrow*).

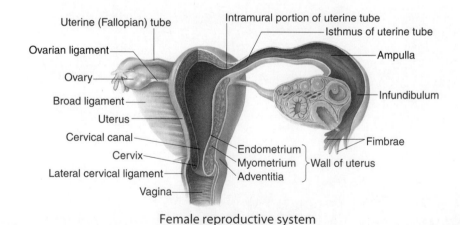

Female reproductive system

KEY					
B	basal layer	GL	gland	OL	outer longitudinal muscle
BV	vascular supply	IL	inner longitudinal muscle	St	stroma
En	endometrium	L	lumen	SV	stratum vasculare
Ep	epithelium	MC	middle circular muscle		
F	functional layer	My	myometrium		

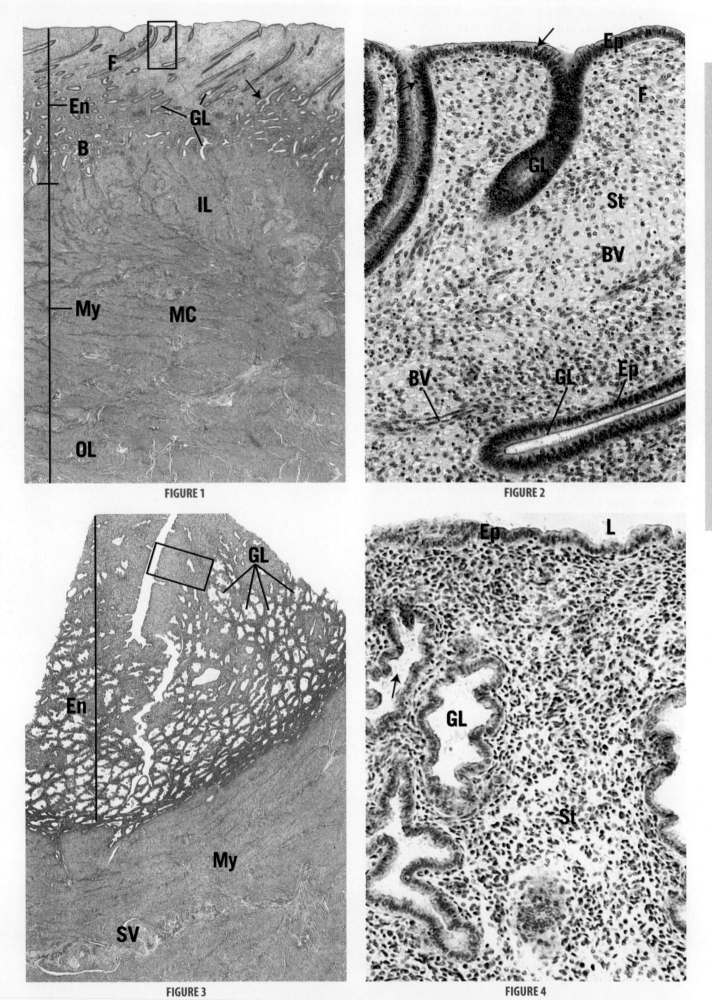

PLATE 17-5 · Uterus

FIGURE 1

FIGURE 2

FIGURE 3

FIGURE 4

PLATE 17-6 · Uterus

FIGURE 1. Uterus. Midluteal phase. Human. Paraffin section. ×270.

During the midluteal phase, the endometrial **glands** (GL) become quite tortuous and corkscrew-shaped, and the simple **columnar cells** (CC) accumulate glycogen (*arrow*). Observe that during this phase of the endometrium, the glycogen is basally located, displacing the **nucleus** (N) toward the center of the cell. Note also that the **stroma** (St) is undergoing a decidual reaction in that some of the connective tissue cells enlarge as they become engorged with lipid and glycogen. A **helical artery** (HA) is evident as several cross sections.

FIGURE 2. Uterus. Late luteal phase. Human. Paraffin section. ×132.

During the late luteal phase of the endometrium, the glands assume a characteristic ladder (or sawtooth) shape (*arrows*). The simple columnar **epithelial cells** (CC) appear pale, and interestingly, the position of the glycogen is now apical (*arrowheads*) rather than basal. The apical location of the glycogen imparts a ragged, torn appearance to the free surface of these cells. Note that the **lumina** (L) of the glands are filled with a glycogen-rich, viscous fluid. Observe also that the **stroma** (St) is infiltrated by numerous **leukocytes** (Le).

FIGURE 3. Uterus. Menstrual phase. Human. Paraffin section. ×132.

The menstrual phase of the endometrium is characterized by periodic constriction and sequential opening of **helical arteries** (HA), resulting in ischemia with subsequent necrosis of the superficial aspect of the functional layer. Due to these spasmodic contractions, sudden spurts of arterial blood detach **necrotic fragments** (NF) of the superficial layers of the endometrium that are then discharged as menstrual flow. The endometrial stroma becomes engorged with blood, increasing the degree of ischemia, and eventually, the entire functional layer is desquamated. Observe that the **lumen** (L) no longer possesses a complete epithelial lining (*arrowheads*). The *boxed area* is presented at a higher magnification in Figure 4.

FIGURE 4. Uterus. Menstrual phase. Human. Paraffin section. ×270.

This photomicrograph is a higher magnification of the *boxed area* of Figure 3. Observe that some of the endometrial **glands** (GL) are torn and a **necrotic fragment** (NF) has been detached from the **functional layer** (F) of the endometrium. The **stroma** (St) is infiltrated by leukocytes, whose dense **nuclei** (N) mask most of the endometrial cells. Note that some of the endometrial cells are still enlarged, indicative of the decidual reaction.

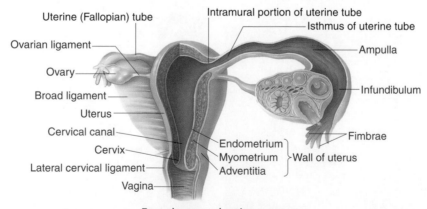

Female reproductive system

KEY							
CC	columnar cell	**HA**	helical artery	**N**	nucleus
F	functional layer	**L**	lumen	**NF**	necrotic fragment
GL	gland	**Le**	leukocyte	**St**	stroma

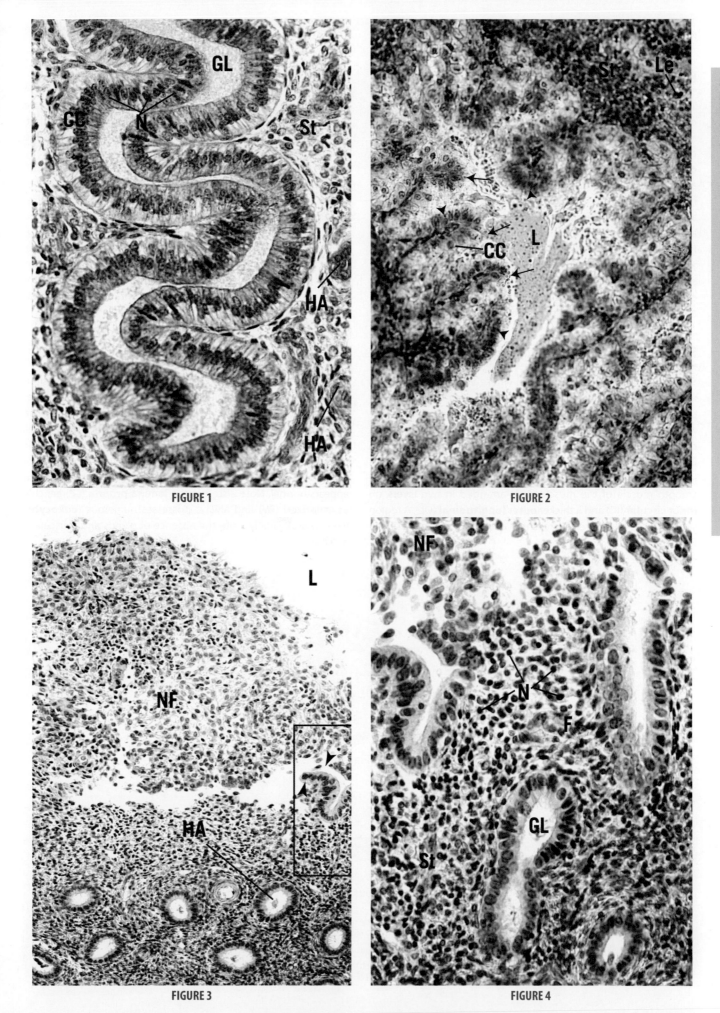

FIGURE 2

FIGURE 3

FIGURE 4

PLATE 17-6 • Uterus

PLATE 17-7 · Placenta and Vagina

FIGURE 1. Placenta. Human. Paraffin section. ×132.

The human placenta is intimately associated with the uterine endometrium. At this junction, the **decidua basalis** (DB) is rich in clumps of large, round to polygonal **decidual cells** (DC), whose distended cytoplasm is filled with lipid and glycogen. Anchoring **chorionic villi** (AV) are attached to the decidua basalis; other villi are blindly ending in the **intervillous space** (IS). These are the most numerous and are referred to as **terminal villi** (TV), most of which are cut in cross or oblique sections. These villi are freely branching and, in the mature placenta, are smaller in diameter than in the immature placenta. *Inset*. **Placenta. Human. Paraffin section.** ×270. Note that the **decidual cells** (DC) are round to polygonal in shape. Their **nuclei** (N) are more or less centrally located, and their cytoplasm appears vacuolated due to the extraction of glycogen and lipids during histologic preparation.

FIGURE 2. Placenta. Human. Paraffin section. ×270.

Cross sections of **terminal villi** (TV) are very simple in the mature placenta. They are surrounded by the **intervillous space** (IS) that, in the functional placenta, is filled with maternal blood. Hence, the cells of the villus act as a placental barrier. This barrier is greatly reduced in the mature placenta, as presented in this photomicrograph. The external layer of the terminal villus is composed of **syncytial trophoblasts** (ST), whose numerous **nuclei** (N) are frequently clustered together as **syncytial knots** (SK). The core of the villus houses numerous fetal **capillaries** (Ca) that are located usually in regions of the villus void of syncytial nuclei (*arrowheads*). Larger fetal **blood vessels** (BV) are also found in the core, surrounded by **mesoderm** (Me). The cytotrophoblasts and phagocytic Hofbauer cells of the immature placenta mostly disappear by the end of the pregnancy.

FIGURE 3. Vagina. l.s. Monkey. Plastic section. ×14.

The vagina is a fibromuscular tube, whose **vaginal space** (VS) is mostly obliterated since its walls are normally in contact with each other. This wall is composed of four layers: **mucosa** (Mu), **submucosa** (SM), **muscularis** (M), and **adventitia** (A). The mucosa consists of an **epithelium** (Ep) and underlying **lamina propria** (LP). Deep to the mucosa is the submucosa, whose numerous large blood vessels impart to it an erectile tissue appearance. The smooth muscle of the muscularis is arranged in two layers, an **inner circular** (IC) and a thicker **outer longitudinal** (OL). A region similar to the *boxed area* is presented at a higher magnification in Figure 4.

FIGURE 4. Vagina. l.s. Human. Paraffin section. ×132.

This photomicrograph is a higher magnification of a region similar to the *boxed area* in Figure 3. The stratified squamous nonkeratinized **epithelium** (Ep) of the vagina is characterized by the empty appearance of the cells, comprising most of its thickness. This is due to the extraction lipids and glycogen during histologic preparation. Observe that the cells in the deeper aspect of the epithelium possess fewer inclusions; therefore, their cytoplasm appears normal. Note also that the **lamina propria** (LP) is richly **vascularized** (BV) and always possesses numerous **leukocytes** (Le) (*arrows*). Finally, note the absence of glands and muscularis mucosae.

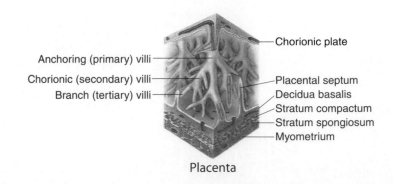

Anchoring (primary) villi
Chorionic (secondary) villi
Branch (tertiary) villi

Chorionic plate
Placental septum
Decidua basalis
Stratum compactum
Stratum spongiosum
Myometrium

Placenta

KEY								
A	adventitia		**IC**	inner circular muscle		**N**	nucleus	
AV	anchoring chorionic villus		**IS**	intervillous space		**OL**	outer longitudinal muscle	
BV	blood vessel		**Mu**	mucosa		**SK**	syncytial knot	
Ca	capillary		**Le**	leukocyte		**SM**	submucosa	
DB	decidua basalis		**LP**	lamina propria		**ST**	syncytial trophoblast	
DC	decidual cell		**M**	muscularis		**TV**	terminal villus	
Ep	epithelium		**Me**	mesoderm		**VS**	vaginal space	

PLATE 17-7 • Placenta and Vagina

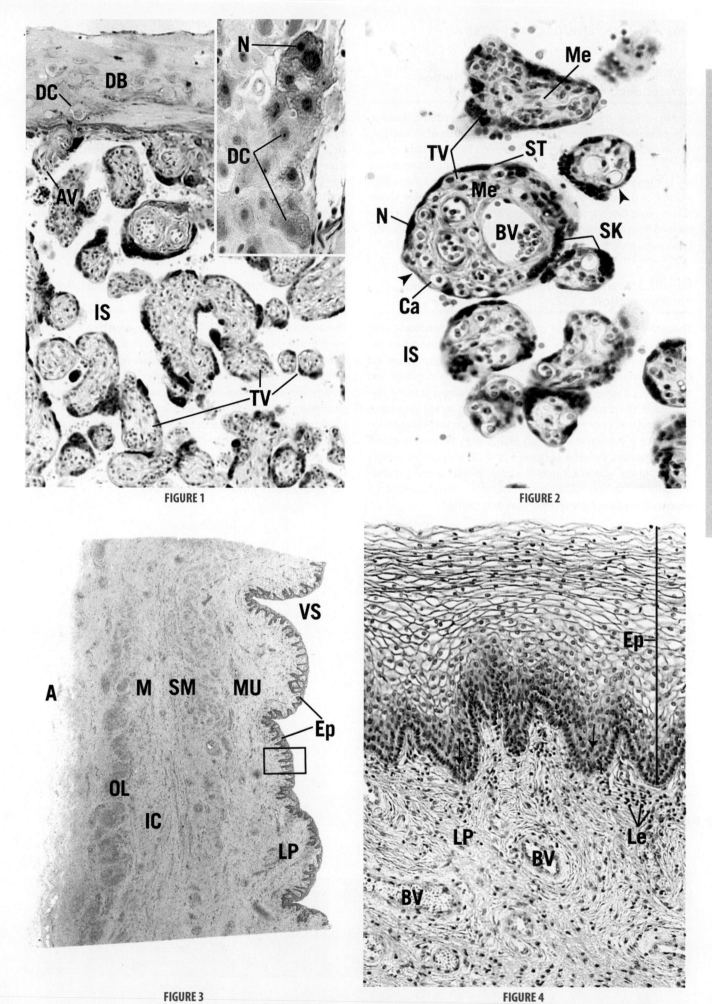

FIGURE 1

FIGURE 2

FIGURE 3

FIGURE 4

PLATE 17-8 · Mammary Gland

FIGURE 1. Mammary gland. Resting. Human. Paraffin section. ×132.

The mammary gland is a modified sweat gland that, in the resting stage, presents **ducts** (D) with occasional **buds of alveoli** (BA) branching from the blind ends of the duct. The remainder of the breast is composed of **dense collagenous connective tissue** (dCT) interspersed with lobules of fat. However, in the immediate vicinity of the ducts and buds of alveoli, the **connective tissue** (CT) is more loosely arranged. It is believed that this looser CT is derived from the papillary layer of the dermis. Compare this photomicrograph with Figure 2.

FIGURE 2. Mammary gland. Lactating. Human. Paraffin section. ×132.

During pregnancy, the **ducts** (D) of the mammary gland undergo major development, in that the buds of alveoli proliferate to form lobules (Lo) composed of numerous alveoli (Al). The interlobular **connective tissue** (CT) becomes reduced to thin sheets in regions; elsewhere it maintains its previous character to support the increased weight of the breast. Observe that the CT in the immediate vicinity of the ducts and lobules (*arrows*) retains its loose consistency. Compare this photomicrograph with Figure 1.

FIGURE 3. Mammary gland. Lactating. Human. Paraffin section. ×132.

The active mammary gland presents numerous **lobules** (Lo) of **alveoli** (Al) that are tightly packed so that the **connective tissue** (CT) elements are greatly compressed. This photomicrograph clearly illustrates the crowded nature of this tissue. Although this tissue bears a superficial resemblance to the histology of the thyroid gland, the presence of ducts and branching alveoli (*arrows*), as well as the lack of colloid material, should assist in distinguishing this tissue as the active mammary gland. *Inset.* **Mammary gland. Active. Human. Paraffin section.** ×270. Observe the branching (*arrows*) of this alveolus, some of whose simple cuboidal **epithelial cells** (Ep) appear vacuolated (*arrowheads*). Note also that the **lumen** (L) contains fatty secretory product (**milk**).

FIGURE 4. Mammary gland. Nipple. Human. Paraffin section. ×14.

The large, conical nipple of the breast is covered by a thin **epidermis** (Ed), composed of stratified squamous keratinized epithelium. Although the nipple possesses neither hair nor sweat glands, it is richly endowed with **sebaceous glands** (SG). The dense irregular collagenous **connective tissue** (CT) core displays numerous longitudinally positioned lactiferous ducts that pierce the tip of the nipple to convey milk to the outside. The lactiferous ducts are surrounded by an extensive network of **smooth muscle** fibers (SM) that are responsible for the erection of the nipple, elevating it to facilitate the suckling process. The region immediately surrounding the nipple is known as the **areola** (Ar).

KEY

AL	alveolus	**D**	duct	**L**	lumen
Ar	areola	**DcT**	dense connective tissue	**Lo**	lobule
BA	buds of alveoli	**Ed**	epidermis	**SM**	smooth muscle
CT	connective tissue	**Ep**	epithelium	**SG**	sebaceous gland

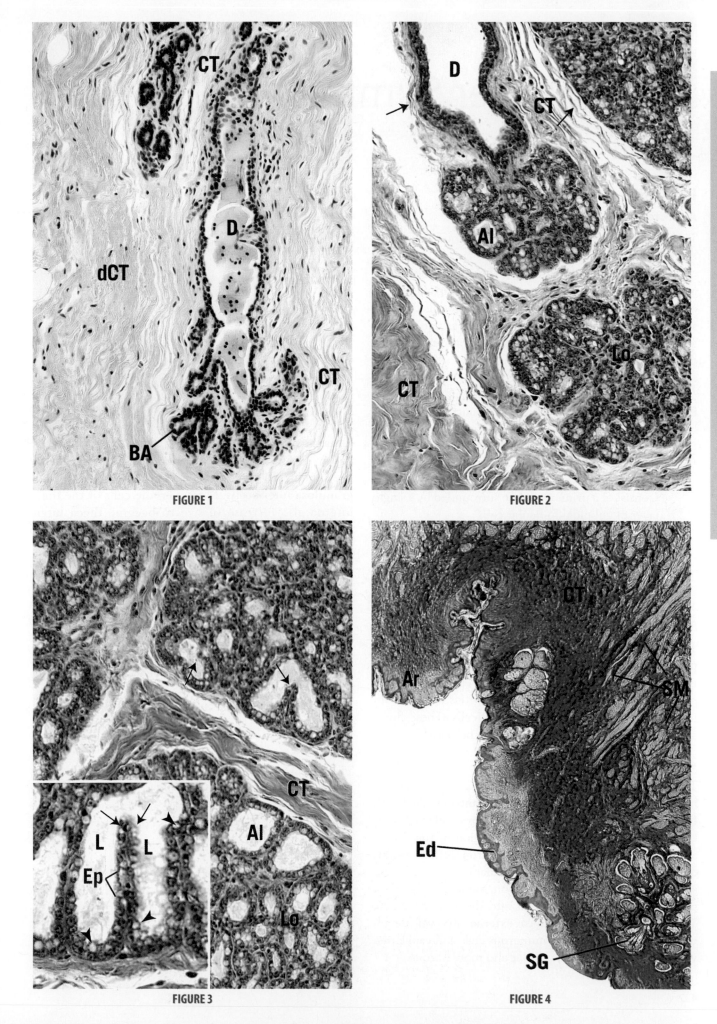

PLATE 17-8 · Mammary Gland

FIGURE 1

FIGURE 2

FIGURE 3

FIGURE 4

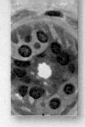

Chapter Summary

I. OVARY

A. Cortex

The **cortex** of the **ovary** is covered by a modified mesothelium, the **germinal epithelium**. Deep to this simple cuboidal to simple squamous epithelium is the **tunica albuginea**, the fibrous connective tissue capsule of the ovary. The remainder of the ovarian connective tissue is more cellular and is referred to as the **stroma**. The cortex houses ovarian **follicles** in various stages of development.

1. Primordial Follicles

Primordial follicles consist of a **primary oocyte** surrounded by a single layer of flattened **follicular (granulosa) cells**.

2. Primary Follicles

a. Unilaminar Primary Follicles
Consist of a **primary oocyte** surrounded by a single layer of cuboidal **follicular cells**

b. Multilaminar Primary Follicles
Consist of a **primary oocyte** surrounded by several layers of **follicular cells**. The **zona pellucida** is visible. The **theca interna** is beginning to be organized.

3. Secondary (Vesicular) Follicle

The **secondary follicle** is distinguished from the primary multilaminar follicle by its larger size, by a well-established **theca interna** and **theca externa**, and especially by the presence of **follicular fluid** in small cavities formed from intercellular spaces of the **follicular cells**. These fluid-filled cavities are known as **Call-Exner bodies**.

4. Graafian (Mature) Follicles

The **Graafian follicle** is very large; the Call-Exner bodies have coalesced into a single space, the **antrum**, filled with **follicular fluid**. The wall of the antrum is referred to as the **membrana granulosa**, and the region of the oocyte and follicular cells jutting into the antrum is the **cumulus oophorus**. The single layer of follicular cells immediately surrounding the oocyte is the **corona radiata**. Long apical processes of these cells extend into the **zona pellucida**. The **theca interna** and **theca externa** are well developed; the former displays numerous cells and capillaries, whereas the latter is less cellular and more fibrous.

5. Atretic Follicles

Atretic follicles are in the state of degeneration. They are characterized in later stages by the presence of **fibroblasts** in the follicle and a degenerated oocyte.

B. Medulla

The **medulla** of the ovary is composed of a relatively loose fibroelastic connective tissue housing an extensive **vascular** supply, including spiral arteries and convoluted veins.

C. Corpus Luteum

Subsequent to the extrusion of the **secondary oocyte** with its attendant **follicular cells**, the remnant of the **Graafian follicle** becomes partly filled with blood and is known as the **corpus hemorrhagicum**. Cells of the **membrana granulosa** are transformed into large **granulosa lutein cells**. Moreover, the cells of the **theca interna** also increase in size to become **theca lutein cells**, although they remain smaller than the **granulosa lutein cells**.

D. Corpus Albicans

The **corpus albicans** is a **corpus luteum** that is in the process of involution and hyalinization. It becomes fibrotic, with few **fibroblasts** among the intercellular materials. Eventually, the corpus albicans will become **scar tissue** on the ovarian surface.

II. GENITAL DUCTS

A. Oviduct

1. Mucosa

The **mucosa** of the oviduct is highly folded in the **infundibulum** and **ampulla**. It is composed of a loose, cellular connective tissue, **lamina propria**, and a **simple columnar epithelial** lining. The epithelium is composed of **peg cells** and **ciliated cells**.

2. Muscularis

The **muscle coat** is composed of an **inner circular** and an **outer longitudinal smooth muscle layer**.

3. Serosa

The oviduct is invested by a **serosa**.

B. Uterus

1. Endometrium

The **endometrium** is subdivided into a **basal** and a **functional layer**. It is lined by a **simple columnar epithelium**. The **lamina propria** varies with the phases of the menstrual cycle.

a. Follicular Phase

The **glands** are straight and display mitotic figures, and the helical arteries grow into the functional layer.

b. Luteal Phase

Glands become tortuous, and the **helical arteries** become coiled. The **lumina** of the glands accumulate **secretory products**. **Fibroblasts** enlarge and accumulate glycogen.

c. Menstrual Phase

The **functional layer** is desquamated, and the lamina propria displays extravasated blood.

2. Myometrium

The **myometrium** is thick and consists of three poorly delineated **smooth muscle** layers: **inner longitudinal**, **middle circular**, and **outer longitudinal**. During pregnancy, the myometrium increases in size as a result of hypertrophy of existing muscle cells and the accumulation of new smooth muscle cells.

3. Serosa

Most of the uterus is covered by a **serosa**; the remainder is attached to surrounding tissues by an **adventitia**.

C. Placenta

1. Decidua Basalis

The **decidua basalis**, the maternally derived **endometrial layer**, is characterized by the presence of large, glycogen-rich **decidual cells**. **Coiled arteries** and straight **veins** open into the labyrinth-like **intervillous spaces**.

2. Chorionic Plate and Villi

The **chorionic plate** is a region of the **chorionic sac** of the fetus from which **chorionic villi** extend into the intervillous spaces of the **decidua basalis**. Each villus has a core of **fibromuscular connective tissue** surrounding **capillaries** (derived from the umbilical vessels). The villus is covered by **trophoblast cells**. During the first half of pregnancy, there are two layers of trophoblast cells, an inner cuboidal layer of **cytotrophoblasts** and an outer layer of **syncytiotrophoblasts**. During the second half of pregnancy, only the **syncytiotrophoblasts** remain. However, at points where chorionic villi are anchored into the decidua basalis, **cytotrophoblasts** are present.

D. Vagina

1. Mucosa

The vagina is lined by a **stratified squamous nonkeratinized epithelium**. The **lamina propria**, composed of a **fibroelastic connective tissue**, possesses no glands. The **mucosa** is thrown into longitudinal folds known as **rugae**.

2. Submucosa

The **submucosa** is also composed of a fibroelastic type of connective tissue housing numerous blood vessels.

3. Muscularis

The **muscularis** is composed of interlacing bundles of **smooth muscle fibers**. Near its external orifice, the vagina is equipped with a **skeletal muscle sphincter**.

4. Adventitia

The vagina is connected to surrounding structures via its **adventitia**.

E. Mammary Glands

1. Resting Gland

The **resting gland** is composed mainly of **dense irregular collagenous connective tissue** interspersed with lobules of **adipose tissue** and numerous **ducts**. Frequently, at the blind ends of ducts, **buds of alveoli** and attendant **myoepithelial cells** are present.

2. Lactating Gland

The **mammary gland** becomes active during pregnancy and lactation. The expanded **alveoli** that form numerous lobules are composed of **simple cuboidal cells**, resembling the thyroid gland. However, the presence of **ducts** and **myoepithelial cells** provides distinguishing characteristics. **Alveoli** and the **lumen** of the ducts may contain a fatty secretory product.

3. Areola and Nipple

The **areola** is composed of thin, **pigmented epidermis** displaying large **apocrine areolar glands**. Additionally, **sweat** and large **sebaceous glands** are also present. The **dermis** presents numerous **smooth muscle fibers**. The **nipple** possesses several minute pores representing the distal ends of **lactiferous ducts**. These ducts arise from **lactiferous sinuses**, enlarged reservoirs at the base of the nipple. The **epidermis** covering the nipple is thin, and the dermis is richly supplied by **smooth muscle fibers** and **nerve endings**. Although the nipple possesses no hair follicles or sweat glands, it is richly endowed with **sebaceous glands**.

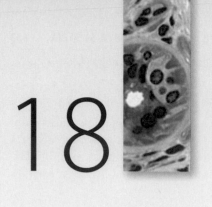

18 MALE REPRODUCTIVE SYSTEM

The male reproductive system (see Graphic 18-1) consists of the two testes (the male gonads), a system of genital ducts, accessory glands, and the penis. The male reproductive system functions in the formation of spermatozoa, the elaboration of male sex hormones, and the delivery of male gametes into the female reproductive tract.

TESTES

Each **testis** is an oval structure housed in its separate compartment within the scrotum. The **tunica albuginea**, the fibromuscular connective tissue capsule of the testis, is thickened at the **mediastinum testis**, from which septa are derived to subdivide the testis into approximately 250 small, incomplete compartments, known as the **lobuli testis**.

- Each lobule houses one to four highly tortuous **seminiferous tubules** that function in the production of **spermatozoa**.
- The highly vascular connective tissue surrounding the seminiferous tubules houses **Leydig's cells (interstitial cells of Leydig)**.
- The wall of the seminiferous tubule is composed of the **seminiferous epithelium** lining its lumen and a slender connective tissue **tunica propria**.
  - The **seminiferous epithelium** is several cell layers thick and is separated from the tunica propria by a basement membrane.
    - The **basal cells** of this epithelium, composed of Sertoli cells and three types of spermatogonia, **dark type A**, **pale type A,** and **type B spermatogonia**, sit on the basement membrane.
      - **Sertoli cells** (see Table 18-1) are supporting cells that form tight junctions with each other

subdividing the lumen of the seminiferous tubule into a **basal compartment** and an **adluminal compartment**, thus establishing a **blood-testis barrier** that protects the developing germ cells and spermatozoa from an autoimmune response.
      - **Spermatogonia** are responsible for spermatogenesis.
    - The cells of the adluminal compartment are **primary spermatocytes**, **secondary spermatocytes**, **spermatids**, and **spermatozoa**.
  - The **tunica propria** of the seminiferous tubule of humans is composed of slender type I collagen fibers interspersed with **fibroblasts** and, perhaps, some **myocytes**.

Spermatogenesis

Spermatogenesis, the process of producing haploid male gametes, is dependent on several hormones that are released at puberty from the adenohypophysis, including **luteinizing hormone (LH)**, **prolactin**, and **follicle-stimulating hormone (FSH)** (see Graphic 18-2). In the mature male, approximately 300 million spermatozoa are produced daily.

- **Prolactin** induces the interstitial cells of Leydig to express **LH receptors**.
  - LH binds to its receptors on the Leydig cells prompting these cells to secrete **testosterone**.
- **FSH** causes **Sertoli cells** to produce **adenylate cyclase**, which, via a cAMP intermediary, stimulates the production of **androgen binding protein (ABP)**.
  - ABP binds with and maintains a high enough concentration of **testosterone** and **dihydrotestosterone** (a transformation product of testosterone by the enzyme **5α reductase**) in the seminiferous epithelium for spermatogenesis to occur.
- **Testosterone** acts as a **negative feedback** for LH release, and **inhibin**, produced by Sertoli cells, inhibits the release of FSH,
- **Activin**, also produced by Sertoli cells, enhances FSH release.
- For spermatogenesis to proceed normally, the testes must be maintained at 35°C, the temperature inside the **scrotum**, a level that is slightly *below* normal body temperature.

Spermatogenesis takes 74 days to be completed, and it occurs in a cyclic but asynchronous fashion along the length of the seminiferous tubule. These **cycles of the seminiferous epithelium** consist of repeated aggregates of cells in varying stages of development. Each aggregate is composed of groups of cells that are connected

TABLE 18-1 • Functions of Sertoli Cells	
During Gestation	**After Puberty**
Synthesize and release antimullerian hormone to suppress the formation of the female genital system and support the development of the male genital system	Physical and nutritional support of developing germ cells Synthesize and release testicular transferrin to transfer iron from serum transferrin to developing germ cells Synthesize and release ABP* Establish blood-testis barrier Phagocytose cytoplasm shed during spermiogenesis Synthesize and release inhibin Secrete fructose-rich medium to provide nutrients for spermatozoa released into the male genital ducts

*ABP, androgen binding protein

to one another by **intercellular bridges**, forming a synchronized syncytium that migrates toward the lumen of the seminiferous tubule as a unit. The three phases of spermatogenesis are **spermatocytogenesis**, **meiosis**, and **spermiogenesis**.

- **Spermatocytogenesis** is a process involving *mitosis*, in which **pale type A spermatogonia** divide to form two types of spermatogonia, more pale type A as well as **type B** spermatogonia, both of which are diploid.
  - **Dark type A spermatogonia** represent a reserve population of cells that normally do not undergo cell division, but when they do, they form pale type A spermatogonia.
  - Type B spermatogonia divide via mitosis to form diploid **primary spermatocytes**. All spermatogonia are located in the **basal compartment**, whereas primary spermatocytes migrate into the **adluminal compartment**.
- **Meiosis phase** starts when primary spermatocytes (**4CDNA** content) undergo the first meiotic division, forming two short-lived **secondary spermatocytes** (**2CDNA** content).
  - Secondary spermatocytes do not replicate their DNA but immediately start the second meiotic division, and each forms two **haploid (N) spermatids**.
- **Spermiogenesis** (Graphic 18-2) is the process of cytodifferentiation of the spermatids into spermatozoa and involves no cell division.
  - The spermatid loses much of its cytoplasm (which is phagocytosed by Sertoli cells), forms an **acrosomal granule**, a long **cilium**, and associated **outer dense fibers** and a **coarse fibrous sheath**.
  - The **spermatozoon** that is formed and released into the lumen of the seminiferous tubule is **nonmotile** and is incapable of fertilizing an ovum.
  - The spermatozoa remain immotile until just before they leave the epididymis. They become capable of fertilizing once they have been **capacitated** in the female reproductive system.

GENITAL DUCTS

A system of **genital ducts** conveys the spermatozoa and the fluid component of the semen to the outside.

- The **seminiferous tubules** are connected by short, straight tubules, the **tubuli recti**, to the **rete testis**, which is composed of labyrinthine spaces located in the **mediastinum testis**.
- From the rete testis spermatozoa enter the first part of the epididymis, the 15 to 20 **ductuli efferentes** that lead into the **ductus epididymis**.

- The **head of the epididymis** is composed of the ductuli efferentes,
- The **body and tail of the epididymis** are 5 m long and are highly folded and form the ductus epididymis (Graphic 18-1).
- The wall of the epididymis is composed of a **smooth muscle coat** surrounding a loose connective tissue and a **pseudostratified stereociliated epithelium** that lines the lumen, where the epithelium is separated from the connective tissue by a basement membrane.
- The epithelium is composed of short **basal cells** and tall **principal cells**.
  - The **basal cells** are regenerative cells.
  - The **principal cells** sport stereocilia (long, nonmotile microvilli) that phagocytose cytoplasmic remnants from spermiogenesis, phagocytose luminal fluid, and synthesize and release **surface-activated decapacitation factor (glycerophosphocholine)**.
- Spermatozoa become **motile** near the end of the body of the epididymis.
- The head of spermatozoa pick up **surface-activated decapacitation factor** from the fluid present in the lumen of the epididymis, which prevents them from being able to fertilize an ovum until that factor is removed from their plasma membrane in the female genital tract.

The thick, muscular **ductus deferens,** the continuation of the tail of the epididymis, passes through the inguinal canal, as a part of the spermatic cord, to gain access to the abdominal cavity.

- Just prior to reaching the prostate gland, the **seminal vesicle** empties its secretions into the ductus deferens, which terminates at this point.
- The continuation of the ductus deferens, known as the **ejaculatory duct**, enters the **prostate gland**, which delivers its secretory product into the ejaculatory duct.
  - The right and left **ejaculatory ducts** empty into the **urethra**, which conveys both urine and **semen** to the outside.
- The **urethra**, which passes through the length of the penis, has three regions: **prostatic, membranous,** and **cavernous (spongy)** portions.

ACCESSORY GLANDS

The three **accessory glands** of the male reproductive system, which supply the fluid component of semen, are the two **seminal vesicles** and the **prostate gland**. Additionally, a pair of small **bulbourethral glands** deliver their viscous secretions into the cavernous (spongy) urethra that lubricates the urethra.

- Each **seminal vesicle**, a long, narrow gland that is highly folded on itself, produces a rich, nutritive substance with a characteristic yellow color that supplies a fructose-rich secretion for the spermatozoa.
- The **prostate gland** is composed of numerous individual glands that surround, and whose ducts pierce, the wall of the urethra. These glands are distributed in three regions of the prostate and are therefore categorized as **mucosal**, **submucosal**, and **external (main) prostatic glands**.
  - The **secretion** of the prostate gland is a whitish, thin fluid containing **fibrinolysin**, **citric acid**, **serine protease (prostate-specific antigen, PSA)**, and **acid phosphatase**.
  - **Prostatic concretions** are frequently found in the lumina of the prostate gland.

PENIS

The **penis**, the male organ of copulation, is normally in the flaccid state. During erotic stimulation, however, its three cylindrical bodies of erectile tissues become distended with blood. The fluid turgid pressure within the vascular spaces of the erectile tissues greatly enlarges the penis, causing it to become erect and hard. Subsequent to ejaculation or the termination of erotic stimulation, detumescence follows and the penis returns to its flaccid state.

Erection and Ejaculation

The **penis,** during **copulation,** delivers spermatozoa-containing **semen** to the female reproductive tract. It is also the excretory organ for urine. The penis is covered by skin and is composed of three **erectile bodies**, the two **corpora cavernosa** and the ventrally positioned **corpus spongiosum (urethrae)**.

- Each erectile body, housing large, endothelially lined **cavernous spaces**, is surrounded by a thick connective tissue capsule, the **tunica albuginea**.
  - The erectile bodies are supplied by **helicine arteries** that are usually bypassed via arteriovenous shunts, maintaining the penis in a flaccid state.
  - **Parasympathetic impulses** to these shunts cause vasoconstriction, directing blood into the helicine arteries and thus into the cavernous spaces.
  - The erectile bodies (especially the corpora cavernosa) become engorged with blood, and the penis becomes **erect**.

Subsequent to ejaculation or in the absence of continued stimulation, parasympathetic stimulation ceases; blood flow to the helicine arteries is diminished; blood slowly leaves the cavernous spaces; and the penis returns to its flaccid condition.

- **Ejaculation** is the forceful expulsion of **semen** from the male reproductive tract.
  - The force required for ejaculation is derived from rhythmic contraction of the thick smooth muscle layers of the **ductus (vas) deferens** and the rapid contraction of the **bulbospongiosus muscle**.
- Each ejaculate contains spermatozoa suspended in **seminal fluid**.
- The accessory glands of the male reproductive system, the **prostate** and **bulbourethral glands**, as well as the **seminal vesicles** (and even the glands of Littré) contribute to the formation of the fluid portion of semen.
- Secretions of the **bulbourethral glands** lubricate the urethra, whereas secretions of the prostate assist the spermatozoa in achieving motility by neutralizing the acidic secretions of the ductus deferens and of the female reproductive tract.
- Approximately 70% of the fluid portion of the semen is due to the secretions of the seminal vesicles.

CLINICAL CONSIDERATIONS

Cryptorchidism

Cryptorchidism is a developmental defect in which one or both testes fail to descend into the scrotum. When neither descends, it results in sterility because normal body temperature inhibits spermatogenesis. Usually, the condition can be surgically corrected; however, the patient's sperm may be abnormal.

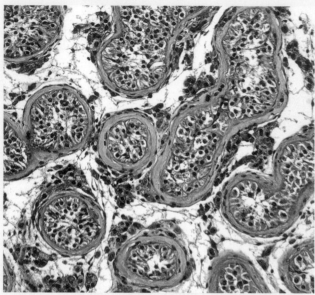

This figure is from the testis of a postpubertal patient demonstrating the absence of spermatogenesis in the seminiferous tubule as well as a very thick, hyalinized basement membrane. (Reprinted with permission from Rubin R, Strayer D, et al., eds. Rubin's Pathology. Clinicopathologic Foundations of Medicine, 5th ed., Baltimore: Lippincott Williams & Wilkins, 2008, p. 763.)

Vasectomy

Vasectomy is a method of sterilization that is performed by making a small slit in the wall of the scrotum through which the ductus deferens is severed.

A normal **ejaculate** averages about 3 mL of semen that contains 60 to 100 million spermatozoa per mL. It is interesting to note that about 20% of the ejaculated spermatozoa are abnormal and 25% immotile. An individual producing less than 20 million spermatozoa per milliliter of ejaculate is considered **sterile**.

Benign Prostatic Hypertrophy

The prostate gland undergoes hypertrophy with age, resulting in benign prostatic hypertrophy, a condition that may constrict the urethral lumen resulting in difficulty in urination. At age 50, about 40% of the male population is affected, and at age 80, about 95% of the male population is affected by this condition.

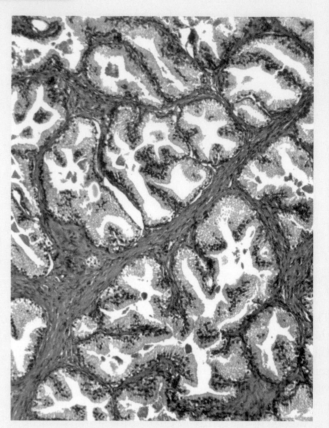

This photomicrograph is from a patient with nodular hyperplasia of the prostate. Observe that the gland is displaying cellular hypertrophy of the epithelium whose folding, in places, partially occludes its lumen. (Reprinted with permission from Rubin R, Strayer, D, et al., eds. Rubin's Pathology. Clinicopathologic Foundations of Medicine, 5th ed., Baltimore: Lippincott Williams & Wilkins, 2008, p. 774.)

Adenocarcinoma of the Prostate

Adenocarcinoma of the prostate affects about 30% of the male population over 75 years of age. Although this carcinoma is slow growing, it may metastasize to the bone. Analysis of elevated levels of **prostate-specific antigen** (**PSA**) in the bloodstream is utilized as an early diagnostic test for prostatic cancer. Biopsy is required for accurate diagnosis.

Testicular Cancer

Testicular cancer affects mostly men younger than 40 years of age. It is discovered on palpation as a lump in the scrotum. If the lump is not associated with the testis, it is usually benign, whereas if it is associated with the testis it is usually malignant; therefore, a lump noticed on the testis, whether or not it is painful, should be examined by a physician. Frequently, individuals with testicular cancer present with elevated blood **alpha-fetoprotein** and **human chorionic gonadotropin** levels.

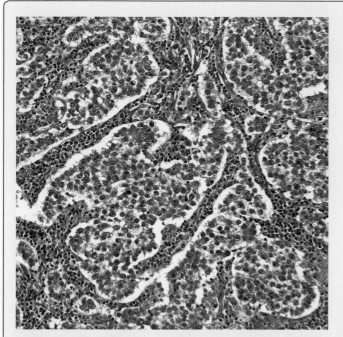

This figure is from the testis of a patient with a form of a testicular cancer known as seminoma. Observe the clusters of tumor cells with large nuclei. These cells are enveloped by a connective tissue septum that appears quite cellular due to the lymphocytic infiltration. (Reprinted with permission from Rubin, R, Strayer, D, et al., eds. Rubin's Pathology. Clinicopathologic Foundations of Medicine, 5th ed., Baltimore: Lippincott Williams & Wilkins, 2008, p. 769.)

Balanoposthitis

Accumulation of a thick, yellowish-white exudate underneath the foreskin of uncircumcised men can be a breeding ground for yeast and bacteria that, if not cleaned, may cause inflammation of the foreskin, known as **posthitis**, as well as inflammation of the glans penis, known as **balanitis**. When the two occur together, the condition is known as **balanoposthitis**. The condition may be accompanied by redness, pain, and itching as well as a swelling of the glans with a concomitant stricture of the urethra.

Phimosis

Phimosis, a tight foreskin that cannot easily be pulled over the glans penis, is a normal condition in uncircumcised infants, but in mature men, the condition can be very painful and may result in interference with urination and sexual activity. As the penis becomes erect, the foreskin cannot expand to accommodate the increase girth and may result in balanoposthitis and urinary tract infections. Circumcision can usually alleviate this condition.

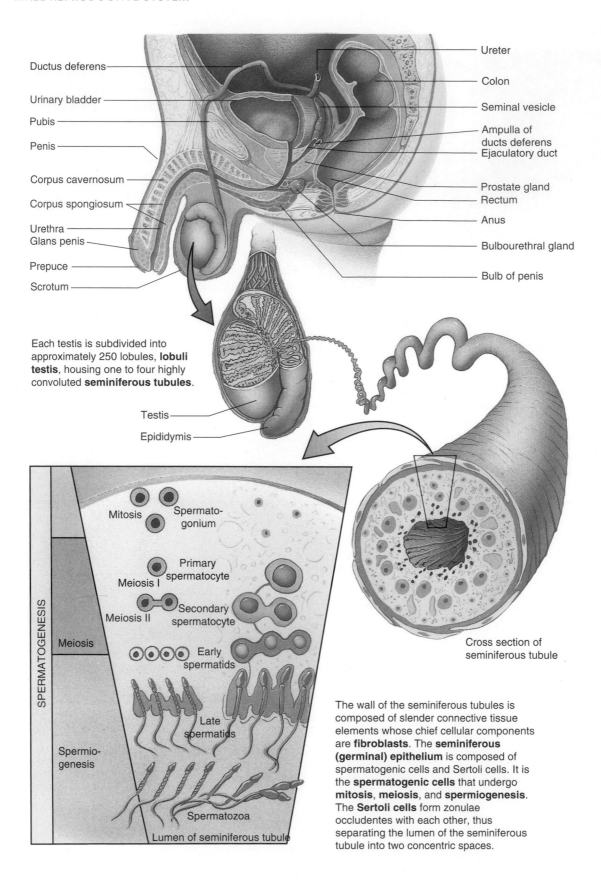

Ductus deferens

Urinary bladder

Pubis

Penis

Corpus cavernosum

Corpus spongiosum

Urethra

Glans penis

Prepuce

Scrotum

Ureter

Colon

Seminal vesicle

Ampulla of ducts deferens

Ejaculatory duct

Prostate gland

Rectum

Anus

Bulbourethral gland

Bulb of penis

Each testis is subdivided into approximately 250 lobules, **lobuli testis**, housing one to four highly convoluted **seminiferous tubules**.

Testis

Epididymis

SPERMATOGENESIS

Mitosis

Spermato-gonium

Primary spermatocyte

Meiosis I

Secondary spermatocyte

Meiosis II

Meiosis

Early spermatids

Late spermatids

Spermio-genesis

Spermatozoa

Lumen of seminiferous tubule

Cross section of seminiferous tubule

The wall of the seminiferous tubules is composed of slender connective tissue elements whose chief cellular components are **fibroblasts**. The **seminiferous (germinal) epithelium** is composed of spermatogenic cells and Sertoli cells. It is the **spermatogenic cells** that undergo **mitosis, meiosis,** and **spermiogenesis**. The **Sertoli cells** form zonulae occludentes with each other, thus separating the lumen of the seminiferous tubule into two concentric spaces.

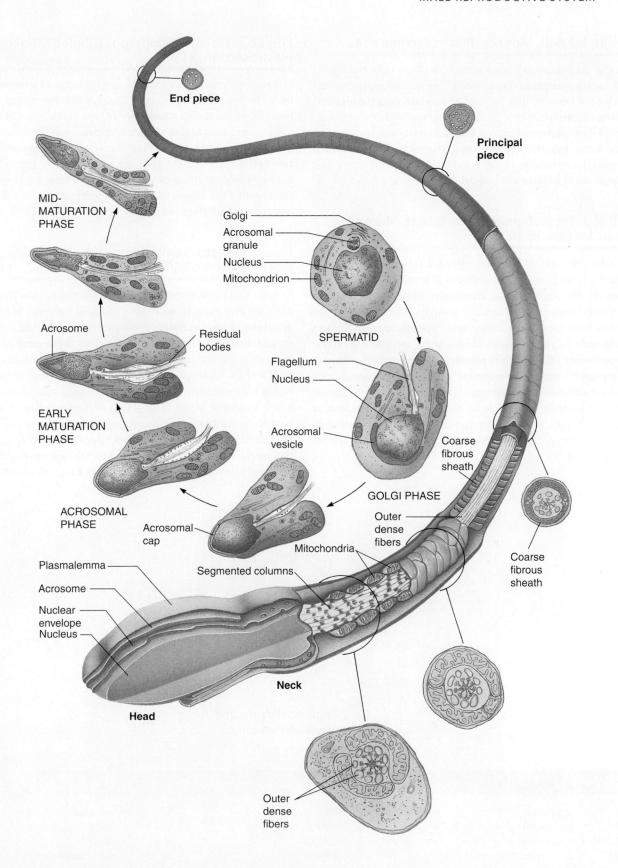

End piece

Principal piece

MID-MATURATION PHASE

Golgi

Acrosomal granule

Nucleus

Mitochondrion

Acrosome

Residual bodies

SPERMATID

Flagellum

Nucleus

Acrosomal vesicle

Coarse fibrous sheath

EARLY MATURATION PHASE

ACROSOMAL PHASE

Acrosomal cap

GOLGI PHASE

Outer dense fibers

Mitochondria

Coarse fibrous sheath

Plasmalemma

Segmented columns

Acrosome

Nuclear envelope

Nucleus

Neck

Head

Outer dense fibers

PLATE 18-1 · Testis

FIGURE 1. Testis. Monkey. Plastic section. ×14.

This low magnification photomicrograph of the testis displays its thick **tunica albuginea** (TA) as well as the slender **septa** (Se) that attach to it. Observe that sections of **seminiferous tubules** (ST) present various geometric profiles, attesting to their highly convoluted form. Note that each **lobule** (Lo) is densely packed with seminiferous tubules, and the connective tissue stroma (*arrows*) occupies the remaining space. A region similar to the *boxed area* is presented at a higher magnification in Figure 2.

FIGURE 3. Testis. Seminiferous tubule. Monkey. Plastic section. ×540.

The adjacent walls of two **seminiferous tubules** (ST), in close proximity to each other, are composed of **myoid cells** (MC), **fibroblasts** (F), and fibromuscular **connective tissue** (CT). The stratified **seminiferous epithelium** (SE) is separated from the tubular wall by a basal membrane (*arrowheads*). **Spermatogonia** (Sg) and **Sertoli cells** (SC) lie on the basal membrane and are in the **basal compartment** (BC), whereas **primary spermatocytes** (PS), secondary spermatocytes, **spermatids** (Sp), and **spermatozoa** (Sz) are in the **adluminal compartment** (AC). Observe that the **lumen** (L) of the seminiferous tubule contains spermatozoa as well as cellular debris discarded during the transformation of spermatids into spermatozoa. Compare the cells of the seminiferous epithelium with those of Figure 4.

FIGURE 2. Testis. Seminiferous tubules. Monkey. Plastic section. ×132.

This photomicrograph is a higher magnification of a region similar to the *boxed area* of Figure 1. Observe that the **tunica vasculosa** (TV) of the **tunica albuginea** (TA) is a highly vascular region (*arrows*) and that **blood vessels** (BV) penetrate the lobuli testis in connective tissue **septa** (Se). The walls of the **seminiferous tubules** (ST) are closely apposed to each other (*arrowheads*), although in certain regions the cellular **stroma** (St) is evident. Observe that the **lumen** (L) of the seminiferous tubule is lined by a stratified **seminiferous epithelium** (SE).

FIGURE 4. Testis. Seminiferous tubule. Monkey. Plastic section. ×540.

Observe that the fibromuscular walls of the two tubular cross sections are very close to each other (*arrows*); however, in regions, **arterioles** (A) and **venules** (V) are evident. The **Sertoli cells** (SC) may be recognized by their pale nuclei and dense **nucleoli** (n). In comparing the **seminiferous epithelia** (SE) of the tubules in the right and left halves of this photomicrograph, as well as those of Figure 3, it should be noted that their cellular compositions are different, indicative of the cyclic stages of the seminiferous epithelium. Note also that three types of spermatogonia are recognizable by their nuclear characteristics: **dark spermatogonia A** (Ad) possessing dark, flattened nuclei; **pale spermatogonia A** (Ap) with flattened pale nuclei; and **spermatogonia B** (B) with round nuclei.

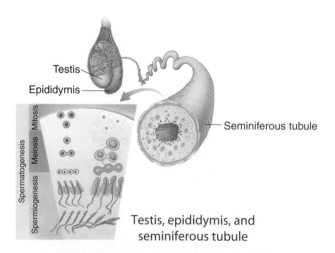

Testis, epididymis, and seminiferous tubule

KEY

A	arterioles	L	lumen	Sp	spermatid
AC	adluminal compartment	Lo	lobule	ST	seminiferous tubules
Ad	dark spermatogonia A	MC	myoid cell	St	stroma
Ap	pale spermatogonia A	n	nucleoli	Sz	spermatozoa
B	spermatogonia B	PS	primary spermatocyte	TA	tunica albuginea
BC	basal compartment	SC	Sertoli cell	TV	tunica vasculosa
BV	blood vessel	SE	seminiferous epithelium	V	venule
CT	connective tissue	Se	septum		
F	fibroblast	Sg	spermatogonia		

PLATE 18-1 · Testis

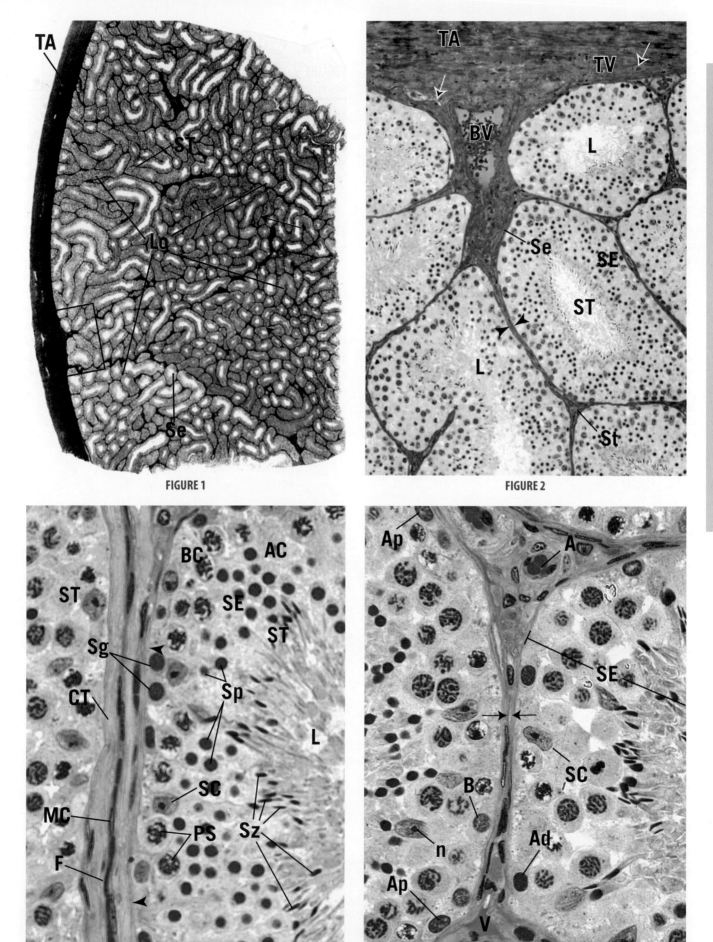

FIGURE 1

FIGURE 2

FIGURE 3

FIGURE 4

PLATE 18-2 · Testis and Epididymis

FIGURE 1. Interstitial cells. Testis. Monkey. Plastic section. ×270.

The **stroma** (St) surrounding **seminiferous tubules** (ST) possesses a rich **vascular supply** (BV) as well as extensive **lymphatic drainage** (LV). Much of the vascular elements are associated with the endocrine cells of the testis, the **interstitial cells of Leydig** (IC), which produce testosterone. *Inset.* **Interstitial cells. Testis. Monkey. Plastic section.** ×540. The **interstitial cells** (IC), located in small clumps, are recognizable by their round-to-oval **nuclei** (N) and the presence of lipid (*arrow*) within their cytoplasm.

FIGURE 3. Ductuli efferentes. Human. Paraffin section. ×132.

The first part of the epididymis, the **ductuli efferentes** (De), receives **spermatozoa** (Sz) from the rete testis. The lumina of the ductuli are lined by a simple columnar **epithelium** (Ep), composed of tall and short cells, which are responsible for the characteristic fluted (uneven) appearance of these tubules. The thick fibroelastic **connective tissue** (CT) wall of the ductuli houses numerous smooth muscle cells (SM).

FIGURE 2. Rete testis. Human. Paraffin section. ×132.

The **rete testis** (RT), located in the **mediastinum testis** (MT), is composed of labyrinthine, anastomosing spaces lined by a simple cuboidal **epithelium** (Ep). The dense collagenous **connective tissue** (CT) of the mediastinum testis is evident, as are the profiles of **seminiferous tubules** (ST). Spermatozoa gain access to the rete testis via the short, straight **tubuli recti** (TR).

FIGURE 4. Ductus epididymis. Monkey. Plastic section. ×132.

The **ductus epididymis** (DE) may be distinguished from the ductuli efferentes with relative ease. Note that the **nuclei** (N) of the pseudostratified **epithelial lining** (Ep) are of two types, oval and round, whereas those of the ductuli are round. Observe that the lumen contains numerous **spermatozoa** (Sz) and that the epithelium sits on a basal lamina. The connective tissue wall of the ductus epididymis may be differentiated easily from its circularly arranged **smooth muscle coat** (SM).

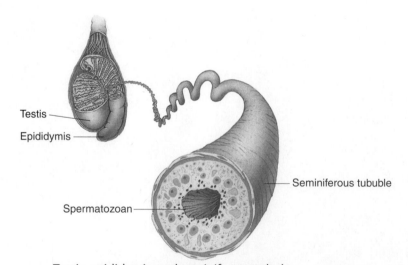

Testis

Epididymis

Seminiferous tubule

Spermatozoan

Testis, epididymis, and seminiferous tubule

KEY					
BV	blood vessel	**IC**	interstitial cells of Leydig	**SM**	smooth muscle
CT	connective tissue	**LV**	lymphatic vessels	**ST**	seminiferous tubules
DE	ductus epididymis	**MT**	mediastinum testis	**St**	stroma
De	ductuli efferentes	**N**	nuclei	**Sz**	spermatozoa
Ep	epithelium	**RT**	rete testis	**TR**	tubuli recti

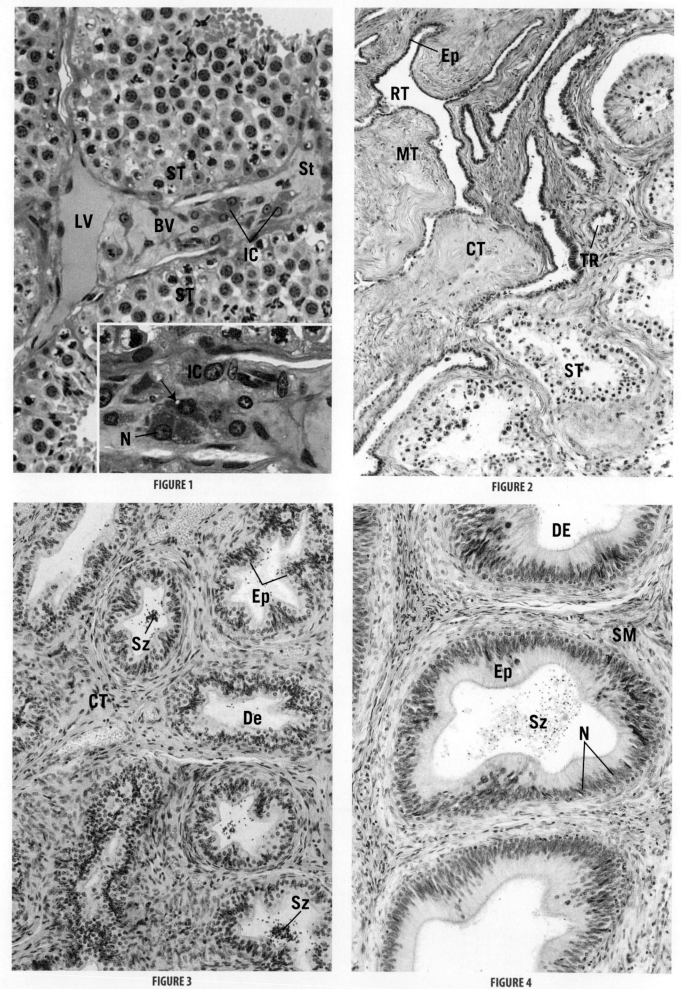

PLATE 18-2 · Testis and Epididymis

FIGURE 1

FIGURE 2

FIGURE 3

FIGURE 4

PLATE 18-3　•　Epididymis, Ductus Deferens, and Seminal Vesicle

FIGURE 1. Ductus epididymis. Monkey. Plastic section. ×270.

The pseudostratified stereociliated columnar **epithelium** (Ep) lining the lumen of the ductus epididymis is composed of two types of cells: short **basal cells** (BC), recognizable by their round nuclei, and tall columnar **principal cells** (PC), whose oval nuclei display one or more **nucleoli** (n). The **smooth muscle** (SM) cells, composing the wall of the epididymis, are circularly oriented and are surrounded by **connective tissue** (CT) elements. *Inset.* **Ductus epididymis. Monkey. Plastic section.** ×540. Observe the round nuclei of the **basal cells** (BC) and oval nuclei of the **principal cells** (PC). Clumped stereocilia (*arrows*) extend into the **spermatozoa** (Sz)-filled lumen.

FIGURE 2. Ductus deferens. Monkey. Plastic section. ×132.

The ductus deferens is a thick-walled, muscular tube that conveys spermatozoa from the ductus epididymis to the ejaculatory duct. The thick, muscular coat is composed of three layers of smooth muscle: **outer longitudinal** (OL), **middle circular** (MC), and **inner longitudinal** (IL). The fibroelastic **lamina propria** (LP) receives its **vascular supply** (BV) from vessels (*arrow*) that penetrate the three muscle layers. A pseudostratified columnar **epithelium** (Ep) lines the spermatozoa-filled **lumen** (L). *Inset.* **Ductus deferens. Monkey. Plastic section.** ×270. A higher magnification of the pseudostratified columnar **epithelium** (Ep) displays the presence of **stereocilia** (Sc).

FIGURE 3. Seminal vesicle. Human. Paraffin section. ×132.

The paired seminal vesicles are elongated tubular glands whose ducts join the ductus deferens just prior to the beginning of the ejaculatory ducts. The highly folded **mucous membrane** (MM) of the seminal vesicle is composed of pseudostratified **epithelium** (Ep) with a thin **connective tissue core** (CT). The folded membrane anastomoses with itself, partitioning off small spaces (*asterisks*) that, although continuous with the central lumen, appear to be discrete regions. A region similar to the *boxed area* is presented at a higher magnification in Figure 4.

FIGURE 4. Seminal vesicle. Monkey. Plastic section. ×540.

This photomicrograph is a higher magnification of a region similar to the *boxed area* of the previous figure. Note that the tall **columnar cells** (CC) have basally located, round **nuclei** (N) and that their cytoplasm displays secretory granules (*arrows*). Short **basal cells** (BC) are occasionally present, which may function as regenerative cells for the epithelium. The secretory product is released into the **lumen** (L) as a thick fluid that coagulates in histological sections. Observe the presence of numerous **capillaries** (C) in the connective tissue core deep to the epithelium. Although **spermatozoa** (Sz) are frequently noted in the lumen of the seminal vesicles, they are not stored in this structure.

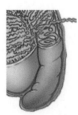

KEY					
BC	basal cell	**L**	lumen	**PC**	principal cell
BV	blood vessel	**LP**	lamina propria	**Sc**	stereocilia
C	capillaries	**MC**	middle circular muscle layer	**SM**	smooth muscle
CC	columnar cell	**MM**	mucous membrane	**Sz**	spermatozoa
CT	connective tissue	**N**	nucleus		
Ep	epithelium	**n**	nucleoli		
IL	inner longitudinal muscle layer	**OL**	outer longitudinal muscle layer		

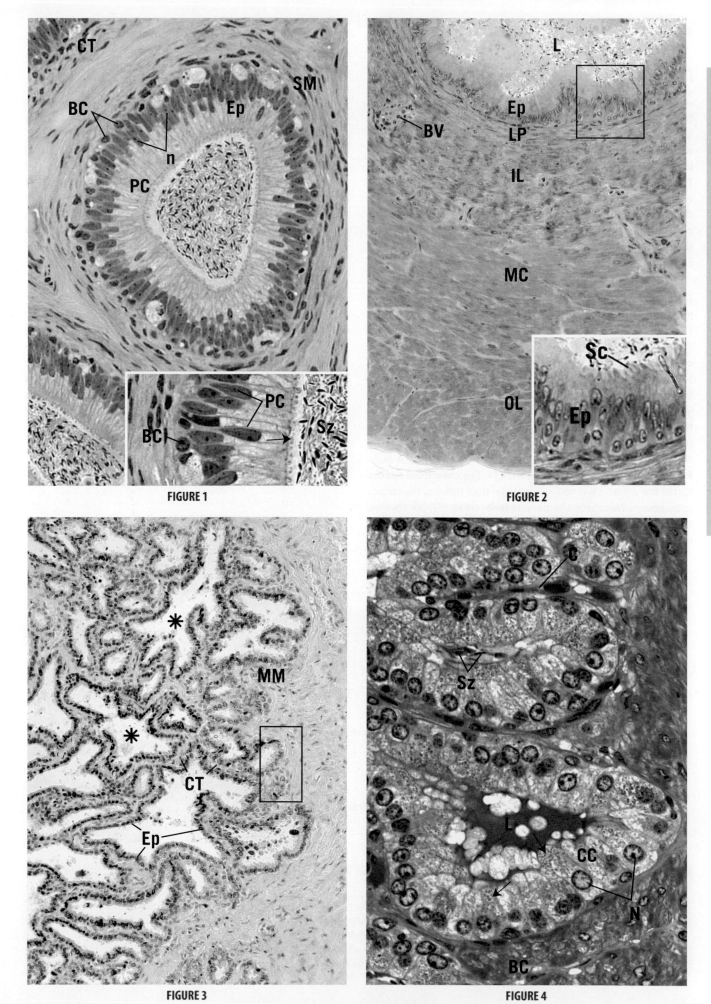

PLATE 18-3 • Epididymis, Ductus Deferens, and Seminal Vesicle

FIGURE 1

FIGURE 2

FIGURE 3

FIGURE 4

PLATE 18-4 · Prostate, Penis, and Urethra

FIGURE 1. Prostate gland. Monkey. Plastic section. ×132.

The prostate gland, the largest of the male reproductive accessory glands, possesses a thick fibroelastic connective tissue capsule with which the connective tissue **stroma** (St) is continuous. Note that the stroma houses **smooth muscle** (SM) and blood vessels. The secretory portion of the prostate gland is composed of individual glands of varied shapes but consisting of a simple cuboidal-to-low columnar type of **epithelium** (Ep), although regions of pseudostratified columnar epithelia are readily apparent. A region similar to the *boxed area* is presented at a higher magnification in Figure 2.

FIGURE 3. Penis. Human. x.s. Paraffin section. ×14.

The penis is composed of three erectile bodies: the two corpora cavernosa and the corpus spongiosum. The cross section of the **corpus spongiosum** (CS) displays the **urethra** (U), which is surrounded by **erectile tissue** (ET), whose irregular, endothelially lined **cavernous spaces** (Cs) contain blood. The spongy tissue is surrounded by the thick, fibrous **tunica albuginea** (TA). The three cavernous bodies are surrounded by a looser connective tissue sheath to which the skin (removed here) is attached. The *boxed area* is presented at a higher magnification in Figure 4. *Inset.* **Penis. Human. x.s. Paraffin section.** ×14. The **cavernous spaces** (Cs) of the corpus cavernosum are larger than those of the corpus spongiosum. Moreover, the **fibrous trabeculae** (FT) are thinner, resulting in the corpora cavernosa becoming more turgid during erection than the corpus spongiosum.

FIGURE 2. Prostate gland. Monkey. Plastic section. ×540.

This photomicrograph is a higher magnification of a region similar to the *boxed area* of the previous figure. Observe that the fibroelastic connective tissue **stroma** (St) presents numerous **blood vessels** (BV) and **smooth muscle cells** (SM). The parenchyma of the gland is composed of **columnar cells** (CC) as well as short **basal cells** (BC). Note that the dome-shaped apices (*arrows*) of some of the columnar cells appear to protrude into the lumen, which contain a **prostatic concretion** (Pc). The number of these concretions, which may calcify, increases with age.

FIGURE 4. Urethra. Human. Paraffin section. ×132.

This photomicrograph is a higher magnification of the *boxed area* of the previous figure. Note that the spongy **urethra** (U) is lined by a pseudostratified columnar **epithelium** (Ep) surrounded by a loose **connective tissue sheath** (CT), housing a rich **vascular supply** (BV). The entire urethra is enveloped by the **erectile tissue** (ET) of the corpus spongiosum. Additionally, the mucous **glands of Littré** (GL) deliver their secretory product into the lumen of the urethra, lubricating its epithelial lining.

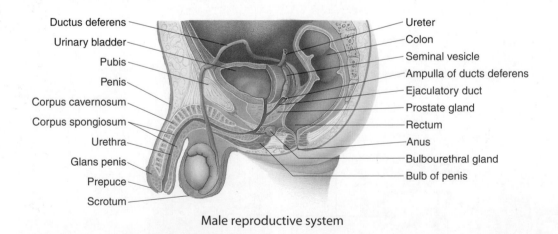

Male reproductive system

KEY							
BC	basal cell	CT	connective tissue	Pc	prostatic concretion
BV	blood vessel	Ep	epithelium	SM	smooth muscle
CC	columnar cell	ET	erectile tissue	St	stroma
CS	corpus spongiosum	FT	fibrous trabeculae	TA	tunica albuginea
Cs	cavernous space	GL	glands of Littré	U	urethra

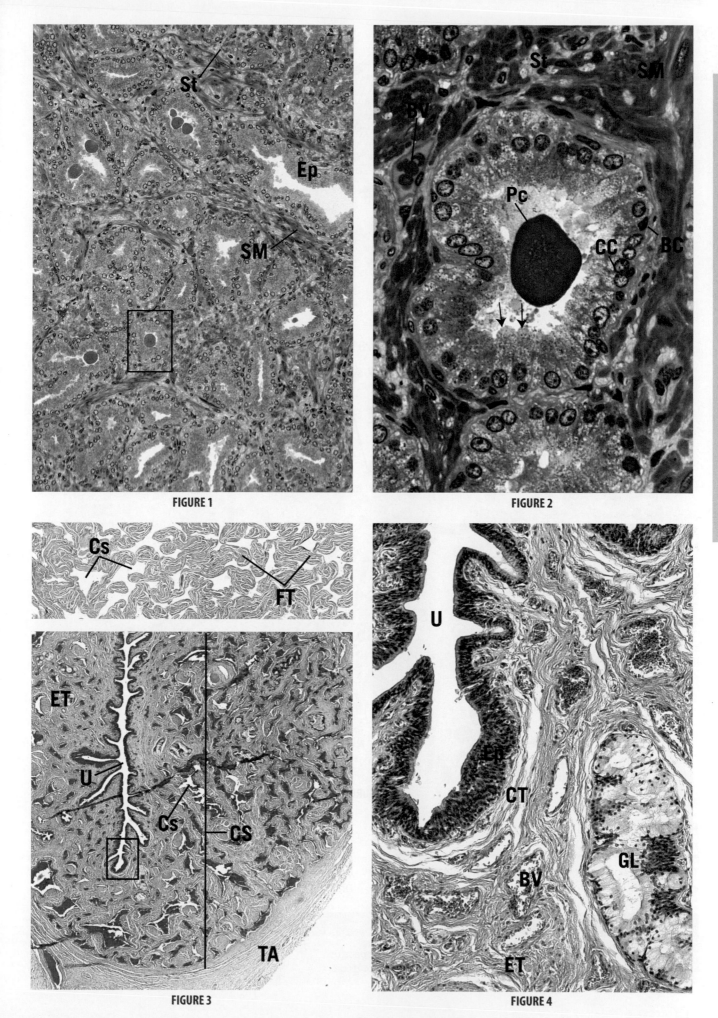

PLATE 18-4 • Prostate, Penis, and Urethra

FIGURE 1

FIGURE 2

FIGURE 3

FIGURE 4

PLATE 18-5 · Epididymis, Electron Microscopy

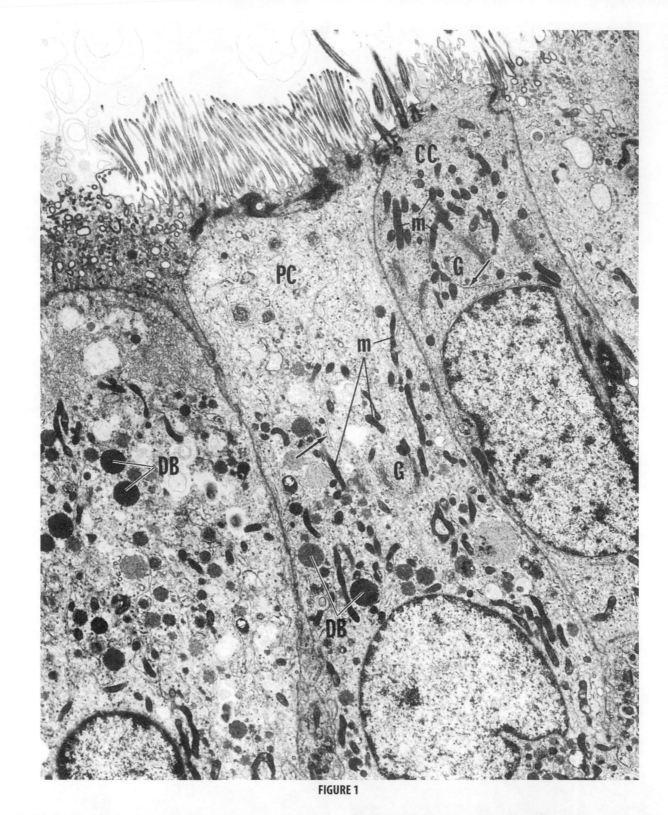

FIGURE 1

FIGURE 1. Epididymis. Rabbit. Electron microscopy. ×7,200.

The epithelial lining of the rabbit ductuli efferentes is composed of two types of tall columnar cells: **principal cells** (PC) and **ciliated cells** (CC). Note that both cell types possess numerous organelles, such as **Golgi** (G), **mitochondria** (m), and rough endoplasmic reticulum (*arrows*). Additionally, principal cells contain **dense bodies** (DB), probably a secretory material. (Courtesy of Dr. R. Jones.)

KEY

CC	ciliated cell	G	Golgi apparatus	PC	principal cell
DB	dense bodies	m	mitochondrion		

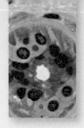

Chapter Summary

I. TESTES

A. Capsule

The fibromuscular connective tissue **capsule** of the testes is known as the **tunica albuginea**, whose inner vascular layer is the **tunica vasculosa**. The capsule is thickened at the **mediastinum testis** from which **septa** emanate, subdividing the testis into approximately 250 incomplete **lobuli testis**, with each containing one to four **seminiferous tubules** embedded in a connective tissue **stroma**.

B. Seminiferous Tubules

Each highly convoluted **seminiferous tubule** is composed of a fibromuscular **tunica propria**, which is separated from the **seminiferous epithelium** by a **basal membrane**.

1. Seminiferous Epithelium

The **seminiferous epithelium** is composed of sustentacular **Sertoli cells** and a stratified layer of developing **male gametes**. Sertoli cells establish a blood-testis barrier by forming occluding junctions with each other, thus subdividing the seminiferous tubule into **adluminal** and **basal compartments**. The basal compartment houses **spermatogonia A** (both **light** and **dark**), **spermatogonia B**, and the basal aspects of Sertoli cells. The adluminal compartment contains the apical portions of Sertoli cells, **primary spermatocytes**, **secondary spermatocytes**, **spermatids**, and **spermatozoa**.

2. Tunica Propria

The **tunica propria** consists of loose collagenous connective tissue, **fibroblasts**, and **myoid cells**.

C. Stroma

The loose vascular connective tissue **stroma** surrounding seminiferous tubules houses small clusters of large, vacuolated-appearing endocrine cells, the **interstitial cells** (of Leydig).

II. GENITAL DUCTS

A. Tubuli Recti

Short, straight tubes, the **tubuli recti**, lined by **Sertoli-like cells** initially and **simple cuboidal epithelium** later, connect the seminiferous tubules to the **rete testis**.

B. Rete Testis

The **rete testis** is composed of cuboidal cell–lined labyrinthine spaces within the **mediastinum testis**.

C. Epididymis

1. Ductuli Efferentes

The **ductuli efferentes** compose the **head of the epididymis**, whose lumina are lined by **simple columnar** (tall ciliated and low nonciliated) **epithelium**. The walls of the ductules consist of fibroelastic connective tissue and **smooth muscle cells**.

2. Ductus Epididymis

The **ductus epididymis** comprises the **body** and **tail** of the epididymis. Its lumen is lined by a **pseudostratified** type of **epithelium** composed of short **basal** and tall **principal cells** bearing **stereocilia** (long microvilli). The epithelium is separated by a **basal membrane** from the connective tissue wall that houses **smooth muscle cells**.

D. Ductus (Vas) Deferens

The enlarged continuation of the ductus epididymis, the **ductus deferens**, is a highly muscular structure. The **mucosal lining** of its small **lumen** is composed of **pseudostratified stereociliated epithelium** lying on a thin fibroelastic **lamina propria**. Its thick, muscular coat is composed of three layers of **smooth muscle**: an **inner** and **outer longitudinal** and a **middle circular** layer. A loose, fibroelastic **adventitia** surrounds the outer longitudinal muscle layer.

III. ACCESSORY GLANDS

A. Seminal Vesicles

As the **seminal vesicles**, two highly convoluted tubular structures, join the ductus deferens, they form the paired **ejaculatory ducts**. The highly folded **mucous membrane** of the seminal vesicle is composed of a **pseudostratified epithelium**, whose columnar cells are interspersed with short **basal cells**, sitting on a fibroelastic **lamina propria**. The muscular coat is composed of **inner circular** and **outer longitudinal** layers of **smooth muscle** and is invested by a fibrous **adventitia**.

B. Prostate Gland

The ejaculatory ducts join the urethra as these three structures traverse the substance of the **prostate gland**, whose capsule is composed of fibroelastic connective tissue and **smooth muscle cells**. The dense **stroma** of the gland is continuous with the capsule. The **parenchyma** of the prostate is composed of numerous individual glands disposed in three layers: **mucosal**, **submucosal**, and **external (main)**. The **lumina** of these three groups drain into three systems of **ducts** that lead into the expanded **urethral sinus**. The folded mucosa of the glands is composed of **simple cuboidal** to **columnar** (with regions of pseudostratified columnar) **epithelia** supported by fibroelastic vascular **stroma** displaying **smooth muscle cells**. Frequently, the lumina of the glands of older men possess round-to-ovoid **prostatic concretions** that are often lamellated and may become calcified.

C. Bulbourethral Glands

Each small **bulbourethral (Cowper's) gland** possesses a thin connective tissue **capsule** whose septa subdivide the gland into **lobules**. The **cuboidal-to-columnar cells** lining the lumen of the gland possess flattened, basally located **nuclei**. The main **duct** of each gland delivers its mucous secretory product into the **cavernous (spongy) urethra**.

IV. PENIS

The **penis**, ensheathed in **skin**, possesses a thick, collagenous capsule, the **tunica albuginea**, that encloses the three cylindrical bodies of **erectile tissue**. The two dorsally positioned **corpora cavernosa** are incompletely separated from each other by **septa** derived from the tunica albuginea. The **corpus cavernosum urethrae (corpus spongiosum)** contains the spongy portion of the **urethra**. The vascular spaces of the erectile tissues are lined by **endothelium**.

V. URETHRA

The male **urethra** is subdivided into three regions: **prostatic**, **membranous**, and **spongy (penile)** urethra.

A. Epithelium

The **prostatic portion** is lined by **transitional epithelium**, whereas the **membranous** and **spongy portions** are lined by **pseudostratified-to-stratified columnar epithelium**. The **spongy urethra** frequently displays regions of **stratified squamous epithelium**. **Goblet cells** and **intraepithelial glands** are also present.

B. Lamina Propria

The **lamina propria** is composed of a type of **loose connective tissue** housing **elastic fibers** and **glands of Littré**. **Smooth muscle**, oriented longitudinally and circularly, is also evident.

19 SPECIAL SENSES

CHAPTER OUTLINE

The organs of special senses include the gustatory, olfactory, visual, auditory, and vestibular systems. The gustatory apparatus, consisting of taste buds, is discussed in Chapter 13, and the olfactory epithelium is treated in Chapter 12. This chapter details sensory endings: the microscopic morphology of the eye, involved with visual sensations, and the ear, involved with auditory and vestibular sensations.

SENSORY ENDINGS

Sensory endings are located at the terminus of dendrites. These specialized receptors (see Table 19-1) are members of the general somatic or general visceral afferent pathways and are:

- specialized to respond to stimuli, such as pressure, touch, temperature, and pain, on the external surface of the body (exteroceptors); additionally, there are special senses of sight and hearing as well as smell and taste
- incorporated into muscles and tendon to perceive the localization of the body in three-dimensional space (proprioceptors), and
- distributed within organs to monitor the activity of these organs as components of the general visceral afferent pathways.

EYE

The **eye** is a sensory organ whose **lens** focuses rays of light originating in the external environment onto photosensitive cells of the **retina** (see Graphic 19-1). The intensity, location, and wavelengths of the transmitted light are partially processed by the retina, and the assembled information is transmitted, via the **optic nerve**, for further processing and interpretation by the visual cortex of the brain as three-dimensional color images of the external milieu.

- Because the eyes are set apart and because their visual fields overlap, such three-dimensional imaging becomes possible.
- Each eyeball (bulb, globe), protected by the eyelids, is movable by means of a group of **extrinsic skeletal muscles** that insert into its fibrous outer tunic, thus assisting in suspending it in its bony orbit and directing the pupil to the most advantageous position for perceiving the image viewed.

Three coats constitute the wall of the bulb: the outer fibrous tunic, the middle vascular tunic (uvea), and the inner retinal tunic.

- The **fibrous tunic (corneoscleral layer)** is composed of the opaque, white **sclera** that covers the posterior aspect of the bulb and the transparent **cornea** that covers the anterior one-sixth of the eyeball.
  - The junction between the sclera and the cornea is known as the **limbus**.
- The **vascular tunic** consists of several regions: the anteriorly positioned **iris** and **ciliary body** and the posteriorly located, highly vascular and pigmented **choroid**.
  - **Melanocytes** located in the epithelium and stroma of the iris block light from passing through the iris, except at the pupil.
  - Additionally, **eye color** is related to the abundance of melanin produced by these melanocytes:
  - A large amount of melanin imparts dark eyes, whereas less melanin renders the eyes light in color.
  - **Intrinsic smooth muscles,** represented by the **sphincter pupillae** and **dilatator pupillae muscles,** adjust the aperture of the **iris**.
  - The **ciliary smooth muscles** alter tension of the suspensory (zonular) fibers anchored in the lens and thus alter the shape of the lens (accommodation) for near and far vision.
- The innermost **retinal tunic** is composed of 10 layers responsible for photoreception and impulse generation (see Table 19-2). The two deepest layers, the retinal pigment epithelium and the layer of rods and cones, bear the major responsibility for photoreception. **Retinal pigment epithelium** functions in **esterifying vitamin A** and transporting it to the rods and cones, **phagocytosing** the shed tips of rods and cones, and **synthesizing melanin**, which absorbs light after rods and cones have been stimulated.
  - **Rods** are sensitive to low light intensity and possess many flattened discs containing **rhodopsin** (an integral membrane protein, **opsin**, bound to **retinal**, the aldehyde form of **vitamin A**) in their outer segment.
    - When light is absorbed by rhodopsin, it dissociates into **retinal** and **opsin** (bleaching), permitting diffusion of bound Ca^{2+} into the outer segment.
    - Excess levels of Ca^{2+} hyperpolarize the cell by closing Na^+ channels, thus preventing the entry of Na^+ into the cell.
    - The electrical potential thus generated is relayed to other rods via gap junctions and then along the pathway to the optic nerve.
    - Dissociated retinal and opsin reassemble, and the Ca^{2+} ions are recaptured, establishing a normal resting potential.
  - **Cones**, sensitive to light of high intensity, producing **greater visual acuity**, are much more numerous

TABLE 19-1 • Specialized Receptors, Their Function and Location

Receptor	Type	Function and Location
Peritrichial nerve endings	Nonencapsulated	Are nonmyelinated and have no associated Schwann's cells. Most are coupled with hair follicles and react to the hair's motion. The sensation is interpreted as touch or being tickled.
Merkel's discs	Nonencapsulated	Mechanoreceptors located in the stratum basale of the epidermis.
Meissner's corpuscles	Encapsulated	Located in the dermal papillae of the dermis and respond to touch sensations
Pacinian corpuscles	Encapsulated	Resemble an onion since epithelioid cells form concentric layers around a naked nerve ending. These corpuscles, located in the hypodermis, mesocolon, and mesentery, respond to vibration, pressure, and deep touch.
Ruffini's endings	Encapsulated	Are composed of highly branched nerve termini surrounded by fibroblast-like cells. They respond to pressure and stretch and are located in nail beds, periodontal ligament, dermis of the skin, and capsules of joints.
Krause's end bulbs	Encapsulated	These spherical capsules containing a naked nerve ending are located in the connective tissues just deep to the epithelium, capsules of joints, peritoneum, and in the dermis of skin. Their function is not known.
Muscle spindles	Encapsulated	Described in the chapter on Muscle. They function in proprioception. They respond to alteration in the length and rate of change in muscle and thus function in proprioception.
Golgi tendon organs	Encapsulated	Described in the chapter on Muscle. Respond to changes in the tension and the rate of tension change around a joint, thus function in proprioception.
Thermoreceptors	Nonencapsulated	They are assumed to be naked nerve endings located in the epidermis that respond to temperature. Their morphology is not known.
Nociceptors	Nonencapsulated	Branched naked nerve endings located in the epidermis. They are stimulated by extremes in temperature, by damage to the epidermis and underlying structures, as well as by certain chemicals as pain sensation.

TABLE 19-2 • Layers of the Retina

Layer	Description
Pigment epithelium	Synthesizes melanin that absorbs light that activated rods and cones; phagocytoses the shed tips of rods and cones; estrifies vitamin A
Layer of rods and cones	Photosensitivity; rods are sensitive to low light intensity, and cones are sensitive to bright light and perceive color.
External limiting membrane	Zonulae adherentes formed between the photoreceptor cells and Müller cells (therefore, it is not a true membrane)
Outer nuclear layer	Houses the nuclear regions of rods and cones
Outer plexiform layer	Region of synapse between axons, photoreceptor cells, and dendrites of horizontal and bipolar cells
Inner nuclear layer	Houses the nuclear regions of Müller, bipolar, amacrine, and horizontal cells
Inner plexiform layer	Region where synapses occur among axons and dendrites of amacrine, bipolar, and ganglion cells
Ganglion cell layer	Region of the cell bodies of multipolar neurons as well as neuroglial cells
Optic nerve fiber layer	Region where the unmyelinated axons of ganglion cells join to form the optic nerve. Once the fibers pierce the sclera, they become myelinated.
Inner limiting membrane	Composed of the expanded terminal processes of Müller cells and their basal lamina

than rods, and they produce **iodopsin**, the photopigment responsible for distinguishing color. Three different moieties of opsin are sensitive to either red, green, or blue light.

- ■ The mechanism of transducing photoenergy into electrical energy for transmission to the brain via the optic nerve is similar to that described in the rods.

○ Rods and cones are either stimulated (on) or inhibited (off) by light, that is, they indicate the location of a light pixel and, in the case of cones, its color.

- ■ Dendrites of 10 different types of **bipolar cells** receive information from the rods and cones, and then this information is conveyed by the axons of the bipolar cells into specific strata of the **inner plexiform layer** of the retina.
- ■ The further transmission of the impulses is monitored and modulated by one or more of the 27 types of **amacrine cells**, whose axons can span several millimeters or just a few micrometers of the retinal expanse.
- ■ The outer layer of the retina contains 12 types of **ganglion cells** whose interactions with bipolar cells and amacrine cells result in the transmission of 12 different moving images (a continuous moving stream that resembles but is not created frame by frame) of the same scene via the optic nerve to the visual cortex of the brain for further analysis, assembly, and interpretation.
- ■ These moving images are very different from each other, in that some consist of highlights, others consist of line drawings of outlines, and still others generate shadows.
- ■ It is the function of the visual cortex to assemble these movies into the world that we recognize.

It must be stressed that this is a simplified description of some of the current concepts of vision that will certainly be modified as more information is gained from research in this field.

○ An additional type of ganglion cells, which make up less than 3% of the ganglion cell population, appear to function in the establishment of the circadian rhythm.

- ■ These ganglion cells possess the light-sensitive pigment **melanopsin** that responds to blue light even in individuals who are blind.
- ■ The axons of these ganglion cells project to the suprachiasmatic nucleus, the region of the brain responsible for the regulation of circadian rhythm.

- ■ It appears, then, that the suprachiasmatic nucleus receives information from these specialized ganglion cells of the retina as to when there is daylight.

The **optic disc**, the region where the optic nerve exits the eyeball, contains neither cones nor rods; consequently, it represents and is called a **blind spot**. Just lateral to the blind spot is the **fovea centralis**, a depression in the retina. The fovea contains mostly cones that are packed so tightly that not all layers of the retina are present. **Visual acuity** is the greatest in the fovea centralis.

- **Accessory structures** of the eye include the conjunctiva, eyelids, and lacrimal gland.
  ○ The **conjunctiva** is a transparent mucous membrane that lines the eyelids and reflects onto the eyeball.
  ○ The **eyelids** contain modified sebaceous glands, the **meibomian glands**, which are responsible for altering the surface tension of the watery tears, thus slowing evaporation.
  ○ The **lacrimal glands** secrete tears, a complex fluid composed of water, proteins, salts, peptides, and other organic molecules which keep the conjunctiva and cornea moist.
    - ■ **Tears** also contain **lysozyme**, an antibacterial enzyme.
  ○ The additional components of the interior of the eyeball are the **aqueous humor**, a fluid; the **vitreous body**, a gel; and the **lens**, all of which serve as parts of the refractive media.
    - ■ The aqueous humor, located in the posterior and anterior chambers of the eye, and the vitreous body, located behind the lens of the eye, are also important in providing nutrients to the avascular lens and cornea.

EAR

The **ear** functions in the reception of sound as well as in the perception of the orientation of the head and therefore the body in relation to the directional forces of gravity (see Graphic 19-2). To perform both functions of hearing and equilibrium (balance), the ear is subdivided into the external, middle, and inner ears.

- The **external ear** is composed of a cartilaginous, skin-covered **auricle** (pinna) and the **external auditory meatus**, with its cartilaginous outer and bony inner aspects, whose internal extent is separated from the middle ear by the thin **tympanic membrane**.
- The **tympanic cavity** of the **middle ear** houses the three **auditory ossicles**, connected in series to each other: the outermost **malleus** (hammer), the middle

incus (anvil), and the innermost **stapes** (stirrup). This cavity is connected to the **nasopharynx** via the cartilaginous **auditory (eustachian) tube**, which permits equalization of atmospheric pressures on either side of the tympanic membrane. Sound waves are funneled by the auricle to the **tympanic membrane**, whose vibrations are amplified and transmitted by the movements of the three bony ossicles to the **oval window** of the inner ear's **cochlea**.

- The **bony labyrinth** of the **inner ear**, subdivided into the **semicircular canals**, **vestibule**, and **cochlea**, is filled with **perilymph**. Loosely contained within it and all of its subdivisions is the endolymph-containing **membranous labyrinth**.

  ○ Movements of the fluid environment within this system are perceived by apical "hairs" of specialized sensory cells contained within the membranous labyrinth and ultimately transduced to electrical impulses for transmission to the brain.

  ○ The **saccule** and **utricle**, specialized structures of the membranous labyrinth in the vestibule, contain **type I** and **type II hair cells** (**neuroepithelial cells** containing many **stereocilia** and a single **kinocilium**), whose free ends are embedded in the **otolithic membrane** containing calcium carbonate crystals known as **otoliths (otoconia)**.

    ▪ **Static equilibrium** and **linear acceleration** are determined by movements (or the lack of movements) in the stereocilia or kinocilia of these hair cells.

    ▪ Threshold bending of the stereocilia or kinocilia will depolarize the hair cells, which, in turn, relay (via neurotransmission) information to the processes of primary vestibular neurons located in Scarpa's ganglion.

  ○ **Semicircular ducts**, specializations of the membranous labyrinth in the semicircular canals, contain **neuroepithelial hair cells** located in the **cristae ampullares** (sensory regions) of the **ampullae**.

    ▪ Free ends of these hair cells have stereocilia that are embedded in a viscous glycoprotein known as the **cupula**.

    ▪ Movement of the endolymph bathing the cupula depolarize the hair cells, which, in turn, alter the activity in the synaptic endings associated with the base of the hair cells.

    ▪ This process is sensitive to **rotational acceleration** in any of the three directions of orientation of the semicircular canals.

    ▪ Thus, these structures are responsible for the vestibular sensations of balance and orientation.

TABLE 19-3 • Cells of the Spiral Organ of Corti

Cells	Function
Border cells	Support the inner aspect of the organ of Corti
Cells of Böttcher	Unclear
Cells of Claudius	Unclear
Cells of Hensen	Support the outer aspect of the organ of Corti
Inner hair cells	Transduction of impulses to bipolar cells of the spiral ganglion
Inner pillar cells	Form the medial wall of the inner tunnel and support the hair cells
Inner phalangeal cells	Surround and support the inner hair cells
Outer hair cells	Transduction of impulses to bipolar cells of the spiral ganglion
Outer phalangeal cells	Support the outer hair cells and their associated nerve fibers
Outer pillar cells	Form the lateral wall of the inner tunnel and support the hair cells

○ The **endolymphatic sac** (terminal end of the **endolymphatic duct**) contains phagocytic cells in its lumen and may function in **resorption of endolymph**.

○ The **cochlear duct (scala media)** contains the **spiral organ of Corti**, which is bordered by the **scala vestibuli** and the **scala tympani** (both scalae contain perilymph and communicate at the **helicotrema**).

○ The **vestibular membrane** located between the scala vestibuli and the cochlear duct functions to maintain the **high ion gradient** between the perilymph and endolymph.

  ▪ The **spiral organ of Corti** (see Table 19-3), sitting on the **basilar membrane**, contains, among other supporting cells, neuroepithelial **inner** and **outer hair cells** whose free ends are embedded in the gel-like **tectorial membrane**.

    - Sound transmission/conduction via the tympanic membrane and ossicles to the oval window sets waves translated to the oval window and sets the perilymph of the scala tympani in motion, which displaces the basilar membrane, thus moving the hair cells but not the tectorial membrane.

- Bending of the hair cells causes them to release neurotransmitter substance, exciting the **bipolar cells** of the spiral ganglion, resulting in transmission of the impulse to higher centers of the brain.
- Although the basilar membrane vibrates at many frequencies, certain regions vibrate optimally at specific frequencies.

- For example, low-frequency sound waves are detected farther away from the oval window.
- It should be noted that loud sounds, such as those at rock concerts, create a great deal of energy within the hearing mechanism, such that it may take 2 or 3 days for the energy to be completely dissipated and the buzzing to stop.

CLINICAL CONSIDERATIONS

Blue Eye Color

Until approximately 6,000 to 10,000 years ago, every human being had brown eyes; then, a small mutation in the switch that turned off OCA2 gene resulted in the inability of that individual to manufacture P protein in the iris. Protein P is involved in melanin formation; thus, the person with this particular mutation was able to synthesize melanin normally except in the iris, and instead of having brown eyes, that person's eyes were blue. Thus, it is believed that all blue-eyed individuals are descendants of that one person born in that era.

Myopia and Hyperopia

As an individual ages, the longitudinal axis of the eye changes, as may the curvature of the cornea, and the lens, instead of focusing the image on the retina, focuses it either in front of the retina (**myopic vision**) or behind the retina (**hyperopic vision**). The condition may be corrected with lenses (eyeglasses or contact lenses) or by refractive surgery, assisting the lens in focusing on the retina.

Glaucoma

Glaucoma is a condition of high intraocular pressure caused by an obstruction that prevents the aqueous humor from exiting the anterior chamber of the eye. If left untreated, the pressure damages the optic nerve to such an extent that blindness may result.

Cataract

Cataract, a common condition of aging, is caused by excessive UV radiation and by pigments and other substances accumulating in the lens, making it opaque and thus impairing vision. This condition may be corrected by excising the lens and replacing it with a plastic lens.

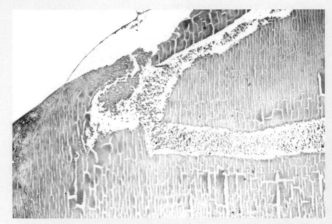

This photomicrograph is from the lens of an older patient who presented with age-related cataract. Observe the presence of cortical extracellular clefts and globules. (Reprinted with permission from Mills SE, Carter, D, et al., eds. Sternberg's Diagnostic Surgical Pathology, 5th ed., Philadelphia: Lippincott Williams & Wilkins, 2010, p. 981.)

Detached Retina

Detached retina may result from a trauma in which the neural and pigmented layers of the retina become separated, resulting to ischemic damage to the neurons. This condition may cause partial blindness, but it may be corrected by surgical intervention.

Retinoblastoma

Retinoblastoma is a malignancy of the very young child, usually detected at about 2 years of age, although at the time of diagnosis the child may be 5 or 6 years old. Approximately a third of the cases have familial components, but at least 60% occur without a familial incidence. The tumor appears white with regions of calcification and yellow foci of necrosis. The tumor may spread by individual cells invading the optic nerve as well as the choroid. The patient has to lose the eyeball to prevent metastasis.

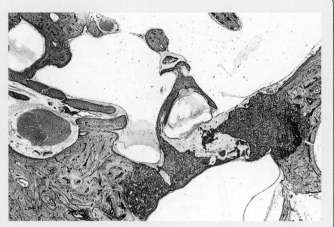

Observe that the footplate of the stapes is fixed to the densely sclerotic bone forming the perimeter of the oval window. (Reprinted with permission from Mills SE, Carter D, et al., eds. Sternberg's Diagnostic Surgical Pathology, 5th ed., Philadelphia: Lippincott Williams & Wilkins, 2010, p. 944.)

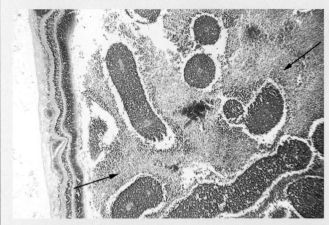

This photomicrograph is from the eyeball of a child with retinoblastoma. Observe the relatively normal retina on the left-hand side of the image. The arrows indicate regions of necrosis in a field of perivascular tumor cells. (Reprinted with permission from Mills SE, Carter, D, et al., eds. Sternberg's Diagnostic Surgical Pathology, 5th ed., Philadelphia: Lippincott Williams & Wilkins, 2010, p. 982.)

Conductive Hearing Loss

Conductive hearing loss may arise from a middle ear infection (otitis media), an obstruction, or otosclerosis of the middle ear.

Nerve Deafness

Nerve deafness results from a lesion in the cochlear portion of the vestibulocochlear nerve (cranial nerve VIII). This condition may be the result of disease, prolonged exposure to loud sounds, and/or drugs.

Ménière's Disease

Ménière's disease is an inner ear disorder characterized by symptoms such as hearing loss due to excess fluid accumulation in the endolymphatic duct, vertigo, tinnitus, nausea, and vomiting. In severe cases, surgical treatment may be required.

Acoustic Neuroma

The condition known as **acoustic neuroma** is a benign tumor whose cells of origin are the Schwann cells of the vestibulocochlear nerve (cranial nerve VIII). It is manifested by loss of hearing, loss of balance, vertigo, and tinnitus. If the tumor is not treated early enough, it may involve other cranial nerves in its vicinity. Recent studies suggest the possibility that long-term exposures to the electromagnetic radiation emitted by cell phones may be a causative factor in the development of acoustic neuroma in susceptible individuals.

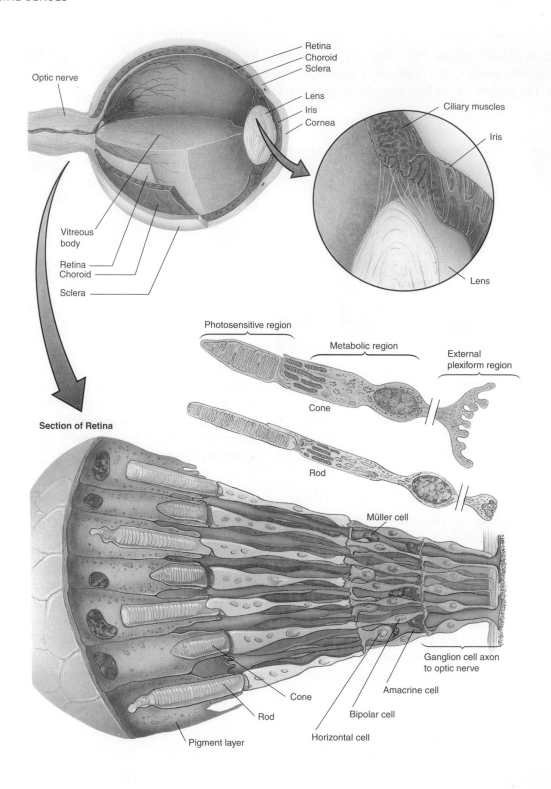

Optic nerve

Retina
Choroid
Sclera

Lens
Iris
Cornea

Ciliary muscles

Iris

Lens

Vitreous body

Retina
Choroid

Sclera

Section of Retina

Photosensitive region

Metabolic region

External plexiform region

Cone

Rod

Müller cell

Ganglion cell axon to optic nerve

Amacrine cell

Cone

Bipolar cell

Rod

Horizontal cell

Pigment layer

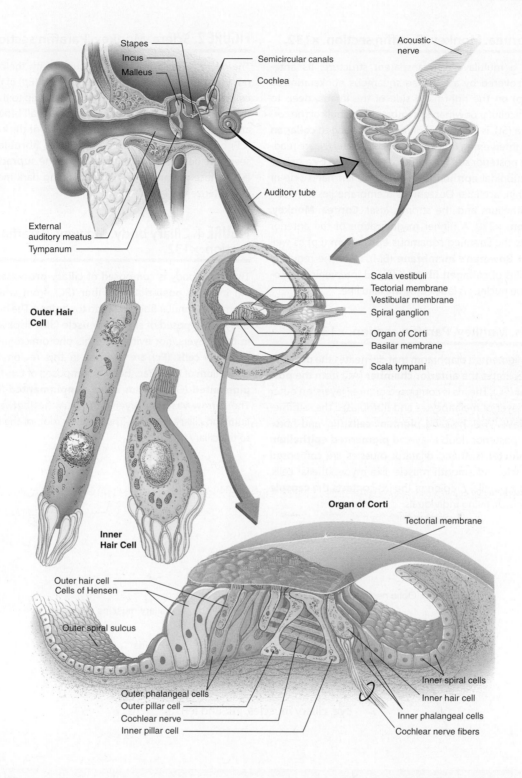

Stapes
Incus
Malleus
Semicircular canals
Cochlea
Acoustic nerve
Auditory tube
External auditory meatus
Tympanum

Scala vestibuli
Tectorial membrane
Vestibular membrane
Spiral ganglion
Organ of Corti
Basilar membrane
Scala tympani

Outer Hair Cell

Inner Hair Cell

Organ of Corti
Tectorial membrane

Outer hair cell
Cells of Hensen
Outer spiral sulcus
Outer phalangeal cells
Outer pillar cell
Cochlear nerve
Inner pillar cell
Inner spiral cells
Inner hair cell
Inner phalangeal cells
Cochlear nerve fibers

PLATE 19-1 • Eye, Cornea, Sclera, Iris, and Ciliary Body

FIGURE 1. Cornea. Monkey. Paraffin section. ×132.

The cornea is a multilayered, transparent structure. Its anterior surface is covered by a stratified squamous nonkeratinized **epithelium** (Ep) on the right-hand side of the image, deep to which is a thin, acellular Bowman's membrane. The bulk of the cornea, the **stroma** (St), is composed of regularly arranged **collagen fibers** (CF) and intervening fibroblasts, whose **nuclei** (N) are readily evident. The posterior surface of the cornea is lined by a simple squamous-to-cuboidal **epithelium** (Ep) on the left-hand side of the image. A thin, acellular Descemet's membrane lies between the simple epithelium and the stroma. *Inset.* **Cornea. Monkey. Paraffin section.** ×270. A higher magnification of the anterior surface displays the stratified squamous **epithelium** (Ep) as well as the acellular **Bowman's membrane** (BM). Note the regularly arranged bundles of **collagen fibers** (CF) and intervening **fibroblasts** (F), whose nucleus is labeled by the lead line.

FIGURE 3. Iris. Monkey. Paraffin section. ×132.

The **iris** (I) is a pigmented diaphragm that delineates the **pupil** (P) of the eye. It separates the **anterior chamber** (AC) from the **posterior chamber** (PC). The iris is composed of three layers: an outer discontinuous layer of melanocytes and fibroblasts; the intermediate **fibrous layer** (FL), housing **pigment cells** (Pc) and fibroblasts; and the posterior double-layered **pigmented epithelium** (PEp). The **sphincter** (sM) and dilatator muscles are composed of smooth muscle and smooth muscle–like myoepithelial cells, respectively. The pupillary region of the iris contacts the **capsule** (Ca) of the **lens** (L) in living individuals.

FIGURE 2. Sclera. Monkey. Paraffin section. ×132.

The sclera is similar to and continuous with the cornea, but it is not transparent. Note that the **epithelium** (Ep) of the conjunctiva covers the anterior surface of the sclera. Deep to the epithelium is the loose **episcleral tissue** (ET), whose small **blood vessels** (BV) are evident. The **stroma** (St) is composed of thick **collagen fiber** (CF) bundles, between which numerous **fibroblasts** (F) can be seen. The deepest layer of the sclera is the **suprachoroid lamina** (SL), whose **melanocytes** (M) containing dark melanin pigment characterize this layer.

FIGURE 4. Ciliary body. Monkey. Paraffin section. ×132.

The ciliary body is composed of **ciliary processes** (CP), projecting into the **posterior chamber** (PC), from which suspensory ligaments (zonular fibers) extend to the lens. The bulk of the ciliary body is composed of **smooth muscle** (SM) disposed more or less in three layers, not evident in this photomicrograph. Numerous **pigment cells** (Pc) are present in this region. Note that the epithelium of the ciliary body is composed of two layers: an **outer pigmented** (OP) and an **inner nonpigmented** (IN) epithelium. The narrow **vascular layer** (VL) intervenes between the epithelium and ciliary muscles. The base, or root, of the iris is anchored to the ciliary body.

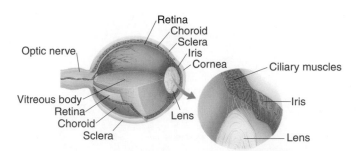

Eye, ciliary muscles, iris, and lens

KEY

AC	anterior chamber	FL	fibrous layer	Pc	pigment cells
BM	Bowman's membrane	I	iris	PEp	pigmented epithelium
BV	blood vessel	IN	inner nonpigmented layer	SEp	squamous epithelium
Ca	capsule	L	lens	SL	suprachoroid lamina
CF	collagen fibers	M	melanocytes	SM	smooth muscle
CP	ciliary process	N	nucleus	sM	sphincter muscle
Ep	epithelium	OP	outer pigmented layer	St	stroma
ET	episcleral tissue	P	pupil	VL	vascular layer
F	fibroblasts	PC	posterior chamber		

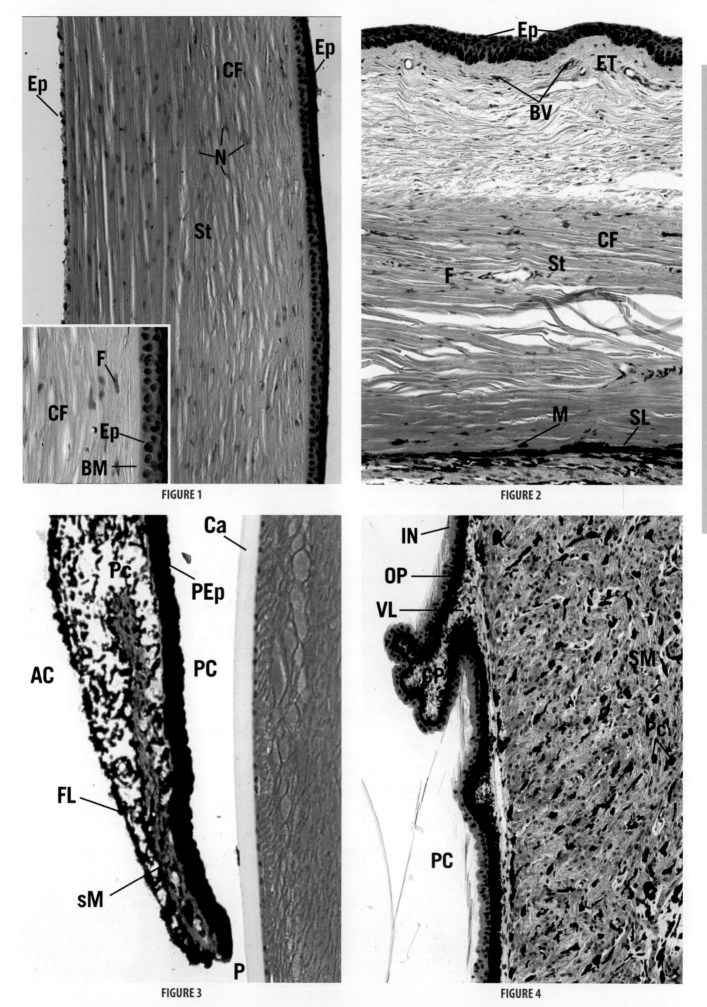

PLATE 19-1 • Eye, Cornea, Sclera, Iris, and Ciliary Body

FIGURE 1

FIGURE 2

FIGURE 3

FIGURE 4

PLATE 19-2 • Retina, Light and Scanning Electron Microscopy

FIGURE 1. Tunics of the eye. Monkey. Paraffin section. ×14.

This survey photomicrograph is of an anterolateral section of the globe of the eye, as evidenced by the presence of the **lacrimal gland** (LG). Note that the three layers of the globe of the eye are extremely thin in relation to its diameter. The **sclera** (S) is the outermost layer. The pigment **choroid** (Ch) and multilayered **retina** (Re) are easily distinguishable even at this low magnification. The **posterior compartment** (PCo) lies behind the lens and houses the vitreous body. A region similar to the *boxed area* is presented at a higher magnification in Figure 2.

FIGURE 3. Rods and cones. Monkey. Scanning electron microscopy. ×6,300.

This scanning electron micrograph of the monkey retina displays regions of several **cones** (C) that display their thicker morphology and wider nuclear zone and of a few **rods** (R) whose diameter is narrower, with a thinner nuclear zone. The inner segments of the **lamina of rods and cones** (2), **external limiting membrane** (3), and outer nuclear layer (4) are clearly recognizable. The microvilli (Mv) noted in the vicinity of the external limiting membrane belong to Müller's cells, which were removed during specimen preparation. Observe the longitudinal ridges (*arrows*) along the surface of the inner segments. (From Borwein B, Borwein D, Medeiros J, McGowan J. The ultrastructure of monkey foveal photoreceptors, with special reference to the structure, shape, size, and spacing of the foveal cones. Am J Anat 1980;159:125–146.)

FIGURE 2. Retina. Pars optica. Monkey. Paraffin section. ×270.

The pars optica of the retina is composed of 10 distinct layers. The **pigment epithelium** (1), the outermost layer, is closely apposed to the vascular and pigmented **choroid** (Ch). Various regions of the **rods** (R) and **cones** (C) characterize the next four layers. These are the **lamina of rods and cones** (2), **external limiting membrane** (3), **outer nuclear layer** (4), and **outer plexiform layer** (5). The **inner nuclear layer** (6) houses the cell bodies of various associative glial (Müller's) and neural cells. The **inner plexiform layer** (7) is a region of synapse formation, whereas the **ganglion cell layer** (8) houses the cell bodies of multipolar neurons and associated neuroglia. The centrally directed (toward the central nervous system) fibers of these ganglion cells form the **optic nerve fiber layer** (9), whereas the **inner limiting membrane** (10) is composed of the expanded processes of Müller's cells along the inner surface of the eye. A region similar to the *boxed area* is presented in Figure 3, a scanning electron micrograph of the rods and cones.

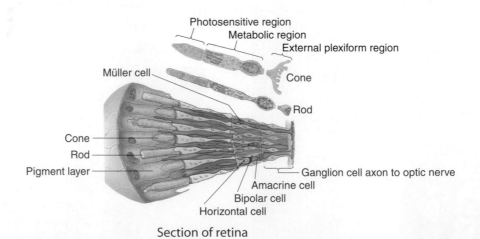

Section of retina

KEY							
1	pigment epithelium	7	inner plexiform layer	LG	lacrimal gland
2	lamina of rods and cones	8	ganglion cell layer	Mv	microvilli
3	external limiting membrane	9	optic nerve fiber layer	PCo	posterior compartment
4	outer nuclear layer	10	inner limiting membrane	R	rods
5	outer plexiform layer	C	cones	Re	retina
6	inner nuclear layer	Ch	choroid	S	sclera

PLATE 19-2 · Retina, Light and Scanning Electron Microscopy

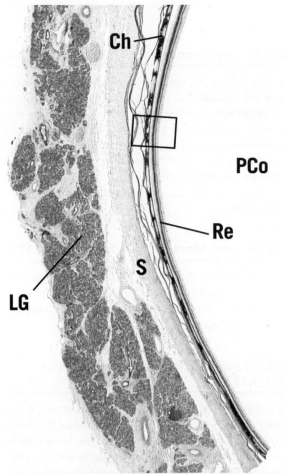

FIGURE 1

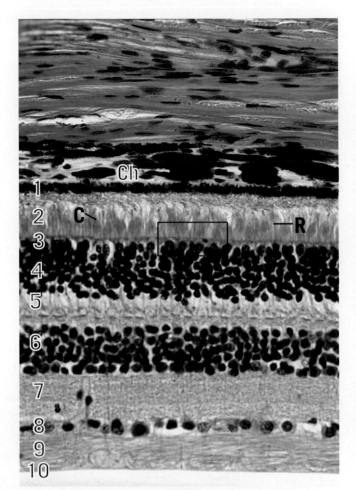

FIGURE 2

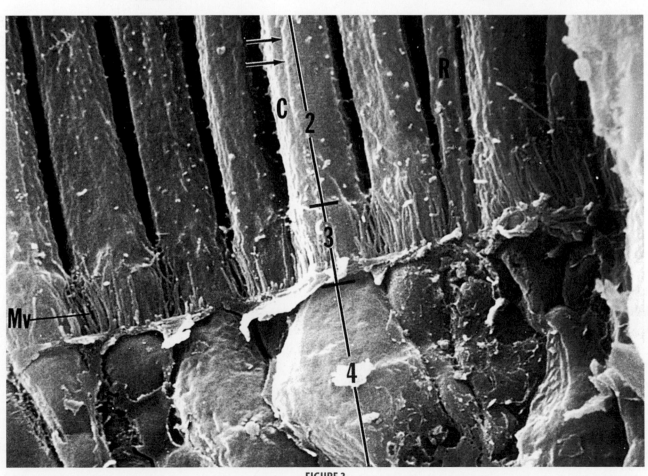

FIGURE 3

PLATE 19-3 • Fovea, Lens, Eyelid, and Lacrimal Glands

FIGURE 1. Fovea centralis. Monkey. Paraffin section. ×132.

The retina is greatly reduced in thickness at the **fovea centralis** (FC) of the macula lutea. This is the region of greatest visual acuity, and **cones** (C) are the only photoreceptor cells in this area. Note that the retinal layers present are the **pigmented epithelium** (1), **lamina of cones** (2), **external limiting membrane** (3), **outer nuclear layer** (4), **outer plexiform layer** (5), **ganglion cell layers** (8), and **inner limiting membrane** (10). Due to the presence of numerous melanocytes, the vascular **choroid** (Ch) appears dark.

FIGURE 3. Eyelid. Paraffin section. ×14.

The external aspect of the eyelid is covered by thin **skin** (Sk). The deep surface of the eyelid is lined by a stratified columnar epithelium, the **palpebral conjunctiva** (pC). The substance of the eyelid is formed by the thick connective tissue **tarsal plate** (TP) and **tarsal glands** (TG). Two skeletal muscles are associated with the upper eyelid, the circularly disposed **orbicularis oculi** (OO) and the longitudinally oriented levator palpebrae superioris. Although the latter muscle is not present in this photomicrograph, its connective tissue aponeurosis is evident (*arrow*). Eyelashes and the sebaceous **ciliary glands** (CG) are present at the free end of the lid.

FIGURE 2a. Lens. Monkey. Paraffin section. ×132.

The lens is a biconvex, flexible, transparent disc covered by a homogenous **capsule** (Ca), deep to which lies the simple cuboidal lens **epithelium** (Ep). The fibers (*arrows*), constituting the bulk of the lens, are composed of closely packed, hexagon-shaped cells whose longitudinal axes are oriented parallel to the surface. The lens is avascular, hence the absence of blood vessels. *Inset.* **Lens. Monkey. Paraffin section.** ×270. Note the presence of the homogeneous **capsule** (Ca) overlying the simple cuboidal lens **epithelium** (Ep).

FIGURE 2b. Lens. Monkey. Paraffin section. ×132.

The equator of the lens displays the presence of younger cells that still possess their **nuclei** (N) and organelles but lose them as these cells mature. Note the **suspensory ligaments** (SL), **capsule** (Ca), and the lens **epithelium** (Ep).

FIGURE 4. Lacrimal gland. Monkey. Paraffin section. ×132.

Lacrimal glands are compound tubuloalveolar glands, separated into lobes and **lobules** (Lo) by **connective tissue** (CT) elements. Since these glands produce a lysozyme-rich, watery secretion, they are composed of numerous **serous acini** (SA), as evidenced by the round, basally located **nuclei** (N) of the secretory cells.

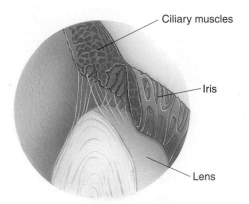

Ciliary muscles, iris, and lens

KEY							
1	pigmented epithelium	Ca	capsule	OO	orbicularis oculi
2	lamina of cones	Ch	choroid	pC	palpebral conjunctiva
3	external limiting membrane	CG	ciliary gland	SA	serous acini
4	outer nuclear layer	CT	connective tissue	Sk	skin
5	outer plexiform layer	EP	epithelium	SL	suspensory ligaments
8	ganglion cell layer	FC	fovea centralis	TG	tarsal glands
10	inner limiting membrane	Lo	lobule	TP	tarsal plate
C	cones	N	nucleus		

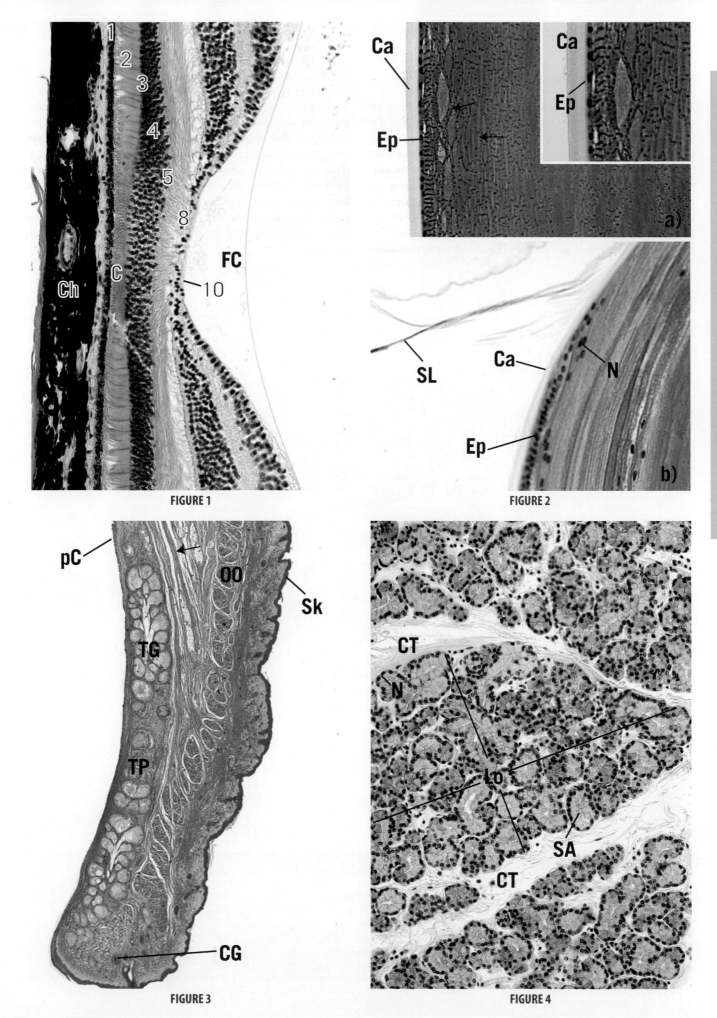

PLATE 19-3 · Fovea, Lens, Eyelid, and Lacrimal Glands

FIGURE 1

FIGURE 2

FIGURE 3

FIGURE 4

FIGURE 1. Inner ear. Paraffin section. ×21.

This photomicrograph is a survey section of the petrous portion of the temporal bone displaying the various components of the inner ear. At the extreme right, note that the spirally disposed **bony cochlea** (BC) encases the endolymph-filled **cochlear duct** (CD) and the perilymph-filled **scala tympani** (ST) and **scala vestibuli** (SV). The apex of the cochlea displays the **helicotrema** (H), the space through which perilymph may be exchanged between the scala tympani and the scala vestibuli. Innervation to the **spiral organ of Corti** (OC), located within the cochlear duct, is derived from the **spiral ganglion** (SG), housed in the **modiolus** (M). Two cranial nerves, **vestibulocochlear** (VN) and **facial** (FN), are evident in this photomicrograph. The **vestibule** (V), as well as sections of the **ampullae** (A) of the semicircular canals containing the **crista ampullaris** (CA), is clearly recognizable. Finally, note one of the **auditory ossicles** (AO) of the middle ear. *Inset.* **Crista ampullaris. Paraffin section.** ×132. The **crista ampullaris** (CA) is housed within the expanded **ampulla** (A) of each semicircular canal. **Nerve fibers** (NF) enter the connective tissue core of the crista and reach the neuroepithelial **hair cells** (HC) that are supported by **sustentacular cells** (SC). Kinocilia and microvilli of the hair cells extend into the gelatinous **cupula** (Cu) associated with the crista.

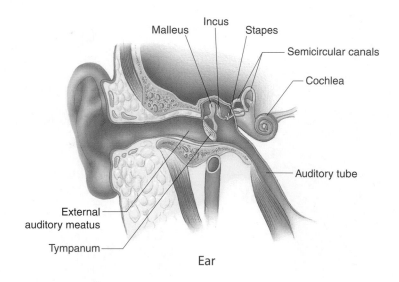

Malleus Incus Stapes

Semicircular canals

Cochlea

Auditory tube

External auditory meatus

Tympanum

Ear

KEY

A	ampulla	**FN**	facial nerve	**SC**	sustentacular cells
AO	auditory ossicle	**H**	helicotrema	**SG**	spiral ganglion
BC	bony cochlea	**HC**	hair cells	**ST**	scala tympani
CA	crista ampullaris	**M**	modiolus	**SV**	scala vestibuli
CD	cochlear duct	**NF**	nerve fibers	**V**	vestibule
Cu	cupula	**OC**	spiral organ of Corti	**VN**	vestibulocochlear nerve

PLATE 19-4 · Inner Ear

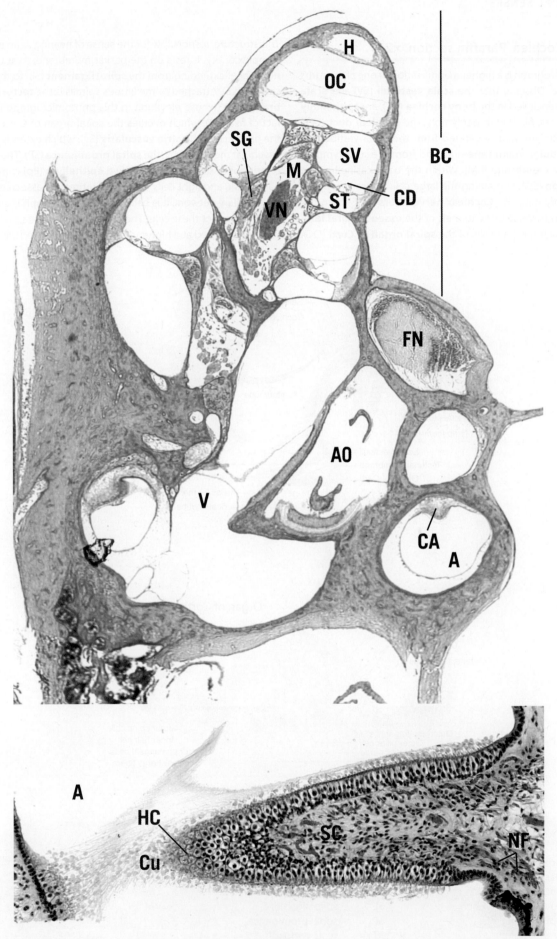

FIGURE 1

PLATE 19-5 · Cochlea

FIGURE 1. Cochlea. Paraffin section. ×211.

This photomicrograph is a higher magnification of one of the turns of the cochlea. Observe that the **scala vestibuli** (SV) and **scala tympani** (ST), enclosed in the **bony cochlea** (BC), are **epithelially** (Ep) lined spaces, filled with perilymph. The **cochlear duct** (CD), filled with endolymph, is separated from the scala vestibuli by the thin **vestibular membrane** (VM) and from the scala tympani by the **basilar membrane** (BM). Within the bony casing lies the **spiral ganglion** (SG), containing the large cell bodies (*arrows*) of primary sensory neurons. **Cochlear nerve fibers** (CNF) from the spiral ganglion traverse bony tunnels of the **osseous spiral lamina** (OL) to reach the hair cells of the **spiral organ of Corti** (OC).

This structure, responsible for the sense of hearing, is an extremely complex entity. It rests on the basilar membrane, a taut, collagenous sheet extending from the **spiral ligament** (SL) to the **limbus spiralis** (LS). Attached to the limbus spiralis is the **tectorial membrane** (TM) (whose elevation in this photomicrograph is an artifact of fixation), which overlies the spiral organ of Corti. Observe the presence of the **stria vascularis** (Sv), which extends from the vestibular membrane to the **spiral prominence** (SP). The stria vascularis possesses a pseudostratified **epithelium** (Ep) composed of basal, dark, and light cells, which are intimately associated with a rich capillary network. It is believed that endolymph is elaborated by some or all of these cells. The morphology of the spiral organ of Corti is presented at a higher magnification in Plate 19-6.

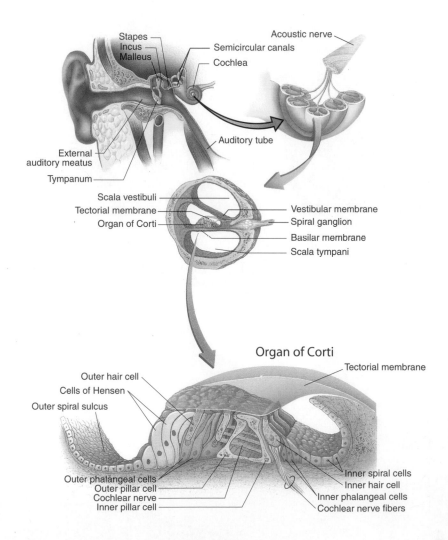

KEY							
BC	bony cochlea	**OC**	spiral organ of Corti	**SV**	scala vestibuli
BM	basilar membrane	**OL**	osseous spiral lamina	**Sv**	stria vascularis
CD	cochlear duct	**SG**	spiral ganglion	**TM**	tectorial membrane
CNF	cochlear nerve fibers	**SL**	spiral ligament	**VM**	vestibular membrane
Ep	epithelium	**SP**	spiral prominence		
LS	limbus spiralis	**ST**	scala tympani		

PLATE 19-5 • Cochlea

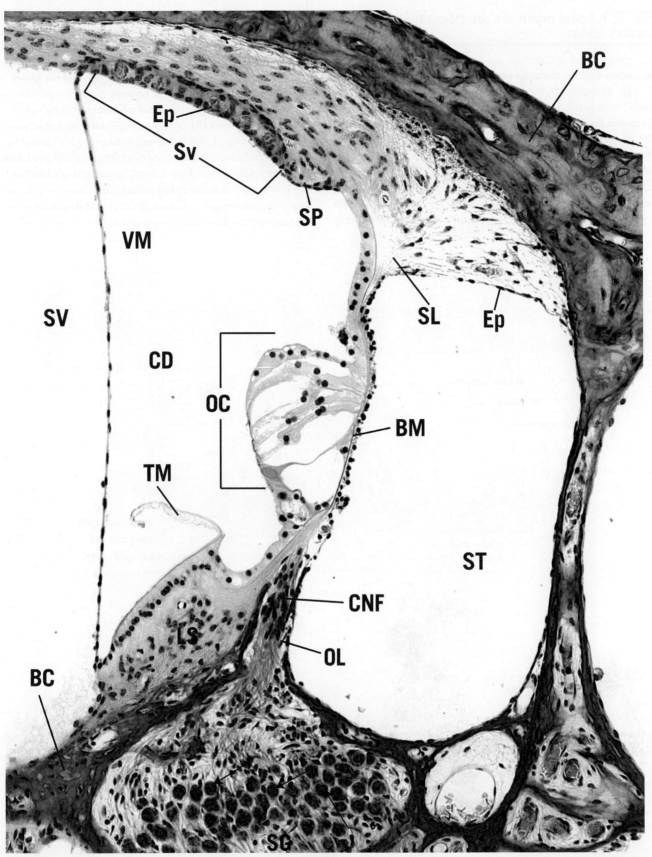

FIGURE 1

PLATE 19-6 · Spiral Organ of Corti

FIGURE 1. Spiral organ of Corti (Montage). Paraffin section. ×540.

The spiral organ of Corti lies on the **basilar membrane** (BM), whose two regions, the **zona pectinata** (ZP) and the **zona arcuata** (ZA), are delineated by the base of the **outer pillar cells** (OPC). The basilar membrane extends from the **spiral ligament** (SL) to the **tympanic lip** (TL) of the limbus spiralis. The **tectorial membrane** (TM) is anchored to the **vestibular lip** (VL) of the limbus spiralis. The tectorial membrane forms a roof over the **internal spiral sulcus** (IS). Observe the **cochlear nerve fibers** (CNF) traversing the tunnels of the **osseous spiral lamina** (OL). The lateral wall of the internal spiral sulcus is formed by the single row of **inner hair cells** (IH), flanked by the **inner phalangeal cells** (IPh) and **border cells**

(Bc). The floor of the internal spiral sulcus is formed by **inner sulcus cells** (IC). Proceeding laterally, the **inner pillar cell** (IPC) and **outer pillar cell** (OPC) form the **inner tunnel of Corti** (ITC). The **spaces of Nuel** (SN) separate the three rows of **outer hair cells** (OH) from each other and from the outer pillar cells. Fine **nerve fibers** (NF) and **phalangeal processes** (PP) traverse these spaces. The outer hair cells are supported by **outer phalangeal cells** (OPh). The space between the **cells of Hensen** (CH) and the outermost row of outer phalangeal cells is the **outer tunnel** (OT). Lateral to the cells of Hensen are the darker staining, deeper positioned **cells of Böttcher** (CB) and the lighter staining, larger **cells of Claudius** (CC), which enclose the **outer spiral sulcus** (OSS). Note that the space above the spiral organ of Corti is the **cochlear duct** (CD), whereas the space below the basilar membrane is the scala tympani.

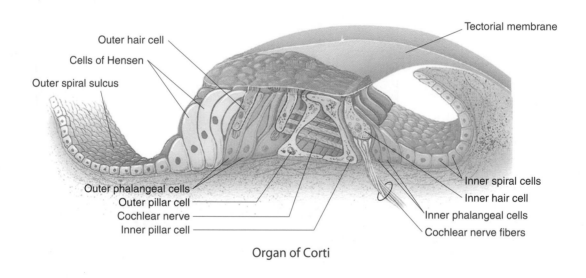

Outer hair cell

Cells of Hensen

Outer spiral sulcus

Tectorial membrane

Outer phalangeal cells

Outer pillar cell

Cochlear nerve

Inner pillar cell

Inner spiral cells

Inner hair cell

Inner phalangeal cells

Cochlear nerve fibers

Organ of Corti

KEY

Bc	border cells	IPh	inner phalangeal cells	PP	phalangeal processes
BM	basilar membrane	IS	internal spiral sulcus	SL	spiral ligament
CB	cells of Böttcher	ITC	inner tunnel of Corti	SN	spaces of Nuel
CC	cells of Claudius	NF	nerve fibers	TL	tympanic lip
CD	cochlear duct	OH	outer hair cells	TM	tectorial membrane
CH	cells of Hensen	OL	osseous spiral lamina	VL	vestibular lip
CNF	cochlear nerve fibers	OPC	outer pillar cells	ZA	zona arcuata
IC	inner sulcus cells	OPh	outer phalangeal cells	ZP	zona pectinata
IH	inner hair cells	OSS	outer spiral sulcus		
IPC	inner pillar cells	OT	outer tunnel		

PLATE 19-6 • Spiral Organ of Corti

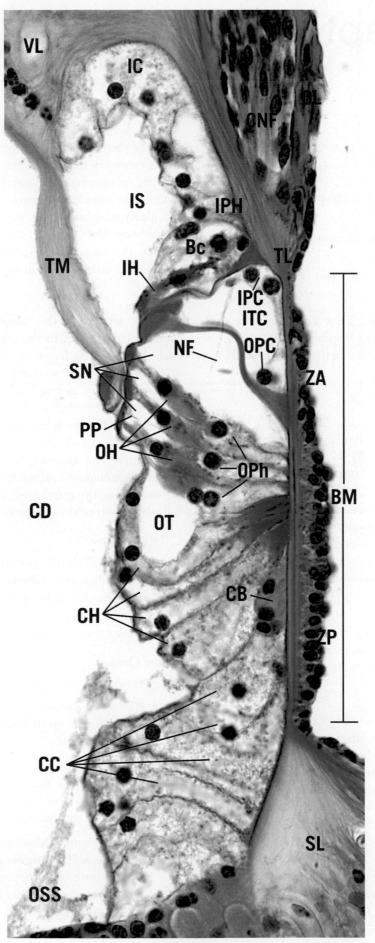

FIGURE 1

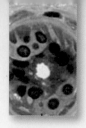

Chapter Summary

I. EYE

A. Fibrous Tunic

1. Cornea

The **cornea** is composed of five layers. From superficial to deep, they are the following:

    a. Stratified squamous nonkeratinized epithelium

    b. Bowman's Membrane
        The outer, homogeneous layer of the stroma

    c. Stroma
        A transparent, dense, regular, collagenous connective tissue housing **fibroblasts** and occasional **lymphoid cells**, comprising the bulk of the cornea

    d. Descemet's Membrane
        A thick, basal lamina

    e. Corneal Endothelium
        Not a true endothelium, a simple **squamous-to-cuboidal epithelium**

2. Sclera

The **sclera**, the white of the eye, is composed of three layers: the outer **episcleral tissue** housing blood vessels; the middle **stroma**, composed of dense, regular, collagenous connective tissue; and the **suprachoroid lamina**, a loose connective tissue housing **fibroblasts** and **melanocytes**.

B. Vascular Tunic

The **vascular tunic (uvea)** is a pigmented, vascular layer housing smooth muscles. It is composed of the **choroid membrane**, the **ciliary body**, and the **iris**.

1. Choroid Membrane

The **choroid membrane** is composed of four layers. The **suprachoroid layer** is shared with the sclera and houses **fibroblasts** and **melanocytes**. The **vascular** and **choriocapillary layers** house larger vessels and capillaries, respectively. The **glassy membrane** (of Bruch), interposed between the choroid and the retina, is composed of basal lamina, collagen, and elastic fibers.

2. Ciliary Body

The **ciliary body** is the region of the vascular tunic located between the **ora serrata** and the iris. The ciliary body is composed of the numerous, radially arranged, **aqueous humor–forming ciliary processes** that together compose the **ciliary crown** from which **suspensory ligaments** extend to the lens. Three layers of **smooth muscle**, oriented more or less meridianally, radially, and circularly, function in visual accommodation. The **vascular layer** and **glassy membrane** of the choroid continue into the ciliary body. The inner aspect of the ciliary body is covered by the inner nonpigmented and outer pigmented layers of the **ciliary epithelium**.

3. Iris

The **iris**, separating the **anterior** from the **posterior chamber**, is attached to the ciliary body along its outer circumference. The free edge of the iris forms the **pupil** of the eye. The iris is composed of three layers: the outer (frequently incomplete) **simple squamous epithelial layer**, a continuation of the corneal epithelium; the intermediate **fibrous layer**, composed of the nonvascular **anterior stromal** and vascular **general stromal layers** that house numerous **melanocytes** and **fibroblasts**; and the posterior **pigmented epithelium**. The **sphincter** and **dilator muscles** of the pupil are composed of myoepithelial cells derived from the pigmented epithelium.

C. Retinal Tunic

The **retinal tunic**, the deepest of the three layers, consists of the **pars iridica**, **pars ciliaris**, and **pars optica**. The last of these is the only region of the retina that is sensitive to light, extending as far anteriorly as the **ora serrata**, where it is continuous with the pars ciliaris.

1. Pars Optica

The **pars optica** is composed of 10 layers.

    a. Pigment Epithelium
        The **pigment epithelium** is attached to the choroid membrane

    b. Lamina of Rods and Cones
        The **outer** and **inner segments** of the photoreceptor cells form the first layer; the remainder of these cells constitutes the next three layers

    c. External Limiting Membrane
        The **external limiting membrane** is not a true membrane. It is merely a junctional specialization between the photoreceptor cells and processes of **Müller (supportive) cells**

d. Outer Nuclear Layer

The **outer nuclear layer** houses the cell bodies (and nuclei) of the photoreceptor cells. At the **fovea centralis**, only cones are present

e. Outer Plexiform Layer

The **outer plexiform layer** is the region of synapse formation between the **axons** of photoreceptor cells and the processes of **bipolar** and **horizontal cells**

f. Inner Nuclear Layer

The **inner nuclear layer** houses the **cell bodies of Müller, amacrine** (associative), **bipolar,** and **horizontal cells**

g. Inner Plexiform Layer

The **inner plexiform layer** is the region of synapses between **dendrites** of **ganglion cells** and **axons** of **bipolar cells.** Moreover, processes of **Müller** and **amacrine cells** are also present in this layer

h. Ganglion Cell Layer

The **ganglion cell layer** houses the **cell bodies of multipolar neurons,** which are the final link in the neuronal chain of the retina, and their **axons** form the optic nerve. Additionally, **neuroglia** are also located in this layer

i. Optic Nerve Fiber Layer

The **optic nerve fiber layer** is composed of the **unmyelinated axons** of the **ganglion cells,** which are collected as the optic nerve

j. Inner Limiting Membrane

The **inner limiting membrane** is composed of the expanded terminal processes of **Müller cells**

2. Pars Ciliaris and Pars Iridica Retinae

At the **pars ciliaris** and **pars iridica retinae,** the retinal layer has been reduced to a thin epithelial layer consisting of a columnar and a pigmented layer lining the ciliary body and iris.

D. Lens

The **lens** is a biconvex, flexible, transparent disc that focuses the incident rays of light on the retina. It is composed of three layers, an elastic **capsule** (basement membrane), an anteriorly placed **simple cuboidal epithelium,** and **lens fibers,** modified epithelial cells derived from the **equator** of the lens.

E. Lacrimal Gland

The **lacrimal gland** is external to the eye, located in the superolateral aspect of the orbit. It is a **compound tubuloalveolar gland,** producing a lysozyme-rich serous fluid with an alkaline pH.

F. Eyelid

The **eyelid** is covered by **thin skin** on its external aspect and by **conjunctiva,** a mucous membrane, on its inner aspect. A thick, dense, fibrous connective tissue **tarsal plate** maintains and reinforces the eyelid. Associated with the tarsal plate are the **tarsal glands,** secreting an oily sebum that is delivered to the margin of the eyelid. Muscles controlling the eyelid are located within its substance. Associated with the eyelashes are **sebaceous glands.** Ciliary glands are located between eyelashes.

II. EAR

A. External Ear

1. Auricle

The **auricle** is covered by thin skin and is supported by highly flexible **elastic cartilage plate.**

2. External Auditory Meatus

The **external auditory meatus** is a **cartilaginous tube** lined by skin, containing **ceruminous glands** and some fine **hair.** The skin of the external meatus is continuous with the external covering of the tympanic membrane. In the medial aspect of the meatus, the cartilage is replaced by **bone.**

3. Tympanic Membrane

The **tympanic membrane** is a thin, taut membrane separating the external from the middle ear. It is lined by **stratified squamous keratinized epithelium** externally and low **cuboidal epithelium** internally and possesses a core of **collagen fibers** disposed in two layers.

B. Middle Ear

The **middle ear** is composed of the **simple cuboidal epithelium**–lined **tympanic cavity** containing the three ossicles (**malleus, incus,** and **stapes**). The tympanic cavity communicates with the nasopharynx via the cartilaginous and bony **auditory tube.** The medial wall of the middle ear communicates with the inner ear via the **oval (vestibular)** and **round (cochlear) windows.**

C. Inner Ear

1. Cochlea

The bony **cochlea** houses the endolymph-filled **cochlear duct** that subdivides the perilymph-filled cochlea into the superiorly positioned **scala vestibuli** and the inferiorly located **scala tympani.**

a. Cochlear Duct

The **cochlear duct** houses the **spiral organ of Corti** that lies on the **basilar membrane.** The spiral organ of Corti is composed of **cells of**

Claudius, cells of Böttcher, and cells of Hensen, all of which assist in the formation of the **outer tunnel** along with the **outer hair cells** and **outer phalangeal cells**. The **tectorial membrane** lies over the outer hair cells as well as the **inner hair cells**, thus forming the **internal spiral tunnel**. The region between the inner and outer hair cells is occupied by **pillar cells**, which assist in the formation of the **inner tunnel (of Corti)**. The **stria vascularis** constitutes the outer wall of the cochlear duct. Nerve fibers lead to the **spiral ganglion** (housing pseudounipolar cells) in the **modiolus**.

b. Membranous Labyrinth

The **membranous labyrinth** is composed of the **utricle**, the **saccule**, and the three **semicircular canals**.

1. Utricle and Saccule

The **utricle** and **saccule** are both filled with **endolymph** and house **maculae**. Each **macula** is composed of simple **columnar epithelium** composed of two cell types, neuroepithelial **hair cells** and **supporting cells**. The free surface of the macula displays the **otolithic membrane**, housing small particles called **otoliths**.

2. Semicircular Canals

The three **semicircular canals** are oriented perpendicular to each other. The **ampulla** of each canal houses a **crista**, a structure similar to a macula, composed of neuroepithelial **hair cells** and **supporting cells**. A gelatinous **cupula** is located at the free surface of the crista, but it contains no otoliths.

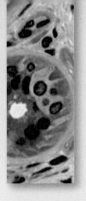

Appendix

The light microscopic study of cells, tissues, and organs requires that the material to be examined be sectioned thinly enough to permit light to penetrate it and that the light be sufficient to be collected by the lenses of the microscope and to reach the retina of the examiner. Moreover, the tissue has to maintain its natural, living characteristics; otherwise, the viewer will have a distorted picture of the tissue. Over the years, numerous procedures were developed and refined to make sure that there is a close resemblance between the image under the microscope and the properties of the tissue while it was in its living state. These procedures include fixation, dehydration, clearing, embedding, sectioning, mounting, staining, and the affixing of a coverslip over the section.

- **Fixation** is the use of chemicals that inhibits tissue necrolysis and prevents alteration of its normal morphology. For light microscopy, the fixative of choice is neutral buffered formalin, although many other fixatives are commonly used.
- **Dehydration** and **clearing** are accomplished by using an increasing concentration of ethanol (from 50% to 100%) followed by a clearing agent such as Xylene to make the tissue transparent and miscible with an embedding material.
- **Embedding** and **sectioning** is the process that permeates the tissue with an agent, such as **paraffin** or a **plastic polymer**, that can be sliced into sections thin enough to be transparent to visible light. Tissues embedded in paraffin are usually sectioned 5 to 10 μm in thickness, whereas those embedded in plastic are sectioned much thinner (≤0.1 μm). Many other embedding media and sectioning techniques are also available.
- Sections obtained from paraffin or plastic blocks are **mounted** on glass slides coated with an adhesive material, such as albumin, to ensure that the sections adhere to the glass slides.
- **Staining** of the sections is necessary because the optical densities of the various tissue elements are so similar that they are indistinguishable from one another without being treated with various dyes. Because many of the stains used are water miscible, the sections must be deparaffinized and rehydrated before they can be stained.
- The stained sections have to be dehydrated once again to permit them to be made permanent by the placing and affixing of a **coverslip** over the tissue section.

Terminology of Staining

Frequently, when staining histological sections, a **principal stain** is used in conjunction with a **counterstain**, a contrasting color that stains those components of the tissue that are not stained well with the principal stain. Usually, the stains are either **acidic (anionic)** or **basic (cationic)** and are attracted to those components of the cell or tissue that are basic or acidic, respectively. Therefore, the acidic components of the cell, such as nucleic acids, attract the basic stains and are said to be **basophilic**. Those components of the cell whose pH is greater than 7, such as many cytoplasmic proteins, attract acidic stains and are said to be **acidophilic**.

Common Stains Used in Histology

Although a great number of histologic and histopathologic stains have been developed, only the most commonly used stains are listed in this Appendix.

479

Hematoxylin and Eosin

Hematoxylin, in conjunction with the counterstain eosin, is one of the most commonly used stains in histological and histopathological preparations. Hematoxylin is a basic stain that dyes nuclei, nucleoli, and ribosomes blue to purple in color. Eosin stains basic components of the cell, including myofilaments of muscle, pink to light red in color. Red blood cells stain orange to bright red in color. Additionally, extracellular matrix proteins, such as collagen, are also stained pink to light red.

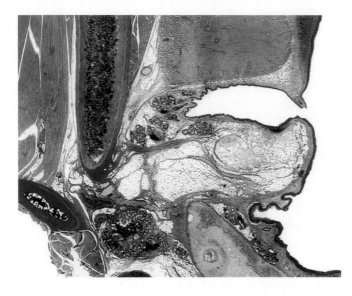

Wright Stain

Wright stain and the related Giemsa stain are designed specifically for staining cells of blood. It stains erythrocytes salmon pink; nuclei of leukocytes and granules of platelets stain dark blue to purple, whereas the specific granules of eosinophils stain salmon pink, and those of basophils stain dark blue to black. The cytoplasm of lymphocytes and monocytes stains a light blue in color.

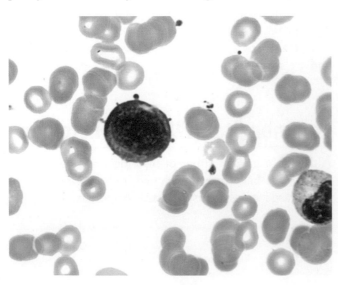

Weigert Method for Elastic Fibers and Elastic van Gieson Stain

Weigert method and van Gieson stain for elastic fibers are both used commonly to stain elastic fibers. They both dye elastic fibers dark blue to black. Since nuclei also stain dark gray to black, the fibroblasts present among the elastic fibers are very difficult to see.

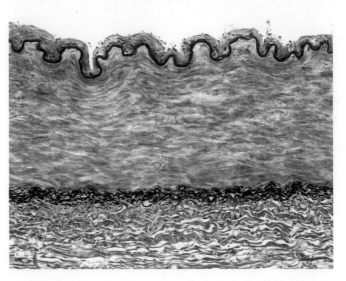

Silver Stain

Silver stain uses silver salts in solution that precipitate out as silver metal on the surfaces of type III collagen fibers (reticular fibers), staining them black. Some cells, such as diffuse neuroepithelial cells, also stain with silver stains and were called argentaffin or argyrophilic cells. Their granules stain brown to black with silver stains.

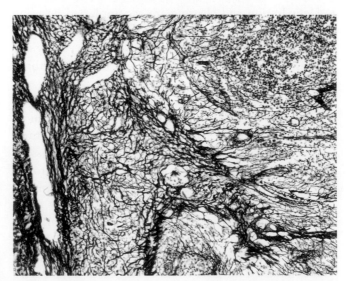

Iron Hematoxylin

Iron ammonium sulfate is a mordant (used to ensure strong adherence of the hematoxylin to the tissue) permitting very good visualization of cell membranes and membrane complexes, such as terminal bars, cross striations of skeletal and cardiac muscle, as well as intercalated discs of cardiac muscle.

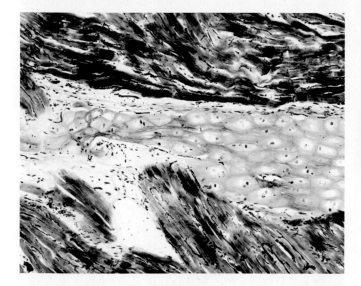

Bielschowsky Silver Stain

Bielschowsky stain uses silver salts to permeate the tissue, and then the silver is reduced so that it stains dendrites and axons black. The surrounding tissues are golden brown yellow with a tinge of red in the cytoplasm, and the nucleoli are black.

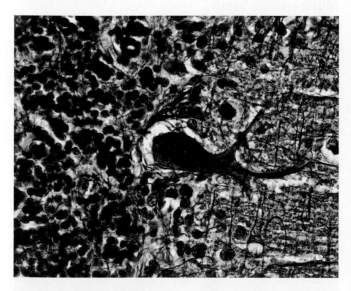

Masson Trichrome

As the name implies, this stain produces three colors and is used to differentiate collagen of connective tissues from muscle and other living cells. Depending on the variant used, collagen is stained blue or green, muscle cells are red, cytoplasm of non-muscle cells are a pink to light red, and nuclei stain black. (Reprinted with permission from Mills SE, Carter D, et al., eds. Sternberg's Diagnostic Surgical Pathology, 5th ed., Philadelphia: Lippincott, Williams & Wilkins, 2010. p. 1694.)

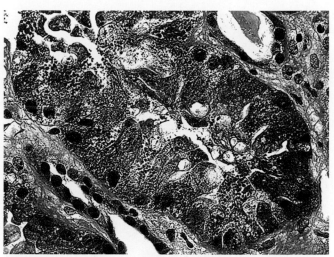

Periodic Acid-Schiff Reaction (PAS)

PAS reaction stains glycogens, glycoproteins, mucins, and glycolipids. Thus, basement membranes stain pinkish red, whereas mucins of goblet cells and of mucous salivary glands stain a deep red to magenta. (Reprinted with permission from Mills SE, ed. Histology for Pathologists, 3rd ed., Philadelphia: Lippincott, Williams & Wilkins, 2007. p. 608.)

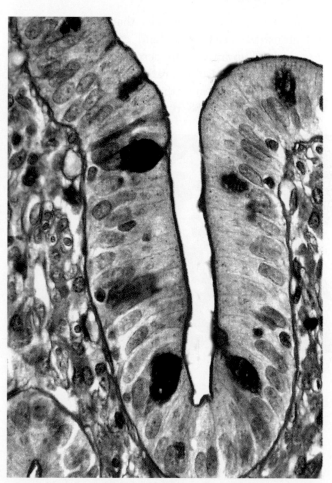

Alcian Blue

Alcian blue is specific for staining mucins, glycoproteins, and the matrix of cartilage blue in color, whereas the cytoplasm stains a light pink and nuclei stain red. (Reprinted with permission from Mills SE, ed. Histology for Pathologists, 3rd ed., Philadelphia: Lippincott, Williams & Wilkins, 2007. p. 415.)

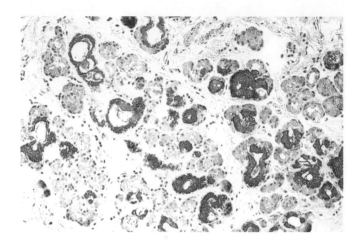

von Kossa Stain

von Kossa stain uses silver salts that become reduced to demonstrate calcification and calcified tissues that stain black. (Reprinted with permission from Rubin R, Strayer D, et al., eds. Rubin's Pathology. Clinicopathologic Foundations of Medicine, 5th ed., Baltimore: Lippincott, Williams & Wilkins, 2008, p. 1113.)

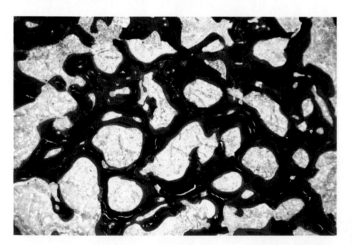

Sudan Red

Sudan red is used to stain lipids, phospholipids, lipoproteins, and triglycerides, all of which stain an intense red with this dye. (Reprinted with permission from Rubin R, Strayer D, et al., eds. Rubin's Pathology. Clinicopathologic Foundations of Medicine, 5th ed., Baltimore: Lippincott Williams & Wilkins, 2008, p. 239.)

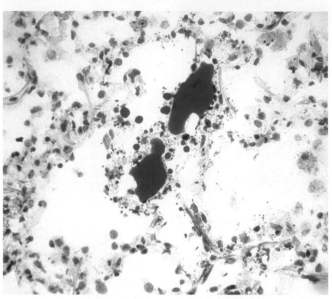

Mucicarmine Stain

As its name implies, mucicarmine is used to localize mucin, which it stains a deep red color. The cytoplasm appears a light, salmon pink, nuclei are stained bluish black, and connective tissue is stained a yellowish-orange color. (Reprinted with permission from Rubin R, Strayer D, et al., eds. Rubin's Pathology. Clinicopathologic Foundations of Medicine, 5th ed., Baltimore: Lippincott, Williams & Wilkins, 2008, p. 541.)

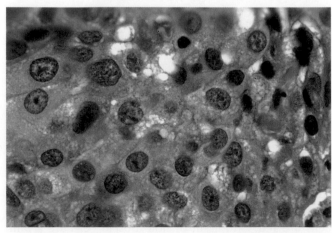

Safranin-O

Safranin-O is used to localize granules of mast cells, cartilage matrix, and mucin of goblet cells, all of which stain orange to red. Nuclei appear dark blue to black. (Reprinted with permission from Mills SE, ed. Histology for Pathologists, 3rd ed., Philadelphia: Lippincott, Williams & Wilkins, 2007. p. 111.)

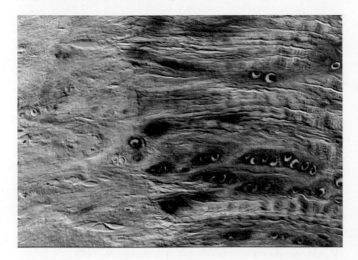

Toluidine Blue

Toluidine blue is a metachromatic stain in that it changes color with specific substances, such as the granules of mast cells and cartilage matrix, both of which stain a reddish-purple color. It acts as a normochromatic stain in that acidic components of the cell, such as ribosomes and nuclei, stain blue. Toluidine blue is especially useful in staining thin, plastic-embedded tissue sections. (Reprinted with permission from Mills SE, ed. Histology for Pathologists, 3rd ed., Philadelphia: Lippincott, Williams & Wilkins, 2007. p. 204.)

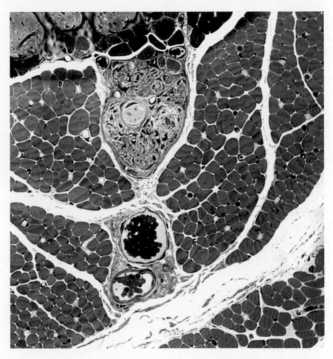

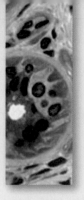

Index

(Note: Page numbers in *italics* denotes figures and those followed by "*t*" denotes tables)

PROPERTY OF LIBRARY
SOUTH UNIVERSITY CLEVELAND CAMPUS
WARRENSVILLE HEIGHTS, OH 44128

RRS1211